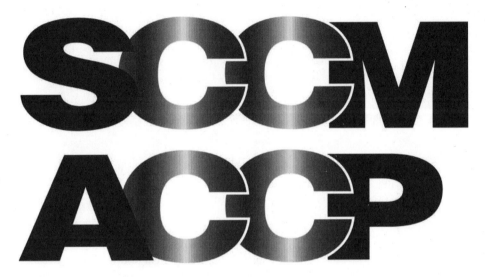

4th Combined Critical Care Course

2002 Course Directors

Jesse B. Hall, MD, FCCP, FCCM
Professor of Medicine/Anesthesia/Critical Care Medicine
Department of Medicine
University of Chicago
Chicago, IL, USA

Eugene B. Freid, MD, FCCM
Associate Professor of Anesthesiology & Pediatrics
Department of Anesthesiology
University of North Carolina
Chapel Hill, NC, USA

The views expressed herein are those of the authors and do not necessarily reflect the views of the American College of Chest Physicians or the Society of Critical Care Medicine.

Use of trade names or names of commercial sources is for information only and does not imply endorsement by the American College of Chest Physicians or the Society of Critical Care Medicine.

The authors and the publisher have exercised great care to ensure that drug dosages, formulas, and other information presented in this book are accurate and in accord with the professional standards in effect at the time of publication. Readers are, however, advised to always check the manufacturer's product information sheet that is packaged with the respective products to be fully informed of changes in recommended dosages, contraindications, and the like before prescribing or administering any drug.

Managing Editor: Stacy L. Wilhite

Printed in the United States of America
First Printing, July 2002

Society of Critical Care Medicine
701 Lee Street, Suite 200
Des Plaines, IL, USA 60016
Phone 847.827.6869
Fax 847.827.6886
www.sccm.org

American College of Chest Physicians
3300 Dundee Road
Northbrook, IL USA 60062-2348
Phone 847.498.1400
Fax 847.498.5460
www.chestnet.org

International Standard Book Number: 0-936145-03-x

CONTRIBUTORS

Richard K. Albert, MD, FCCP
Professor and Vice Chair for Educational Affairs
University of Colorado Health Sciences Center
Director, Department of Medicine
Denver Medical Center
Denver, CO, USA

Joshua O. Benditt, MD
Director of Respiratory Care Services
Division of Pulmonary and Critical Care Medicine
University of Washington School of Medicine
Seattle, WA, USA

Thomas P. Bleck, MD, FACP, FCCM, FCCP
The Louise Nerancy Eminent Scholar in Neurology
Professor of Neurology, Neurological Surgery, and
Internal Medicine
Director, Neuroscience ICU
Department of Neurology
University of Virginia Medical Center
Charlottesville, VA, USA

Mary L. Brandt, MD
Professor of Surgery and Pediatrics
Department of Pediatric Surgery
Baylor College of Medicine
Houston, TX, USA

R. Phillip Dellinger, MD, FCCP, FCCM
Director, Section of Critical Care Medicine
Rush Medical College
Cook County Hospital and Rush-Presbyterian-St.
Luke's Medical Center
Chicago, IL, USA

Todd Dorman, MD, FCCM
Associate Professor
Departments of Anesthesiology/Critical Care
Medicine, Medicine, Surgery, and Nursing
The Johns Hopkins Hospital
Baltimore, MD, USA

David J. Dries, MSE, MD, FCCP, FCCM
John F. Perry, Jr., Professor
Department of Surgery
University of Minnesota
Director of Academic Programs
Regions Hospital
St. Paul, MN, USA

Gregory T. Everson, MD, FACP
Professor of Medicine
Director of Hepatology
Medical Director of Liver Transplantation
University of Colorado School of Medicine
Denver, CO, USA

Jesse B. Hall, MD, FCCP
Professor of Medicine, Anesthesia,
and Critical Care
The University of Chicago
The Pritzker School of Medicine
Chicago, IL, USA

Steven M. Hollenberg, MD, FCCP, FCCM
Director, Vascular Physiology Research Laboratory
Associate Director, MICU
Assistant Professor of Medicine
Sections of Cardiology/Critical Care
Rush-Presbyterian-St. Luke's Medical Center
Chicago, IL, USA

George H. Karam, MD, FCCP
Professor of Medicine
LSU School of Medicine, New Orleans
Head, Department of Medicine
Earl K. Long Medical Center
Baton Rouge, LA, USA

John P. Kress, MD, FCCP
Assistant Professor of Medicine
Section of Pulmonary and Critical Care
University of Chicago
Chicago, IL, USA

James A. Kruse, MD, FCCM
Professor of Medicine
Wayne State University School of Medicine
Chief, Pulmonary/Critical Care Medicine
Department of Medicine
Detroit Receiving Hospital
Detroit, MI, USA

Laurent Lewkowiez, MD
Assistant Professor of Medicine
Denver Health and Hospitals
University of Colorado Health Sciences Center
Denver, CO, USA

Stuart L. Linas, MD
Professor of Medicine
Rocky Mountain Professor of Renal Research
University of Colorado Health Sciences Center
Chief, Renal Division
Denver Medical Center
Denver, CO, USA

Judith A. Luce, MD
Director, Oncology Services
San Francisco General Hospital
Associate Professor of Medicine
University of California, San Francisco,
* School of Medicine*
San Francisco, CA, USA

Margaret M. McQuiggan, MS, RD, CSM
Clinical Dietician Specialist
Memorial Hermann Hospital
Houston, TX, USA

Frederick A. Moore, MD, FCCM
James H. "Red" Duke, Jr. Professor and
* Vice Chairman*
Department of Surgery
University of Texas - Houston Medical School
Medical Director of Trauma Services
Memorial Hermann Hospital
Houston, TX, USA

Richard S. Muther, MD
Medical Director
Division of Nephrology
Research Medical Center
Kidney Associates of Kansas City, P.C.
Kansas City, MO, USA

Michael S. Niederman MD, FCCM
Division of Pulmonary/CCM
Winthrop University Hospital
Mineola, NY, USA

Gregory A. Schmidt, MD, FCCP
Professor of Clinical Medicine and Clinical
Anesthesia & Critical Care
University of Chicago
Chicago, IL, USA

James K. Stoller, MD, FCCP
Vice Chairman
Division of Medicine
Head, Section of Respiratory Therapy
Department of Pulmonary/Critical Care Medicine
The Cleveland Clinic Foundation
Cleveland, OH, USA

Jeanine P. Wiener-Kronish, MD, FCCP
Professor of Anesthesia and Medicine
Vice-Chair, Department of Anesthesia,
* Critical Care, and Perioperative Care*
Investigator, Cardiovascular Research Institute
University of California, San Francisco,
* School of Medicine*
San Francisco, CA, USA

Janice L. Zimmerman, MD, FCCP, FCCM
Professor of Medicine
Baylor College of Medicine
Associate Chief, Medical Service
Ben Taub General Hospital
Houston, TX, USA

STATEMENT OF FACULTY FINANCIAL DISCLOSURE

The American College of Chest Physicians (ACCP) and the Society of Critical Care Medicine (SCCM) endorse the Standards of the Accreditation Council for Continuing Medical Education (ACCME) whereby faculty members at this education event should disclose significant relationships with commercial companies whose products or services are discussed in their educational presentation. For faculty members, significant relationships include receiving commercial company research grants, consultancies, honoraria and travel, or other benefits or having a self-managing equity interest in a company. Disclosure of a relationship is not intended to suggest or condone a bias in any presentation, but is made to provide participants with information that might be of potential importance to their evaluation of a presentation.

The following faculty members have indicated to the ACCP and the SCCM that no significant relationships exist with any company/organization whose products or services may be discussed during their presentation.

Richard K. Albert, MD
Joshua Benditt, MD
Mary L. Brandt, MD
Todd Dorman, MD, FCCM
Gregory T. Everson, MD
James Forrester, MD
Eugene B. Freid, MD, FCCM
Jesse B. Hall, MD, FCCP, FCCM
Steven Hollenberg, MD, FCCP, FCCM
John P. Kress, MD
James A. Kruse, MD, FCCM
Stuart Linas, MD
Richard S. Muther, MD
Gregory A. Schmidt, MD, FCCP
James K. Stoller, MD
Jeanine P. Wiener-Kronish, MD
Janice L. Zimmerman, MD, FCCP, FCCM

The following faculty members have disclosed significant relationships exist with the following company/organization whose products or services may be discussed during their presentation. Company names appear as provided by the presenter.

Thomas Bleck, MD, FCCP, FCCM
Alsius Corporation, Ortho-MacNeil, Pfizer

Shannon Carson, MD
Eli Lilly

R. Phillip Dellinger, MD, FCCM
Aventis Speakers' Bureau

David Dries, MD, FCCM
Eli Lilly, Wyeth-Ayerst

George Karam, MD
Merck, Pfizer, Wyeth-Ayerst

Judith Luce, MD
National Cancer Institute, Avon Foundation

Frederick A. Moore, MD, FCCM
Novartis

Michael S. Niederman, MD, FCCM
Bayer, Bristol Myers, Elon, Pfizer, Pharmacia

The following faculty have not filed a disclosure statement with the American College of Chest Physicians or the Society of Critical Care Medicine at the time of printing of the syllabus:

Laurent Lewkowiez, MD

TABLE OF CONTENTS

TACHYARRHYTHMIAS, DIAGNOSIS AND MANAGEMENT

Laurent Lewkowiez, MD

Objectives

- To understand the basic mechanisms of arrhythmias
- To understand the basic types of supraventricular arrhythmias and their treatments
- To understand the basic assessment of wide complex tachycardias
- To understand the basic management of atrial fibrillation
- To understand the basic treatment of ventricular tachycardia and fibrillation.

Key Words: Orthodromic reciprocating tachycardia, AV nodal reentrant tachycardia, Atrial flutter, Atrial fibrillation, WPW syndrome, Ventricular tachycardia, Ventricular fibrillation

Table of Abbreviations

ORT	Othodromic Reciprocating Tachycardia
AVNRT	AV Nodal Reentrant Tachycardia
AV node	Atrioventricular node
WPW	Wolf Parkinson White syndrome
PAC	Premature Atrial Contraction
INR	International Normalized Ratio
RF	Radiofrequency ablation
MI	Myocardial Infarction
bpm	Beats per minute
msec	Millisecond
TEE	Transesophageal Echo

INTRODUCTION

The assessment, diagnosis, and management of tachyarrhythmias is a complex and sometimes difficult task. These arrhythmias, however, share many basic similarities. When approached with a logical and organized algorithm they may be accurately diagnosed and managed successfully. It is helpful to separate supraventricular arrhythmias from ventricular arrhythmias as they have markedly different treatment and risks of death.

The mechanisms of arrhythmia vary between abnormal automaticity, triggered arrhythmias, and reentry arrhythmias. Abnormal automaticity is defined as automatic impulse generation from cells that do not normally demonstrate this behavior or when the automaticity of these cells overtakes the sinus node, the primary site of automatic depolarization.

Triggered arrhythmias are generally due to secondary depolarizations that arise early during repolarization or immediately following repolarization. They typically are described as early afterdepolarization, the presumptive cause of Torsades de Pointes, and delayed after depolarizations, the presumptive cause of digoxin toxicity induced proarrhythmia.

Reentry is the most commonly encountered mechanism of arrhythmia. The primary requirements of reentrant arrhythmias are an area of slow or delayed conduction, an anatomical or functional separate path of conduction, and unidirectional block.

Clinically arrhythmias caused by various mechanisms act quite differently with pharmacologic and electrical intervention. Automatic arrhythmias are usually either transiently suppressed by external stimulation, as in pacing, or are unaffected. In general, they cannot be pace terminated or terminated with electrical cardioversion and are frequently resistant to pharmacological therapy. They are amenable to catheter ablation. Reentry arrhythmias are amenable to pace termination, cardioversion, ablation, and pharmacological intervention. Finally, the activity of triggered arrhythmias, although difficult to prove in vivo, behaves in a fashion that is somewhere in between that of automatic and reentrant arrhythmias.

SUPRAVENTRICULAR TACHYCARDIAS

Diagnosis

Supraventricular tachycardias are a common clinical problem. The electrocardiogram (ECG) is the cornerstone of diagnosis. In particular, it should be appreciated that the zones of transition frequently lead to the diagnosis of the underlying arrhythmia. These zones are typically onset, termination, and slowing or bundle branch block during tachycardia. It is at these points that information regarding the arrhythmia is acquired. During the tachycardia, it is difficult to know if the atria are driving the ventricles or vice versa.

Types

The types of supraventricular tachycardia (SVT) and their prevalence are dependent on the age of the population studied. In young infants and children, atrial tachycardia and junctional tachycardia are common. In adolescents and adulthood, the majority of SVT is of the reentrant variety. Approximately 90% of regular narrow complex tachycardias are of reentrant etiology. The common supraventricular arrhythmias and their prevalence in adults includes: AV nodal reentrant tachycardia 60%; orthodromic reciprocating tachycardia (ORT) 30%; and atrial tachycardia 10%. Approximately 2 to 5% of SVT is due to the well-publicized Wolff Parkinson White Syndrome (WPW).

The clinical importance in their differentiation is mainly in determining the response to various pharmacological interventions and to catheter based interventions. Supraventricular tachycardias are best assessed by the relationship of the P wave to the R wave. If the P wave is closer to the previous R wave then the subsequent R wave the arrhythmia is considered a short RP tachycardia. If the P wave is closer to the subsequent R wave then the arrhythmia is considered a long RP tachycardia.

SHORT RP TACHYCARDIAS

AV Nodal Reentrant Tachycardia

AV nodal reentrant tachycardia (AVNRT) is a narrow complex tachycardia where the two pathways involved are thought to be within the AV node itself or limited to the perinodal tissue. One pathway has fast conduction and the other pathway conducts slowly.

The onset of this arrhythmia, when captured, frequently begins with a premature atrial contraction (PAC) which conducts with a dramatically lengthened PR interval. This electrocardiographic finding is the surface manifestation of a block in forward conduction down the usual fast conducting AV nodal pathway and subsequent conduction down a slowly conducting AV nodal pathway found in these patients. The onset of this arrhythmia requires the recovery of the fast conducting pathway allowing for retrograde conduction. This completes the circuit and meets the requirements for reentry.

AVNRT is characterized on ECG by a very short RP conduction interval with a retrograde P wave only visible in one-third of the cases. In these cases, close inspection in lead V1 for a pseudo R and inferior leads for a pseudo S wave may be confirmatory. In the remaining two-thirds of the cases the P wave is buried within the QRS complex.

AVNRT is extremely responsive to AV nodal blocking agents and may be acutely terminated with vagal maneuvers in about one-third of the cases. They are nearly always responsive to Adenosine, beta blockers, or calcium channel blocker therapy acutely. However, medical therapy is rarely 100% effective and recurrences are the norm. Catheter ablation of this arrhythmia is 95% successful with major complications occurring in less than 1% of cases.

Orthodromic Reciprocating Tachycardia

Orthodromic Reciprocating Tachycardia (ORT) is also a short RP and narrow complex tachycardia. Anterograde *(forward)* conduction occurs via the normal AV nodal conduction system with retrograde conduction via a concealed accessory pathway. The RP interval is forcibly longer than with AVNRT because it requires some conduction through the ventricle prior to returning up the accessory pathway.

Patients with the WPW syndrome frequently present with ORT as a narrow complex tachycardia without evidence of pre-excitation. Importantly, if the associated tachycardia rate slows with the onset of a bundle branch block, then this is a strong indicator that the associated tachycardia is ORT with the accessory pathway located on the side of the associated bundle branch block.

Because ORT it is obligated to use the AV node for anterograde conduction, it is amenable to AV nodal blocking agents for acute and chronic therapy. Although ORT utilizes an accessory pathway, its lack of forward conduction allows the safe use of AV nodal blocking agents in distinction to WPW syndrome. However, pharmacological therapy is frequently less than adequately effective and recurrences on medical therapy are common. This arrhythmia is also very amenable to catheter ablation, which has a 95% success rate and low complication rate.

LONG RP TACHYCARDIAS

Long RP tachycardias are less commonly encountered. They include sinus tachycardia, sinus node reentrant tachycardia, syndrome of inappropriate sinus tachycardia, atrial tachycardia. Some include atrial flutter, although the flutter wave generally falls midway between the R wave complexes. Other less common arrhythmias that also present as long RP tachycardias include atypical AVNRT, permanent form of junctional reciprocating tachycardia (PJRT) *(an ORT with a slowly conducting retrograde only accessory pathway)*, and rarely junctional tachycardia.

Sinus Tachycardia

Sinus tachycardia is generally described as a long RP tachycardia, usually in response to physiologic etiologies such as pain or hypovolemia. The P wave morphology is generally upright in leads I, II, and AVF, which

is consistent with its origin at the superior vena cava (SVC) and right atrial junction with subsequent spread laterally and inferiorly. This is differentiated from Sinus Node Reentrant tachycardia by its onset and termination rather than P wave morphology, which are similar.

Sinus Node Reentrant Tachycardia

Sinus node reentrant tachycardia has an abrupt onset and termination rather than gradual onset and termination as in sinus tachycardia. It is amenable to calcium channel blockers, such as diltiazem and verapamil, and adenosine for acute termination, but is much less well controlled by beta blocker therapy. In addition, it has been successfully treated with catheter ablation.

Syndrome of Inappropriate Sinus Tachycardia

The syndrome of inappropriate sinus tachycardia is generally diagnosed by history and holter after excluding other causes of resting sinus tachycardia. It presents with typical sinus complex and a lower heart rate not below 130bpm. It frequently presents in young women. It is treated with beta blocker therapy although high doses have been needed for control. Catheter ablation of this arrhythmia has met with disappointing results due to a high rate of recurrence.

Atrial Tachycardia

Atrial tachycardia is generally described as a long RP tachycardia and with heart rate between 150 and 250 bpm. It may, however, present as a short RP tachycardia when associated with first degree AV block, although this is rare. As implied by its name, this arrhythmia generally does not require AV nodal or infranodal tissue for its maintenance. The P wave complex is generally different from that of sinus origin. The PR interval is greater than 0.12 msec, which differentiates this arrhythmia from junctional tachycardia with retrograde conduction. The origin of the atrial tachycardia may be inferred with some accuracy by evaluating its morphology in leads V1 and AVL. An upright P wave in lead V1 and negative wave in AVL implies a left atrial tachycardia, while the reverse implies a right atrial source.

The diagnosis of atrial tachycardia, aside from its electrocardiographic appearance, may be aided by the use of adenosine. If intravenous adenosine leads to AV block with continued atrial arrhythmia, then ORT is excluded and AVNRT is significantly less likely. The response of Sinus tachycardia to adenosine is one of general slowing or transient arrest. However, in some published series, as many as 70-80% of atrial tachycardia may also be transiently terminated with adenosine.

The mechanism of atrial tachycardia is frequently related to associated co-morbidities. Patients with increased cathecholamine state may present with automatic and triggered mechanisms. Patients with previous cardiac surgery may present more often with scar reentry tachycardia. The arrhythmia circumnavigates the surgical scar, forming separate functional or anatomic limbs of the tachycardia. Slow conduction and unidirectional block induced by a premature beat, completes the triad leading to reentry.

Therapy for atrial tachycardia is complex and controversial. Automatic atrial tachycardia frequently found in children may spontaneously regress. Atrial tachycardia in adults is frequently treated with antiarrhythmic therapy. Rate control of these rhythms may be difficult despite use of calcium channel blockers and beta blockers. The use of digoxin may exacerbate triggered causes of atrial tachycardia. Class IA agents such as Procainamide and class IC agents such as flecainide and propafenone may be utilized in patients without structural heart disease or coronary artery disease. However, the GI side effects of procainamide as well as frequent association with drug induced lupus limits its utility. Class III agents, such as sotalol and amiodarone, are utilized frequently in these patients for rhythm control as well. However, the need to initiate sotalol as an in-patient in order to observe for dramatic QT prolongation and the potential for Torsades de Pointes, combined with the high side effect profile of amiodarone, limits enthusiasm for their use. Factors such as co-morbidities, drug side effects, reluctance to lifelong drug therapy, and the fact that the drugs are only moderately

effective have led many to pursue abalation therapy. Catheter ablation has up to an 80% cure rate.

Atrial Flutter

A related arrhythmia to reentrant atrial tachycardia is the commonly encountered arrhythmia of atrial flutter. Atrial flutter generally has an atrial rate of between 250 and 350 bpm and ventricular rates generally in the 150 or 75 bpm range. Occasionally, atrial flutter presents with a variable ventricular response. Atrial flutter typically rotates in a counterclockwise fashion around the right atrium bounded anteriorly by a narrow isthmus of tissue located between the tricuspid valve and posteriorly by the Eustachian ridge. Typically, it has negative saw tooth pattern in inferior leads II and AVF and positive flutter waves in lead VI. It may occasionally travel in a clockwise rotation with reversed ECG presentation but with an identical atrial rate.

The treatment of atrial flutter is similar to that of atrial fibrillation, however rate control in flutter is substantially more difficult to obtain. Atrial flutter may respond to DC cardioversion or may be pace terminated by pacing in the atrium at increasing rates above that of the intrinsic arrhythmia. Atrial flutter may be associated with a lower rate of thromboembolism than atrial fibrillation. However is has been associated with multiple documented episodes of stroke following cardioversion. The indications for anticoagulation are considered the same as for atrial fibrillation. Radiofrequency ablation, which targets the isthmus of tissue, is highly effective in patients with primarily atrial flutter without concomitant atrial fibrillation. When bi-directional conduction block is obtained in the isthmus *(inability to conduct in the isthmus)* typical atrial flutter is no longer possible. The success rate of atrial flutter ablation is in the 80 to 90% range in experienced hands.

WPW Syndrome

Wolff Parkinson White (WPW) syndrome is estimated to be present in 0.3% of the population with estimated risk of sudden death of one per 1000 patient years. As previously mentioned WPW syndrome may present with the narrow complex tachycardia ORT. However, much of the discussion regarding this syndrome is associated with atrial fibrillation and will be further discussed in that section below. WPW syndrome may also present as a regular wide complex tachycardia, indicating anteriograde conduction over the accessory pathway. The differentiation of the wide complex manifestations of this syndrome is beyond the scope of this discussion.

The electrocardiographic presentation of WPW syndrome is an accelerated AV conduction with a short PR interval and a QRS duration greater than 120 msec *(3 small boxes on ECG)* with an abnormal bizarre initial upstroke and frequently abnormal repolarization. In addition, patients with WPW syndrome frequently have pseudo infarction on ECG secondary to their abnormal origin of ventricular depolarization.

The cause of this abnormal ventricular depolarization is due to the presence of one or more accessory pathways. These accessory pathways are small bands of tissue that failed to separate during development allowing continued electrical conduction between the atria and ventricles at sites other than at the AV node. The accessory pathway conduction circumvents the usual conduction delay between the atria and ventricles that occurs within the AV node. This leads to early eccentric activation of the ventricles with subsequent fusion with the usual AV nodal conduction. These pathways may allow rapid conduction from the atria to the ventricle, which may predispose patients to a risk of sudden death from ventricular fibrillation.

ATRIAL FIBRILLATION

Atrial fibrillation is the most common arrhythmia affecting between 2 to 4% of the population. Its prevalence increases markedly with age, increasing to up to 5 to 10% of the population over age 80 years of age. Atrial fibrillation remains one of the more complex and challenging cardiac arrhythmias to manage. It is associated with significant co-morbidities and an increased risk of death. Patients with atrial fibrillation have 2 times the mortality of those

without atrial fibrillation. Symptoms may range from none to syncope, dizziness, palpitations, worsening heart failure, and angina.

Atrial fibrillation is characterized by a lack of organized atrial activity on surface ECG manifesting as a lack of clear P waves between QRS complexes. It also presents with an irregular ventricular response.

The mechanisms of atrial fibrillation are now more clearly understood and new management strategies are continually evolving. Atrial fibrillation has now been shown to be due to multiple reentrant wavelets conducting between the right and left atrium. Factors that increase the number of wavelets that can exist at any one-time increase the likelihood that atrial fibrillation will be sustained. Likewise, factors that diminish the number of wavelets increase the likelihood that atrial fibrillation will spontaneously terminate. Thus, increased atrial size, slow intra-atrial conduction, and a shortened atrial refractory period all lead to an increased number of wavelets and increase the likelihood that atrial fibrillation will be sustained. Conversely, pharmacological treatment frequently prolongs the refractory period of atrial tissue. A prolonged refractory period increases the path length of the reentrant wavelet thereby decreasing the number of possible wavelets that can occupy the atria. This renders the arrhythmia more likely to self terminate. Nonpharmacologic treatment of atrial fibrillation with a catheter and the surgical maze procedures aim to electrically isolate the atria into small areas that are not capable of maintaining numerous wavelets thereby preventing maintenance of atrial fibrillation.

Management of atrial fibrillation involves more than symptom relief. Atrial fibrillation is known to be associated with increased risk of stroke and death. The risk of thromboembolism in nonanticoagulated patients is between 5 and 6% per year but may be as high as 20% in certain populations, including the elderly and those with certain valvular lesions *(i.e., mitral stenosis)*. In addition, atrial fibrillation with rapid ventricular response has been shown to lead to a tachycardia-mediated cardiomyopathy *(a rate induced form of progressive left ventricular dysfunction)* that is reversible if maintenance of sinus rhythm and/or rate control are performed. Improvement in left ventricular function has been shown to occur both with pharmacological control as well as after AV nodal ablation with pacing in patients with tachycardia-induced cardiomyopathy.

Acute Management of Atrial Fibrillation

Acute management of atrial fibrillation initially focuses on rate control, and anticoagulation. Rate control may usually be obtained through the use of calcium channel blockers, beta blockers, Amiodarone, and rarely with digoxin alone to slow the ventricular response. The use of acute beta blocker therapy for rate control in patients with left ventricular dysfunction and decompensated congestive heart failure should be avoided. In these patients, calcium channel blockers may be used cautiously. Digoxin and amiodarone may be particularly effective in light of their lack of negative inotropic effect. Patients with duration of atrial fibrillation less than 48 hours may generally undergo DC cardioversion to normal sinus rhythm with minimal risk of thromboembolism. The rate of embolism with cardioversion within 48 hours without prior anticoagulation is estimated to be approximately 0.8%. Pharmacologic therapy for acute conversion to sinus rhythm may also be performed within 48 hours. After that time, conversion should only be performed with extreme caution unless previous anticoagulation has been documented. Cardioversion may be performed in extreme cases such as severe refractory congestive heart failure, intractable angina, or refractory hypotension when ventricular response cannot be controlled. These cases are, however, extremely rare.

Patients not anticoagulated with atrial fibrillation that has lasted greater than 48 hours may undergo TEE *(transesophageal echo)* and subsequent cardioversion if no thrombus is seen within the left atria or appendage followed by anticoagulation for at least 1 month as an alternative to prolonged preconversion anticoagulation. This method has demonstrated a low incidence of thromboembolism in a small pilot study, with a larger study comparing conventional anticoagulation to transesophageal guided cardioversion with short-term

anticoagulation. Regardless of prior anticoagulation 4 weeks of anticoagulation is required with INR of two to three. This is to prevent formation of thrombus and embolization prior to recovery of normal atrial function.

- It is important to realize, prior to initiation of immediate cardioversion, that in patients with paroxysmal atrial fibrillation 50% of patients will spontaneously convert without electrical or pharmacological intervention.

- Digoxin, which in the past was heavily used for the prevention and conversion of atrial fibrillation, is ineffective at either and may actually be profibrillatory by shortening the atrial refractory period

- After cardioversion, calcium channel blockers have been shown to decrease the incidence of early recurrence of atrial fibrillation. Certain studies have shown a greater propensity of spontaneous conversion with beta blocker therapy compared to calcium channel blocker therapy.

Chronic Management of Atrial Fibrillation

Chronic therapy of atrial fibrillation may focus on rhythm or rate control as well as anticoagulation.

Patients with atrial fibrillation, paroxysmal or sustained, with the presence of diabetes, hypertension, valvular heart disease, congestive heart failure, hyperthyroid state, or age greater than 65 should be anticoagulated to decrease the risk of thromboembolism chronically.

The fervor with which maintenance of sinus rhythm is pursued should be based on the severity of symptoms as well as the associated co-morbidities *(e.g., congestive heart failure).*

Chronic ventricular rate control similar to acute treatment may generally be successfully obtained in atrial fibrillation with calcium channel blockers, diltiazem, and verapamil or beta blockers such a esmolol, metoprolol, atenolol or propranolol.

Digoxin was traditionally used in the past but is mainly effective in bed bound patients and is easily overcome with sympathetic stimulation. Digoxin is particularly helpful in patients presenting with congestive heart failure due to left ventricular dysfunction in which the negative inotropic effects of beta blockers and calcium channel blockers may be detrimental. In patients where digoxin, calcium channel blockers, and beta blocker therapy are ineffective or inapplicable, Amiodarone may be used a for rate control and to aid in future maintenance of sinus rhythm. This is particularly helpful in congestive heart failure but is unlikely to acutely convert the patient.

The benefit of chronic maintenance of sinus rhythm versus ventricular rate control alone is still an unsettled debate. Numerous clinical risk factors mitigate against the successful maintenance of sinus rhythm. Prolonged atrial fibrillation enlarged left atrial size > 5.0 cm, and advanced age all make lasting sinus rhythm less likely. However, at least 1 attempt at cardioversion and maintenance of sinus rhythm should be entertained. Preliminary results from studies comparing rhythm versus rate control have thus far failed to show benefit.

Pharmacologic Maintenance of Sinus Rhythm

In patients in whom maintenance of sinus rhythm is desired and pharmacological assistance is required a variety of antiarrhythmic drugs may be helpful; however, the patients underlying co-morbidities are important in selection of the appropriate drug class. Maintenance of sinus rhythm with pharmacological therapy is similar among class I and III drugs. Average recurrence of atrial fibrillation approaches 50% as opposed to 80% for placebo at 1 year.

Some evidence exists that amiodarone, a class III drug, may have slightly higher success rate, as may dofetilide a new class III drug. Both Amiodarone and dofetilide have been shown to also be safe in coronary artery disease and left ventricular dysfunction. Class 1 C agents, such as flecainide and propafenone, are safe in the absence of structural heart disease and coronary artery disease. Many experts have touted these to be the drugs of choice in patients with atrial dysrrhythmias without structural heart disease. However, these drugs have the ability to convert atrial fibrillation to atrial flutter with 1 to 1 ventricular conduction. This can lead to extremely rapid ventricular rates and subsequent cardiovascular collapse. Therefore with class IC drugs an AV nodal blocking agent should also be used. Exercise testing while on medication is advocated by some as use dependence associated with these drugs *(increasing drug effect at increasing heart rates)* can lead to proarrhythmia at rapid heart rates.

It is important to realize that reversion to atrial fibrillation on medical therapy does not represent failure. Indeed, if the patient symptomatically improves and remains in sinus rhythm for a reasonable period of time, (determined by the willingness of the physician and patient to undergo subsequent cardioversion) recurrent cardioversion and pharmacological maintenance are a reasonable treatment plan.

In patients where pharmacological maintenance of sinus rhythm is ineffective and rate control is inadequate for symptom relief new therapies are on the horizon. The success of the surgical Maze procedure approaches a 90% freedom from recurrent atrial fibrillation. The Maze procedure involves a thoracotomy with substantial morbidity and a mortality of approximately 2%. This has led to investigation for percutaneous Maze, which appear difficult.

There is new enthusiasm for focal atrial fibrillation ablations. In atrial fibrillation ablations focal initiating areas, which are frequently found in the pulmonary veins, are ablated with a catheter approach. These procedures appear promising alternative to medical therapy.

Rate Control in Atrial Fibrillation

Rate control with AV nodal blocking agents is relatively effective for control of symptoms in many patients. Amiodarone may be considered for rate control in patients with severe left ventricular dysfunction who do not tolerate the negative inotropic effect of calcium channel blockers and beta blockers. In some patients, maintenance of sinus rhythm is not feasible and AV nodal blockade with adequate rate control is impossible to obtain through pharmacological treatment. For such patients, several non-pharmacological treatments are available.

Significant experience with AV nodal ablation and subsequent pacemaker implantation has demonstrated significant improvement in symptoms but the need for anticoagulation is not avoided as the atrial fibrillation continues. In addition an increased incidence of sudden death has been noted immediately after ablation, which is thought to be due to pause dependent arrhythmic death secondary to Torsades de Pointes. Long-term outcomes in these patients has been shown to be similar to medical therapy with regard to mortality with improved quality of life and symptoms.

Management of Atrial Fibrillation with WPW

Management of atrial fibrillation in a patient with WPW syndrome is a special situation. The use of AV nodal blocking agents as the primary therapy for rate control should be avoided because they may paradoxically increase AV nodal conduction and heart rate due to removal of a concealed retrograde conduction in the accessory pathway. This may lead to an increased rate of ventricular response, ventricular fibrillation, and/or possibly death.

Intravenous Procainamide or Ibutilide is the initial drug of choice to slow conduction down the accessory pathway and to facilitate possible conversion and maintenance of sinus rhythm. Intravenous Amiodarone is the drug of choice in patients with a rapid ventricular response with diminished left ventricular function and/or heart failure. DC cardioversion should be undertaken in patients with a rapid ventricular response with symptomatic hypotension.

All atrial fibrillation patients with symptomatic WPW syndrome should undergo electrophysiologic evaluation. Patients with rapid ventricular conduction over the accessory pathway at a rate greater than 240 bpm and any preexcited ventricular complex with a RR interval shorter than 250 msec may be at increased risk of sudden death as compared to the general population and should undergo RF *(radiofrequency)* ablation. Patients with symptomatic WPW syndrome without the above findings should also be studied and ablated rather than treated medically if inducible

arrhythmias utilizing the pathway are found. Asymptomatic patients with WPW syndrome do not in general require electrophysiologic study unless they are in high-risk professions such as airline pilot or professional climber.

WIDE COMPLEX ARRHYTHMIAS

The assessment of wide complex tachyarrhythmias can be confusing and challenging. The diagnosis of wide complex tachycardia is a ventricular rate above 100 beats per minute and QRS duration greater than 120 msec. The differential diagnosis of wide complex tachyarrhythmia is ventricular tachycardia, supraventricular tachycardia with bundle branch block or with functional bundle branch block *(aberrancy),* and pre-excited tachycardias with anterograde accessory pathway conduction with a supraventricular arrhythmia. Metabolic disorders, such as extreme hyperkalemia, and occasionally large anterior myocardial infarction may mimic wide complex arrhythmias. The majority of patients seen with wide complex tachycardias present with sinus tachycardia and bundle branch block. Higher risk populations, which includes patients with depressed left ventricular function and patients with previous myocardial infarction, overwhelmingly present with ventricular arrhythmias as a cause of their wide complex tachyarrhythmias. Indeed, diagnosis by history in these patients has been shown to work nearly as well as more complex algorithms.

The necessity in differentiating supraventricular tachycardia (SVT) with bundle branch block from ventricular tachycardia (VT) is that it avoids delays in appropriate therapy and avoids use of contraindicated medications, such as verapamil, which was used historically with SVT. Verapamil has precipitated numerous episodes of hemodynamic collapse in patients with VT. Evaluation by a 12 lead ECG determines whether the wide complex is typical for a bundle branch block. If the complex is not typical for a bundle branch block then the diagnosis defaults to ventricular tachycardia. Although this sounds simple, the algorithms developed may be complicated and cumbersome.

THE BRUGADA CRITERIA

A frequently used diagnostic algorithm by Brugada incorporates many previously published morphology criteria in a stepwise algorithm and has been demonstrated to be very sensitive and specific in the absence of preexisting intraventricular conduction abnormalities. Wide complex tachycardias are divided into right and left bundle branch type. If the complex is upright in lead V1 of a standard 12 lead ECG then it is defined as a right bundle branch type. If the complex is negative in lead V1 then it is defined as a left bundle branch type. *See Table I below.*

Table I. Diagnosis of wide QRS complex tachycardia

Diagnosis Of Wide QRS Complex Tachycardia With A Regular Rhythm

Step 1. Is there absence of an RS complex in all precordial leads V1 – V6?

If yes, then the **rhythm is VT.**
- Sens 0.21 Spec 1.0

Step 2. Is the interval from the onset of the R wave to the nadir of the S wave greater than 100 msec in **any** precordial leads?

If yes, then the **rhythm is VT.**
- Sens 0.66 Spec 0.98

Step 3. Is there AV dissociation?

If yes, then the **rhythm is VT.**
- Sens 0.82 Spec 0.98

Step 4. Are morphology criteria for VT present? *See Table II.*

If yes, then the **rhythm is VT.**
- Sens 0.99 Spec 0.97

Table II. Morphology criteria for ventricular tachycardia

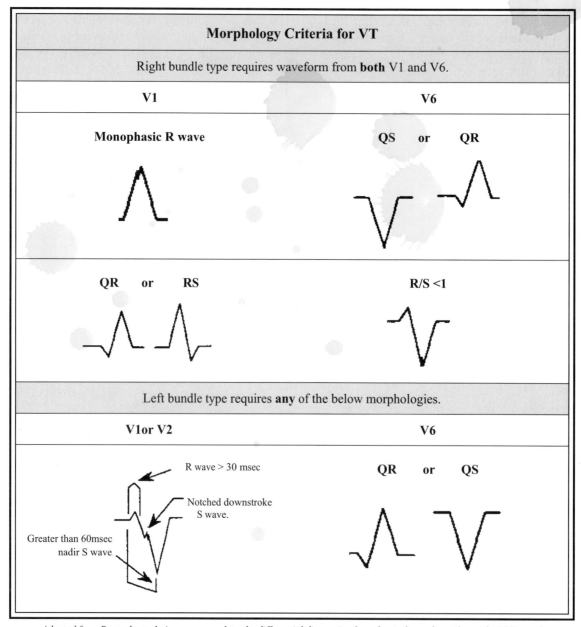

Adapted from Brugada et al. A new approach to the differential diagnosis of regular tachycardia with a wide QRS complex. Circulation 1991; 83:1649-59.

Once the diagnosis of ventricular tachycardia is made therapy depends on the clinical condition of the patient and the presence or absence of left ventricular dysfunction. If the patient is unstable then DC cardioversion is indicated. If the patient appears stable with minimal symptoms, without heart failure or angina and adequate blood pressure, then pharmacological treatment may be utilized. The choice of agent depends greatly on the presence or absence of left ventricular dysfunction.

NEW ACLS GUIDELINES

There have been significant changes in published guidelines for Adult Cardiac Life Support (ACLS) regarding monomorhpic venrticular tachycardia and ventricular fibrillation. The results of out-of-hospital arrest trials have shown significant efficacy for amiodarone. Multiple studies have shown a neutral mortality or trend towards benefit in patients who are treated with amiodarone post MI as well as patients with CHF, particularly in the nonischemic population. As a result, amiodarone has replaced many formerly heavily utilized antiarrhythmics as the primary therapy. In addition it should be noted that the use of combination antiarrhythmic therapy is strongly discouraged because of a proarrhythmic potential and limited efficacy.

New emphasis in the ACLS guidelines is placed on the differentiation of treatment in patients with normal left ventricular function and those with diminished function. For patients with depressed left ventricular function, amiodarone is the agent of choice. In patients with preserved left ventricular function and wide complex arrhythmia of unknown etiology or VT, acceptable choices of therapy include DC cardioversion, amiodarone, or procainamide.

For every tachyarrhythmia, amiodarone may be used as a primary or secondary choice. Lidocaine is now considered secondary in therapy as a result of its limited effectiveness in ventricular tachycardia in nonischemic tissue.

For wide complex tachycardias, DC cardioversion is a universally acceptable treatment option and should be considered the primary choice. Proper sedation should always be provided prior to cardioversion. DC cardioversion is always indicated for unstable rhythms.

Polymorphic VT *(where the ventricular complex changes morphology or axis throughout the arrhythmia)* as well as Ventricular fibrillation should receive prompt rapid treatment with DC cardioversion. The pharmacologic treatment of choice is intravenous Amiodarone administered as a 150 mg bolus over 10 minutes, but it has been successfully used for out-of-hospital arrests with a 300 mg intravenous bolus. These rhythms are generally the result of severe metabolic disturbance and cardiac ischemia. However, polymorphic VT is rarely associated with a prolonged QT interval presenting as Torsades de Pointes.

VENTRICULAR TACHYCARDIA IN PATIENTS WITH NORMAL LEFT VENTRICULAR FUNCTION

In addition to monomorphic ventricular tachycardia (*ventricular complexes are stable from beat to beat with regard to morphology*) due to coronary artery disease and nonischemic cardiomyopathies, ventricular tachycardia also occurs rarely in patients without structural heart disease. These ventricular tachycardias frequently present as palpitations and extremely rarely as sudden death. The morphology may be a left bundle branch type in patients with right ventricular outflow-tract tachycardia. This type of VT is adenosine sensitive and responds to calcium channel blockers and occasionally beta blockers. It frequently is erroneously diagnosed as being from a supraventricular origin. Right bundle branch morphology VT originating from the left ventricle may also present in patients without structural heart disease. This type of VT is verapamil responsive. Both types of VT are also amenable to catheter ablation, which has a curative rate of greater than 90%.

Torsades de Pointes

Torsades de Pointes has been described as appearing to twist around it's baseline. It is polymorphic VT defined by its association the QT segment prolongation. This rhythm is adversely affected by bradycardia and is frequently pause dependent (*initiated after a pause*). An assessment should be made for causative agents, which include many noncardiac medications. In addition, many antiarrhythmics that prolong cardiac repolarization such as Vaughn Williams Class I A and Class III drugs will exacerbate this arrhythmia.

Most cases of Torsades de Pointes are acquired by a combination of iatrogenic prolongation of ventricular repolarization from drugs (*see Table III*), hypokalemia, or hypomagnesemia and an underlying mild repolarization abnormality.

Since the QT interval lengthens with decreasing heart rate, a measurement of a rate independent QT interval may be calculated. The standard correction for rate is the QT interval by divided the square root of the RR interval measured in milliseconds. The presence of a corrected QT interval of greater than 440-450 msec should be considered abnormal. Patients with QT intervals corrected for rate greater than 500 and certainly 600 msec have been shown to be at increased risk for Torsades de Pointes.

Treatment of acquired long QT syndrome leading to Torsades de Pointes consists of removal of offending agents or conditions. Further therapy includes treatment with intravenous magnesium, which prevents the onset of Torsades de Pointes. Temporary pacing or administration of isoproterenol increases the underlying heart rate and shortens the QT interval, diminishing the risk of arrhythmia.

Congenital Long QT Syndrome

Some patients present with syncope or sudden death and are found to have pause dependent polymorphic VT, Torsades de Pointes and a prolonged QT interval without any offending agent or condition . These patients have congenital long QT syndrome. The majority of patients with congenital long QT Syndrome have Long QT syndrome 1 (LQT1). These patients have an abnormality in a potassium ion channel. This leads to prolonged ventricular repolarization and an increased risk of sudden death, particularly with exercise. Patient's with long QT syndrome 3 (LQT3) have have an abnormality involving a sodium channel also leading to prolonged repolarization and increased risk of death. These patients paradoxically have an increased risk of death while sleeping. Therapy for congenital long QT syndrome patients with symptoms of dizziness, syncope or sudden death is considered to consist of beta blocker therapy and pacing. Some advocate a left stellate ganglionectomy in addition.

Many experts feel that the addition of ICD (Implantable cardiodefibrillator) rather than surgery in combination with beta blocker

therapy is optimum. Beta blocker therapy has been shown to decrease their risk of death by approximately 50%. In addition it is felt that pacing also reduces mortality by approximately 25%. Beta blocker therapy is particularly effective for LQTI patients, and a smaller subgroup of patients with a potassium channel abnormality known as Long QT2. Patients with LQT3 do not respond to beta blocker therapy and this may explain why some patients in the past appeared to benefit from beta blockers, while others in the population did not. These patients may be treated with some efficacy using mexilitine (a sodium channel blocker) but would also require an ICD if syncope or sudden death has occurred.

Sudden Death in Patients with Normal Left Ventricular Function

In addition to long QT syndrome, patients with normal left ventricular function may also present with ventricular fibrillation, and cardiac arrest. This patient population includes some rare syndromes of which you should be aware. The Brugada syndrome is characterized by syncope and sudden death. These patients frequently present with electrocardiographic findings consistent with incomplete right bundle branch block ST elevations in leads V1 and V2 that may be exacerbated with intravenous procainamide and flecanide. These drugs increase the degree of ST segment elevation. The degree of ST segment elevation may also vary over time. This may complicate the diagnosis as at times patients may have a normal resting ECG. Treatment in patients with cardiac arrest or syncope with the above ECG finding consists of ICD implantation.

Right Ventricular Dysplasia

Right Ventricular dysplasia is a common cause of arrest in young patients, particularly in Europe. The electrocardiographic presentation is delayed right ventricular activation presenting as incomplete or complete right bundle branch block. An epsilon wave seen as a positive deflection following the R wave and deep T

Table III. QT Prolonging or Torsadogenic Drugs

The following drugs have been shown to prolong the QT interval or have documented clinical Torsades de Pointes reported in the literature

Amantadine	Chloralhydrate	Disopyramide	Flecanide	Isradapine	Pentamidine
Quetiapine	Sparfloxacin	Tizanide	Fluoxetine	Ketaconazole	Pimozide
Aminophylline	Chloroquine	Dofetilide	Foscarnet	Levofloxacin	Probucol
Quinidine	Sumatriptan	Trimethorprim	Fosphentoin	Levomethadyl	Erythromycin
Amiodarone	Ciprofloxacin	Sulfa	Gatifloxin	Mesoridazine	Zolmitriptan
Risperdone	Tacrilimus	Doxepine	Halofantrine	Moexitine/Hctz	Felbamate
Barium	Cisapride	Venlafaxine	Haloperidol	Moxifloxicin	Clarithromycin
Salmeterol	Tamoxifen	Droperidol	Ibutilide	Naratripan	Terfenadine
Bepridil	Sertraline	Vistaril	Imipramine	Nicardipine	Desipramine
Thioridazine	Chlorpromazine	Sotalol	Indipamide	Octreotide	

wave inversion in the anterior precordium are classic ECG findings. The diagnosis is commonly confirmed with an MRI revealing fatty infiltration of the right ventricle. It may also be confirmed with echocardiography although it is insensitive, or right ventricular angiography. It presents with ventricular arrhythmias originating from the right ventricle and is exacerbated by exercise. Although Sotalol has been shown to be effective at suppressing inducible arrhythmias with right ventricular dysplasia, ICD therapy is recommended. Patients occasionally die from progressive right ventricular mechanical failure.

Hypertrophic Cardiomyopathy

Sudden death or syncope in patients with significant left ventricular hypertrophy should alert the physician to the possibility of hypertrophic cardiomyopathy. These patients are frequently asymptomatic prior to their arrest, which is frequently related to exertion. This syndrome accounts for the majority of sudden cardiac death in young adults in the US. Risks for sudden death among patients with suspected hypertrophic cardiomyopathy are extreme ventricular hypertrophy, exertional hypotension, documented nonsustained VT, and previous syncope and family history of sudden death. Implantable cardiodefibrillators have been shown to be effective therapy, however, screening and appropriate selection of asymptomatic patients remains problematic.

IMPLANTABLE CARDIODEFIBRILLATOR

Since 1983 with the FDA approval of implantable cardiodefibrillators (ICDs) for human use, the indications for ICD implantation continue to expand. Technical advances allow increasing ease of implantation with diminishing size. ICDs are now almost entirely nonthoracotomy placed and the risk of death with implantation is under 1%. They frequently include many of the features of pacemakers including dual chamber pacing and sensing. They may have rate responsive abilities in addition to impressive intracardiac electrogram monitoring, including some holter abilities. In addition, they have complex algorithms that aid in decreasing spurious electrical therapy for rapid SVT, which may overlap in rate with dangerous ventricular arrhythmias. ICDs are extremely effective at preventing arrhythmic death. Many studies report arrhythmic risk of death to be reduced to 2% per year. Increasing evidence is mounting as to the superiority of ICD therapy in patients with cardiac arrest and inducible ventricular arrhythmias with coronary artery disease.

The Amiodaraone Versus the Implantable Defibrillator (AVID) study demonstrated the superiority of ICD in patients with cardiac arrest, poorly tolerated VT, with ejection fraction of less than 35%. In addition primary prevention studies in high risk patients *(e.g., Ejection fraction less than 40% and coronary artery disease, found to have with inducible arrhythmias in electrophysiology study)* have demonstrated the benefit of ICD over medical therapy with dramatic reduction in overall mortality. Patients receiving ICDs in this population achieved relative mortality reductions approaching 50%! Recent data has also demonstrated benefit of ICD in primary prevention of sudden death in patients with severely reduced ejection fraction (<30%), and history of previous MI compared to conventional therapy.

As a result of these advances and the increase in implantation, the critical care physician is increasingly likely to encounter patients with ICDs and ICD related complications and/or emergencies. In order to understand the emergency one must realize that the ICD mainly treats arrhythmias based on the ventricular rate. Preprogrammed heart rate zones trigger the device to intervene with therapy such as automatic pacing or low or high energy shocks. Complex algorithms to prevent therapy for SVT and atrial fibrillation exist but are not always utilized due to fear of withholding appropriate therapy for ventricular arrhythmias which could be misclassified as SVT or sinus tachycardia.

Complications Associated with ICDs

Complications of ICD therapy include, inappropriate shocks secondary to lead fracture, atrial fibrillation with rapid ventricular response, failure to treat secondary to undersensing, inappropriate therapy due to oversensing of intrinsic cardiac signal or external noise such as electronic theft devices. Patients receiving more than two to three ICD discharges in a 24 hour period should be treated as a medical emergency.

Treatment

ICD shocks are extremely painful and can be very traumatic which can result in posttraumatic stress disorder. Patients presenting with incessant shocks that are appropriately delivered should be admitted to intensive care unit. They frequently require sedation and antiadrenergic therapy as well as antiarrhythmic therapy and correction of any underlying electrolyte abnormalities. A search for exacerbating conditions such as congestive heart failure or increasing ischemia should be

undertaken. An emergent consultation with an electrophysiologist should be obtained to interrogate the device for the possibility of malfunction. If an electrophysiology consultation is not available and the patient appears to be receiving spurious shocks without evidence of ventricular arrhythmia then the placement of a strong magnet over the device will impede its ability to sense, which will prevent further device intervention.

Trouble Shooting

In patients where the device fails to terminate arrhythmias, one should look for migration of the ventricular lead or pharmacologic causes of increased defibrillation threshold such as amiodarone or certain class I agents *(e.g., flecainide)*. If a device completes all of it's therapy without termination of the arrhythmia, it will generally not reinitiate therapy unless sinus rhythm has been redetected. Occasionally, in patients with incessant arrhythmias, the device will terminate the arrhythmia with each output however the reinitiation of arrhythmia occurs before success has been detected. In this situation the device may withhold further therapy after completion of the maximal number of interventions.

For ineffective defibrillation from a device, patients should be externally defibrillated. Paddles or patches should not be placed directly on the device. Subsequent to external defibrillation, the device should be interrogated to ensure that no changes in programming occurred.

Problems Associated with Tests/Procedures in ICD patients.

Patients with ICDs are problematic with regard to various tests and procedures. In general, with few exceptions, patients with ICDs should not undergo MRI tests. The strong magnetic field will impair the sensing ability of the device and may damage internal circuits.

Electrocautery during surgery frequently will be interpreted by the device as a rapid tachyarrhythmia. This leads to inappropriate discharges to the patient with disconcerting but harmless shocks to the surgeon. Patients with

ICD frequently must have their device detection algorithms turned off or placed on monitor during surgery if electrocautery is planned. The problem of electrical oversensing is increased in pacer dependent patients with ICDs that also function as pacemakers. In these patients, a temporary pacer may need to be placed in asynchronous mode during electrocautery since electrocautery will lead to inhibition of pacing and possible asystole. If only limited electrocautery is needed, then monitoring the patient's rhythm for prolonged pauses may suffice with limitation on the length of surgical RF application.

Finally, as patients receiving ICDs frequently have other severe comorbid diseases and end of life issues frequently arise. If a patient is clearly terminal or the decision to withdraw care has been made, it is reasonable to turn off the ICD to avoid therapy for terminal arrhythmias. The device must be removed prior to cremation to avoid explosion of the battery. Due to the complex and specialized nature of ICDs and their programming, the input of an electrophysiologist should be obtained as soon as possible.

CONCLUSION

The diagnosis of tachyarrhythmias depends heavily on ECG assessment. Treatment depends mainly on differentiation of supraventricular and ventricular arrhythmias as well as the presence or absence of left ventricular dysfunction. Patients with unstable rhythms should immediately undergo DC cardioverson or defibrillation. Patients with stable symptoms may be treated with pharmacologic therapy. Patients with stable ventricular arrhythmias should still be considered for electrical therapy due to its low risk of proarrhythmia.

Class IA drugs such as procainamide, quinidine, dysopyramide, class IC drugs such as propafenone, and flecainide should be avoided in patients with left ventricular dysfunction and/or coronary artery disease due to their increased mortality with their use. In this population, amiodarone is the pharmacologic treatment of choice.

Once the ventricular arrhythmia is controlled, ICD therapy is frequently indicated. ICDs are more effective at preventing death in patients with depressed left ventricular function with previous arrest and/or sustained monomorphic VT with coronary artery disease. Patients with supraventricular tachycardia may be controlled with a variety of antiarrhythmics and AV nodal blocking agents. An increasing number of patients are definitively treated with catheter ablation.

Atrial fibrillation continues to be troublesome but new catheter based modalities promise to offer new therapeutic options in the near future. Until then, rate control and rhythm control remain reasonable treatment strategies depending on patient symptoms. Patients with moderate or high risk for thromboembolism including diabetics, hypertension, valvular disease, congestive heart failure, previous stroke or age greater than 65 should be anticoagulated with coumadin to reduce the risk of stroke with target INR of 2.0 to 3.0.

Patients with WPW syndrome should be screened for symptoms. Asymptomatic patients generally do not need further evaluation. Patients with palpitations or syncope should undergo electrophysiologic study with ablation for inducible arrhythmias or rapid accessory pathway conduction faster than 250bpm.

REFERENCES

1. The Antiarrythmics Versus Implantable Defibrillators (AVID) Investigators: A Comparison of antiarrythmic drug therapy wit implantable defibrillators in patients resuscutated from near fatal ventricular arrythmia. *N Engl J Med* 1997; 337:1576-83 *First major study to demonstrate benefit of ICD over Drugs in patients with sustained arrhythmias, or arrest.*

2. Brugada P, Brugada J, et al: A new approach to the differential diagnosis of a regular tachycardia with a wide QRS complex. *Circulation* 1991; 83:1649-1659 *A classic article illustrating an algorithmic and reproducible approach to differentiating wide complex tachycardia.*

3. Cardiac Arrhythmia suppression Trial (CAST) Investigators: Preliminary report:

Effect Of Encainide And Flecainide On Mortality. *In:* A Randomized Trial Of Arrhythmia

4. Suppression After Myocardial Infarction. *N Engl J Med* 1989; 321:406-412
Seminal study that showed dramatically increased mortality in patients treated with encainide and flecanide in a post-MI. population despite arrhythmia suppression.

5. Effect of prophylactic amiodarone on mortality after acute myocardial infarction and in congestive heart failure: meta-analysis of individual data from 6500 patients in randomised trials. Amiodarone Trials Metap analysis Investigators. *Lancet* 1997; 350:1417-24
A meta-analysis suggesting the Amiodarone improves survival after MI and in congestive heart failure.

6. Fuster V, et al: ACC/AHA guidelines for the Management of Atrial Fibrillation. *Circulation* 2001; 104:2118-2150
Current updated recommendations for management of atrial fibrillation.

7. Gregoratos G, Cheitlin, et al: ACC/AHA guidelines for implantation of cardiac pacemakers and antiarrhythmic devices: *J Am Coll Cardiol* 1998; 31:1175-209.
Review of indications for implantation of pacemakers and ICD.

8. Guidelines 2000 for Cardiopulmonary Resuscitation and Emergency Cardiovascular Care. *Circulation* 2000; 102:08
Updated Guidelines for resuscitation and their explanation of supportive data.

9. Moss, et al: Prophylactic Implantation of Defibrillator in Patients with Myocardial infarction and reduced ejection fraction. *N Engl J Med* 2002; 346:877-883
Study revealing primary prevention mortality benefit of ICD versus control in depressed LV function and previous MI without arrhythmia induction.

10. Myerburg RJ, et al: Interpretation of outcomes of Antiarrhythmic Clinical trials. *Circulation* 1998; 97:1514-1521
An excellent discussion on confounding factors that influence the design and interpretation of antiarrhythmic studies.

11. Prystowsky EN, Benson W, Fuster V, et al: Management of Patients with atrial Fibrillation. *Circulation* 1996; 93:1262-1277
An exhaustive review on the subject of atrial fibrillation.

12. Singh Bramah N, et al: Current Antiarrhythmic Drugs: An overview of Mechanism of action and potential clinical utility. *J Cardoivasc Electrophysiol* 1999; 2:283-301
An excellent review of the mechanism of action and application of current antiarrhythmics.

13. Torp-Pedersen C, Moller M, Bloch-Thomsen PE, et al: Dofetilide in patients with congestive heart failure and left ventricular dysfunction. Danish Investigation of Arrhythmia and Mortality on Dofetilide Study Group. *N Eng J Med* 1999; 341:857-65
Dofetilide had no adverse mortality effect in group of patients with congestive heart failure.

14. Wellens HJJ, et al: The value of the electrocardiogram in the differential diagnosis of a tachycardia with a widened QRS complex. *Am J Med* 1978; 64:27-33.
Another classic article helping to differentiate ventricular tachycardia from abberancy.

BRADYCARDIA, DIAGNOSIS AND MANAGMENT

Laurent Lewkowiez, MD

Objectives

- To describe the cardiac conduction system and its vascular supply
- To describe the mechanisms leading to bradycardia
- To describe various causes of symptomatic bradycardia, as well as their treatment

Key Words*:* Sinus node, AV node, His Purkinje system, sick sinus syndrome, chronotropic incompetence, complete heart block, atrial fibrillation

TABLE OF ABBREVIATIONS

AMI	acute myocardial infarction
AV block	atrioventricular block
AV node	atrioventricular node
BBB	bundle branch block
LAD	left anterior descending artery
MI	myocardial infarction
PDA	posterior descending artery
SA node	sinoatrial node

INTRODUCTION

Bradycardia is defined as a heart rate below 60 beats per minute. The causes of bradycardia are numerous. Bradycardia may be a normal underlying rhythm for many, or it may herald impending conduction failure and/or syncope or sudden death. It may be intrinsic or extrinsic relating to disease processes or drug effects. Bradyarrhythmia may be due to failure of impulse formation or failure of impulse conduction. The significance of the underlying bradycardia must be closely scrutinized as to its contribution to symptoms and/or pathology, because its relation to symptoms and significance are frequently far from straightforward.

THE CARDIAC CONDUCTION SYSTEM

The cardiac conduction system is comprised of the sinus node (SA node), the atrioventricular node (AV node), the His bundle, and the His Purkinje system, which includes the left and right bundle branches. The SA node is located at the junction of the superior vena cava and right atrium. It initiates the normal heartbeat with rapid rate of depolarization. The vascular supply to the sinus node is provided by the right coronary artery in 55% of the population, the circumflex coronary artery in 35% of the population, and both in 10% of the population. The sinus node is innervated heavily by both parasympathetic as well as sympathetic nerves, which exert a profound effect on its underlying rate of depolarization.

The AV node is located in the anterior interatrial septum superior and anterior to the coronary sinus. The vascular supply of the AV node is provided by the AV nodal artery, which is supplied by the right coronary artery in 85% of the population and the circumflex in 15 % of the population. In addition, septal perforators from the left anterior descending artery frequently supply the AV node. The AV node is also extensively innervated by both sympathetic and parasympathetic inputs. Importantly, the conduction of the AV node is decremental. This trait causes the refractoriness of the AV node to increase with increasing stimulation, allowing the AV node to limit input into the ventricular chamber, which protects against ventricular fibrillation.

The His Purkinje system is comprised of the bundle of His, the right and left bundle branches, and the distal purkinje fibers. The common His bundle is immediately anterior to the AV node and dives into the central fibrous body. The His bundle divides into the right and left bundle branch systems. The vascular supply of the His bundle is dually supplied by both anterior and posterior septal perforators. The right bundle branch travels along the interventricular septum in the subendocardium towards the base of the anterior papillary muscle. It receives its blood supply from both the AV nodal artery and anterior septal perforators from the left anterior descending artery (LAD). The left bundle branch is not as well defined. It is more of a fan-like structure that is roughly divided into a left anterior fascicle and left posterior fascicle. The anterior fascicle passes anteriorly toward the left anterior papillary muscle of the left ventricle. The left posterior fascicle passes posterio-medially along the interventricular septum toward the posterior papillary muscle. Blood supply to the left anterior fascicle is derived from septal perforators from the LAD. Septal perforators from both the LAD and the posterior descending artery (PDA) feed the left posterior fascicle, which is the larger of the 2.

BRADYCARDIA

The etiology of bradyarrhythmias may be divided into extrinsic or intrinsic types. Abnormal impulse formation or conduction due to drugs, systemic diseases, or due to effects from extracardiac pathology is termed extrinsic in nature. Processes involving abnormalities in cardiac impulse formation and conduction due to primary cardiac degeneration or damage are termed intrinsic in nature. The vast majority of bradyarrhythmias are due to SA node dysfunction and/or AV nodal block, due to either intrinsic or extrinsic causes.

EXTRINSIC CAUSES OF BRADYCARDIA

Drugs

The extrinsic causes of bradyarrhythmias are varied and most frequently involve the effects of drugs that suppress sinus node and AV nodal function (Table 1) Toxic doses of beta-blockers, calcium channel blockers, and digoxin frequently precipitate symptomatic bradycardia. Therapeutic doses of these same drugs can cause symptomatic bradycardia in patients with underlying SA node and/or AV node disease. Digoxin toxicity may

present with multiple cardiac rhythms. These rhythms include atrial arrhythmias with AV nodal block, regularization of atrial fibrillation, accelerated junctional tachycardia, and ventricular tachycardia. With the presentation of atrial arrhythmias, such as atrial tachycardia with AV block, one must initially consider digoxin toxicity, particularly in the elderly and in patients with renal dysfunction. However, many Class I and III antiarrhythmics predispose patients to sinus node dysfunction and AV conduction block, especially when subclinical underlying disease is present. In particular, Amiodarone and Sotalol are known for exacerbating these conditions. Other drugs that are not primarily used for cardiac rate control express significant effects on cardiac impulse formation and conduction, particularly when underlying cardiac disease is already present. These include many centrally acting antihypertensives that diminish central sympathetic output such as Reserpine, alphamethlydopa, and Clonidine. In addition, many antidepressants, antipsychotics, and antiseizure medications also may exert negative effects on the SA and/or AV nodal function, including tricyclic antidepressants, thioridazine, phenothiazines, Lithium, Dilantin, and carbamazapine. Exposure to organophosphates and cholinesterase inhibitors may also present with bradyarrhythmia.

Reflexes

Bradyarrhythmias associated with significant symptoms may frequently be secondary to vagally mediated reflexes. The most common vagal reflex is neurocardiogenic syncope, which occurs frequently in young, otherwise healthy, individuals. Neurocardiogenic syncope presents as a sudden loss of consciousness *(syncope)* with dramatic episodes of bradycardia and occasionally asystole precipitated by upright posture, which is frequently associated with a prodrome of nausea or sensation of heat. Syncope may also occur without dramatic bradycardia when predominant vasodepressor component is causative. These episodes are usually diagnosed clinically, but may also be diagnosed with upright tilt table may also be diagnosed with upright tilt table

Table 1. Extrinsic causes of bradyarrhythmias

Drugs

B-blocking agents   Amiodarone
Calcium channel blockers   Cimetidine
Lithium   Sotalol
Digoxin   Reserpine
α-2 agonists   Propoxyhene
Tricyclic antidepressants   Alphamethyldopa
Cholinergic agents   Organophosphate overdose
Chloraquine   Cholinestease inhibitors
Class I antiarrhythmic agents   Phenothiazenes
Amatadine   Thioridazine
Carbamazapine   Phenytoin

Situational Reflex Bradycardia

Neurocardiogenic syncope   Pain syncope
Maxilofacial reflex   Defacation syncope
Micturition syncope   Vomiting
Oculocardiac reflex   Swallow syncope
Cough syncope

Infection

Viral	*Bacterial*	*Parasitic*
Varicella	Endocarditis	Chagas Disease
Mononucleosis	Dyptheria	
Hepatitis	Lyme Disease	
Mumps		
Rubella		
Rubeola		
RSV		

Metabolic

Hypokalemia, hyperkalemia, hypothyroidism, hyperthyroidism, hypercalcemia, hypoxia, Hypermagnesemia

Rheumatologic

Systemic lupus erythmatosis, rheumatoid arthritis, Reiter's syndrome, systemic sclerosis

Infiltrative Processes

Sarcoid, amyloid

Other

Obstructive sleep apnea, myotonic dystrophy, congenital heart block, postoperative heart block, hypothyroidism testing. Treatment may include: tilt training, anti-cholinergics, Midodrine, beta blocker therapy, salt therapy, fludricortisone, SSRI inhibitors, and occasionally with rate drop pacing. Other reflexes that may also present with bradycardia are situational reflexes such as micturition syncope, cough syncope, defecation syncope, swallow syncope, pain syncope, vomiting induced syncope, the maxillofacial reflex during surgery, and the occulocardiac reflex. Bradyarrhythmias, of special concern are associated with intracranial pathology such as hemorrhage, large stroke, and elevated intracranial pressure. Reflex tachycardia and bradycardia may also be seen following spinal cord trauma for up to four to six weeks post injury.

Metabolic

Metobolic disturbance are also a common and generally reversible cause of bradycardia. In particular hypoxia, hyperkalemia, hypokalemia, hypercalcemia and hypermagnesemia should be sought. Hypo and hyperthyroidism should also be ruled out, particularly in the elderly.

Rheumatologic

Rheumatologic diseases can cause of bradycardia and heart block. Although all connective disease processes may, on occasion, involve the cardiac conduction system, overt conduction disorders with these disease processes is the exception rather than the rule. However, Rheumatoid arthritis (RA), systemic lupus erythmatosis (SLE), Systemic sclerosis all rarely present with AV block, with RA patient presenting with up to 10 % of some form of conduction block due to some involvement of the conduction system with Rheumatoid nodules. Reiters syndrome deserves special note as heart block may be present in up to 25% of cases. Sarcoid also will frequently present with some form of conduction block and/or delay in addition to increased risk of sudden death due to ventricular arrhythmia.

Infection

Infectious causes of bradycardia and heart block are uncommon in the western world with exceptions. Although viral myocarditis is common, and most commonly caused by coxackie B virus, permanent heart block is uncommon although transient block is not. Other viral causes of bradycardia are, mononucleosis, mumps, rubella, rubeola, RSV, and Varicella. Bacterial causes of bradycardia are uncommon but can occur with local extension of endocarditis involving the cardiac conduction system. Diptheria, rickettsial diseases, fungal and helminthic infections infrequently cause AV block. Of note in Central and South America is trypanosomiasis, which generally is associated with cardiomyopathy and ventricular arrhythmia, may also present with conduction disorders. In the Northeast U.S. a concern is the spirochetal disease of Lyme disease which causes a significant incidence of AV block. Patients with Lyme disease may develop cardiac involvement in up to 10% of cases, with AV block the most common presentation, usually occurring within the first 5 months of tick bite. Typically conduction block is transient except on occasion.

Other

Other unusual causes of bradycardia are trauma, postoperative heart block particularly after AV valve repair or replacement, and muscular myotonic dystrophy.

INTRINSIC CAUSES OF BRADYCARDIA

Intrinsic causes of bradycardia include degeneration of the cardiac conduction system with fibrotic replacement of the SA node, Lev's disease *(the spread of fibrosis and calcification from the adjacent cardiac skeleton)*, Lenegre's disease *(an idiopathic fibrotic degeneration of the His purkinje system)*, ischemia, and infarction. The infranodal conduction system is particularly susceptible to infarction due to its discrete location and its function as the only electrical connection between the atria and the ventricles.

Sinus Node Dysfunction

Sinus node dysfunction, also known as sick sinus syndrome, is a common disorder that encompasses patients with tachycardia–bradycardia syndrome, chronotropic incompetence, and inappropriate bradycardia. This spectrum of disorders has been increasing in prevalence among the elderly. Occurrence is estimated to be 1 in 600 among those over age 65. Sinus node dysfunction accounts for greater than 50% of pacemaker implantation in western countries. It may present as a failure of adequate impulse generation *(ie. sinus arrest or sinoatrial block)* or as an abnormal transmission within the atria, which may lead to atrial arrhythmias and fibrillation. Presentation also occurs as excessive overdrive inhibition by arrhythmias, which may lead to prolonged sinus pauses and inability to achieve adequate heart rate with exertion.

Common causes of SA node dysfunction include many of the medications previously mentioned. *See Table 2.* These medications are frequently necessary for treatment of other co-morbidities in elderly patients, which would be a reasonable indication for pacemaker implantation. Metabolic disturbances, especially hyperkalemia, and endocrine disorders such as hyper- and hypothyroidism may also lead to or exacerbate SA node dysfunction. Incidences of sinus arrest, severe sinus bradycardia, and AV block have been well documented to occur in patients with obstructive sleep apnea. Such incidences have also been documented to resolve with successful treatment of the sleep apnea. One must be particularly cautious when diagnosing SA node and AV node dysfunction in the young. Brodski et al documented significant episodes of high-grade AV block, sinus pauses, and sinus arrest in asymptomatic male medical students by 24-hour monitoring. Among well-trained athletes, a resting sinus bradycardia and a junctional rhythm with sinus suppression are generally regarded as normal.

Intrinsic Causes of Sinus Node Dysfunction

Fibrotic degeneration of the SA node in the elderly is common and likely is responsible for a large portion of SA node dysfunction, as is underlying coronary disease. As both of these processes occur with increasing incidence with the elderly, their separation as to a cause of SA node dysfunction is difficult. The diagnosis of Sinus node dysfunction remains inexact. Practically speaking, however, sinus pauses

greater than three seconds while awake are relatively rare and may trigger further evaluation. First degree sinus node block cannot be discerned from a surface ECG. Wenckebach periodicity to sinus block can be seen as a shortening of the PP interval prior to loss of P wave. Chronotropic incompetence also lacks an accepted definition but some use the inability to achieve 90% of age predicted maximal heart rate as a definition. In tachycardia-bradycardia syndrome patients manifest both atrial arrhythmias and excessive sinus node suppression. These patients are at increased risk of co-morbidity secondary to thromboembolism.

The diagnosis of Sinus node dysfunction is clinical with symptoms of fatigue, dizziness, presyncope, syncope, and exercise intolerance with or without the symptoms of transient tachycardia. It is supported by findings of sinus bradycardia, exit block, or arrest while awake and is frequently associated with intermittent atrial fibrillation. Symptoms are frequently intermittent and evaluation with continuous loop monitors, and implantable loop monitors may be required. Intracardiac evaluation of sinus node function with the perfomance of sinus node recovery time after rapid atrial pacing has relatively good specificity within the 90% range with sensitivity in the 60 to 70 % range. The evaluation with exercise treadmill testing may be very helpful for the diagnosis of chronotropic incompetence.

Treatment of sinus node dysfunction is directed at alleviation of symptoms as well as preventing complications of the syndrome. In previous studies, dual chamber pacing reduced risk of new onset atrial fibrillation from 5% per year to 1.2 % per year. Thromboembolism with incidence of nearly 15% at 38 months was reduced to 1.6% in atrial paced patients. In review of multiple non-randomized studies, atrial based pacing reduced the incidence of atrial fibrillation by 74% in comparison to ventricular pacing; however, anticoagulation with atrial fibrillation is still necessary. Treatment with pacing is extremely effective when bradyarrhythmias are causative for symptoms. *See Table 3.* In addition, rate adaptive pacing may be extremely effective at treatment for chronotropic incompetence. The removal of offending extrinsic drug effect may significantly improve symptoms. However,

Table 2. Drugs affecting sinus node function

Amiodarone	Reserpine
Flecanide	β-blockers
Propafanone	Pindolol
Sotalol	Acebutalol (less so, secondary to ISA)
Procainamide	Verapamil
Disopyramide	Diltiazem
Quinidine (less frequently)	Cimetidine
Alphamethyldopa	Phenytoin
Clonidine	Carbamazapine
Lithium	

improvement of mortality due to pacing in sinus node dysfunction has not been proven. Catheter ablation of focal atrial arrhythmias may have a larger role in the future with the advent of spatial mapping systems and pulmonary vein ablation.

AV CONDUCTION DISTURBANCES

AV conduction involves conduction from the atrium through the AV node, common His bundle and bundle branch system. A conduction block that occurs in the AV node and common His bundle will result in complete AV block. A conduction block that occurs below the His bundle will result in either bundle branch block or a fascicular block with AV conduction maintained through the remaining fascicles unless extensive infranodal conduction disease exists. Similar to the SA node, both extrinsic and intrinsic causes of conduction block may occur. In addition, because these specialized areas of conduction are discretely defined anatomically, they are susceptible to injury from trauma and, even more common, from infarction and ischemia. The location of the conduction block can frequently be determined by examining the remaining pattern of cardiac activation and/or the etiology of the block. The prognostic significance of the conduction block depends upon the location of the disturbance, nodal versus infranodal, as well as the etiology. Atrioventricular block located in the supra nodal or nodal region generally does not progress rapidly to complete heart block. However, an AV block located in the infra nodal region may frequently demonstrate unpredictable conduction

due to an all or nothing conduction, which may rapidly progress to complete heart block. In addition, an escape rhythm with nodal block is generally located in the AV junction, which has a stable escape rate between 40 to 60 bpm. Escape rhythms originating below the AV junction generally have a much slower escape rate and are frequently unreliable.

Atrial Fibrillation

Special consideration must be given to bradycardia associated with an underlying atrial fibrillation. A conservative approach should be entertained when evaluating pauses in this population because heart rate variability among patients with atrial fibrillation exceeds that of sinus rhythm dramatically. Implantation of pacemakers for symptomatic bradycardia in this condition is relatively common; however, a review of holter data on asymptomatic patients with atrial fibrillation revealed frequent and prolonged pauses. Pauses greater than two seconds was found to occur in 2/3[rds] of the patients and pauses greater than three seconds in 20% of the patients. Therefore, daytime pauses up to 2.8 seconds and nighttime pauses up to four seconds during atrial fibrillation may be considered within normal limits.

1st Degree AV Block

By definition, 1st degree AV block represents a PR interval greater than 200 msec *(equal to one large block on ECG at standard speed 25 mm/sec)*. There is maintenance of AV conduction with each beat. In general, first degree AV block is due to delayed AV nodal conduction, although, it may also be due in part to slow intra-atrial conduction and occasionally to delayed conduction below the AV node when a wide ventricular complex is seen.

2ⁿᵈ Degree AV Block

Second degree AV block implies continued conduction of supraventricular stimuli to the ventricle with some organized atrial activation that fails to conduct to the ventricle. There are two distinct subtypes.

Mobitz Type I Pattern (Wenckebach)

Mobitz Type I *(Wenckebach)* appears as a progressive conduction delay prior to the blocked beat. It presents with a lengthening PR interval. The greatest increment in PR prolongation is seen in the second PR interval in a classic Wenckebach sequence. The degree of lengthening between atrial and ventricular depolarization lessens with each beat, resulting in a narrowing of the RR interval. The PR interval usually shortens after the blocked beat and the pattern may repeat itself. A classic Wenckebach pattern presents only 30% of the time. Wenckebach periodicity more commonly presents as an atypical Wenckebach pattern where the PR prolongation may not be progressive or may be variable due to the additional effect of sinus arrhythmia. The presence of a Wenckebach conduction block, classic or atypical, generally implies that the AV node is the site of the block. However, a block in the His Purkinje system may occasionally, but rarely does, present in this fashion when significant disease is present. The underlying ventricular complex is generally narrow unless underlying bundle branch block or intraventricular conduction delay is present.

Mobitz Type II

Mobitz Type II block is defined as AV nodal conduction with intermittent failure to conduct without evidence of progressive PR interval prolongation prior to block. Mobitz type II block is most often associated with His-purkinje disease. The QRS complex is usually wide.

2 to 1 AV block

Block location in 2:1 AV block cannot be known with certainty. Certain findings, however, may suggest nodal or infranodal AV block. An underlying narrow complex rhythm suggests nodal disease although His bundle disease can not be excluded. A PR interval that is greater than 300msec suggests an AV nodal location of the block. AV block associated with slowing sinus rate suggests a vagally mediated etiology also suggesting AV nodal level of block.

3ʳᵈ Degree AV Block (Complete Heart Block)

Third Degree AV Block or Complete heart block occurs when atrial and ventricular activity are independent with atrial activity faster than ventricular activity. The location of the block, though generally infranodal, may be implied by the width of the QRS escape rhythm. A rate of 40 to 60 bpm is consistent with a junctional or AV nodal escape rhythm. A wide complex rhythm that is less than 40 bpm suggests an infranodal level of block.

BRADYCARDIA WITH ACUTE MI

Acute myocardial infarction presents with significant bradyarrhythmias approximately 25 to 30% of the time. Forty percent of these bradyarrhythmias are sinus bradycardia. Twenty percent present as a junctional rhythm and 15% present as an idioventricular rhythm. Junctional and ventricular escape rhythms occur with failure of higher pacemaker sites. The remaining 35% are due to AV block, 27% of which are 1ˢᵗ or 2ⁿᵈ degree AV block and 8% are complete heart block.

The location and pathophysiology of the AV block as well as the symptom status of the patient are essential considerations in the decision to proceed with temporary pacing and/or aggressive pharmacologic therapy. Patients with acute inferior MI and AV block frequently have AV nodal ischemia with high levels of local adenosine, causing AV block. This generally is responsive to pharmacologic therapy such as Atropine or Methylxanthines

Table 4. Risk scale for complete heart block with acute myocardial infarction

Conduction Defect	Points
First-degree AV block	1
Second-degree type I, II	1
Right bundle branch block	1
Left bundle branch block	1
Left anterior fascicular block	1
Left posterior fascicular block	1

Risk Score for Complete Heart Block

Score	Heart Block
0	1.2%
1	7.8%
2	25%
3 or more	$\geq 36.4\%$

Adapted from Lamas, MD. Et al: Am J Cardiol 1986; 57.

and the long-term prognosis for recovery of conduction is quite good.

Acute necrosis of the AV node is rare due to the dual blood supply from the LAD and right coronary artery distributions. In contrast, high grade AV block in acute anterior MI is typically associate with necrosis of the local conduction system. Patients with AV block and anterior MI have increased mortality due to complications of the conduction block and due mainly to their larger extent of infarction. The AV block in these patients rarely responds to pharmacologic therapy and generally would benefit from prophylactic temporary pacing and have indication for permanent pacing.

Risk Progression for Complete Heart Block

The risk of progression to complete heart block in acute myocardial infarction may be predicted by scoring based on the presenting underlying conduction disease. *See Table IV.* The risk of progression to complete heart block in acute myocardial infarction depends upon the extent of infranodal conduction defects as opposed to symptoms. The survival of patients with acute myocardial infarction and AV block is determined largely by the extent of myocardial damage and the degree of infra nodal

conduction system disease. This is due to the unfavorable short and long-term prognosis of patients with acute MI and intraventricular conduction defects with the exception of left anterior fascicular block. The increased risk of death is not necessarily due to AV block; although, risk of block in these patients is increased as shown in Table III. Pacing in these patients is aimed at treating AV block and reducing the risk of sudden death. Reduction in mortality with pacing in these patients is felt to be masked by increases in mortality due to the extensive area of infarction and thus is still recommended.

THERAPY FOR AV BLOCK WITH ACUTE MI

Therapy for AV block which accompanies acute MI is guided by the etiology and location of the AV block (nodal or infranodal), type of MI (anterior or inferior), and associated symptoms. For inferior MI and nodal AV block, Atropine is an excellent initial therapy particularly in the first 6 hours of presentation. Doses should be administered in 0.5 mg increments with a maximal dose of 0.04mg/kg. Doses less than 0.5 mg should be avoided due to risk of paradoxical bradycardic response. Increasing emphasis is being placed on the use of temporary transcutaneous pacing in light of the low risk of complication and a relatively high effectiveness. Patches may be placed prophylacticaly on patients that are considered to have only a moderate risk of development of AV block. Transcutaneous patches also may be placed and utilized while waiting for placement of temporary transvenous pacemaker. Indications for temporary transvenous pacemaker placement include: symptomatic bradycardia, unresponsiveness to pharmacological therapy, alternating bundle branch block, bifascicular block with 1st degree AV block, and Mobitz type II 2nd degree block. Access should generally be obtained via the right internal jugular or left subclavian vein in order to reduce the risk of complication and to ensure safe placement and stability. An adequate pacing safety margin of three times adequate pacing safety margin of three times threshold is recommended. See Table V for therapeutic summary.

Table 5. Treatment indications for various bradyarrhythmias

I.	**Placement of a Transcutaneous Patch in Acute Myocardial Infarction**	
	A. Class I	1. Symptomatic sinus bradycardia
		2. Mobitz type II block
		3. Third-degree AV block
		4. Alternating bundle branch block and/or RBB with alternating left anterior fascicular and left posterior fascicular block
		5. Newly acquired bifascicular block
		6. RBB and first-degree AV block
II.	**Indications for Atropine with Bradycardia and Acute Myocardial Infarction**	
	A. Class I	1. Symptomatic bradycardia with heart rate < 50 beats/min associated with hypotension, ischemia, or a ventricular escape rhythm
		2. Asystole
		3. Symptomatic AV block at the AV nodal level type I, second-degree AV
	B. Class III	1. AV block at an infranodal level, AV block either second-degree type II or third-degree, or AV block with a wide-complex rhythm due to myocardial infarction
		2. Asymptomatic sinus bradycardia
III.	**General Indications for Permanent Pacing**	
	A. Class I	1. Third-degree AV block at any level when associated with symptoms
		2. Asystole ≥ secs or or escape rate < 40 beats/min in an awake, symptom-free patient
		3. After an AV junctional ablation
		4. Postoperative AV block that is not expected to resolve
		5. Neuromuscular disease with AV block, such as myotonic dystrophy, Kearns-Sayre syndrome, Erbs dystrophy, and peroneal muscular atrophy
		6. Second-degree AV block, regardless of location, with symptoms
		7. Intermittent third-degree AV block with bifascicular or trifascicular block
		8. Type II second-degree AV block with bifascicular or trifascicular block
	B. Class III	1. Asymptomatic first-degree AV block
		2. Asymptomatic type I second-degree AV block not known to be intra- or infraHisian
		3. AV block expected to resolve
		4. Bifascicular block without AV block or symptoms.
		5. Bifascicular block with first-degree AV block, without symptoms
IV.	**Permanent Pacing after Acute Phase of Myocardial Infarction**	
	A. Class I	1. Persistent second-degree AV block in the His-Purkinje system with bilateral BBB or third-degree AV block
		2. Transient advanced second- or third-degree infranodal block AV block with associated BBB. If site uncertain, EPS may be indicated.
		3. Persistent and symptomatic second- and third-degree AV block
	B. Class III	1. Transient AV block in the absence of intraventricular conduction defects
V.	**Indications for Transvenous Pacing in Acute Myocardial Infarction**	
	A. Class I	1. Asystole
		2. Symptomatic bradycardia including hypotension with first-degree AV block unresponsive to atropine
		3. Bilateral BBB (alternating BBB, or right BBB with alternating LAFB or LPFB)
		4. New or indeterminant age bifascicular block with first-degree AV block
		5. Mobitz type II second-degree AV block
	B. Class III	1. First-degree AV block
		2. Type I second-degree AV block with normal hemodynamics
		3. Accelerated idioventricular rhythm
		4. BBB or fascicular block known to exist before myocardial infarction

AV, atrioventricular; BBB, bundle branch block.

CONCLUSION

The evaluation and treatment of bradycardia is, to a large extent, determined by the company it keeps. In the emergency department only 15% of bradyarrhythmias are due to primary conduction system disorders. Elderly patients are much more likely to present with primary conduction disorders and are much less likely to respond to pharmacologic therapy. The clinician must astutely assess the etiology of bradycardia as to extrinsic or intrinsic causes as well as the location of the conduction defect (Sinus, AV nodal, or His purkinje system) in order to assess the reversibility and risk of progression to a life threatening rhythm. In addition, one must be cognizant that bradycardia is a frequent finding in asymptomatic individuals and may be unassociated with the patients presenting symptoms. There are few indications for permanent pacing in an asymptomatic individual. However, symptomatic bradycardia, regardless of location, which is unlikely to resolve and not due to an easily reversible cause is an indication for pacing. Bradycardia occurring during sleep alone should prompt investigation for obstructive sleep apnea but is not an indication for pacing. In symptomatic individuals where the relationship to bradycardia is unclear, loop monitor, or implantable loop monitor may be helpful in discerning cause and effect. Patients presenting with AV block and infranodal conduction disease are at greater risk to progress to complete heart block. Patients with sick sinus syndrome will likely benefit from dual chamber pacing to reduce the risk of thromboembolism as well as symptomatic improvement. Finally, in patients with neurocardiogenic or vagally mediated bradycardia should avoid the aggravating stimulus. In those patients where the aggravating stimulus is unavoidable, such as upright posture, treatment with various pharmacologic therapy, tilt training, and rate drop pacing appear effective and promising.

REFERENCES

1. ACC/AHA Guidelines of Implantation of Cardiac Pacemakers and Antiarrhythmia Devices. *J Am Coll of Cardiol* 1998; 31:1175-1209
   A complete review of indications for implantation of permanent pacing devices and anti tachycardic devices.

2. Anderson HR, Nielsen JC et al: Long term follow up of patients from a randomized trial of atrial versus Ventricular pacing for Sick Sinus Syndrome. *Lancet* 1997; 350:1210-1216
   Trial documenting benefits of atrial pacing versus ventricular pacing in patients with sick sinus syndrome with reduced mortality, reduced atrial fibrillation, and reduced incidence of thromboembolism.

3. Brady WJ, JR: Evaluation and Management of Bradyarrhythmias in the Emergency Department. *Emerg Med Clin of North Am* 1998; 16:361-387
   A thorough review of the various causes of bradycardia, as well as a reasonable discussion of their therapy.

4. Brodsky M: Arrhythmias Documented by 24 hours Continuous Electrocardiographic Monitoring in 50 Male Medical Students without apparent Heart Disease. *Am J Cardiol* 1977; 39:390-395
   An important paper revealing the range of rhythm disturbances found in healthy volunteers by holter moniter.

5. Lamas G, et al: A simplified Method to Predict Occurrence of Complete Heart Block During Acute Myocardial Infarction. *Am J Cardiol* 1986; 57:1213-1218

6. Mangrum MJ, Dimarco J: The Evaluation and Management of Bradycardia. *N England J Med* 2000; 342:703-709
   An excellent review of bradycardia, its classification and management.

7. Prystowsky EN, et al: Management of Patients with atrial Fibrillation. *Circulation* 1996; 93:1262-1277
   An excellent thorough review of this extensive subject including pathophysiology, treatment options, and a critical review of current data regarding anticoagulation and rhythm and rate control.

8. Ryan JT, et al: 1999 update: ACC/AHA guidelines for the Management of Patients with Acute myocardial Infarction. *Circulation* 1999; 100:1016-1030
   Discussion of Post MI management

including discussion regarding acute and chronic pacing post MI.

9. Stegman S, Burrroughs J, Henthorn R, et al: Asymptomatic Bradyarrhythmias as a Marker of Sleep Apnea. *Pace* 1996; 19; 899-90
A discussion of marked rhythm disturbances noted in patients with sleep apnea

PERIOPERATIVE EVALUATION AND MANAGEMENT OF PULMONARY DISEASE

Todd Dorman, MD, FCCM

Objectives

- To review anesthetic interactions with the pulmonary system
- To review how to preoperatively assess risk in patients with pulmonary disease
- To review postoperative respiratory dysfunction

Key Words: Pulmonary disease, risk assessment, preoperative evaluation

INTRODUCTION

The major focus of this chapter will be on important perioperative pulmonary issues. These include effects of anesthetic agents on the respiratory system, risk factors for perioperative pulmonary complications, and postoperative pulmonary dysfunction. Finally, I will present some strategies for improved outcomes in defined patient populations.

PERIOPERATIVE PULMONARY RISK AND COMPLICATIONS

Effects of Anesthetics on the Respiratory System

Classically, anesthetic agents are credited with producing consistent respiratory system effects. However, since the studies that have shown these effects were not controlled for surgery, it remains unclear as to how much of these effects are independently associated with the provision of anesthesia. Intellectually this is important, as there might be interactions between anesthetic agents and the surgical stress response that are either negative or synergistic in nature.

With that clarification in mind, there are a host of respiratory system changes that have been ascribed to anesthetics and to general anesthesia in particular. An understanding of these effects is required in order to preoperatively assess patient risks and the likelihood of developing a postoperative complication. It has been shown that the volatile anesthetic agents impair lung immune function principally by decreasing mucociliary function and alveolar macrophage quantity and activity (1). General anesthesia with volatile anesthetics has also been demonstrated to increase alveolar-capillary permeability, inhibit surfactant release, and to potentially alter responsiveness to circulating endogenous substances (2). Finally, a decrease in FRC of between 15 to 20% and a decrease in thoracic cavity volume is seen rapidly after the induction of general anesthesia (3). The net effect of these changes is to cause atelectasis and an increased ventilation-perfusion mismatch, clinically seen as a widened alveolar-arterial gradient and often as frank hypoxemia. Consequently, these patients commonly require supplemental oxygen and positive end-expiratory pressure (PEEP) postoperatively to overcome these effects. Time on t-piece should be avoided as it may lead to a worsening of their inherent postoperative pathophysiologic state.

It should be mentioned that not all the effects of general anesthesia on the respiratory system are detrimental. In fact, volatile anesthetics are the most potent bronchodilators available (4). Since the provision of volatile anesthetics usually requires an endotracheal tube (ETT), which can be seen by the body as a foreign object worsening bronchospasm, the provision of this form of therapy cannot be undertaken lightly. However, given the rise in death rate from asthma in this country, one might speculate that volatile anesthetics are underutilized in this patient population.

Many of these effects are either not seen in patients who have surgery under regional techniques or are seen in a significantly attenuated degree. Consequently, depending on the surgical procedure, it is often best to avoid general anesthesia; however, no blanket recommendation can be made. Combined anesthetics where regional and general techniques are combined are commonly utilized but not well evaluated for impact on perioperative pulmonary risk. In fact, it is best left to the discretion of the anesthesiologist providing the anesthetic.

Common Postoperative Pulmonary Changes

As stated above, numerous perioperative changes in the pulmonary system can be easily demonstrated. The most important changes are the decrements in lung volumes, diaphragmatic function, and an attenuated ventilatory response to hypercarbia and hypoxia. These changes collectively increase the risk of postoperative hypoxemia and diminish the ability of the clinician to recognize its existence.

Forced vital capacity and FRC are reduced to almost 40% of baseline values in the immediate postoperative period, and do not recover fully for almost 2 weeks. This places FRC at or below closing volume in many patients, and consequently leads to an increased risk of pulmonary complications. Postoperatively, the diaphragm lacks the ability to generate a normal amount of force after upper abdominal and thoracic surgery (3). This effect is not explained by residual neuromuscular blockade, nor does pain management correct it. Volatile anesthetics blunt the ventilatory response to hypercarbia and hypoxia.

Concentrations as low as 0.1 MAC have been demonstrated to alter ventilatory responsivity. Consequently, patients may not demonstrate the classic clinical signs of hypercarbia and hypoxia (i.e., tachypnea, tachycardia), and thus these patients may be at a further increased risk for complications including cardiopulmonary arrest, especially once discharged from the postanesthesia care unit (PACU).

Risk Factors for Perioperative Pulmonary Complications

Somewhere between 30 and 80% of patients will suffer a postoperative pulmonary complication. In 1968, Wightman evaluated 785 patients and determined that those that smoked, had COPD, or were > 70 years of age had an increase in postoperative productive cough fever, or new auscultatory findings (5). Upper abdominal or thoracic procedures were associated with a 20-fold increase in postoperative pulmonary complications. More recently in a study by Pederson, the following relative risks of developing a postoperative pulmonary complication were determined (6).

It appears from studies like these that the common risk factors for postoperative pulmonary complications can be summarized best by stating increasing age, upper abdominal or thoracic surgery, delirium, or CVA, emergency surgery, or prior lung disease, specifically COPD and smoking. A recent risk index for predicting postoperative pneumonia has been published but not yet studied with

Table 1. Relative risks of developing a postoperative pulmonary complication.

Risk Factor	Relative Risk
Age > 70 yrs	7.46
Age 50-69 yrs	4.14
Major abdominal surgery	3.90
Emergency surgery	3.49
COPD	3.13
Age 30-49 yrs	2.29
GA > 180 mins	1.52

COPD, chronic obstructive pulmonary disease; GA, general anesthesia.

interventions aimed to reduce pneumonia in high-risk patients (7). Although each study tends to define complications differently, the most commonly evaluated complications include hypoxemia, bronchospasm, atelectasis, respiratory failure, pneumonia, and acute respiratory distress syndrome (ARDS). Pulmonary embolism is typically not included as a postoperative pulmonary complication.

Preoperative Assessment of Patients at Risk for Pulmonary Complications

Unfortunately, the optimal preoperative risk assessment test has not been determined. What is clear from the literature is that clinical variables are superior to spirometry in predicting postoperative pulmonary complications. In fact, in one study those patients not taking bronchodilators and with a normal chest x-ray (CXR) suffered no postoperative pulmonary complications, while those both on bronchodilators and having an abnormal CXR had a 33% rate of complications.

Historically, we were taught that patients with forced expiratory volumes at 1-second (FEV_1) less than 1 liter were unacceptable risks for surgery. Recently, studies involving lung reduction surgery patients has taught us that even those with the most severe lung disease (average FEV_1 < 0.68 liters) may actually benefit from some surgical procedures. These findings further emphasize that no test has been established as a gold standard for determining postoperative risk.

Patients with Asthma

Although bronchospasm clearly increases a patient's perioperative risk, no controlled study has been able to show that there is a risk reduction by controlling bronchospasm. That being said, if a patient has severe bronchospasm under anesthesia, possibly related to the endotracheal tube being perceived as a foreign object, one may not be able to adequately ventilate or oxygenate the patient. This situation, commonly referred to as "rock bag," is obviously life threatening. Consequently, inhaled beta-2 agonists and steroids are the mainstay of both prophylaxis and treatment. In fact, steroids are probably the

most useful strategy. In commonly used doses (i.e., 40mg prednisone for 2 days preoperatively), there is no increase in postoperative complications such as infection or wound healing (8,9).

Patients with COPD

Perioperative pulmonary complications are common in patients with COPD. History and physical exam are the most important components of the preoperative evaluation of these patients. Spirometry does not have a role in the routine preoperative evaluation of these patients (10). Pharmacologic management with inhaled bronchodilators and/or steroids is frequently useful. Theophylline can be of some use, but its usefulness is limited in the perioperative period because of its propensity to initiate or aggravate arrhythmias. Preoperative physical therapy and exercise may be the most useful adjuvant for risk limitation. Arterial blood gases should not be routinely ordered. Room air oxygen saturation and history and physical exam are still the mainstays of preoperative evaluation for these patients. A preoperative CXR is only required for patients with severe COPD or if age > 65.

Patients with Cigarette Smoking

Whether the patient has documented COPD or merely smokes, smoking cessation is beneficial. Patients with > 20-pack/year smoking histories are at an increased risk for postoperative pulmonary complications. When smokers stop smoking at least 48 hours preoperatively, their carboxyhemoglobin levels normalize, some cilia begin to beat again, and the cardiovascular effects of nicotine are abolished. If they can stop for 2 weeks preoperatively, then their sputum volume will be reduced. Ideally they should refrain from smoking for 8 weeks preoperatively, as the studies have shown that it requires this duration of cessation to lower risk (11). In fact, a recent report in patients having a pneumonectomy demonstrated that smoking cessation for less than 1 month as compared to greater than 1 month was associated with a significant increase in the rate of pneumonia, ARDS, and death (12). Finally, in those patients who have acutely stopped smoking, consideration for nicotine withdrawal in the postoperative period must be undertaken.

Patients with Sleep Apnea

The importance of sleep apnea in the perioperative period is poorly understood. Essentially no information exists. Patients who have a documented or undocumented history of sleep apnea will likely see a worsening of this postoperatively. At present, most centers do not routinely monitor these patients, while a few centers do place these patients in monitored beds for the night of surgery (see Figure 1). Oxygen therapy and/or CPAP should be considered for several days postoperatively, as they may be at risk of developing more severe episodes of desaturation. Whether episodes of desaturation from obstructive sleep apnea are wholly or partially responsible for episodes of postoperative hypertension or myocardial ischemia is only speculative at this time.

Postoperative Respiratory Dysfunction

Postoperative respiratory dysfunction is invariably present in postoperative patients. In the majority of patients, it has limited clinical significance. In contrast, postoperative respiratory failure can be a devastating complication that increases mortality, length of stay, and cost.

Respiratory failure requiring mechanical ventilatory support is both a clinical and a physiologic diagnosis. The most commonly quoted physiologic parameters consistent with respiratory failure are listed below. One is cautioned that despite adequately appearing parameters, some patients will require ventilatory support based purely upon their clinical appearance. In addition, patients often require ventilatory support because of non-respiratory organ system failure or dysfunction despite an adequately functioning respiratory system.

HOW TO OPTIMIZE OUTCOME AND AVOID INTUBATION

Although it would be wonderfully easy if the evidence clearly supported that regional anesthesia was associated with fewer postoperative complications and thus was associated with an improved outcome to date, no such clear evidence exists. Well done clinical trials are sorely needed in this domain, especially for high-risk patients. The type of surgical procedure or approach may also have impact on the rate of complications. Adequate pain management strategies may be useful. Avoiding intermittent nurse-administered dosing and utilizing patient controlled techniques is beneficial. However, one must always remember to evaluate pain at both rest and with activity when determining the quality of pain control. Regional techniques, especially those that avoid opioids, may be particularly useful for those patients with CO_2 retention at baseline. As simple as it seems, oxygen therapy has been associated with a reduction in postoperative complications including a reduced rate of nausea and vomiting, surgical wound infections, and heart rate.

Consequently, it appears that the best strategies for limiting postoperative pulmonary complications include smoking cessation, bronchodilators, steroids, pulmonary rehabilitation and exercise training (early ambulation), lung expansion techniques (incentive spirometry), and supplemental oxygen.

Some commonly deployed strategies that have fallen from favor include: intermittent positive pressure breathing (IPPB), continuous positive airway pressure (CPAP), and chest physiotherapy. Although these do increase the hands-on therapy the patient receives, they are quite labor intensive, are uncomfortable for the patient, and have been shown to not be cost-effective when deployed across all postoperative patients. Bilevel positive airway pressure (BiPAP) does allow the clinician to set differing levels of support for inspiration and expiration resulting in improved tidal volumes and functional residual capacity. However, to date there is a paucity of data supporting its use in postoperative patients. Similar to CPAP, an

Adult OSA post-op Disposition Decision Tree

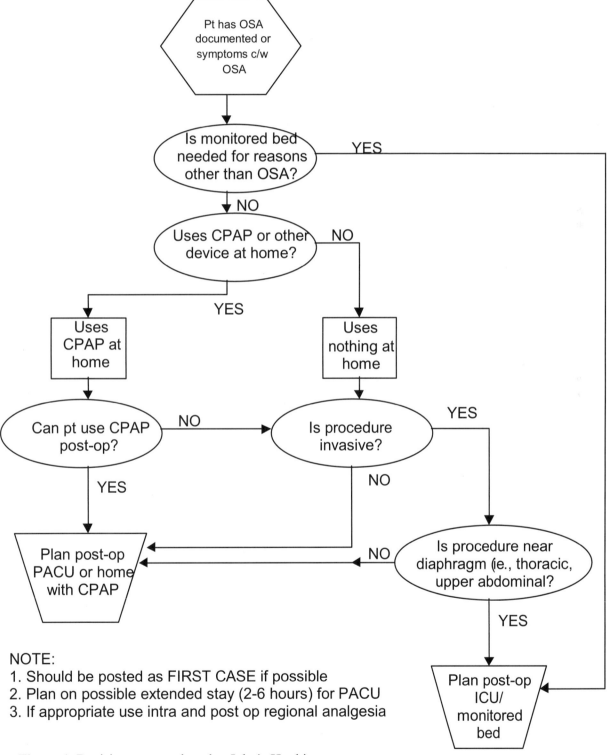

NOTE:
1. Should be posted as FIRST CASE if possible
2. Plan on possible extended stay (2-6 hours) for PACU
3. If appropriate use intra and post op regional analgesia

Figure 1. Decision tree employed at John's Hopkins.

Table 2. Commonly quoted physiologic parameters consistent with respiratory failure

Parameter	Normal	Failure
Respiratory rate (breaths/min)	12-18	> 35
Inspiratory force (cm H_2O)	-75 to -125	< -25
Vital capacity (mL/kg)	65-75	< 15
FEV_1 (mL/kg)	50-60	< 10
Compliance (mL/cm H_2O)	> 100	< 30
PaO_2 (torr)	80-95	< 70
A-aDO_2 (torr)	25-65	> 450
Qs/Qt (%)	5-8	> 15-20
$PaCO_2$ (torr)	35-45	> 55
VD/VT (%)	20-30	> 60

FEV_1, forced expiratory volume in 1 second; A-aDO_2, alveolar/arterial oxygen tension difference; Qs/Qt, physiologic shunt fraction; VD/VT, physiologic deadspace ratio.

appropriate mask fit is required which may be uncomfortable for the patient or frankly may not be attainable if a nasogastric tube is in place. Leak compensation is now available on many devices and should overcome this limitation. These noninvasive techniques have been shown to have a role in the management of specific patient types (e.g., pulmonary edema), but they require experienced staff support as the literature also seems to point to the fact that patients who fail these devices do worse overall.

Mechanical Ventilation

Ventilator Management

No one mode of ventilatory support has been proven to provide improved outcome for all patients with postoperative respiratory failure. The 2 most commonly utilized modes of invasive ventilatory support are synchronized intermittent mandatory ventilation (SIMV) and assist-control ventilation (A/C). The initial mode of choice and subsequent management mode are both dependent upon the integration of the patient's clinical condition, the disease state initiating the need for mechanical ventilation, and local preferences and resources.

Ventilatory management requires the physician to independently assess oxygenation, ventilation, and patient comfort, and then integrate these considerations into a unified ventilator management strategy. Merely standing at the bedside and trying to breathe in the same manner the patient is being ventilated will often identify whether the support level the patient is receiving is adequate. Initial respiratory rate and tidal volume settings should always provide for adequate ventilation (CO_2 removal) appropriate for the patient's metabolic state. Too often initial settings are inadequate and the patient's acidosis is worsened because the initial settings do not take into account the degree of metabolic acidosis that requires compensation. Initial oxygen settings should always include 100% oxygen that can then be weaned by either monitoring continuously oxygen saturation or by arterial blood gases. Most institutions utilize PEEP in low levels (< 5 cm H_2O) as part of initial settings. PEEP is then usually titrated up as needed to improve oxygenation and to enable the fractional inspired oxygen concentration (FiO_2) to be weaned toward nontoxic levels (< 0.55). PEEP is commonly underutilized in postoperative patients as they routinely develop posterior-basilar atelectasis and seemingly would benefit from higher PEEP levels and possibly short inspiratory holds/pauses. Some patients inherently exhibit intrinsic PEEP or because of less than ideal inspiratory to expiratory (I:E) ratio develop intrinsic PEEP. In these patients it is often useful to monitor total PEEP. Although many centers favor inverse ratio ventilation (IRV & PCIRV) in difficult-to-oxygenate patients, it has been shown that IRV merely trades extrinsic PEEP for higher levels of total PEEP.

Table 3. Criteria for determining readiness for extubation

Parameter	Value
PaO_2 on FIO_2	> 80 torr on < 0.6
$PaCO_2$	< 45 torr
Respiratory rate	< 35 breaths/min
Tidal volume	> 5 mL/kg
Vital capacity	> 10 mL/kg
Minute ventilation	< 10 L/min
Negative inspiratory force (NIF)	-20 cm H_2O or more negative
Rapid shallow breathing index	< 80

Recent trends in ventilatory management include utilization of high levels of PEEP under the theory that these higher levels better keep airways open and avoid repetitive opening and closing alveolar injury (13). Data in acute lung injury patients also implies that through the use of lower tidal volumes (< 6 cc/kg) and higher PEEP levels, systemic cytokine concentrations are reduced as well as possibly the incidence of multiple organ dysfunction. Some centers utilize static pressure-volume curves to try to determine the optimal PEEP. Unfortunately, this strategy has not been proven to alter outcome. Use of lower lung volume strategies is highly recommended in patients with acute lung injury. The tidal volume should start at 6 cc/kg and plateau pressure monitored. The TV should be progressively reduced further to lower the inspiratory plateau pressure to < 30 cm H_2O (14). Concomitantly, the rate may need to be increased in order to enhance minute ventilation. These lower lung volume management strategies often lead to some degree of carbon dioxide retention, termed "permissive hypercapnia." The respiratory acidosis that results should not be treated with bicarbonate unless the pH is extremely low (< 7.10). A recent trial of low lung volume strategy coupled with higher PEEPS has been stopped secondary to no difference between that strategy and low lung volume with "standard" PEEP (personal communication with ARDS network). Currently, partial liquid ventilation, high frequency oscillatory ventilation, and rescue steroid strategies are being investigated. Finally, although proponents of extracorporeal membrane oxygenation (ECMO) do exist,

insufficient evidence exists to supports its use in adults.

Weaning and Extubation

No single method of weaning has been proven to outperform other methods of weaning. Most experts would agree that when patients are ready to wean they will wean. Irrespective of mode of ventilation, most weaning occurs in the same sequence. Initially, FiO_2 is weaned to 40% or less, then PEEP is weaned to minimal and then either rate is weaned or if low rate and pressure support (PS) are the management mode, then PS is weaned. Numerous criteria have been established to determine if the patient is ready for the terminal weaning event, extubation (Table 3).

In addition to ensuring that the patient meets these or similar extubation criteria, one should ensure that the patient is awake, alert, and able to protect his/her airway. If there is any risk of airway edema, a cuff test should be performed to assess for an inspiratory and expiratory leak off mechanical ventilation. Secretions should be minimal or at a minimum not copious or tenacious and should be improving. Hemodynamic and metabolic stability should also exist prior to extubation. Finally, extubation should not occur either during or immediately prior to other possible stressors such as hemodialysis or transportation to tests.

ANNOTATED REFERENCES

1. Kotani N, Lin CY, Wang JS: Loss of alveolar macrophages during anesthesia and operation in humans. *Anesth Analg* 1995; 81:1255-62

2. Tobin WR, Kaiser HE, Groeger AM: The effects of volatile anesthetic agents on pulmonary surfactant function. *Vivo* 2000; 14:157-63

3. Tokics L, Hedenstierna G, Strandberg A: Lung collapse and gas exchange during general anesthesia: Effects of spontaneous breathing, muscle paralysis, and positive end-expiratory pressure. *Anesthesiology* 1987; 66:157-167

4. Brown RH, Mitzner W, Zerhouni E: Direct in vivo visualization of bronchodilation induced by inhalational anesthesia using high-resolution computed tomography. *Anesthesiology* 1993; 78:295-300

5. Wightman JA: A prospective survey of the incidence of postoperative pulmonary complications. *Br J Surg* 1968; 55:85-91

6. Pedersen T, Viby-Mogensen J, Ringsted C: Anaesthetic practice and postoperative pulmonary complications. *Acta Anaesthesiol Scand* 1992; 36:812-8

7. Arozullah AM, Khuri SF, Henderson WG: Development and validation of a multifactorial risk index for predicting postoperative pneumonia after major noncardiac surgery. *Ann Intern Med* 2001; 135:847-857

8. Kabalin CS, Yarnold PR, Grammer LC: Low complication rate of corticosteroid-treated asthmatics undergoing surgical procedures. *Arch Intern Med* 1995; 155:1379-84

9. Warner DO, Warner MA, Barnes RD: Perioperative respiratory complications in patients with asthma. *Anesthesiology* 1996; 85:460-7

10. Preoperative pulmonary function testing. American College of Physicians. *Ann Intern Med* 1990; 112:793-4

11. Warner DO, Warner MA, Offord KP: Airway obstruction and perioperative complications in smokers undergoing abdominal surgery. *Anesthesiology* 1999; 90:372-9

12. Vaporciyan AA, Merriman KW, Ece F: Incidence of major pulmonary morbidity after pneumonectomy: Association with timing of smoking cessation. *Ann Thorac Surg* 2002; 73:420-6

13. Kollef, MH, Schuster DP: The Acute Respiratory Distress Syndrome. *New Engl J Med* Jan 5, 1995; 332(1):27-37

14. Ventilation with lower tidal volumes as compared with traditional tidal volumes for acute lung injury and the acute respiratory distress syndrome. The Acute Respiratory Distress Syndrome Network. *New Engl J Med* 2000 May 4; 342(18):1301-8

15. Jayr C, Thomas H, Rey A: Postoperative pulmonary complications. Epidural analgesia using bupivacaine and opioids versus parenteral opioids. *Anesthesiology* 1993; 78:666-76

16. Ballantyne JC, Carr DB, deFerranti S: The comparative effects of postoperative analgesic therapies on pulmonary outcome: Cumulative meta-analyses of randomized, controlled trials. *Anesth Analg* 1998; 86:598-612

17. Greif R, Akca O, Horn EP: Supplemental perioperative oxygen to reduce the incidence of surgical-wound infection. Outcomes Research Group. *N Engl J Med* 2000; 342:161-7

18. Nomori H, Kobayashi R, Fuyuno G: Preoperative respiratory muscle training. Assessment in thoracic surgery patients with special reference to postoperative pulmonary complications. *Chest* 1994; 105:1782-8

PERIOPERATIVE EVALUATION AND MANAGEMENT OF CARDIOVASCULAR DISEASE

Todd Dorman, MD, FCCM

Objectives

- To review the key components of the surgical stress response and how they impact cardiovascular outcomes
- To review how to preoperatively assess risk in patients with cardiovascular disease
- To review how to appropriately evaluate patients with cardiovascular disease with the goals of risk minimization and high quality outcomes.

Key Words: Cardiovascular disease, risk assessment, preoperative evaluation

INTRODUCTION

Some of the most challenging patients seen in the intensive care unit (ICU) are those that present postoperatively. These patients not only find themselves in the midst of a critical illness, but are simultaneously experiencing pathophysiologic effects of the surgical stress response. A thorough understanding of how to best preoperatively evaluate and risk assess these patients so they might be optimized upon entry into their critical illness phase is well within the scope of the intensivist. Furthermore, a clear understanding of these evaluations and their potential limitations is required in order to provide optimal postoperative care.

Disorders of the cardiovascular system are commonly seen in the perioperative period. Disorders related to congenital and contractile heart diseases are important but outside the scope of this chapter. With regard to evaluating patients with or at risk of cardiovascular disease, this chapter will focus on those patients with ischemic heart disease. Finally, I will present some strategies for improved outcomes in this patient population.

SURGICAL STRESS RESPONSE

Before we can proceed with discussing the important perioperative cardiovascular processes, a brief review of the surgical stress response is required. The surgical stress response is a graded neuroendocrine response to surgical trauma (1). In other words, the bigger the threat or insult the bigger is the neuroendocrine response. Direct correlation between the magnitude of the stress response and perioperative pathophysiologic events has been well established (1). Furthermore, the stress response follows a reproducible cycle of events. Consequently, when patients "fall off" the curve this typically represents an interceding event such as sepsis.

In response to tissue injury the anterior pituitary secretes ACTH, GH, prolactin, and endorphin; the posterior pituitary secretes AVP, and the adrenal secretes cortisol and epinephrine. The sympathetic nervous system becomes hyperactive as well and large increases in circulating norepinephrine have been demonstrated (Table 1). This surgical stress response is a primordial response that is related to the classic fight or flight response. In addition to the classic concepts of rises in epinephrine (adrenaline), the rationale for these neuroendocrine changes includes analgesia, hypercoagulability, conservation of fluid and mobilization of metabolic substrate. The fact that these neuroendocrine changes occur is intellectually stimulating, but for our patients what is important is the fact that these changes are associated with clinically relevant perioperative events. The physiologic effects of these neuroendocrine changes includes tachycardia, tachyarrythmias, hypertension, myocardial ischemia, congestive heart failure, hypokalemia, hypomagnesemia, infections, hyperglycemia, hypermetabolism, fluid and electrolyte shifts, altered immune function and hypercoagulability (2).

Table 1. Neuroendocrine changes of the surgical stress response

Organ	Hormone
Anterior pituitary gland	Increased ACTH
	Increased GH
	Increased prolactin
	Increased endorphin
	Decreased TSH
Posterior pituitary gland	Increased AVP
Autonomic nervous system	Increased norepinephrine
Adrenal gland	Increased cortisol
	Increased epinephrine

Modern anesthetic management significantly attenuates the intraoperative stress response. In fact, a well-controlled anesthetic prevents most of these stress related neuroendocrine changes such that these changes usually do not start to occur until emergence. Consequently, the highest risk period for most patients is during the first 3 postoperative days. Control of this response postoperatively requires strategies that either diminish the production of these neuroendocrine factors (i.e., regional blocks, centrally acting alpha-2 agonists) or block the end organ effects of these factors (i.e., beta-blockers). Which of these strategies is better has not yet been determined, although the benefits of beta-blockers have been well elucidated (3, 4, 5). The final important point regarding the surgical stress response is that this reproducible programmed response to surgical stress follows a predictable time course. For example, epinephrine is known to precipitously rise around the time of emergence from an anesthetic, peak, and then return to normal levels usually by 12 hours postoperatively. Whereas norepinephrine rises at the same time, but once it peaks it will plateau for potentially 3 days and then return to baseline levels. This surgical stress response is so predictable that deviation from these set patterns can be utilized as evidence of intercurrent events such as infectious complications or myocardial ischemia.

ISCHEMIC HEART DISEASE

There are approximately 27 million non-cardiac surgeries in this country per year (6). Of these, it is estimated that between 1 and 1.5 million have known coronary artery disease, and an additional 3 to 4 million have greater than 3 risk factors (see Eagle criteria Table 2) (7). Understanding how patients with either known or suspected ischemic heart disease are evaluated preoperatively is important in understanding how to provide care for these patients postoperatively in and beyond their ICU stay.

Risk Assessment

Overall anesthetic-related risk has diminished from 1 in 1,000 cases to approximately 1 in 400,000 cases over the last 20 years. This is a safety record unparalleled in medicine. Despite this improvement, perioperative risk persists. Basic preoperative risk assessment requires that the clinician appreciate that total risk is the sum of the patient's disease-based risk times the physiologic impact of the surgical stress response for that particular case (Figure 1). Patient disease-based risk is usually stratified by the American Society of Anesthesiologists physical status class. Class 1 patients, defined by no organic disease, have a mortality rate

$$\text{\textbf{Patient Disease}} \quad \text{X} \quad \text{\textbf{Surgical Stress}} \quad = \quad \textbf{RISK}$$

Figure 1. Perioperative risk is the sum of the risks from the patient's medical condition, surgical procedure, and the elicited surgical stress response.

between 0 and 0.4%. Class 2 patients, defined by known organic disease without functional impairment, have a mortality rate between 0.5 and 2%. Class 3 patients, defined by organic disease with definitive systemic involvement producing functional impairment, have a mortality rate between 5-10%. Class 4 patients, defined by severe disease that is life threatening, have a mortality rate of approximately 75%. Class 5 patients are defined as moribund on entry to the OR and thus are not expected to survive the operation (8). In addition to this simple, yet highly predictive stratification, patients are further classified as either elective or emergent. Emergency status then conveys an increase in risk of 2-3 times the baseline risk. The severity (magnitude and duration) of the surgical stress response can also be stratified. Cataract and other peripheral procedures produce almost no discernable stress response. Bladder and lower abdominal procedures produce less of a response than upper abdominal procedures and thoracic procedures produce a greater stress response than upper abdominal procedures (Figure 2) (1). Anesthetics represent such a small fraction of risk they are not routinely considered.

Cardiovascular risk assessment has classically utilized 3 risk assessment tools. The Goldman criteria, established in the late 1970s, did try to provide a risk stratification model for clinicians (Table 2) (9). In an attempt to improve upon this index, Detsky published the Modified Multifactorial Index in 1986 (Table 2) (10). These criteria try to more clearly define risk by substratifying several of the symptom complexes. Finally, Eagle et al suggested in 1989 that the major risk factors simply included age > 70, history of angina, history of ventricular ectopic activity requiring treatment,

diabetes on therapy and Q-waves on ECG (Table 2) (7). These criteria have been adopted by the American Heart Association (AHA) and are incorporated into their algorithm for preoperative assessment of the patient with heart disease for noncardiac surgery (11, 12). The most recent version of the ACC/AHA guideline divides the risk factors into 3 categories. The major risk factors include unstable coronary syndromes (acute or recent MI or Canadian anginal class III or IV), decompensated heart failure, significant arrhythmias (high-grade AV block, symptomatic ventricular arrhythmias, or supraventricular arrhythmias with uncontrolled rate), and severe valvular disease. The intermediate risk factors include Canadian anginal class I or II, previous MI or pathologic Q-wave, compensated CHF, IDDM, or renal insufficiency. The minor risk factors include advanced age, abnormal ECG, rhythm other than sinus, low functional capacity (inability to climb one flight of stairs with a bag of groceries), history of stroke, or uncontrolled systemic hypertension. The importance of functional capacity is best demonstrated by the fact that patients classified as high risk but who are asymptomatic and can run for 30 minutes daily may need no further evaluation. The guidelines further stress that completely sedentary patients without a history of cardiovascular disease but who have other risk factors may indeed need further preoperative evaluation. From available literature it appears that a cut-off of about 4 metabolic equivalents (MET) of activity represents the transition from poor functional capacity to acceptable functional capacity. Four METS is approximately equivalent to doing light housework while greater than 4 METS

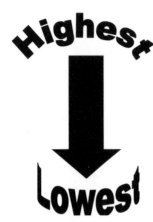

Aortic Procedures
Intrathoracic
Orthopedic
Infrainguinal
Vascular
Head & Neck
Carotid
TURP

Figure 2. Not all surgical procedures equal risk. The above figure demonstrates the relative relationship of a variety of common surgical procedures.

Table 2: Commonly Used Risk Criteria

Goldman risk factors	Detsky risk factors	Eagle risk factors
Age > 70 years (5)	Age > 70 years (5)	Age > 70 years
MI < 6 months (10)	MI < 6 months (10) MI > 6 months (5)	Q-wave on ECG
S3 gallop or JVD (11)	Pulmonary edema in the last week (10) Pulmonary edema—ever (5)	History of angina
Important valvular aortic stenosis (3)	Critical aortic stenosis (20)	
Non-sinus rhythms PACs or > 5 PVCs/min (7)	Non-sinus rhythms, PACs or > 5 PVCs/min (5)	History of PVCs requiring therapy
PO2 < 60 or PCO2 > 50 mmHg, K < 3.0, HCO3 < 20 mEq/L, BUN > 50 or Cr > 3.0 mg/dl, abnormal SGOT, signs of chronic liver disease, or patients bedridden from chronic cardiac disease (3)	Angina class 3/unstable (10) Angina class 4 (20)	Diabetes on therapy/
Intraperitoneal, intrathoracic or aortic operation (3)	Poor general medical condition (5)	
Emergency operation (4)	Emergency operation (10)	

The numbers in parentheses in the Goldman and Detsky columns are the points assigned to each risk group. These points are then summed to determine the patient's risk level. Eagle's risk factors are not assigned points, and the number of factors is merely counted. JVD, jugular venous distention; MI, myocardial infarction; PAC, premature atrial contraction; PVC, premature ventricular contraction.

starts at being able to walk on level ground at a speed of at least 4 mph. In addition to these cardiovascular risk factors, one must also consider other organ system diseases that may complicate cardiovascular management. These disorders include but are not limited to severe obstructive or restrictive pulmonary disease, uncontrolled IDDM, significant azotemia, and hemorrhagic disorders.

Risk in Patients with Previous MI

The risk of a perioperative myocardial infarction (MI) in a patient with a history of a recent MI appears to be related to the time interval between the recent MI and the proposed surgical procedure. Historically, it was believed that within the first 3 months after an MI the risk of a subsequent perioperative MI was 30%. This risk fell to 15% if the time interval was between 3 and 6 months and then fell further to 5-6% for those whose MI was greater than 6 months prior to the proposed procedure. These risk percentages were based on 149 patients studied over 17 years. In 1983, Rao et al reevaluated this risk relationship and concluded that the risk was closer to 6% for those whose recent MI was in the last 3 months. This risk level fell to 2% for those between 3 and 6 months, and was < 2% for those after 6 months (13). Although these are the commonly quoted (and tested) risk percentages, these do not take into account that the functional status of a patient after an inferior MI is different than after an anterior MI, and not all anterior MIs are equivalent. In fact, our recommendations are that if the case is urgent or life threatening, then proceed no matter the time frame between the MI and the proposed case. If the case is purely elective and can be postponed, then delaying the case until some period after 3 months should be considered. If the case is elective but waiting is not an option (i.e., resectable tumor), then consider proceeding for those with return of good functional status or angiography for those in question. One should always keep in mind that the stress response induced by some procedures is less than the stress of driving to have the procedure performed.

What Testing Should Be Initiated?

For patients either at risk or those scheduled to have vascular surgery, the AHA/ACC guidelines recommend either a dipyridamole thallium or a dobutamine stress echocardiogram as a risk assessment tool (11,12). Unfortunately, the clinical efficacy of this recommendation has yet to be determined. For such tests to be truly useful as preoperative screening tools they must have a high positive predictive value so that we do not cancel cases and expose patients needlessly to additional tests when in fact they would never have had an event. In fact, the positive predictive value of each of the tests is quite low, in the < 25% range, making none of the tests quite as useful as we would like. If a preoperative cardiovascular assessment test is indicated, then a dobutamine stress echocardiogram is probably the more useful test. Baseline cardiac function is provided as well as response to tachycardia. Furthermore, the response to dobutamine more closely mimics the heart rate, blood pressure, and inotropic changes seen during the perioperative period. Some investigators have even recommended that for patients with class 1 or 2 angina, or for those merely at risk that the perioperative period might serve as the most cost-effective stress test available (6). These investigators would caution us to remember that those patients with class 3 or 4 angina, and clearly anyone with either unstable or crescendo angina, must be evaluated prior to proceeding to the OR, unless the case is absolutely emergent.

Management of Patients With or at Risk of Ischemic Heart Disease

Patients should continue their inotropic and antiarrythmic medications up to and including the day of surgery. Aspirin, if being taken for angina or cerebrovascular symptoms, can be continued throughout the perioperative period without significantly increasing the risk of either perioperative bleeding or transfusion requirements. However, given the inherent risks of some surgical procedures, the surgeon should be involved in the decision to continue or withhold aspirin perioperatively. Beta-blockers should not only be continued throughout the perioperative period, consideration for initiating beta-blocker therapy should be strongly entertained if the patient is not already on this class of medications. The study by Mangano et al has clearly shown that patients who receive perioperative beta-blocker therapy have better long-term outcome (14). An additional important study that has demonstrated the benefit of aggressive beta-blockade in the perioperative period is the work by Poldermans et al. This study compared 59 patients that received bisoprolol to 54 patients that did not prior to vascular surgery. All patients in both groups had more than 1 risk factor and all had positive dobutamine stress exams. A reduction in mortality from 17% in the control group to 3.4% in the treatment group was realized. In addition, a reduction of non-fatal MIs was achieved (17% reduced to 0%). These studies utilized aggressive preoperative beta-blockade, something that many anesthesiologists remain uncomfortable with. We presently beta-block patients intraoperatively with short acting agents and begin longer acting agents once the period of rapid fluid shifts has started to subside postoperatively. This strategy also permits us to more safely utilize beta-blockers in a broader population of patients including those that have a history of asthma or bronchoreactive COPD. I strongly recommend one continuously evaluates compliance with beta-blocker administration aiming for > 85% compliance.

Valvular Heart Disease

The basic preoperative evaluation of patients with known or suspected valvular heart disease is not very much different from the routine evaluation of such patients. Identifying the valvular lesion by stethoscopy and history is the first step. This is usually followed by quantifying the severity of that valvular lesion with echocardiography. Although an understanding of all valvular lesions is required to provide care to this potentially complex group of patients, one particular valvular lesion requires special attention because the risk associated with it is commonly misunderstood. Aortic stenosis offers unique challenges during the perioperative period, especially when the valve area is significantly reduced and the

stenosis is designated as critical. Furthermore, an understanding of both the valve area (severity of valvular lesion) and the valvular gradient (marker of LV function) are required. Too often consultants believe that a regional anesthetic would be safer for a patient with critical aortic stenosis when in fact nothing could be further from the truth. The profound combined preload and afterload reduction seen with spinal and epidural approaches makes them inherently dangerous for patients that require high diastolic blood pressure. Although a safe regional anesthetic in such patients can be accomplished by a highly seasoned anesthesiologist, the most common approach is to avoid the risks associated with hemodynamic pertubations from regional techniques and to provide a stable general anesthetic period.

Management of Patients with Arrhythmias

Given the clear data on the ability of beta-blocker withdrawal to induce life-threatening arrhythmias, all patients that chronically receive these medications should continue them throughout the perioperative period and should always take them on the morning of surgery with a sip of water less than 25 cc. Given the potent anti-arrhythmic effects of beta-blockers, in addition to the previously discussed anti-ischemic benefits, these agents stand out as therapeutic agents especially for supraventricular tachyarrythmias (SVT). Beta-blocker treatment has been associated with slightly faster rate control for postoperative SVT and a significantly higher rate of conversion to sinus rhythm. In patients that cannot tolerate beta-blockade because of demonstrated complications such as wheezing or a fall in cardiac performance, then calcium channel blockers become a reasonable class of agents with diltiazem more commonly utilized because of its lower negative inotropic effect. The newer anti-arrhythmics such as ibutilide and amiodarone have limited roles as primary therapeutic agents as this time secondary to their side effects but might have a significant role (i.e., amiodarone) in maintaining sinus rhythm after cardioversion in these patients. The role of magnesium remains unclear. It appears that high plasma levels of magnesium are required for it to function as an anti-arrhythmic, but given its low cost and low rate of toxicity it seems prudent to maintain most patients in the high-normal range during the perioperative period. Ventricular tachyarrythmias are managed the same in the perioperative period as they are for other patients. Ischemic etiologies must be considered and electrolytes corrected. Ultimately, defibrillation and potent anti-arrhythmics may be required.

Patients with a history of bradycardia offer a different challenge during the perioperative period. Their tachycardiac threshold for ischemia may be at a lower and undefined rate. Given their low basal rate, aggressive beta-blockade may not be neither necessary nor prudent. Temporary pacemakers may be required during the perioperative period, as some patients will experience bradycardic rhythms perioperatively, most commonly of the nodal variety. Patients who require pacemakers at baseline will require these pacemakers to be identified and evaluated within the 6 months prior to surgery. The electrocautery devices utilized during surgery can reprogram or disable some pacemakers so a clear understanding of the make and type of pacemaker is required, as well as access to experts in pacemaker programming. Automated implantable cardiac defibrillators (AICD) must be turned off immediately preoperative and then reprogrammed immediately postoperatively. If this is not accomplished, electrical devices utilized in the operating room, like the electrocautery, can reprogram the device or cause the device to deliver shocks despite ongoing normal cardiac rhythms potentially causing fatal arrhythmias. Then, because the device was either reprogrammed or disabled by the electrical impulse, it would not be available to help defibrillate the patient. When these devices are combined AICD–pacemaker, then the pacemaker function should remain turned on while the AICD is temporarily disabled and restarted postoperatively.

Other Methods for Controlling the Stress Response That Can Improve Outcome

Previously, I mentioned that besides beta-blockers, alternate strategies for modulation of stress response included approaches that diminish the production of these neuroendocrine factors such as temperature control, regional blocks, and centrally acting alpha-2 agonists. Hypothermia has been shown to be a stimulator for the secretion of catecholamines. When patients were randomized to routine attempts to maintain temperature and convective warming, those patients that received convective warming had epinephrine levels that barely changed from baseline, whereas the control patients experienced almost a tripling of their epinephrine levels. Convective warming also reduced the magnitude of the rise seen in norepinephrine levels from a 3-fold rise to barely a 20% increase. Furthermore, Kurz et al demonstrated that maintenance of a temperature of 36.6°C versus 34.7°C was associated with a 3-fold reduction in infectious complications and a reduction in length of stay. To summarize the hypothermia literature, it has been demonstrated that hypothermia potentiates the catecholamine response to surgery. The higher catecholamine concentrations exacerbate vasoconstriction and reduce tissue paO2. Finally, perioperative warming decreases wound infections by preventing hypothermia-mediated tissue hypoxia.

The alpha-2-agonists have been extensively studied for their ability to reduce the surgical stress response. Clonidine has been studied in its IV, PO, and dermal patch preparations, and appears to be effective in all forms. In a study done by Dorman et al, the use of perioperative clonidine compared to placebo reduced the magnitude of the increase in perioperative plasma epinephrine and norepinephrine concentrations by almost 50%. These reductions were correlated with beta perioperative heart rate and blood pressure control. Other alpha-2-agonists like dexmedetomidine and mivazoral are under investigation for their potential use in the perioperative period.

The debate regarding the potential benefits of regional anesthesia versus general anesthesia rages onward. It is clear from the literature that epidural and spinal anesthetics help ablate the catecholamine response to lower extremity revascularization, as well as modify the cortisol and glucose response to surgical stress. Several older studies seemed to demonstrate a benefit of these regional techniques for patients undergoing hip replacement surgery. In this population, a lower incidence of DVT and subsequent PE is felt to be associated with the control of the central aspects of the stress response seen when these regional techniques are deployed. In patients undergoing radical retropubic prostatectomy, the data seem to demonstrate a slight reduction in blood loss and transfusion requirements in patients that receive a regional anesthetic as compared to those receiving a general anesthetic with positive pressure ventilation. Otherwise, no conclusive data exists for the claim that regional anesthesia is either safer or better. Recently, a controversial meta-analysis was published which on first pass seemed to show for the first time that regional was indeed significantly better across the board. Unfortunately, numerous methodological flaws make interpretation of this study quite difficult.

The Importance of Volume Status Perioperatively

Maintenance of euvolemia throughout the perioperative period is extremely important and can be quite difficult. In order for patients to tolerate induction of general anesthesia or the initiation of a major neuraxial regional block, hypovolemia must be avoided. If the patient is hypovolemic, then they will not tolerate the deleterious effects of either anesthetic type and profound hypotension will ensue. During the case, especially those with an open body cavity like exploratory laporotomies, patients will third-space into the environment significant fluid quantities. These patients will require approximately 10 mL/kg/hr of crystalloid in addition to maintenance fluids and blood loss replacement. For a 70 kg patient having a 5-hour major abdominal case, this can amount to 5-7 liters of fluid and if there is any blood loss, this total can easily rise to 10 liters. These volumes over relatively short periods are not excessive and in fact, if patients are not this well resuscitated then they will either be at risk of hypotension and organ hypoperfusion during the case or shortly thereafter. The third spacing that these patients experience does not stop once the

abdomen is closed. Cytokines appear to be responsible for the ongoing capillary leak that these patients experience. This intense third-spacing can persist for 24 hours but usually subsides by 12 hours postoperatively. Although this postoperative capillary leak does not seem to require the same volume of fluid replacement as that which occurs intraoperatively, it can approach that volume in some patients especially those not well resuscitated intraoperatively. Once the capillary leak subsides, fluids can be reduced to minimal volumes. Once minimal volumes have been tolerated as exhibited by the maintenance of heart rate, mean arterial pressure, pulse pressure, and urine output, then judicious diuresis might be indicated. It is an extremely rare patient, probably in the range of < 1%, that requires diuretics on the day of a surgical procedure or within 12 hours of most surgical procedures.

ANNOTATED REFERENCES

1. Chernow B, Alexander HR, Smallridge RC et al: Hormonal responses to graded surgical stress. *Arch Intern Med* 1987; 147:1273-1278

2. Weissman C: The metabolic response to stress: An overview and update. *Anesthesiology* 1990; 73:308-327

3. Dorman T, Clarkson K, Rosenfeld BA: Effects of clonidine on prolonged postoperative sympathetic response. *Crit Care Med* 1997; 25:1147-1152

4. Parker SD, Breslow MJ, Frank SM: Catecholamine and cortisol responses to lower extremity revascularization: Correlation with outcome variables. *Crit Care Med* 1995; 23:1954-1961

5. Breslow MJ, Jordan DA, Christopherson R: Epidural morphine decreases postoperative hypertension by attenuating sympathetic nervous system hyperactivity. *JAMA* 1989; 261:3577-3581

6. Rosenfeld BA, Breslow MJ, Dorman T: Postoperative management strategies may obviate the need for most preoperative cardiac testing. *Anesthesiology* 1996; 84:1266-1268

7. Eagle KA, Boucher CA: Cardiac risk of noncardiac surgery. *N Engl J Med* 1989; 321:1330-1332

8. Forrest JB, Rehder K, Goldsmith CH, et al: Multicenter study of general anesthesia. I. Design and patient demography. *Anesthesiology* 1990; 72:252-61

9. Goldman L, Caldera DL, Nussbaum SR: Multifactorial index of cardiac risk in noncardiac surgical procedures. *N Engl J Med* 1977; 297:845-50

10. Detsky AS, Abrams HB, Forbath N: Cardiac assessment for patients undergoing noncardiac surgery. A multifactorial clinical risk index. *Arch Intern Med* 1986; 146:2131-4

11. Palda VA, Detsky AS: Guidelines for assessing and managing the perioperative risk from coronary artery disease associated with major noncardiac surgery Part I. *Ann Intern Med* 1997; 127:309-312

12. Palda VA, Detsky AS: Perioperative assessment and management of risk from coronary artery disease Part II. *Ann Intern Med* 1997; 127:313-328

13. Rao TL, Jacobs KH, El-Etr AA: Reinfarction following anesthesia in patients with myocardial infarction. *Anesthesiology* 1983; 59:499-505

14. Mangano DT, Layug EL, Wallace A: Effect of atenolol on mortality and cardiovascular morbidity after noncardiac surgery: Multicenter Study of Perioperative Ischemia Research Group. *N Engl J Med* 1996; 335:1713-20

15. Kurz A, Sessler DI, Lenhardt R: Perioperative normothermia to reduce the incidence of surgical-wound infection and shorten hospitalization. Study of Wound Infection and Temperature Group. *New Engl J Med* 1996; 334

16. Rodgers A: Reduction of postoperative mortality and morbidity with epidural or spinal anaesthesia: Results from overview of randomised trials. *BMJ* 2000; 321

17. Pasternack PF, et al: The hemodynamics of beta-blockade in patients undergoing abdominal aortic aneurysm repair. *Circulation* 1987; 76

18. Balser JR, et al: Beta-adrenergic blockade accelerates conversion of postoperative supraventricular tachyarrhythmias. *Anesthesiology* 1998; 89

19. Poldermans D, et al: The effect of bisoprolol on perioperative mortality and myocardial infarction in high-risk patients undergoing vascular surgery. *New Engl J Med* 1999; 341

20. Epstein J, Breslow MJ: The stress response of critical illness. Critical Care Clinics. 15(1): January 1999

21. Dorman T, et al: Effects of clonidine on prolonged postoperative sympathetic response. *Crit Care Med* 1997; 25

22. Breslow MJ, et al: Determinants of catecholamine and cortisol responses in lower extremity revascularization. *Anesthesiology* 1993; 79

23. Frank SM, et al: The catecholamine, cortisol, and hemodynamic responses to mild perioperative hypothermia. *Anesthesiology* 1995; 82

24. Tsukada K, et al: Pentothal interleukin-6, interleukin-8, and granulocyte elastase activity after elective surgery. *APMIS* 1994; 102

TRANSPLANTATION

Joshua O. Benditt, MD, FCCP

Objectives

- To identify general principles and common themes of organ transplantation
- To review the clinical course and serious complications of liver transplantation
- To identify common problems associated with heart, heart-lung, and lung transplantation
- To outline major complications of kidney and kidney-pancreas transplantation

Key Words: liver transplantation, heart transplantation, heart-lung transplantation, lung transplantation, kidney transplantation, pancreas transplantation

TABLE OF ABBREVIATIONS

ARDS acute respiratory distress syndrome
CMV cytomegalovirus
EBV Epstein-Barr virus
GVHD graft-versus-host disease
HSV herpes simplex virus
IL interleukin
PCP *Pneumocystis carinii* pneumonia
PTLD posttransplant lymphoproliferative disorder
SVR systemic vascular resistance
VZV varicella zoster virus

GENERAL PRINCIPLES

The number of transplants performed each year is increasing steadily. Approximately 23,000 organs were transplanted in the United States in 2000, and nearly 80,000 patients are currently on waiting lists. Intensivists are likely to face transplant-related problems in the preoperative support of transplant candidates with end-stage organ failure, in the routine postoperative care of transplant recipients, and in the management of life-threatening complications of transplantation.

Temporal Organization of Complications

The complications of transplantation are related to the underlying disease and premorbid condition of the patient, the transplant procedure, rejection of the graft or host, and the consequences of immunosuppression. These complications occur in temporal patterns.

Noninfectious problems in the first few weeks after solid organ transplantation include: a) surgical complications; b) graft dysfunction related to ischemia, preservation, and reperfusion; and c) rejection. After the first few months, chronic rejection is a significant problem.

Infectious complications also exhibit temporal patterns. Nosocomial infections are prominent in the early posttransplant course, followed by the reactivation of latent infection in the graft or host and new opportunistic infections related to the intensity and duration of immunosuppression. Staphylococci and Gram-negative bacilli are the most common early bacterial pathogens, followed later by infections caused by *Legionella*, *Nocardia*, *Mycobacteria*, and *Listeria*. Candidiasis and aspergillosis are the major fungal infections occurring in the first few months after transplantation, but reactivation of endemic mycoses and cryptococcosis may present later. Herpes simplex virus (HSV) often reactivates in the initial weeks after transplantation, and Herpesvirus-6 is increasingly recognized 2 to 4 weeks posttransplant. Cytomegalovirus (CMV) and hepatitis C infections typically present after the first month. The peak incidence of Epstein-Barr virus (EBV)-related posttransplant lymphoproliferative disorder (PTLD) is 3 to 6 months after transplant. Dermatomal reactivation of varicella-zoster virus (VZV) also occurs in this time frame. Toxoplasmosis and *Pneumocystis carinii* pneumonia (PCP) may develop after the first posttransplant month.

Immunosuppression

Immunosuppression is required to prevent rejection of the transplanted organ or, in the case of bone marrow transplantation, to prevent graft-versus-host disease (GVHD). The approaches to induction and maintenance immunosuppression, and the treatment of established rejection vary significantly from 1 institution to another. Most centers use a combination of agents in low doses to minimize the toxicity of individual drugs.

Cyclosporine is a fungal cyclic peptide that inhibits transcription of interleukin (IL) 2 and the expression of IL-2 receptors, resulting in blockade of T-cell activation. There are marked individual variations in the absorption and metabolism of cyclosporine; precise timing of dosages and monitoring of drug levels are essential. Cyclosporine is metabolized by the hepatic cytochrome p450 system and is subject to many drug interactions. Drugs that increase cyclosporine levels include erythromycin, ketoconazole, itraconazole, cimetidine, and diltiazam. Agents that decrease cyclosporine levels include phenytoin, phenobarbital, trimethoprim, rifampin, and isoniazid. Important side-effects include nephrotoxicity, hypertension, neurotoxicity (tremors, paresthesias, seizures, etc.), gingival hyperplasia, hyperlipidemia, and hypertrichosis.

Tacrolimus (FK506) is a macrolide that has essentially the same mechanism of action as cyclosporine. In liver, kidney, and lung transplant recipients tacrolimus is more effective than cyclosporine in preventing acute and chronic rejection, and is effective in the treatment of acute rejection. In comparison with cylosporine, tacrolimus is associated with more neurotoxicity, nephrotoxicity, and glucose intolerance but less hypertension, dyslipidemia, gingival hyperplasia, or hirsuitism.

Azathioprine is a purine analog that inhibits lymphocyte proliferation. Leukopenia, hepatitis, and cholestasis are important toxicities. Mycophenolate mofetil is a more selective inhibitor of purine synthesis that appears to be more effective than azathioprine at preventing acute rejection. Diarrhea, emesis, and leukopenia are the principal side-effects of mycophenolate mofetil.

Corticosteroids are nonspecific anti-inflammatory agents that inhibit cytokine production, antigen recognition, and T-cell proliferation. The familiar side-effects of corticosteroids include Cushing's syndrome, hyperglycemia, hyperlipidemia, osteoporosis, myopathy, and cataracts.

Polyclonal and monoclonal antibodies are used to deplete the T cells that mediate acute rejection. Antithymocyte and antilymphocyte globulin may cause serum sickness, thrombocytopenia, and leukopenia. Initial treatment with OKT3, a murine monoclonal antibody to the T-cell receptor, often elicits fever, chills, and a capillary leak syndrome resulting in hypotension and pulmonary edema. OKT3 also increases the risks of CMV infection and EBV-related PTLD. Newer mouse/human chimeric monoclonal antibodies to IL-2 receptors (basiliximab, daclizumab) are associated with less toxicity.

Rejection

Several patterns of rejection have been described in solid organ transplantation. Hyperacute rejection is seen within minutes to hours of transplantation, and is mediated by preformed antibodies that cause vascular injury. The kidney and heart are particularly susceptible, but the liver is resistant to hyperacute rejection. There is no treatment, but this form of rejection often can be avoided by pretransplant cross-matching. Accelerated rejection is an uncommon form of antibody-mediated rejection that is seen several days after transplantation and characterized histologically by vascular necrosis. Acute rejection is the most common cause of graft failure, and is mediated by T cells. Acute rejection may be seen as early as the first week, and any time thereafter. Chronic rejection appears >3 months after transplantation, is characterized by a slowly progressive course associated with histologic fibrosis, and often is refractory to treatment.

Infection

Pretransplant identification of latent infections in the donor and recipient is essential in defining risks. Routine testing includes serologies for CMV, HSV, EBV, VZV, hepatitis A, B, and C, HIV, toxoplasmosis, and relevant endemic mycoses such as histoplasmosis and coccidiomycosis. A tuberculin test should be placed and the chest radiograph evaluated for granulomatous disease. Indolent infection of the oral cavity and sinuses should be excluded, and immunizations should be brought up-to-date. Prophylaxis is effective against many latent and some acquired infections. Routine surveillance is helpful for the preemptive management of CMV infections, and possibly others. Suspected infection should be approached with an assessment of risks and an aggressive effort at specific diagnosis.

CMV is the bane of transplantation. Primary infection occurs when a seronegative patient receives an organ from a seropositive donor; secondary or reactivation infection develops in seropositive recipients. Active infection (viral replication) will develop in most patients at risk, and is diagnosed by antigen detection, nucleic acid identification, or culture. Symptomatic disease develops in 40% to 60% of primary infections and approximately 20% of secondary infections. The manifestations of CMV disease vary with the organ transplanted. The risk of CMV disease is increased in patients who are treated with antithymocyte globulin or OKT3. CMV disease is treated with ganciclovir, with or without CMV immune globulin. CMV disease can be prevented by the use of screened blood products, oral valacyclovir prophylaxis, and by prophylactic or pre-emptive (at the earliest sign of viral replication) treatment with ganciclovir and hyperimmune globulin.

The posttransplant lymphoproliferative disorder is caused by EBV infection and occurs in 6% to 9% of lung transplants, 3% to 5% of heart transplants, 2% to 4% of liver transplants, and <1% of kidney transplants. The risk of PTLD is increased by treatment with anti-T cell antibodies. PTLD presents 6 to 24 weeks after transplantation with an infectious mononucleosis-like syndrome or diverse local manifestations that may involve any lymphatic tissue, the gastrointestinal tract, lungs, kidneys, or brain. The diagnosis is made by demonstrating the EBV genome in association with benign or malignant lymphatic proliferation. Treatment strategies include

reduced immunosuppression, interferon-alpha, and cytotoxic chemotherapy. Local resection may be helpful and there is an uncertain role for acyclovir or ganciclovir.

LIVER TRANSPLANTATION

Perspective

There were 4,954 liver transplants performed in the United States in 2000. The most common indications are chronic active hepatitis C, alcoholic cirrhosis, cryptogenic cirrhosis, primary biliary cirrhosis, and sclerosing cholangitis. For patients transplanted over the last 10 years, graft and patient survivals are 73% and 82%, respectively, at 1 year, and 63% and 73% at 4 years.

Usual Clinical Course

Liver transplant recipients require ICU care for 2 to 4 days after surgery. The cardiac output is generally high and the systemic vascular resistance (SVR) low; circulatory instability is common and usually volume-responsive. Myocardial depression is a poor prognostic sign. Calcium may be depleted by the citrate in blood products. Hyperglycemia is common and potassium levels may be high or low. A mild metabolic acidosis may be present initially, but metabolic alkalosis develops as the liver metabolizes citrate. Deficient clotting factors and thrombocytopenia contribute to a significant bleeding diathesis. Blood products are usually replaced empirically (for evident bleeding and a fall in hematocrit), although many centers monitor coagulation with thromboelastography, a rapid measure of the time to onset of clotting, the rate of clot formation, and maximum clot elasticity. Important signs of a functioning graft are the production of golden brown bile, the restoration of clotting, the absence of a metabolic acidosis, and the resolution of encephalopathy. Patients should be awake and alert within 12 hours. The serum bilirubin may rise initially because of hemolysis, but liver enzymes should fall each day. The prothrombin time and partial thromboplastin time should improve daily and be normal within 72 hours. Most patients can be extubated within 48 hours.

Noninfectious Complications

Hemorrhage in the first 48 hours usually is due to diffuse oozing in the setting of a coagulopathy and is managed with blood products. Later, intra-abdominal bleeding may be related to necrosis of a vascular anastamosis. Gastrointestinal hemorrhage may result from stress ulceration or the development of portal hypertension.

Primary graft failure occurs in 1% to 5% of liver transplants and usually is a consequence of ischemic injury. The signs of graft failure include poor bile formation, metabolic acidosis, and failure to resolve encephalopathy and coagulopathy. The treatment is retransplantation within 48 hours, before brainstem herniation from cerebral edema.

Vascular complications include thromboses of the hepatic artery, hepatic vein, or portal vein. Hepatic artery thrombosis occurs in about 5% of patients and presents in 1 of 4 ways: massive liver necrosis (fever, rising enzymes, deterioration in mental status, renal insufficiency, shock); a bile leak with or without evidence of liver injury; recurrent bacteremia from hepatic abscesses; or as an asymptomatic finding on routine ultrasound. The diagnosis is made by duplex ultrasonography, and the treatment is operative repair or retransplantation. Portal vein thrombosis is less common, and presents with ascites and variceal hemorrhage, with or without graft dysfunction. Hepatic vein thrombosis is rare and presents with liver failure and massive ascites.

Biliary complications occur in up to 28% of patients. Bile leaks are caused by traumatic or ischemic injury to the common bile duct. Biliary obstruction may be caused by kinking or displacement of drainage tubes, dysfunction of the sphincter of Oddi, or strictures. Biliary complications are diagnosed by cholangiography, and are managed with surgical or endoscopic repair.

Acute rejection is the most common cause of liver dysfunction after transplantation. Most patients experience at least 1 episode, usually 4 to 14 days after transplantation. The clinical signs (fever, tenderness and enlargement of graft), and laboratory features (elevated hepatocellular enzymes and bilirubin) are nonspecific. The diagnosis is confirmed with liver biopsy demonstrating mononuclear cell portal infiltration, ductular injury, and venulitis. Most patients respond to pulse steroids or anti-T-cell antibodies. ICU readmission is rarely required.

Common noninfectious pulmonary complications of liver transplantation include atelectasis, pleural effusions, and pulmonary edema. In most cases, preoperative shunting caused by the hepatopulmonary syndrome improves over days to months posttransplant. Respiratory muscle weakness, the abdominal wound, impaired mental status, and severe metabolic alkalosis may contribute to delayed weaning. Acute respiratory distress syndrome (ARDS) occurs in <10% of liver graft recipients, usually as a consequence of sepsis.

Neurologic dysfunction after liver transplantation may be caused by hepatic encephalopathy, hypoglycemia, intracranial hemorrhage, air embolism, drug toxicity, or infection.

Infection

Bacteria are the most important causes of infection after liver transplantation, particularly in the first 6 weeks after grafting. Gram-positive cocci and Gram-negative bacilli are the predominant pathogens, and the site of infection often involves the transplanted liver or the reconstructed biliary tree. Intra-abdominal abscesses, peritonitis, cholangitis, and surgical wound infections are the most common foci of bacterial infection, followed by pneumonia, catheter sepsis, and urinary tract infections. Prophylactic systemic and topical antibiotics are commonly used but are of unproven value.

CMV infection will be evident in approximately 50% of liver transplant recipients, and half of these cases will be symptomatic. A seropositive donor is the most important risk factor for CMV disease. The peak onset of CMV infection is 28 days after transplantation. A mononucleosis-like syndrome characterized by fever, malaise, myalgias, and neutropenia is the most common manifestation. Hepatitis is the most common organ involvement. Anecdotal reports suggest that treatment of CMV disease with ganciclovir is beneficial. CMV disease can be prevented in high-risk patients by long-term (100-day) ganciclovir prophylaxis or by preemptive treatment at the first sign of viral replication. HSV mucositis reactivates in 40% to 50% of seropositive patients and can be prevented or treated with acyclovir.

Fungal infections complicate 10% to 40% of liver transplants, usually in the first 2 months, and are more common than with other organ transplants. Candidemia, from an abdominal or vascular source, is the leading mycosis, followed by pulmonary aspergillosis. Pneumocystis infections are rare in patients receiving prophylaxis.

HEART TRANSPLANTATION

Perspective

There were 2,198 heart transplants performed in the United States in 2000. Ischemic cardiomyopathy, idiopathic cardiomyopathy, and congenital heart disease are the leading indications, together accounting for >80% of procedures. Patient survival is 83% at 1 year, and 72% at 4 years.

Usual Clinical Course

Cardiac function is depressed for several days postoperatively, and the right ventricle recovers more slowly than the left. Cardiac output is initially rate-dependent in the denervated heart, and low-dose isoproterenol or pacing is often required for 2 to 4 days. Patients are routinely extubated within 24 hours and discharged from the ICU within 48 hours.

Noninfectious Complications

The early complications of heart transplantation include those of cardiac surgery in general. Most patients develop left lower lobe atelectasis that may persist for weeks. Pleural, pericardial, and mediastinal fluid collections are common, but hemorrhage is unusual. Pulmonary edema is a frequent occurrence because of pretransplant congestion, postoperative left ventricular dysfunction, and volume overload; heparin-protamine reactions and reperfusion injury may alter lung permeability. Persistent

pulmonary hypertension is an important early problem that may lead to right ventricular failure. Prostaglandin E1, nitric oxide, inotropes, and assist devices may be effective.

Rejection may occur any time after heart transplantation and is diagnosed histologically from routine surveillance endomyocardial biopsies. Clinical signs of rejection such as fever, heart failure, arrhythmias, and pericardial friction rubs are unreliable. The severity of rejection is graded by the degree of lymphocytic infiltration and myocyte necrosis. Mild cases may resolve spontaneously; about one third of patients require treatment for rejection. Most episodes respond to pulse corticosteroids and/or increased doses of cyclosporine. Refractory cases usually respond to anti-T-cell treatment.

Accelerated coronary atherosclerosis is the leading cause of death >1 year after heart transplantation. The cumulative incidence is approximately 10% per annum. Calcium channel blockers and HMG CoA reductase inhibitors may slow the development of allograft vasculopathy.

Infection

Nosocomial bacterial pneumonia, mediastinitis, empyema, and catheter-related infections are common in the first month after transplantation. Gram-negative bacilli and *S. aureus* are frequent pathogens. *Legionella* pneumonia and wound infections are important in the first 3 months after heart transplantation, particularly in hospitals with contaminated water supplies. *Nocardia* infection of the lung may present any time after the first postoperative month, and may disseminate to brain or bone. Atypical mycobacterial infections have been reported in 3% of heart transplant patients, usually involving the lung, mediastinum, or soft tissues.

Aspergillosis is the most common fungal infection after heart transplantation, developing in 5% to 10% of recipients, usually in the first month. The lung is the primary site of infection, but dissemination is evident in half the cases at diagnosis.

Toxoplasmosis is an important consideration when a seronegative recipient receives a heart from a seropositive donor. Primary infection presents 4 to 6 weeks after transplantation with fever and nonspecific signs involving the heart, brain, eyes, lungs, and/or liver; myocardial infection may mimic rejection. The diagnosis is supported by seroconversion and confirmed by the demonstration of tachyzoites in tissue. Treatment with pyrimethamine and sulfadiazine is effective if instituted promptly. Pyrimethamine also may be effective in preventing primary infection. Reactivation of latent toxoplasmosis in seropositive recipients is not clinically significant. PCP develops in 3% of cardiac transplant patients without prophylaxis, but is now rare.

Active CMV infection will develop in most seropositive patients and seronegative recipients of hearts from seropositive donors. One third of these infections will be symptomatic, usually with a mononucleosis-like syndrome. CMV pneumonia develops in 10% of infected patients. Serious morbidity and mortality are largely limited to patients with primary infection. Ganciclovir appears to be effective in the treatment of CMV disease in heart transplant patients. The role of ganciclovir in prophylaxis is uncertain. Reactivation of oral and genital HSV infection is common in the first few months after heart transplantation. VZV typically reactivates in a dermatomal distribution 3 to 6 months after transplantation. HSV and VZV infections usually remain localized and respond to acyclovir.

PTLD develops in 2% to 7% of heart transplant recipients, usually presenting 3 to 6 months after transplantation. PTLD is probably caused by EBV and the risk is markedly increased by treatment with OKT3. Any lymphatic tissue may be involved, as well as the gastrointestinal tract, lungs, kidneys, or brain. Most cases respond to a reduction in immunosuppressive therapy. Resection of localized tumors and treatment with acyclovir may be helpful.

LUNG AND HEART-LUNG TRANSPLANTATION

Perspective

There were 956 lung transplants and 48 heart-lung transplants are performed in the United States in 2000. The leading indications for single-lung transplantation are COPD, idiopathic pulmonary fibrosis, and α-1 antitrypsin deficiency. Double-lung transplants usually are performed mainly for septic lung disease (cystic fibrosis or bronchiectasis). The leading indications for heart-lung transplants are Eisenmenger's complex and primary pulmonary hypertension. The survival rates for grafts and patients following lung transplantation are 73% and 74%, respectively, at 1 year and 47% and 50% at 4 years. The survival of heart-lung transplants is 65% at 1 year and 46% at 5 years.

Usual Clinical Course

Volume overload and pulmonary edema are common early problems. Cardiac function may be impaired if cardiopulmonary bypass was required (all heart-lung transplants, some lung transplants). Cardiac output is rate-dependent in denervated hearts, and responds to isoproterenol. Care must be taken to avoid air trapping in an emphysematous native lung. Independent lung ventilation through a double-lumen endotracheal tube may be necessary in some single-lung transplants to improve ventilation-perfusion matching or reduce air trapping. Most patients can be extubated within 36 hours. Patients receiving single-lung transplants for primary pulmonary hypertension often are heavily sedated for 48 to 72 hours before extubation to reduce pulmonary arterial hypertensive crises. Reflexive coughing is lost in the denervated lung, and pulmonary toilet is critical to secretion management. Lymphatics are severed in the transplanted lung, impairing extravascular fluid clearance and rendering the graft particularly susceptible to edema.

Noninfectious Complications

Hemorrhage early after lung transplantation is usually from the mediastinum or pleura. Bleeding is particularly common in heart-lung transplants because of the extensive mediastinal dissection and the need for heparinization during bypass. Patients with cystic fibrosis also are at increased risk of hemorrhage because pleural adhesions often must be severed to remove the native lungs. Bilateral bronchial anastomoses require less mediastinal dissection and are associated with less bleeding than tracheal anastomoses.

The pulmonary re-implantation response is evident in most patients. This is a form of reperfusion injury that results in noncardiogenic pulmonary edema. The clinical features include alveolar and interstitial infiltrates on chest radiograph, a decline in lung compliance, and impaired gas exchange. The response peaks 2 to 4 days after transplantation and resolves gradually thereafter with careful fluid management and diuresis. The diagnosis is made by the clinical presentation and time course, and the exclusion of infection, rejection, and cardiogenic pulmonary edema.

Airway dehiscence, stenosis, and bronchomalacia were major causes of morbidity and mortality in the early years of lung transplantation. The use of omental wraps or telescoping bronchial anastomoses has markedly reduced the incidence of airway complications. Strictures now develop in about 10% of cases and stents are occasionally required for the management of stenoses.

Phrenic nerve paralysis resulting from thermal or mechanical injury occurs in <5% of patients. The injury is often temporary, with gradual recovery over several weeks.

Acute rejection occurs as early as 3 days after lung transplantation and most patients will experience at least 1 episode within the first postoperative month. Lung rejection is more common than heart rejection in heart-lung transplants. The clinical manifestations are nonspecific and include low-grade fever, dyspnea, cough, fatigue, hypoxemia, a fall in FEV1, and new or changing infiltrates on chest radiograph (the chest x-ray is usually normal when rejection occurs >1 month after transplantation). Infection and edema are the major alternative considerations in the first few weeks after transplantation; later CMV is the principle concern. Bronchoscopy is helpful in excluding infection and confirming rejection. Transbronchial biopsies demonstrate the characteristic perivascular mononuclear infiltrates with a sensitivity of 70% to 90% and specificity of >90%. There may be a role for identifying donor-sensitized lymphocytes by bronchoalveolar lavage. Most patients respond promptly to pulse corticosteroids; nonresponders are treated with anti-T-cell antibodies.

Obliterative bronchiolitis is the major manifestation of chronic rejection in the transplanted lung and a leading cause of late mortality. The incidence of obliterative bronchiolitis increases over time and is found in 60% to 70% of patients that survive for 5 years after transplantation. Repeated episodes of acute rejection and CMV infection are possible risk factors. Obliterative bronchiolitis may present any time after the second postoperative month, with half the cases presenting in the first year. Patients may complain of dyspnea or cough, and chest radiographs are usually normal. The clinical diagnosis hinges on spirometric demonstration of significant declines in FEV1 and FEF25-75. Some centers have found transbronchial biopsies to be helpful. Treatment is with increased immunosuppression, but no strategy has been demonstrated to be effective. Pulmonary function may stabilize with treatment, but rarely improves. The mortality of obliterative bronchiolitis is 40% within 2 years of diagnosis.

Infection

Infection is the leading cause of death after lung transplantation, and most infections are located in the thorax. Most centers advocate an aggressive approach to etiologic diagnosis, relying heavily on bronchoscopy. In single-lung transplant recipients, infection in the native lung is a significant problem.

Bacteria are the most common agents of infection after lung transplantation. Bacterial pneumonia is most frequent in the early postoperative period, but purulent bronchitis often presents weeks to months after transplantation; late bacterial infections are particularly common in patients with obliterative bronchiolitis. Typical nosocomial pathogens are the usual culprits, although native strains of *Pseudomonas cepacia* and *P. aeruginosa* are problematic in patients with cystic fibrosis. Prophylactic broad-spectrum antibiotics are routinely administered for the first 48 to 72 hours after transplantation, empirically or guided by cultures from the donor and recipient respiratory tracts; the validity of this practice has not been tested by controlled trial. Bacterial infections usually respond to antibiotics.

CMV disease is more common in lung allograft recipients than in other solid organ transplant patients. Most seropositive recipients will develop positive blood and bronchoalveolar lavage cultures (active infection) a median of 40 days after transplantation in the absence of prophylaxis, but the risk and severity of symptomatic CMV disease are highest in seronegative patients who receive a lung from a seropositive donor (i.e., those with primary infection). Treatment with OKT3 is an additional risk for CMV disease. CMV pneumonitis is the most common manifestation of CMV disease in lung allograft recipients. The chest radiograph is nonspecific and a positive bronchoalveolar lavage culture is predictive of histologic evidence of infection only in the highest risk patients (seronegative recipient, seropositive donor). Transbronchial biopsies are required to identify viral inclusions and to exclude rejection. Treatment of CMV pneumonitis in lung transplant recipients with ganciclovir is probably effective, but has not been prospectively studied. The direct mortality from CMV disease in treated patients is about 1%, but CMV infection may increase the risk of acute and chronic rejection. Prophylaxis with ganciclovir may be effective in preventing or delaying CMV disease in at-risk patients, but the optimal regimen has not been defined.

HSV mucositis develops in 30% of seropositive lung transplant recipients in the absence of acyclovir prophylaxis, and half of these patients develop pneumonia. Primary HSV infections are rare. Acyclovir appears to be effective in preventing reactivation of HSV. EBV-related posttransplant lymphoproliferative disorder occurs in approximately 6% of lung allograft recipients. The typical case presents within the first 4 months after transplantation with nodular infiltrates in the lung allograft, although any lymphoid tissue may be involved. Most patients respond to a reduction in the immunosuppressive regimen.

Fungal infections occur in 15% to 35% of lung transplant recipients. Candidiasis is the most common mycosis, and may involve the mediastinum, the airway anastomosis, or dissemination from a cutaneous or vascular site.

Invasive aspergillosis typically presents as a focal pneumonia or necrotizing airway infection. The reported mortality of fungal infections after lung transplantation has ranged from 20% to 80%. The roles for antifungal prophylaxis and aggressive treatment of mucosal isolates are unclear.

KIDNEY TRANSPLANTATION

Perspective

There were 8,079 cadaveric donor and 5,293 living donor kidney transplants performed in the United States in 2000. The leading indications are diabetes mellitus, hypertensive nephrosclerosis, and chronic glomerulonephritis. The current survival rates for grafts and patients after cadaveric transplant is 88% and 95% at 1year, respectively; and 67% and 85% at 4 years. After living donor transplants, the survival rates of grafts and patients is 92% and 97% at 1 year, respectively; and 81% and 92% at 4 years. Graft survival is influenced by HLA matching. Postoperatively, urine output, volume status, and electrolytes must be followed closely, but most renal transplant recipients have a stable course and require intensive care for <24 hours.

Noninfectious Complications

Serious noninfectious complications are uncommon after renal transplantation. Volume overload and graft dysfunction occasionally lead to pulmonary edema. Surgical complications such as renal artery thrombosis, renal vein thrombosis, urine leaks, and lymphoceles occur in <5% of patients. Hyperacute rejection from preformed antibodies causes immediate graft failure and is usually detected in the operating room. Acute rejection occurs in 50% to 60% of cases within the first 3 months and is suspected by a rise in creatinine not attributable to cyclosporine toxicity. Acute rejection is empirically treated with corticosteroids; refractory cases are confirmed by renal biopsy. Chronic rejection develops in 8% to 10% of patients and causes steady deterioration of graft function.

Infection

Urinary tract infections are common early after renal transplantation and can be prevented with prophylactic antibiotics. Bacterial infections of the wound, intravenous catheter sites, and the respiratory tract also may complicate the early postoperative course. Opportunistic infections caused by *Legionella*, *Nocardia*, and *Listeria* usually occur 1 to 6 months after transplantation. Fungal infections are less common in renal graft recipients than in other organ transplant patients.

Primary CMV infection develops in 70% to 90% of seronegative recipients of a kidney from a seropositive donor, and 50% to 60% of these patients will be symptomatic. CMV infection develops in 50% to 80% of seropositive recipients and 20% to 40% of these patients will have clinical disease. The onset of infection is usually 1 to 6 months after transplant. The mononucleosis-like CMV syndrome is the most common manifestation of CMV disease in renal transplant recipients; about 25% of symptomatic patients will develop CMV pneumonia. Ganciclovir appears to be effective in treating CMV disease in the setting of renal transplantation.

KIDNEY-PANCREAS TRANSPLANTATION

Perspective

There were 1,346 pancreas transplants performed in the United States in 2000; of these, 911 were in association with kidney transplants for diabetic nephropathy. Pancreas transplantation normalizes glucose metabolism and reduces the recurrence of vascular disease in the renal graft. The exocrine output of the transplanted pancreas is drained to the bladder via a duodenocystostomy. Current survival rates for grafts and patients after pancreas transplantation are 77% and 92% at 1 year, respectively, and 64% and 84% at 4 years.

Usual Clinical Course

Patients require ICU monitoring of fluids and electrolytes, and tight glucose control with an insulin drip to keep the pancreas at rest. Glucose regulation may normalize within hours, but several days are often required for full graft function.

Noninfectious Complications

Complications are more common after kidney-pancreas transplantation than after renal grafting alone. Surgical complications include vascular thrombosis, hematuria, perforation of the duodenal segment, and urethral stricture. Loss of sodium bicarbonate in the urine may cause significant dehydration and metabolic acidosis. Acute pancreatic rejection occurs in >85% of cases, more commonly than kidney rejection, and is more refractory to corticosteroids. Pancreatic rejection is diagnosed by an abrupt fall in urinary amylase; some centers confirm rejection histologically by cystoscopic biopsy. Most cases of pancreatic rejection fail to respond to corticosteroids and require repeated courses of OKT3.

Infection

Infections also are more common in patients with kidney-pancreas transplants than in recipients of a renal allograft alone because of the additional surgery and the need for more immunosuppression. Wound infections, urinary tract infections, and abdominal abscesses caused by bacteria or fungi are particularly frequent in the first month after transplant, but may appear a year or more postoperatively. Active CMV infection will develop in most patients at risk, and the majority of these infections will be symptomatic with a viremic syndrome; hepatitis is the most common site of tissue infection.

REFERENCES

1. Cerra FB, Gruber SA: Critical care of the transplant patient. *Crit Care Clin* 1990; 6:813-1034
   Review articles on many aspects of solid organ transplantation.
2. Ettinger NA, Trulock EP: Pulmonary considerations of organ transplantation. Parts 1-3. *Am Rev Respir Dis* 1990; 143:1386-1405; 144:213-223, 433-451

An excellent review, including discussions of liver, kidney, heart, heart-lung and and marrow transplantation.

3. Judson MA, Sahn SA: The pleural space and organ transplantation. *Am J Respir Crit Care Med* 1996; 153:1153-1165
   A very thorough review of pre- and posttransplant pleural complications associated with marrow and organ transplantation.

4. Rubin RH: Infection in transplantation. *Infect Dis Clin North Am* 1995; 9:811-1092
   Excellent articles covering every aspect of infection in organ and marrow transplantation.

5. Winkel E, DiSesa VJ, Costanzo, MR, et al: Advances in transplantation. *Dis Month* 1999; 45:60-114
   Discussions of heart, pancreas, and liver transplantation.

6. Kron RAF, Wiesner RH, Rettke SR, et al: Symposium on liver transplantation. *Mayo Clin Proc* 1989; 64:84-115, 216-245, 340-359, 424-450, 545-569, 670-707
   A 6-part series including articles on intraoperative and ICU management, infectious complications, and management of rejection.

7. O'Brien JD, Ettinger NA: Pulmonary complications of liver transplantation. *Clin Chest Med* 1996; 17:99-114
   An excellent review, including a discussion of pretransplant considerations.

8. Arcasoy SM, Kotloff RM: Lung transplantation. *N Engl J Med* 1999; 340:1081-1091
   An informative and concise review.

9. Trulock EP: Lung transplantation. *Am J Respir Crit Care Med* 1997; 155:789-818
   A very thorough review based on the Washington University experience.

10. Wood DE, Raghu G: Lung transplantation part II: Postoperative management and results. *West J Med* 1997; 166:45-55
    A good review of postoperative management from the University of Washington perspective.

11. Rowe JM, Ciobanu N, Ascensao J, et al: Recommended guidelines for the management of autologous and allogeneic bone marrow transplantation. *Ann Intern Med* 1994; 120:143-158
    Excellent review of approaches to prevention and treatment of common problems.

12. Armitage JO: Bone marrow transplantation. *N Engl J Med* 1994; 330:827-838
    Concise overview.

13. Sable CA, Donowitz GR: Infections in bone marrow transplant recipients. *Clin Infect Dis* 1994; 18:273-284
    Succinct review.

14. Soubani AO, Miller KB, Hassoun PM: Pulmonary complications of bone marrow transplantation. *Chest* 1996; 109:1066-1077
    A concise but thorough review.

15. Rubenfeld GD, Crawford: Withdrawing life support from mechanically ventilated recipients of bone marrow transplants: A case for evidence-based guidelines. *Ann Intern Med* 1996; 125:625-633
    An analysis of 865 ventilated patients; there were no survivors among those with lung injury and either >4 hours of pressor support or sustained hepatic and renal failure.

COMA AND DELIRIUM

Thomas P. Bleck, MD, FACP, FCCM, FCCP

Objectives

- Understand the anatomic and physiologic determinants of consciousness
- Recognize the need for common definitions of behavior in comatose and delirious patients
- Be able to perform a rapid coma examination
- Develop an initial management approach

Key Words: Coma, stupor, delirium, obtundation, vegetative state, death

INTRODUCTION

'Altered mental status' belongs in the category of terms that are widely understood but lack a consensual definition. In modern multidisciplinary ICUs, the combination of the diseases being managed and the drugs employed for that management results in a large percentage of patients who develop at least a temporary impairment of awareness or behavior. This area has been obscured by the psychiatric redefinition of delirium into a very broad concept which no longer requires agitation for its diagnosis. Intensivists should be aware of this as they interact with their psychiatric and neurologic colleagues.

Definitions

The following definitions are as described by Plum and Posner (1), except as noted.

Confusion: Confused patients are bewildered and often have difficulty following commands. Disorientation to place and time is common ('except in rare instances of acute delirium, disorientation to self is confined to psychologic disturbances'). Memory is disturbed. Drowsiness is prominent and may alternate with nighttime agitation.

Delirium: Delirium is defined as 'a floridly abnormal mental state characterized by disorientation, fear, irritability, misperception of sensory stimuli, and, often, visual hallucinations.' This definition is diagnostically more specific than that of the DSM-IV (2). ('The essential feature of a delirium is a disturbance of consciousness that is accompanied by a change in cognition that cannot be better accounted for by a preexisting or evolving dementia. The disturbance develops over a short period of time, usually hours to days, and tends to fluctuate during the course of the day. There is evidence from the history, physical examination, or laboratory tests that the delirium is a direct physiologic consequence of a general medical condition, substance intoxication or withdrawal, use of a medication or toxin exposure, or a combination of these factors.') Delirium has also been termed 'acute brain failure,' which may be a foreign notion to localizationists but is a valuable tool for communication.

Obtundation: This term is defined as mental blunting, associated with slowed psychological responses to stimulation and an increase in drowsiness and in the number of hours slept.

Stupor: Stupor is described as 'a condition of deep sleep or behaviorally similar unresponsiveness in which the patient can be aroused only by vigorous and repeated stimuli.' This is not sleep from an EEG perspective.

Coma: Coma is 'a state of unarousable psychologic unresponsiveness in which the subjects lie with eyes closed. Subjects in coma show no psychologically understandable response to external stimuli or inner need. They neither utter understandable words nor accurately localize noxious stimuli with discrete defensive movements.'

Vegetative state: A vegetative state is 'the subacute or chronic condition that sometimes emerges after severe brain injury and comprises a return of wakefulness accompanied by an apparent total lack of cognitive function.

An operational definition is that the eyes open spontaneously in response to verbal stimuli. Sleep-wake cycles exist. The patients spontaneously maintain normal levels of blood pressure and respiratory control. They show no discrete localizing motor responses and neither offer comprehensible words nor obey any verbal commands. A *persistent or chronic vegetative state* refers to this condition in its permanent form and designates subjects who survive for prolonged periods (sometimes years) following a severe brain injury without ever recovering any outward manifestations of higher mental activity. In most instances, the vegetative state follows upon a period of sleep-like coma. Nearly all patients in coma begin to awaken within 2 to 4 weeks no matter how severe the brain damage. Although many such patients are akinetic and mute, others with apparently similar degrees of brain damage may be restless, noisy, and hypermobile.' Synonyms include coma vigil, apallic syndrome, cerebral death, neocortical death, total dementia, and akinetic mutism. It is important to recognize that PVS after trauma, especially in the younger patient, does not carry nearly as dismal a prognosis for recovery as does that following anoxia (3).

ICU psychosis: Considerable debate exists about the existence of a specific disorder of behavior or perception related solely to ICU confinement. Opinions vary (even in the same text) from:

> When faced with a patient who is confused and perhaps agitated, the first question must be 'Is the patient delirious?' *The clinician should not attribute the change in mental status to an 'ICU psychosis.'* The brain's response to a physiologic *(sic)* insult, whether metabolic, anoxic, toxic, or infectious, is delirium (4).

to:

> The incidence of abnormal behavior, perception, or cognition in adult patients admitted to an ICU is somewhat disputed, but every observational study has reported some incidence of such abnormalities with the highest estimates placed at 70 percent. These aberrations typically occur after 5 to 7

days of ICU stay, and risk of their development increases with duration of stay. It is perhaps intuitively clear that life in the ICU is sufficiently stressful to result in overt psychiatric consequences for the patient. Physically, the patient often experiences substantial pain. Sleep is unlikely to even approximate the normal architecture, and sleep deprivation is common. Perception is grossly distorted with loss of day-night cycles, immobilization, technology's noise, and overwhelming monotony. Emotionally, the patient must contend with the fear of death, the loss of self-control, the total invasion of privacy, and the dependence on staff and machines to perform even basic bodily functions. This physical and emotional crisis occurs most commonly in conjunction with polypharmacy and neurologic consequences of underlying disease.

Some authors have objected to the use of the term 'ICU psychosis,' largely because it is a convenient catch-all obscuring the identification of specific disorders. Nonetheless, it is our observation that when all organic causes of abnormal mentation described above have been excluded, many patients are encountered with persisting difficulties that do respond to modification of the ICU experience. *We emphasize, however, that this is a diagnosis of exclusion and that other possibilities must be rigorously considered and sought* (5).

Death: Rather than using terms like brain death, I find it more useful to think of death as death, and as being a consequence of either complete cardiopulmonary or complete brain failure. This helps counteract the notion that 'brain death' is somehow less a form of death than cardiopulmonary death. The old distinction of 'death' and 'brain death' is a major stumbling block in the pursuit of organ donation, and to a lesser extent, in the withdrawal of support from dead patients whose bodies are being ventilated and kept perfused with vasopressors.

DIAGNOSING DEATH BY BRAIN CRITERIA

1. *Permissive diagnosis* (a reason sufficient to explain death; failure to meet this criterion

explains almost all cases of recovery after the diagnosis of 'brain death.' Hypothermia and drug intoxication must be excluded or corrected before proceeding, and intact neuromuscular transmission should be demonstrated (spinal reflexes are adequate; in case of question, train-of-four stimulation may be used).

2. *Absence of brainstem reflexes,* usually including:

    a. cervico-ocular

    b. vestibulo-ocular

    c. cough

    d. gag

    e. corneal, and pupillary reflexes

    f. absence of response to noxious stimuli applied to the face.

Apnea testing should be included here but is often listed as a separate criterion. The patient should not breath when the P_aCO_2 is allowed to rise from 40 torr to 60 torr (the British use 50 torr as the target). The patient must be adequately preoxygenated and should receive supplemental oxygen during the test (either 10 cm CPAP or a tracheal catheter supplying a 10 L/min flow).

3. *Confirmatory tests* are not required in most circumstances. The exceptions to this are primarily in circumstances where the examinations stated above cannot be completed (e.g., patients who do not tolerate the apnea test from a cardiovascular standpoint, or whose faces are too swollen to examine their eye movements).The most useful confirmatory test is a nuclide angiogram, butcontrast angiography may also be used.An EEG is not required and is of limited utility; the conditions which render the physical examination unreliable (e.g., hypothermia, hypnosedative drug intoxication) also may make the EEG appear to show cerebral electrical silence.

UNCONSCIOUSNESS

Unconsciousness is produced in 1 of 3 ways: diffuse bilateral involvement of the cerebral hemispheres, injury to the brainstem reticular activating system (RAS), or a combination of focal injuries to the cortex and brainstem. Herniation is a special case of RAS insult, caused by a cerebral space-occupying lesion which produces a mechanical shift of brainstem structures.

Consciousness has 2 necessary components: arousal and content. Specific structures in the central nervous system (CNS) modulate arousal; lesions in these areas render the patient unable to respond in spite of intact sensory afferents. Unconsciousness is the condition in which the patient makes no appropriate responses to stimuli, either external (e.g., pain) or internal (e.g., thirst). This state does not exclude posturing and other reflex movements.

Causes of Unconsciousness

There are a large number of causes of coma, and it is convenient to classify them as those producing diffuse bihemispheric dysfunction versus those with structural lesions producing mass effect. Some of the major causes are shown in shown in Table 1. Non-convulsive status epilepticus may present as unresponsiveness. Subtle signs, such as eyelid fluttering, mild facial twitching, or nystagmus may be the only evidence that the patient is seizing. Similarly, a post-ictal state may show prolonged unresponsiveness, and include focal signs of hemiparesis (Todd's paralysis) or posturing.

Psychiatric conditions mimicking coma include catatonia, conversion reactions, and feigned coma. In these conditions, pupillary responses will be normal, as will ocular movements. The motor examination may demonstrate normal tone in supposedly paretic limbs, and when asleep, the patient will have normal movements.

THE ANATOMY OF CONSCIOUSNESS

Two major neuroanatomic structures are necessary for consciousness: the reticular activating system (RAS) and the cerebral hemispheres. The RAS is primarily responsible for arousal mechanisms, and the hemispheres influence the content of consciousness.

Table 1. Causes of coma

Presentation as diffuse bihemispheric process (usually symmetric, often with intact brainstem reflexes)

DRUG INTOXICATION:
Barbiturates
Opiates
Alcohol
Antidepressants
Benzodiazepines
Sedatives/Tranquilizers
Drugs of abuse
Antipsychotic agents
Anticholinergics
Salicylates

METABOLIC:
Hypo/Hypernatremia
Hypoglycemia
Non-ketotic hyperosmolar coma
Diabetic ketoacidosis
Hypo/hypercalcemia
Hypothyroidism
Uremia
Hepatic encephalopathy
Hypo/hyperthermia
Hypercarbia
Hypoxia

OTHER CAUSES:
Diffuse presentations:
    Toxins, especially carbon monoxide, methanol
    Meningitis/Encephalitis—viral or bacterial
    Sepsis
    Hypertensive encephalopathy
    Subarachnoid hemorrhage (low-grade)
    Head trauma, mild
    Seizures/Post-ictal

Presentation as brainstem process (often asymmetric, impaired brainstem function)
    Brainstem infarction/hemorrhage
    Posterior fossa tumor
    Herniation—from any cerebral space occupying lesion (tumor, stroke, hemorrhage)
    Subarachnoid hemorrhage (higher grades)
    Trauma, severe

The RAS receives input from all major afferent tracts and projects widely to the thalamus, basal forebrain, and the cerebral hemispheres. The crucial segment of the RAS for arousal is between the rostral midbrain and the midpons. Isolated lesions to this portion of the RAS produce coma, whereas lower lesions do not. Damage to the thalamus or hypothalamus can also alter consciousness, which is understandable given the large interconnection between these structures and the RAS, but bilateral involvement is usually required.

Focal lesions in the cerebral cortex tend not to alter arousal but instead affect the content of consciousness. To affect arousal, large areas of both hemispheres need to be involved, either on a structural or metabolic basis. Large focal processes such as tumor or infarction may alter the contralateral hemisphere by pressure effects, or by disrupting circulation or metabolism. Dominant hemisphere lesions may be more significant in affecting arousal than ones in the nondominant hemisphere.

Herniation

Herniation is caused when pressure of a mass lesion forces brain tissue to shift from one intracerebral compartment to another, and it can cause unconsciousness when pressure on the brainstem disrupts the RAS (6). The total volume contained in the cranial vault is limited and a mass lesion must cause some shift of the intracerebral contents. Initially, a mass lesion displaces cerebrospinal fluid, but eventually a limit is reached and intracranial pressure increases. Brain tissue is highly inelastic so this pressure causes herniation.

Central herniation is presumed to be from a pressure cone forcing the brain out towards its only exit, the foramen magnum. Uncal herniation occurs when the medial temporal lobe is forced over the tentorial edge into the space beside the lateral midbrain. This compresses the third cranial nerve and particularly the parasympathetic fibers to the pupil traveling around the outside of the nerve, causing unilateral dilation of the pupil on the side of the lesion, the 'blown pupil.'

Ropper (7) has ascribed many of the signs of herniation to horizontal displacement of the brainstem. Acute pupillary dilation often corrects within minutes of initiating therapy for increased ICP, which is more consistent with lateral displacement than with irreversible uncal herniation.

Downward herniation can distract the basilar artery, which is tethered to the skull base, away from the brainstem and cause hemorrhage or infarction. Eventually, the downward movement increases subtentorial pressure and forces the cerebellar tonsils out the foramen magnum. Tonsillar herniation can also occur if a lumbar puncture is performed on a patient with elevated ICP, generating a large transforamenal pressure gradient. This is often catastrophic, as acute pressure on the medulla causes sudden respiratory arrest. Upward herniation of brainstem structures through the tentorium is possible in the setting of large posterior fossa masses, which increase subtentorial pressure.

Evaluation of Unconsciousness

Evaluation must be rapid since morbidity is often related to how quickly therapy is begun. Many of the diffuse metabolic or toxic causes of coma resolve without long-term CNS damage, whereas acute structural disease, especially if causing herniation, may be rapidly fatal.

A key tenet of the care of the comatose patient is that initial treatment must proceed simultaneously with diagnosis. Acute (over seconds to minutes) coma suggests cerebrovascular disease, either hemorrhagic or ischemic, or cardiac arrest. A recent history of head injury may indicate a subdural or epidural hematoma. A subacute course (many minutes to hours) may suggest intoxication or infection, while a more prolonged period of altered mental status might occur from a CNS tumor or a systemic metabolic disturbance. Weakness or falling to one side suggests a focal lesion. A history of epilepsy may point to a post-ictal state. Witnesses should be carefully questioned about possible toxic ingestion.

Laboratory Studies

Laboratory studies may not aid in acute management but frequently help with assessment later in the patient's course. Serum biochemistry will identify major metabolic derangements, including hypoglycemia, nonketotic hyperglycemia, and diabetic ketoacidosis (8). A complete blood count should be obtained, since either CNS or systemic infections can cause coma. Urinalysis should be routine, as urosepsis may present first as altered mental status, and often occurs without fever in the elderly. Hypothyroidism can cause coma of unknown etiology, so a thyroid-stimulating hormone level needs to be drawn.

A urine toxicological screen for drugs of abuse is almost always needed, since drug overdose is one of the most common causes of coma of unknown etiology (Plum and Posner 1982). Drug abuse is frequently implicated in cases of trauma. Mixed intoxication with combinations of alcohol, barbiturates, opiates, and benzodiazepines may be seen, and the patient should be routinely screened for these agents. Finally, unconsciousness with focal signs can be caused by cocaine intoxication, which can cause cerebral vasculitis and stroke.

Blood gas analysis is necessary to assess hypoxia, hypercarbia, or abnormal pH. Hypoxia may be due to drug intoxication. Particular acid-base abnormalities are often helpful in diagnosing metabolic encephalopathies. Respiratory acidosis, with hypoxia, occurs with hypoventilation from respiratory depressants. Metabolic acidosis may suggest particular toxic ingestions, e.g., salicylates or alcohols, or diabetic ketoacidosis, uremia, sepsis or lactic acidosis. Compensatory respiratory alkalosis can be seen with many of the metabolic acidoses. Pure respiratory alkalosis, with hyperventilation, may suggest psychogenic coma.

EXAMINATION

The neurologic examination is directed to assess the etiology of unconsciousness, the goal being to determine whether there is a bihemispheric process versus an RAS problem, looking particularly for signs of herniation. One neurologic cause of pseudocoma needs to be excluded immediately, the 'locked-in' state (9). In this condition, usually due to pontine infarction or hemorrhage, all cortical control except of vertical gaze is disconnected. Often the patient is only able to look upward, but may not even being capable of opening his/her eyelids. If, on opening the patient's eyelids, he can follow the command to look up, the patient is not comatose but locked-in, and needs studies directed towards identifying a pontine lesion.

Pupillary Responses

The pupils should be examined, preferably with a bright light and with the room darkened. The pupillary light reflex requires both intact sympathetic and parasympathetic systems to dilate and constrict, respectively. The key paradigm to remember is that damage to the midbrain not only affects the RAS, but also pupil reactivity, whereas metabolic disease produces coma, but usually leaves the light reflex intact.

Specific structural lesions produce particular pupillary patterns. *Hypothalamic lesions*, either by direct involvement or secondary to increased pressure from above, interrupt the efferent sympathetic pathways, producing small, reactive pupils. *Unilateral diencephalic dysfunction* may cause a Horner's syndrome of unilateral pupillary constriction and ptosis, which may be an early sign of herniation. *Dorsal midbrain damage* interrupts the parasympathetic efferents, and the pupils become slightly large and unreactive but may spontaneously fluctuate in size (hippus). *Central midbrain lesions* damage both sympathetic and parasympathetic tracts producing fixed, often irregular, midposition pupils. This is most frequently seen in the setting of true

transtentorial herniation and generally implies a poor outcome. *Pontine lesions*, usually hemorrhagic, interrupt the descending sympathetic fibers and irritate the parasympathetic fibers, producing pinpoint pupils. More *caudal* lesions affect only the sympathetic system, again causing a Horner's syndrome. Finally, a unilateral fixed, dilated pupil suggests *third nerve* dysfunction.

Small reactive pupils are the hallmark of drug,(particularly opiate) intoxication and metabolic disease, but there are a few exceptions. The light reflex is usually resistant to metabolic disease, but it may be suppressed in the setting of severe drug overdose, especially from barbiturates. Severe opiate intoxication may mimic the pinpoint pupils of pontine hemorrhage. Anticholinergics may produce large, unreactive pupils associated with altered mental status, as can glutethemide intoxication. Anoxia may cause fixed dilated pupils, which become reactive if cerebral oxygen delivery is restored in time.

Eye Movements

If purposeful movements (such as visual tracking movements looking toward a loud noise) are absent, check for spontaneous roving eye movements. Roving movements are often seen with metabolic encephalopathies. All of these findings imply intact cortical control of the brainstem. A fixed deviation of eyes usually means there is a hemispheral lesion on the side toward which the eyes deviate, often associated with a contralateral hemiparesis. Isolated pontine lesions can cause eye deviation toward the damaged side, associated with an ipsilateral (i.e., contralateral to the pontine lesion). A fixed downward gaze is seen with midbrain compression from above. Inability of one eye to move medially is seen with upper brainstem lesions to the medial longitudinal fasciculus, on the side of the abnormal eye, and is called an internuclear ophthalmoplegia.

If no spontaneous movement is found, the cervico-ocular reflex should be tested (doll's eyes maneuver); an important caveat is to be sure that there is no possibility of a cervical cord or spine lesion prior to testing. The reflex is tested by rapidly turning the head from midline to one side and observing the eye movements. In the intact brainstem, this produces a contralateral conjugate eye movement, the net effect of which is to keep the eyes seemingly fixed on a point in space. After a few moments the eyes should return to midposition. The head should then be turned in the opposite direction to check for symmetry of the response. Failure of the reflex in either direction implies brainstem dysfunction. The reflex also works in the vertical plane and should be tested in a similar fashion. If this maneuver fails or is untestable because of neck injury, the vestibular-ocular reflex may be assessed by caloric testing. This is done by elevating the patient's head to 30 degrees if possible, and rapidly instilling about 50 mL of iced water with a syringe. It is important to first check that the ear canal is clear and that the tympanic membrane is not damaged, a relative contraindication to the test. Cold water instilled against the tympanic membrane produces cooling of the adjacent semicircular canal, increasing the local density of the endolymph and creating a net flow towards the cooler side. This direction of flow mimics head turning away from the stimulated side, and therefore causes reflex slow eye movement towards the stimulus. In an intact brain, the frontal eye fields attempt to override this brainstem-driven tonic eye deviation, producing rapid saccades away from the stimulus (nystagmus), but with cortical damage the eyes will maintain a fixed deviation. Cold caloric testing is a potent stimulus to the brainstem and may produce gaze deviation even when head turning fails to do so. The key observation is that whenever conjugate gaze occurs, regardless of the stimulus, it implies an intact brainstem in the region of the RAS. Eye deviation from hemispheral lesions can usually be overcome by these maneuvers, whereas with pontine lesions the eyes will not cross midline. Total lack of response can be seen with severe brainstem dysfunction, drug ingestion (especially barbiturates, narcotics, and phenytoin), neuromuscular blockade, or bilateral vestibular lesions.

Motor Responses

The patient is observed for spontaneous movement or, if none is present, response to stimulus. The type of motor response and its symmetry provide important clues to assess the location and severity of focal deficits. Any asymmetry of the motor patterns suggests a contralateral focal cerebral lesion. Comatose patients may not show purposeful movements such as reaching for their endotracheal tube or localizing painful stimuli, which requires an intact sensory system, efferent motor system, and cortical processing. Patients who cannot localize pain may withdraw from focal stimuli, again requiring functioning afferent and efferent tracts.

Abnormal motor responses include decorticate and decerebrate posturing. Decorticate posturing consists of flexion of the arms and extension of the legs, while in decerebrate posturing, both the arms and the legs extend. The important principle of localization is that both forms of abnormal posture can occur with hemispheral as well as brainstem lesions. Prognostically, decerebrate is worse than decorticate posturing. Any comatose patient who develops either form of abnormal posturing needs intervention for acute worsening.

Extension of the arms with weak flexion of the legs or absent leg movement implies severe structural damage of the pontine tegmentum. This finding indicates severe brainstem dysfunction and carries a grave prognosis (10). Total loss of tone does not necessarily mean upper brainstem damage and can be associated with spinal cord or medullary transection (spinal shock), peripheral nerve injury or disease, or neuromuscular blockade.

Finally, one must be careful not to confuse reflex activity with other responses. In particular, triple flexion of the lower extremity is a reflex signaling upper motor neuron dysfunction. It may look like spontaneous movement of the leg away from painful stimuli, but it is a reflex; the important finding is that the reflex response is very rapid and stereotyped.

Respiration

Respiration is controlled by brainstem structures with mediation by cortical influences, and specific respiratory patterns have localizing value. Unfortunately, these patterns are often not noticed in patients receiving mechanical ventilatory support. The most common abnormal respiratory pattern is Cheyne-Stokes respiration, in which there is a sequential waxing and waning of tidal volume, including periods of apnea. It can be seen in noncomatose patients with congestive heart failure, hypoxia, or occasionally during normal sleep, and is associated with bihemispheric dysfunction in unconscious patients. Respiratory centers in the brainstem increase or decrease the respiratory rate in response to elevated or lowered $PaCO_2$ levels respectively. There is, however, frontal lobe control such that even with very low $PaCO_2$ levels, respiration does not stop but only slows, with a reduced tidal volume, until the $PaCO_2$ normalizes. When bihemispheric dysfunction is present on a structural or metabolic basis, the modulating influence of the cortex is lost and Cheyne-Stokes respiration is seen.

Damage to the upper brainstem reticular formation is reported to cause sustained hyperventilation, called central neurogenic hyperventilation or central reflex hyperpnea. Tachypnea is often seen in comatose patients, but other causes, particularly hypoxia, neurogenic pulmonary edema, or metabolic disarray are more likely. To diagnose true CNH requires an increased PaO_2, decreased $PaCO_2$, without other metabolic changes or drug intoxication.

Apneustic, cluster, and ataxic breathing are patterns associated with lesions of the mid-lower pons, upper medulla, and caudal medulla respectively, and all provide inadequate ventilation, so mechanical support is needed. With apneusis, a patient has a prolonged inspiratory pause, or respiration may consist of cycles of quick inhalation/pause/exhalation/pause. Cluster breathing consists of several rapid shallow breaths followed by a pause, while ataxic breathing is irregular brief respirations of small, random tidal volumes. Finally, apnea is of poor localizing value and may be seen secondary to cardiac arrest, multifocal brain lesions, drug overdose, spinal cord transection, or primary pulmonary process.

CT Scanning

Any unconscious patient with focal signs will need a CT scan, as many will have potentially treatable problems. The differential diagnosis of coma with focal signs includes tumor, increased ICP, intracranial hemorrhage, CNS infection, and stroke. Unfortunately, some structural lesions may not produce focal signs but only brainstem dysfunction. Because of this, most comatose patients with coma of unknown etiology will need early CT scanning. Any comatose patient may also have fallen, and will be at risk for a traumatic subdural or epidural hematoma in addition to his/her primary problem. Traumatic hematomas may appear after the initial CT, so acute worsening of any patient is an indication for repeat scanning.

Lumbar Puncture and Antibiotics

Other than suspected bacterial meningitis, an LP is needed in any patient for whom the cause of coma is still unknown after initial evaluation to look for nonbacterial meningitis or encephalitis, especially viral or fungal, or occult subarachnoid hemorrhage.

INITIAL MANAGEMENT

Resuscitation

Acute care must always start with basic life support: a patent airway, ventilation, and circulation. An easily reversible cause of coma if treated sufficiently rapidly, is hypoxia secondary to airway obstruction or pulmonary disease. However, central nervous system (CNS) lesions can cause abnormal respiratory patterns as well. Quickly observing the patient's respiratory pattern may help with localization as described above. Comatose patients are frequently intubated for 1 of 2 reasons: ventilatory failure or airway protection. Airway protective reflexes of gagging and coughing may be lost in coma, increasing the risk of aspiration. Also, the tongue and oro-pharynx relax, increasing the chance of airway obstruction. The aspiration risk is increased if gastric lavage is used for suspected toxic ingestion without a cuffed endotracheal tube in place.

Prior to intubation, the stability of the cervical spine must be assessed, particularly in patients with trauma. Also, patients who lose consciousness acutely may fall and injure their cervical spine. Because patients with altered mental status may be unable to tell the examiner about neck pain, all comatose patients should be treated as if they have a neck injury unless a reliable witness can attest to the lack of a fall or other potential for neck injury.

A patient in a hard cervical collar may be difficult to intubate orally, as neck extension cannot and should not be attempted, so nasotracheal intubation may be preferred. The one exception to nasal intubation would be if there is a suspected basilar skull fracture. If raised intracranial pressure (ICP) is at all possible, 100 mg lidocaine or 300 mg thiopental should be administered intravenously 1 minute prior to intubation to blunt the rise in ICP normally associated with intubation.

A key part of the immediate evaluation is the patient's vital signs, which may themselves help decide the cause of unconsciousness. Severe hypotension can be sufficient to cause symptomatic CNS hypoperfusion and should be corrected urgently with fluids and/or vasopressors. Conversely, a severely elevated blood pressure may cause hypertensive encephalopathy, a neurologic emergency requiring rapid treatment.

Urgent Corrective Measures

Hypoglycemia can be catastrophic to the CNS, with degree of injury determined by the length of time and level of the low blood glucose (8). Fingerstick determinations are potentially unreliable, as the glucometers can be less accurate at low values; a measured serum glucose may in reality be much lower than that estimated by fingerstick methods. A fingerstick glucose reading less than 60 mg/dL should prompt urgent replacement of glucose. A dose of 50 mL of D50/W should be given immediately to any patient with coma of unknown etiology. This will produce no detrimental effect on other causes of coma (except Wernicke's encephalopathy, discussed below). Even in the case of hyperglycemic states producing coma, the marginal increase in total body glucose will not adversely affect treatment or generate CNS damage. In the case of hypoglycemia, glucose replacement may produce rapid reversal of unconsciousness.

Prior to giving glucose, thiamine (1 mg/kg IV) must be administered to prevent precipitating acute Wernicke's encephalopathy (confusion, ataxia, and ophthalmoplegia) with

associated necrosis of the midline gray structures leading to permanent memory loss. Alcoholics are at particular risk because of poor general nutrition. Although most patients will not be thiamine deficient, the potentially terrible result if missed makes thiamine administration before giving glucose imperative.

Narcotic overdose is a common cause of coma in emergency room patients, as well as in hospitalized, and, particularly, ICU patients. The classic findings in narcotic intoxication are coma, small reactive pupils, shallow respirations, and hypotension. Unfortunately, not all patients may display these findings. Pupillary responses in particular may be unreliable. Other drug ingestion, e.g., anticholinergics, may mask pupil findings. Hypoxia, brainstem lesions, or barbiturates may also blunt the response. Because the physical signs can be unreliable and narcotic overdose is common, any patient with coma of unknown etiology should be given naloxone 0.2-0.4 mg by slow IV injection.

MANAGEMENT OF SPECIFIC CAUSES (11)

Elevated ICP

If increased ICP is suspected, treatment needs to be initiated immediately, particularly if herniation is identified. The patient's head should be elevated to between 30-45 degrees and, if possible, the neck placed in a neutral position to facilitate venous return. Adequate ventilation and oxygenation are essential, as hypoxia or hypercarbia will increase cerebral blood flow and ICP. Hyperventilation to lower the patient's $PaCO_2$ to approximately 25-30 mmHg will acutely reduce cerebral blood volume and ICP, but this effect is transient, and other interventions to control ICP will need to follow

For severe rises in ICP, mannitol should be administered at a dose of 0.25-0.5 g/kg every 4-6 hours, taking care to correct serum electrolytes, osmolality, and polemic status. The mechanism of action of this agent is uncertain (extracellular space dehydration versus intravascular volume expansion), but its utility is not. Administration of steroids is somewhat controversial, being useful for tumors and abscesses, possibly efficacious in meningitis, and of no benefit in stroke or anoxia. If the cause of coma is unknown and the patient has evidence of increased ICP, an initial IV dose of 4-6 mg dexamethasone may be given empirically while diagnostic studies are undertaken.

Other factors that should be considered in the acute management of ICP include: a) adequate sedation, with the addition of neuromuscular blockade if necessary to stop excess muscle activity, b) low ventilator pressure settings, which allows for good central venous return, and c) suppression of fever, which accelerates cerebral metabolism and thereby raises oxygen consumption, resulting in increased cerebral blood flow and higher ICP. Fever also accelerates neuronal damage from other causes. Finally, care should be taken not to acutely lower blood pressure (unless hypertension is very severe) to maintain cerebral perfusion pressure.

Investigation of the patient with raised ICP requires a CT scan to exclude a space occupying lesion and neurosurgical support if this is found. Alternative considerations requiring specific treatment include cerebrovascular accident, subarachnoid hemorrhage and metabolic encephalopathy.

Drug Intoxication

When drug overdose or toxin ingestion is suspected, activated charcoal at a dose of 50-100 mg should be given to prevent system absorption. Gastric lavage may also be useful and is preferred over emesis. Use of both charcoal and lavage require airway protection, and in patients with mental status changes this usually mandates intubation prior to treatment. For suspected benzodiazepine intoxication, flumazenil given in divided doses up to 1 mg total may produce dramatic arousal, but is contraindicated in cases where tricyclic antidepressants may also have be consumed, as there is an increased risk of seizures and status epilepticus. Flumazenil is also reported to improve mental function transiently in patients with hepatic coma, probably by reversing the GABAergic effect of accumulating endogenous benzodiazepine receptor ligands.

Seizures

Status epilepticus is another cause of coma requiring emergent action. Clinical generalized convulsive status epilepticus (GCSE) is readily recognized, but nonconvulsive status (NCSE) may be difficult to discern. Often the only indication of NCSE may be subtle twitching of individual muscles, particularly the face, rhythmic eye movements, or blinking. Status epilepticus of either type needs rapid treatment both to suppress the seizures and to prevent their recurrence. Lorazepam at 0.1 mg/kg is often effective at terminating seizures. At the same time, 20 mg/kg of phenytoin or fosphenytoin should usually be administered (at a rate no greater than 50 mg/min), with and additional 5 mg/kg to be given if the patient is still seizing. Further therapy may include midazolam, propofol, or high-dose pentobarbital. An emergent EEG is indicated for any patient with suspected NCSE, or a patient being put in drug-induced coma to control seizures.

Meningitis

Emergent antibiotic therapy is indicated for any patient with suspected bacterial meningitis. In this life-threatening illness, treatment should not be delayed to obtain a CT or an LP. Lumbar puncture results will not be significantly compromised if obtained immediately after antibiotic administration.

SUPPORTIVE CARE

Fluid therapy and vital organ support must be ongoing. The unconscious patient is totally dependent on nursing care, with particular attention paid to eye, mouth, and pressure area care. Nutritional requirements will usually be provided enterally.

The unconscious patient may be capable of supporting respiration without mechanical ventilation. However, protection of the airway may not be possible after the cessation of

Table 2. Features associated with a poor prognosis after cardiorespiratory arrest

Decerebrate posturing and rigidity for > 24 hours in nontrauma patients
Decerebrate posturing and rigidity for > 2 weeks in trauma patients
Absent vestibulo-ocular reflex for > 24 hours
Absent pupillary reflexes for > 24 hours in postanoxic brain injury
Absent pupillary reflexes for > 3 days in trauma patients

respiratory support. For this reason an early tracheotomy is useful to provide some airway protection from oropharyngeal secretions.

MONITORING UNCONSCIOUSNESS AND PROGNOSTICATION

The Glasgow Coma scale (GCS) is a common method for monitoring the progress of coma, producing a score between 15 (normal) ands 3 (deep coma), and taking into account eye opening, motor responses, and verbal responses. Frequent assessment of the GCS gives an objective measure of progress. Otherwise, the prognosis deteriorates with the duration of coma; patients with postanoxic coma for 3 days rarely survive without severe disability (12).

Poor prognostic features are listed in Table 2. Outcome from coma is primarily dependent on the cause, assuming that appropriate steps are taken to avoid secondary injury from hypoxia, hypotension, etc. In cases of severe head injury, recent data gives an overall mortality of 37%, and good or moderate outcome at 43% (13). Coma from anoxia is associated with a poor prognosis, with 90% mortality at 1 year if coma lasts more than 6 hours. Septic encephalopathy carries a 35-53% mortality dependent on severity (14). Hepatic coma is associated with good recovery in only 27% of patients (15). Outcome from drug ingestion, if the patient survives until hospitalization, is quite good.

As part of the SUPPORT study, Hamel et al identified day 3 prognostic variables associated with 2-month mortality in a cohort of 596 patients with 'nontraumatic coma' (31% cardiac arrest, 36% ischemic stroke or intracerebral hemorrhage, 33% other causes) (16). The variables included abnormal brainstem response (any of absent pupillary response,

absent corneal response, or absent or dysconjugate roving eye movements), OR=3.2 (1.3-8.1 95% CI), absent verbal response (4.6, 1.8-11.7), absent withdrawal response to pain (4.3, 1.7-10.8), creatinine > 1.5 mg/dL (4.5, 1.8-11.0), and age 70 or older (5.1, 2.2-12.2). Two-month mortality for patients with 4 or 5 risk factors was 97%. Brainstem and motor responses best predicted 2 months death or severe disability; with either an abnormal brainstem response or absent motor response to pain, the rate of death or severe disability at 2 months was 96%.

Somatosensory evoked potentials (SEPs) are useful adjuncts for prognostication (17). A systematic review showed that the positive likelihood ratio, positive predictive value, and sensitivity were 4.04, 71.2%, and 59.0%, respectively, for normal SEPs (predicting favorable outcome), and 11.41%, 98.5%, and 46.2%, respectively, for bilaterally absent SEPs (predicting unfavorable outcome). Twelve of 777 patients were identified with bilaterally absent SEPs who had favorable outcomes. These false positives were typically pediatric patients or had suffered traumatic brain injuries. More exotic techniques hold the promise of greater precision (18), but as of now no technique is completely correct.

REFERENCES

1. Plum F, Posner JB: The Diagnosis of Stupor and Coma. Third Edition. Philadelphia, FA Davis, 1980
   The standard work, and still a treasure trove.
2. Diagnostic and Statistical Manual of Mental Disorders. (DSM-IV). Washington DC, American Psychiatric Association, 1994
3. Bleck TP: Vegetative state after closed-head

injury. *Neurology Chronicle* 1992; 1:10-11
A review of prognostic information.

4. Wise MG, Terrell CD: Delirium, psychotic disorders, and anxiety. *In:* Principles of Critical Care. Hall JB, Schmidt GA, Wood LDH. New York, McGraw-Hill, 1992, pp 1757-1769

5. Pingleton SK, Hall JB: Prevention and early detection of complications of critical care. *In:* Principles of Critical Care. Hall JB, Schmidt GA, Wood LDH. New York, McGraw-Hill, 1992, pp 587-611

6. Bleck TP, Webb AR: The unconscious patient – Causes and Diagnosis. *In:* The Oxford Textbook of Critical Care. Webb AR, Shapiro MJ, Singer M, et al (Eds). Oxford, Oxford University Press, 1999, pp 440-444

7. Ropper AH: Lateral displacement of the brain and level of consciousness in patients with an acute hemispheral mass. *N Engl J Med* 1986; 314:953-968

8. Malouf R, Brust JC: Hypoglycemia: Causes, neurological manifestations and outcome. *Ann Neurol* 1985; 17:421-438

9. Hawkes CH: 'Locked-in' syndrome: Report of 7 cases. *Br Med J* 1974; 4:379-382

10. Turazzi S, Bricolo A: Acute pontine syndromes following head injury. *Lancet* 1977; 2:62-64

11. Bleck TP, Webb AR: The unconscious patient – Management. *In:* The Oxford Textbook of Critical Care. Webb AR, Shapiro MJ, Singer M, et al (Eds). Oxford, Oxford University Press, 1999, pp 444-446

12. Levy DE, Caronna JJ, Singer BH, et al: Predicting outcome from hypoxic-ischemic coma. *JAMA* 1985; 253:1420-1426

13. Chestnut RM, Marshall LF, Klauber MR, et al: The role of secondary brain injury in determining outcome from severe head injury. *J Trauma* 1993; 34:216-222

14. Bolton CF, Young GB, Zochodne DW: The neurological complications of sepsis. *Ann Neurol* 1993; 33:94-100

15. Levy DE, Bates D, Caronna JJ: Prognosis in nontraumatic coma. *Ann Intern Med* 1981; 94:293-301

16. Hamel MB, Goldman L, Teno J, et al: Identification of comatose patients at high risk for death or severe disability. SUPPORT Investigators. Understand Prognoses and Preferences for Outcomes and Risks of Treatments. *JAMA* 1995; 273:1842-1848

17. Carter BG, Butt W: Review of the use of somatosensory evoked potentials in the prediction of outcome after severe brain injury. *Crit Care Med* 2001; 29:178-186

18. Guerit JM: The usefulness of EEG, exogenous evoked potentials, and cognitive evoked potentials in the acute stage of postanoxic and posttraumatic coma. *Acta Neurol Belg* 2000; 100:229-136

HEAD AND SPINAL CORD INJURY

Thomas P. Bleck, MD, FACP, FCCM, FCCP

Objectives

- To understand the role of primary and secondary injuries in head trauma
- To consider the controversies regarding hyperventilation, hypothermia, and cerebral perfusion pressure management in acute head trauma
- To recognize the potential importance of different means of blood pressure support in acute spinal cord injury
- To review the role of methylprednisolone and other agents in the management of acute spinal cord injury

Key Words: cerebral blood flow, cerebral perfusion pressure, cerebral salt wasting, cerebral vasospasm, free radicals, head trauma, hyperventilation, hyponatremia, intracranial pressure, methylprednisolone, nosocomial pneumonia, pulmonary edema, seizures, spinal cord injury, subarachnoid hemorrhage, tirilizad mesylate

TABLE OF ABBREVIATIONS

ADH	antidiuretic hormone
CBF	cerebral blood flow
CK	creatine kinase
CNS	central nervous system
CPP	cerebral perfusion pressure
CSF	cerebrospinal fluid
CT	computed tomography
DAI	diffuse axonal injury
EEG	electroencephalogram
CGS	Glasgow Coma Scale
GI	gastrointestinal
HHT	hypertensive-hypovolemic therapy
ICP	intracranial pressure
MAP	mean arterial pressure
PEEP	positive end-expiratory pressure
SAH	subarachnoid hemorrhage
SSEP	somatosensory-evoked potentials
TCD	transcranial Doppler

INTRODUCTION

Contemporary research into the optimal management of head and spinal cord trauma has generated considerable heat and very little light. This overview will touch on some accepted and some controversial aspects of management. In the interpretation of studies in this area, it is important to recall that most series use the NIH Traumatic Coma Data Bank of the 1970s as a benchmark (1). One of the few solid statements one can make in this area is that everyone's outcomes will be better than the TCDB data, or their own historical controls. This probably reflects the decline of hypoxia and hypotension as causes of secondary injury, and generally higher standards of supportive medical and nursing care. A reasonable prognostic model is available for those inclined toward prognostication (2).

The recently published guidelines for head trauma management (3) represent a very carefully performed evidence-based review of the available literature, and should be studied by anyone caring for these patients. Unfortunately, very few of the important questions about head injury management have been studied in randomized, double-blind trials, so very few actual standards could be developed. The following is a personal view of head injury management in the ICU.

One deplorable trend in this field is the increase in penetrating head injuries in urban areas (4), as well as the continued epidemic of intoxicated drivers and failure to wear seat belts. The vast majority of severe head trauma seen in my institution would be easily preventable.

Pathophysiologic Considerations

Mass Lesions

Masses (in trauma, discrete masses are almost always hematomas) both distort normal structures (brain, cranial nerves, blood vessels,

CSF pathways) and contribute to elevations in intracranial pressure. Epidural hematomas generally occur at sites of skull fractures that lacerate meningeal vessels; the bleeding forms a clot which requires a craniotomy for removal. Chronic subdural hematomas result from torn bridging veins in the subdural space; they are usually liquefied on presentation and can be evacuated via burr holes. In contrast, acute subdural hematomas almost always signify a deceleration injury with a substantial underlying cerebral contusion. The contusion itself swells and acts like a mass but is not separate from the brain substance.

Diffuse Axonal Injury

Older literature stressed the density difference between gray and white matter as the cause of shearing at the gray-white junction during deceleration injuries. While this does occur, and is probably responsible for the petechial and slit hemorrhages that occur in patients suffering this mechanism of injury, it does not appear to be the cause of diffuse axonal injury (DAI), which is a major cause of long-term disability in head-injured patients. In DAI, loss of the axon is an active process that begins with disruption of the microtubular structures at the initial segment and progresses (in humans) for about 24 hours (5). Current theories stress a connection between intracellular calcium toxicity, the resultant mitochondrial dysfunction, and DAI. Intrathecal cyclosporine (given prior to experimental injury) will attenuate or prevent these changes (6).

Intracranial Pressure

Thirty years of research confirms that sustained elevation of intracranial pressure (> 20 mm Hg) is associated with a poor outcome (7). Beyond that, little has been proven regarding the role of ICP elevation itself in affecting prognosis. Patients with other conditions (e.g., pseudotumor cerebri) commonly tolerate much higher ICP levels for months.

The classic teaching (the Monro-Kellie hypothesis) states that the skull is a fixed volume in which brain, blood, and CSF are constrained. An increase in the volume of any 1 component must be balanced by movement of another component out of the skull. This relationship can be overcome by enlarging the skull, e.g., by craniectomy.

In head trauma, the major causes of elevated ICP are mass lesions, hypercarbia, hypoxia, and hyperemia. The need to remove mass lesions that raise ICP or distort brain structures, and to prevent secondary injury due to hypoxia, seem well established. The importance of hyperemia remains debated, in part because of uncertainty about cerebral perfusion and substrate delivery.

Cerebral Perfusion Pressure

The concept of cerebral perfusion pressure (CPP = MAP-ICP) is used as a shorthand method to try to ensure adequate substrate delivery at the tissue level, which is not usually measured directly. Recommendations to maintain CPP at a particular level are based in part on the effects of lowering CPP in normal subjects (e.g., thresholds for clinical and electroencephalographic changes in people whose MAP is reduced, or in animals whose ICP is increased). One school of head trauma management maintains the primacy of CPP and ignores ICP (except for the removal of mass lesions) in favor of elevating MAP (8). A diametrically opposed view suggests that MAP should be lowered to prevent the development of hydrostatic cerebral edema (9).

The contention that increasing MAP produces compensatory cerebral vasoconstriction, and therefore lowers ICP by decreasing cerebral blood volume, depends on intact autoregulation. The degree to which autoregulation remains intact is uncertain, but when hyperemia is present it would appear to be a sign that autoregulation has failed.

The CPP equation is commonly written as CPP =MAP-(the greater of ICP or jugular venous pressure). However, the jugular venous pressure cannot be higher than the ICP, or jugular venous flow would be reversed until the ICP met the JVP.

A recently published parallel study in spinal cord injury patients suggests that aggressive volume and blood pressure support in this group will also improve outcome (10). This study similarly studies from the problem of relying historical controls rather than concurrently randomized controls. It does suggest that vascular disorders affecting vessels from the microvasculature up to the anterior spinal artery may play an important role in secondary injury to the spinal cord, just as hypotension worsens outcome after head trauma. Because hypotension is a ubiquitous problem after cervical spinal cord injuries, there are many opportunities for this damage to be compounded.

A competing theory, espoused by the group in Lund, holds that the arterial pressure head is the driving force for cerebral edema and thus should be lowered (11). As with almost all post-TCDB studies, they claim improved outcome with respect to historical controls. At present, there is no randomized comparison of any of these strategies.

Cerebral Blood Flow

One important observation of the last several years is that a substantial minority of severe head injury patients (GCS scores 3-8) have regionally diminished cerebral blood during the first 24 hours (12-14). Ischemic areas surrounding contusions may be particularly vulnerable (15). Such observations led to a widely cited and rarely read study (16) in which routine hyperventilation without respect to ICP or CPP had an apparently deleterious effect on outcome at 3 months, but not at 1 year. The authors' conclusion should be reviewed by everyone who uses or eschews hyperventilation: "It is concluded that prophylactic hyperventilation is deleterious in head-injured patients with motor scores of 4-5."

The effect of hyperventilation on CBF is not mediated by the $PaCO_2$, but rather by the pH of the extracellular fluid bathing the arterioles. The CNS, in concert with the rest of the body, attempts to restore the pH after we perturb it. The commonly stated maxim that hyperventilation stops working is not strictly true. Rather, the effect of hyperventilation is counterbalanced by: a) continued evolution of the pathologic processes raising ICP in the first place; b) active clearance of bicarbonate from the CSF by the choroid plexus, which lowers the pH despite a constant $PaCO_2$; and occasionally c)

the increase in intrathoracic pressure produced by our attempts to further lower the $PaCO_2$ below about 25 torr.

A system for continuous direct CBF measurement by thermal diffusion is under investigation (17). Other techniques, such as cold xenon CT, radioactive xenon scintigraphy, or PET, only provide data for a narrow temporal window. Jugular venous oxygen measurements are certainly affected by cerebral blood flow but are also altered by many other factors (18).

Glycolysis is also accelerated after severe head trauma (19), although the relationships among this phenomenon, cerebral blood flow, and outcome remain obscure.

Traumatic Subarachnoid Hemorrhage

Although trauma has long been recognized as the most common cause of SAH, the influence of subarachnoid blood on head trauma prognosis and complications is only now becoming apparent (20). Vasospasm does occur in trauma patients with SAH (21), with the potential for delayed ischemic damage. Whether calcium channel manipulations will be helpful remains debated (but is still debated in aneurysmal SAH as well) (22).

Seizures

Acute seizures following head trauma are probably due to a combination of mechanical deformation of neurons and excessive extracellular concentrations of excitatory amino acids (e.g., glutamate) and potassium. There is no clear relationship between early (first week) and later posttraumatic seizures; phenytoin prophylaxis decreases the early ones, but may not have much effect on later seizures (23). Later seizures may be related to hemosiderin deposition in the cortex in addition to the factors producing early seizures.

Anatomic Considerations in Spinal Cord Injury

The susceptibility of the spinal cord to trauma is due to a combination of its relationship to the vertebral bodies, their processes, the intervertebral disks, and the blood vessels. In addition to direct cord trauma, vascular mechanisms should be considered. The patient with an anterior spinal artery infarction will lose motor strength in addition to pain and temperature sensation below the lesion, but will typically retain proprioception.

An important, but commonly overlooked, critical care issue in the care of patients with spinal cord injuries is the role of the parasternal intercostal muscles in ventilation. Patients with lower cervical or upper thoracic cord lesions commonly present with adequate ventilatory parameters, but fail in a few days as they exhaust the ability of their accessory muscles to compensate for the loss of the stenting action of the parasternal intercostals. In some centers, these patients are routinely intubated on admission. We usually wait for an increase in rate and a decline in vital capacity, recognizing that by this time the patient is frequently in a halo vest and is difficult to intubate.

Free Radicals and Excitotoxins

Research into the mechanisms by which trauma damages the nervous system continues apace, with the role of free radicals and excitotoxins as final mediators of injury still appearing important. Trials of free-radical scavengers, such as PEG-SOD (24) and tirilizad mesylate, have been disappointing in head trauma, as have a number of putative excitatory amino acid antagonists.

In spinal cord injury, free-radical scavenging has a more established benefit. The high-dose methylprednisolone trial (NASCIS II) demonstrated a modest improvement in outcome in patients receiving a day of the drug at 30 mg/kg. More recently, NASCIS III demonstrated that high-dose methylprednisolone and tirilizad mesylate were equivalent in their beneficial effects.

EVALUATION

Physical Examination

In addition to the general trauma surveys and the GCS, patients with severe head trauma need careful observation for changes in their neurologic exam which may suggest the

need for treatments beyond the "simple" management of ICP and CPP. In the sedated but unparalyzed patient, changes in eye movements, posturing, and the resting tone of the extremities provide clues regarding the actual consequences of ICP and CPP changes inside the skull. Neuromuscular junction blockade eliminates the exam except for pupillary responses, and should be avoided unless other measures are unable to keep the ICP and CPP in the desired ranges.

Signs of Herniation

Although the classical explanation of cerebral herniation is usually wrong, the observed signs remain extremely important. A third nerve palsy initially develops when the diencephalon is displaced laterally, pulling the midbrain with it and stretching the ipsilateral third nerve between the cavernous sinus and the front of the midbrain. Early in this process, it is often easily reversed. At this time, the mesial temporal structures have not herniated over the tentorial edge; imaging studies show that the perimesencephalic cistern *larger* on the side of the lesion at that point. Later, the temporal lobe may herniate, producing the classic findings ascribed to herniation in earlier studies.

A change for the worse in the patient's exam should lead to consideration of acute interventions to lower ICP, raise CPP, and repeating a CT scan. Since a substantial, even life-threatening, degree of horizontal shift can occur before the ICP rises noticeably, one should not wait for the ICP to go up when the patient develops a third nerve palsy, or a patient previously demonstrating flexor posturing becomes extensor. Although the mechanisms are uncertain, mannitol infusion or brief hyperventilation will often reverse these acute changes and allow time for consideration of more definitive treatment.

Serial examination of the patient with a spinal cord lesion is the only readily available monitor for change in function. The examiner should be familiar with the motor and sensory distributions of the spinal levels in order to detect changes in the extent of cord involvement.

Intracranial Pressure Monitoring and CSF Drainage

The "best" way to monitor and manage elevated ICP is largely a matter of personal preference. Centers that rely on ventriculostomies stress the ability to remove fluid as a means of ICP/CPP control, but keeping these catheters working is often difficult as the brain swells, and the risk of infection is substantial. Parenchymal pressure monitors (e.g., systems by Camino and Codman) are preferred in many centers, but begin to drift from the pressure monitored via ventriculostomy after about 5 days. This seems to reflect gliosis at the tip of the catheter; many change the monitoring device at 5 days if it is still being used for clinical decisions. The older subarachnoid space monitoring devices (Richmond bolts, Philadelphia screws) are rarely used. ICP monitoring is associated with better survival (25), although the observational study demonstrating this did not reveal what aspects of management derived from the ICP data influenced the outcome.

CT Scanning

CT scanning is typically used in the initial evaluation of head injuries, and is certainly the current test of choice for the rapid exclusion of intracranial masses (Table 1). Although magnetic resonance imaging (MRI) is more sensitive and may be a better prognosticator, CT will adequately reveal those lesions that require management. The scan merits repeating if physical exam or ICP changes suggest the possibility of a previously unsuspected mass.

Magnetic Resonance Imaging

MRI has largely replaced myelography in the evaluation of spinal cord injury. It discloses information about the interior of the spinal cord (e.g., contusion, hematomas, edema, ischemia), which is therapeutically and prognostically useful. If MRI is contraindicated, CT myelography is the next best choice.

MRI provides better prognostic information than CT (27), but does not show other problems requiring acute management and is less well suited to detecting bony abnormalities; it is also more difficult to perform in trauma patients. CT remains the study of choice.

Jugular Venous Oxygen Saturation Monitoring

This continues to be an area of controversy. As a technique, it is supposed to measure the oxygen extraction of the brain in a manner analogous to mixed venous oxygen saturation measurements. The proponents of the technique believe that it can be used to determine what modes of therapy are most appropriate for ICP elevations, specifically, whether it is safe to increase the degree of CNS alkalosis by hyperventilation. Its opponents are concerned that a whole-hemisphere measurement of oxygen extraction will be unable to detect focal areas of cerebral ischemia. A multivariate analysis of ICP, MAP, CPP, and jugular venous oxygen saturation revealed that jugular venous saturation did not have an independent effect on outcome (28). It seems reasonable to assume that if increasing alkalosis increases oxygen extraction (or increases the cerebral venous lactate concentration), then the alkalosis should be reversed and another mode of therapy substituted. Whether it is safe to further increase the degree of alkalosis if the extraction does not increase is another matter.

More contemporary thinking about cerebral oxygen utilization in severe head trauma suggests that high SjO_2 values do not indicate hyperemia, but rather failure of oxygen utilization associated with hyperglycolysis (29). This effect is underlined by the understanding that decreased oxygen extraction is itself a marker of poor outcome (30).

Table 1. Marshall classes of head injury by CT, and GOS % from TCBD data

Category	Description	Percent of Patients	Good/moderate	Severe/ Vegetative	Dead
No CT data		2.3	5.9	0.0	94.1
Diffuse injury I	No visible pathology on CT	7.0	61.6	28.8	9.6
Diffuse injury II	Cisterns visible, shift 0–5 mm, no high or mixed density lesion >25 cm^3	23.7	34.5	52.0	13.5
Diffuse injury III (swelling)	Cisterns compressed or absent, shift 0–5 mm, no high or mixed-density lesion >25 cm^3	20.5	16.4	49.7	34.0
Diffuse injury IV (shift)	Shift > 5 mm, no high or mixed density lesion > 25 cm^3	4.3	6.2	37.6	56.2
Evacuated mass lesion	Any lesion surgically evacuated	37.0	22.8	38.4	38.8
Nonevacuated mass	High or mixed-density lesion > 25 cm^3 not surgically evacuated	4.8	11.1	36.1	52.8
Brainstem injury	No brainstem reflexes by physical exam	0.4	0.0	33.3	66.7

It is important to recognize that all subsequent studies have shown improved outcome when compared with the TCDB data; nevertheless, these data demonstrate the relative percentages expected and the value of the CT classification scheme.

Cortical PO$_2$ Monitoring

This is a relatively new technique in the clinical arena. It involves placing a PO$_2$-sensing electrode on the cerebral cortex at the time of a craniotomy. If jugular vein oxygen monitoring can be faulted for overlooking regional abnormalities in perfusion, this technique has the opposite problem: the volume of tissue sampled is very small. Initial reports suggest that it will be a useful technique (31).

Transcranial Doppler Blood Flow Velocity Measurement

This technique is primarily of value for detecting vasospasm related to traumatic SAH. Vasospasm produces an increase in the flow velocity of RBCs in involved arteries, since by Poiseulle's law the velocity increases as the diameter of the vessel decreases. Since elevated ICP can also affect flow velocity, some recommend following the ratio of internal carotid to middle cerebral artery flow velocities.

Electroencephalography and Evoked Potentials

The role of EEG in the workup of suspected seizures is relatively clear, but the utility and indications for continuous EEG monitoring remain to be established. Unsuspected, subclinical seizures have a deleterious effect on outcome in neuro-ICU patients (32). Patients who develop refractory status epilepticus should have continuous EEG monitoring. Subclinical seizures occur in some head trauma patients, but the actual incidence of this problem is just coming into focus; Vespa et al found that 20% of severely traumatized patients had at least brief subclinical seizures (33). Whether the breakdown product of atracurium (laudanosine) is epileptogenic in humans remains untested. In the head trauma patient requiring neuromuscular junction blockade, EEG monitoring can be useful for assessing the degree of cortical function, and for determining whether sedation is needed (and the appropriate dose).

The degree of reactivity on a single EEG in the first 2 days after trauma is an excellent predictor of prognosis (34).

Evoked potential studies are very useful for prognostication in the first few hours following severe head trauma (35). Somatosensory evoked potentials (SSEP) have received the most study; prolongation or loss of the N20 potential (the first cortical component of the median nerve SSEP) is a powerful predictor of outcome. However, even the absence of SSEPs is not completely predictive of poor outcome (36). A recent comprehensive review of this topic is available (37).

Management

Resuscitation and Airway Management

The most important considerations in the prehospital and initial resuscitative phases in head or spinal cord trauma patients are to avoid hypoxia and hypotension (96).

Head trauma patients must be assumed to have a concomitant cervical spine injury until proven otherwise. Intubation is performed with in-line traction to prevent lateral movement. While fiberoptic oral intubation may be mechanically safest, the delay in securing the airway is seldom worthwhile. Nasotracheal intubation is best avoided until basilar skull and cribriform plate fractures can be excluded, which generally means that orotracheal intubation has already been performed.

Intubation of patients with severe head trauma in the field (as opposed to the emergency department) was associated with higher mortality in 1 retrospective study (39). While I suspect this means that the patients who had the most severe injury were chosen for field intubation, and that field intubation was more likely to be successful in the more severely injured patients, this bears further study.

Excluding cervical spine disorders often takes several days in the comatose patient who cannot indicate pain during flexion/extension views of the neck. When such patients are otherwise stable, we employ CT scanning with traction to exclude cervical spine instability.

Posture and Head Position

The standard recommendation, and our usual practice, is to keep these patients sitting up between 30 and 60 degrees above horizontal in hopes of improving their venous return and therefore lowering ICP (40). It is important to remember that in such a patient, the CPP should be calculated based on the MAP *at the level of the ICP measurement*, generally estimated at the ear for parenchymal transducers.

The desirability of the head-up position is not universally accepted. The proponents of CPP-driven management attempt to keep the patient's head at the level of the heart to keep cerebral perfusion maximal. In other conditions associated with ICP elevation, such as hepatic failure, the ICP may actually increase as the head is raised. Thus, at a minimum, the decision to nurse the patient head-up depends on knowing the effect on ICP and CPP in each individual patient.

Intracranial Pressure, Cerebral Perfusion Pressure, and Cerebral Blood Flow Management

Because these factors are so strongly interrelated, the modalities for their management will be discussed together.

Mannitol

Mannitol is usually the first-time drug for lowering ICP. The mechanism by which it works remains debated, but some combination of osmotic removal of ECF, improvement in RBC membrane deformability (and therefore, improved blood rheologic properties), free-radical scavenging, and increased cardiac output due to improved central filling pressures is probably involved. The initial dose is 0.25 g/kg q 4 hours; although an upper limit for the increased osmolality often produced is often given (e.g., 310-320 mOsm/L), there are few data upon which to base such a recommendation.

Hypertonic Saline

Some investigators propose that small quantities of hypertonic saline be used in place of mannitol, claiming a prolonged ICP-lowering effect. This is a promising approach that deserves further study. A recent publication from Croatia suggests that cerebral salt wasting is unexpectedly common in patients with penetrating head trauma (41).

Sedation

Sedative drugs, usually benzodiazepines (typically with a narcotic) or propofol, are frequently used in head injury patients either because these patients appear to be agitated, to lower ICP (either by relieving agitation or by decreasing cerebral metabolism, to which CBF is coupled under autoregulation), or to promote synchrony with the ventilator. Because of cost issues, midazolam and propofol are often eschewed in favor of lorazepam. The perceived advantage of midazolam as an agent whose effects will terminate rapidly is probably lost during infusion's lasting days. Propofol is

probably superior in this regard. However, the circumstances in which the ability to rapidly terminate sedative drug action is clinically important are quite rare. Propofol should not be abruptly terminated due to risk of withdrawal seizures, even after only several hours of infusion.

Some members of the CPP camp attempt not to sedate patients, using the sympathetic nervous system effects of agitation to help raise MAP.

Although it is tempting to try to reverse the effects of benzodiazepines with flumazenil, the likelihood of seizures in this situation makes this process very dangerous.

Analgesia

Morphine and fentanyl are both effective and inexpensive choices for sedation. We tend to favor fentanyl for reasons of less hypotention, less interference with gut motility, and more rapid clearance when the dose is reduced. When patients need "sedation" for a procedure, such as a CT scan, we typically use fentanyl because it can safely be reversed with naloxone if we need to return the patient to baseline for examination.

Mechanical Ventilation and Airway Management

If the ICP and CPP are easily maintained with normo- or only modest hypocarbia (e.g., $PaCO_2$ in the mid-30 torr range), whatever ventilatory mode is best tolerated by the patient is adequate. We tend to use pressure-support ventilation with a back-up rate in such patients not requiring sedation, or even a CPAP circuit, to prevent deconditioning. If sedation (or neuromuscular junction blockade) is required, then we choose SIMV or assist-control.

Although routine hyperventilation may be deleterious and is probably not useful, brief periods of hyperventilation may be lifesaving during impending herniation. Hyperventilation works very rapidly, because CO_2 diffuses very rapidly across the blood-brain barrier.

The optimal weaning strategy for head trauma patients is not established. We decrease pressure support as tolerated, which works in most patients, some of whom are "rested on a rate" at night as they improve. Concurrent chronic obstructive pulmonary disease, reactive airway disease, and pulmonary infections often delay or prolong weaning.

Positive end-expiratory pressure (PEEP) is acceptable as needed to maintain oxygenation (42). Acute respiratory distress syndrome and other conditions which stiffen the lung decrease the transmission of high alveolar pressures to the great veins by virtue of the poor lung compliance they produce. Thus, patients who need high levels of PEEP seldom experience further elevations in ICP when their airway pressures are high. However, patients with relatively normal lung mechanics may exacerbate their intracranial hypertension if one attempts to hyperventilate them profoundly for ICP control, regardless of whether hyperventilation is a performed by increasing the tidal volume (which raises mean intrathoracic pressure directly) or increasing the respiratory rate (which may generate unintended PEEP by stacking breaths).

The time when it is best to perform a tracheostomy in a head injury patient remains to be established. We do so in patients who are ready to be weaned but who do not protect their airways adequately, or who are awakening and are uncomfortable with an endotracheal tube but who are not nearly ready to wean. Percutaneous tracheostomy is increasingly our method of choice.

We routinely perform early tracheostomy on patient with complete cervical cord lesions above C5. Although this may delay a cervical fusion if one is required (due to concern about tracheal secretions infecting an anterior fusion), the risk of hypoxia or death with accidental extubation in these patients argues for an early surgical airway. Those with lesions between C5 and T5 often receive early tracheostomies as well.

Neuromuscular Junction Blockade

The mechanisms by which neuromuscular junction blockade decreases ICP in patients who are already deeply sedated are uncertain. Some improvement in thoracic compliance may play a role, but this often seems inadequate to explain the magnitude of the change.

Cerebrospinal Fluid Drainage

Centers routinely placing ventriculostomy catheters for ICP measurement also use them for ICP control by withdrawing small amounts of CSF when ICP elevations occur. There is a learning curve for the ability to successfully and rapidly place a catheter in the small ventricles often found in head injury patients. If the CT scan reveals hydrocephalus, then a ventriculostomy is the treatment of choice.

High-Dose Barbiturates

When ICP elevation fails to respond to the measures described above, many intensivists have used high-dose barbiturates in the past. This modality is still employed occasionally, although concerns about hypotension have diminished enthusiasm for it. A typical dose would be 5 - 12 mg/kg of pentobarbital as a loading dose, with an infusion starting at 1 mg/kg/hr and increased as necessary for ICP control and as tolerated by the MAP. Although EEG burst-suppression has been used as a marker for the depth of anesthesia (the pattern correlating with the maximal decrease in CBF, and therefore ICP, that can be achieved with barbiturates), we usually follow the ICP and the CPP rather than the EEG (although the neurosurgeons often ask for the EEG).

High-dose barbiturates are potent venodilators and myocardial depressants; these effects result in diminished cardiac output and hypotension. Since this runs counter to the goals of CPP management, these drugs are avoided by its practitioners.

Craniectomy

Craniectomy defeats the Monro-Kellie relationship by making more space for the swollen brain. This treatment was formally introduced in 1971 by Ransohoff and Kjellberg. Recently, Polin and colleagues analyzed our results (but these data are not from a prospective, randomized trial): decompressive bifrontal craniectomy provides a statistical advantage over medical treatment of intractable posttraumatic cerebral hypertension and should be considered in the management of malignant posttraumatic cerebral swelling. If the operation can be accomplished before the ICP value exceeds 40 torr for a sustained period and within 48 hours of the time of injury, the potential to influence outcome is greatest (43).

Compared with hypothermia or high-dose barbiturates, craniectomy represents a more easily tolerated technique for managing ICP. The question of the added value of neuroprotection of the other methods remains to be studied.

Temperature Control

Hypothermia is emerging as a potentially useful modality to manage ICP and to improve outcome in severe head injury (44, 45). Unfortunately, the multicenter trial was stopped early, and showed no benefit (46). Fever control, however, should probably be approached aggressively, since it seems clear that fever raises ICP and cerebral energy expenditure (47), and probably worsens outcome.

Antiseizure Drugs

Presently, most centers use antiseizure prophylaxis for the first week or so after severe head trauma. The available agents vary in their ability to prevent late epilepsy in experimental models, but to date this has not been translated into clinical trial. We use phenytoin as the first agent. If this must be changed because of allergy (or, more commonly, part of an unexplained fever drill), we currently use gabapentin for patients able to absorb drugs from the GI tract—those who can't get phenobarbital or valproate until they can.

Long-term phenytoin use appears to have negative cognitive and behavioral consequences in these patients (49); phenobarbital and the benzodiazepines carry theoretical risks (50). Patients who have seizures after the first week should be treated chronically; we tend to use carbamazepine.

Free-Radical Scavengers

There is yet to be a free-radical scavenger of proven clinical benefit in humans with head injuries. In spinal cord injury, 1 unexpected finding of the NASCIS III trial was the benefit of 48 hours of high-dose methylprednisolone in patients whose steroid regimen was started late.

Nutrition and GI Bleeding Prophylaxis

Despite all of our concerns about the need for nutrition in trauma patients, the optimal strategy remains unproven. We attempt to feed these patients enterally as soon as possible. All tubes are placed through the mouth to decrease the risk of sinusitis. If patients are candidates for tracheostomy, a percutaneous endoscopic gastrostomy is performed as well.

Patients who cannot be fed receive ulcer/gastritis prophylaxis, usually with an H_2 blocker (51). If nonsteroidal anti-inflammatory agents are used, we add misoprostol.

REFERENCES

1. Marshall LF, Becker DP, Bowers SA, et al: The National Traumatic Coma Data Bank. Part 1: Design, purpose, goals, and results. *J Neurosurg* 1983; 59:276–284
2. Signorini DF, Andrews PJ, Jones PA, et al: Predicting survival using simple clinical variables: A case study in traumatic brain injury. *J Neurol Neurosurg Psychiatry* 1999; 66:20–25
3. Brain Trauma Foundation, American Association of Neurological Surgeons, Joint Section on Neurotrauma and Critical Care: Guidelines for the management of severe head injury. *J Neurotrauma* 1996; 13:641–734
4. Stone JL, Lichtor T, Fitzgerald LF, et al: Demographics of civilian cranial gunshot wounds: Devastation related to escalating semiautomatic usage. *J Trauma* 1995; 38:851–854
5. Fitzpatrick MO, Dewar D, Teasdale GM, et al: The neuronal cytoskeleton in acute brain injury. *Br J Neurosurg* 1998; 12:313–317

6. Okonkwo DO, Povlishock JT: An intrathecal bolus of cyclosporin A before injury preserves mitochondrial integrity and attenuates axonal disruption in traumatic brain injury. *J Cereb Blood Flow Metab* 1999; 19:443–451

7. Signorini DF, Andrews PJ, Jones PA, et al: Adding insult to injury: The prognostic value of early secondary insults for survival after traumatic brain injury. *J Neurol Neurosurg Psychiatry* 1999; 66:26–31

8. Rosner MJ, Rosner SD, Johnson AH: Cerebral perfusion pressure: Management protocol and clinical results. *J Neurosurg* 1995; 83:949–962

9. Juul N, Morris GF, Marshall SB, et al: Intracranial hypertension and cerebral perfusion pressure: Influence on neurological deterioration and outcome in severe head injury. The Executive Committee of the International Selfotel Trial. *J Neurosurg* 2000; 92:1-6

10. Vale FL, Burns J, Jackson AB, et al: Combined medical and surgical treatment after acute spinal cord injury: Results of a prospective pilot study to assess the merits of aggressive medical resuscitation and blood pressure management. *J Neurosurg* 1997; 87:239–246

11. Eker C, Asgeirsson B, Grande PO, et al: Improved outcome after severe head injury with a new therapy based on principles for brain volume regulation and preserved microcirculation. *Crit Care Med* 1998; 26:1881-1886

12. Cold GE: Does acute hyperventilation provoke cerebral oligaemia in comatose patients after acute head injury? *Acta Neurochir (Wien)* 1989; 96:100–106

13. Bouma GJ, Muizelaar JP, Stringer WA, et al: Ultra-early evaluation of regional cerebral blood flow in severely head-injured patients using xenon-enhanced computerized tomography. *J Neurosurg* 1992; 77:360–368

14. Skippen P, Seear M, Poskitt K, et al: Effect of hyperventilation on regional cerebral blood flow in head-injured children. *Crit Care Med* 1997; 25:1402–1409

15. McLaughlin MR, Marion DW: Cerebral blood flow and vasoresponsivity within and around cerebral contusions. *J Neurosurg* 1996; 85:871–876

16. Muizelaar JP, Marmarou A, Ward JD, et al: Adverse effects of prolonged hyperventilation in patients with severe head injury: A randomized clinical trial. *J Neurosurg* 1991; 75:731–739

17. Carter LP: Thermal diffusion flowmetry. *Neurosurg Clin North Am* 1996; 7:749–754

18. Robertson CS, Cormio M: Cerebral metabolic management. *New Horiz* 1995; 3:410–422

19. Bergsneider M, Hovda DA, Shalmon E, et al: Cerebral hyperglycolysis following severe traumatic brain injury in humans: A positron emission tomography study. *J Neurosurg* 1997; 86:241–251

20. Taneda M, Kataoka K, Akai F, et al: Traumatic subarachnoid hemorrhage as a predictable indicator of delayed ischemic symptoms. *J Neurosurg* 1996; 84:762–768

21. Romner B, Bellner J, Kongstad P, et al: Elevated transcranial Doppler flow veloci ties after severe head injury: cerebral vasospasm or hyperemia? *J Neurosurg* 1996; 85:90–97

22. Murray GD, Teasdale GM, Schmitz H: Nimodipine in traumatic subarachnoid haemorrhage: A reanalysis of the HIT I and HIT II trials. *Acta Neurochir (Wien)* 1996; 138:1163–1167

23. Temkin NR, Dikmen SS, Wilensky AJ, et al: A randomized, double-blind study of phenytoin for the prevention of posttraumatic seizures. *N Engl J Med* 1990; 323:497–502

24. Young B, Runge JW, Waxman KS, et al: Effects of pegorgotein on neurologic outcome of patients with severe head injury. A multicenter, randomized controlled trial. *JAMA* 1996; 276:538–543

25. Lane PL, Skoretz TG, Doig G, et al: Intracranial pressure monitoring and outcomes after traumatic brain injury. *Can J Surg* 2000; 43:442-448

26. Marshall LF, Marshall SB, Klauber MR, et al: The diagnosis of head injury requires a classification based on computed axial tomography. *J Neurotrauma* 1992; 9 (Suppl 1):S287-292

27. Paterakis K, Karantanas AH, Komnos A, et al: Outcome of patients with diffuse axonal injury: The significance and prognostic value of MRI in the acute phase. *J Trauma* 2000; 49:1071-1075

28. Struchen MA, Hannay HJ, Contant CF, et al: The relation between acute physiological variables and outcome on the Glasgow Outcome Scale and Disability Rating Scale following severe traumatic brain injury. *J Neurotrauma* 2001; 18:115-125

29. Bergsneider M, Hovda DA, Shalmon E, et al: Cerebral hyperglycolysis following severe traumatic brain injury in humans: A positron emission tomography study. *J Neurosurg* 1997; 86:241-251

30. Macmillan CS, Andrews PJ, Easton VJ: Increased jugular bulb saturation is associated with poor outcome in traumatic brain injury. *J Neurol Neurosurg Psychiatry* 2001; 70:101-104

31. van Santbrink H, Maas AI, Avezaat CJ: Continuous monitoring of partial pressure of brain tissue oxygen in patients with severe head injury. *Neurosurgery* 1996; 38:21–31

32. Young GB, Jordan KG, Doig GS: An assessment of nonconvulsive seizures in the intensive care unit using continuous EEG monitoring: An investigation of variables associated with mortality. *Neurology* 1996; 47:83–89

33. Vespa PM, Nuwer MR, Nenov V, et al: Increased incidence and impact of nonconvulsive and convulsive seizures after traumatic brain injury as detected by continuous electroencephalographic monitoring. *J Neurosurg* 1999; 91:750-760

34. Gutling E, Gonser A, Imhof HG, et al: EEG reactivity in the prognosis of severe head injury. *Neurology* 1995; 45:915–918

35. Hutchinson DO, Frith RW, Shaw NA, et al: A comparison between electroencephalography and somatosensory evoked potentials for outcome prediction following severe head injury. *Electroencephalogr Clin Neurophysiol* 1991; 78:228-333

36. Schwarz S, Schwab S, Aschoff A, et al: Favorable recovery from bilateral loss of somatosensory evoked potentials. *Crit Care Med* 1999; 27:182–187

37. Carter BG, Butt W: Review of the use of somatosensory evoked potentials in the prediction of outcome after severe brain injury. *Crit Care Med* 2001; 29:178-186

38. Statham PF, Andrews PJ: Central nervous system trauma. *Baillieres Clin Neurol* 1996; 5:497–514

39. Murray JA, Demetriades D, Berne TV, et al: Prehospital intubation in patients with severe head injury. *J Trauma* 2000; 49:1065-1070

40. Meixensberger J, Baunach S, Amschler J, et al: Influence of body position on tissue-Po_2, cerebral perfusion pressure and intracranial pressure in patients with acute brain injury. *Neurol Res* 1997; 19:249–253

41. Bacic A, Gluncic I, Gluncic V: Disturbances in plasma sodium in patients with war head injuries. *Mil Med* 1999; 164:214–217

42. Cooper KR, Boswell PA, Choi SC: Safe use of PEEP in patients with severe head injury. *J Neurosurg* 1985; 63:552–555

43. Polin RS, Shaffrey ME, Bogaev CA, et al: Decompressive bifrontal craniectomy in the treatment of severe refractory posttraumatic cerebral edema. *Neurosurgery* 1997; 41:84–92

44. Metz C, Holzschuh M, Bein T, et al: Moderate hypothermia in patients with severe head injury: Cerebral and extracerebral effects. *J Neurosurg* 1996; 85:533–541

45. Marion DW, Penrod LE, Kelsey SF, et al: Treatment of traumatic brain injury with moderate hypothermia. *N Engl J Med* 1997; 336:540–546

46. Clifton GL, Miller ER, Choi SC, et al: Lack of effect of induction of hypothermia after acute brain injury. *N Engl J Med* 2001; 344:556-563

47. Matthews DS, Bullock RE, Matthews JN, et al: Temperature response to severe head injury and the effect on body energy expenditure and cerebral oxygen consumption. *Arch Dis Child* 1995; 72:507–515

48. Temkin NR, Dikmen SS, Anderson GD, et al: Valproate therapy for prevention of posttraumatic seizures: A randomized trial. *J Neurosurg* 1999; 91:593-600

49. Dikmen SS, Temkin NR, Miller B, et al:
     Neurobehavioral effects of phenytoin
     prophylaxis of posttraumatic seizures.
     JAMA 1991; 265:1271–1277

50. Goldstein LB: Prescribing of potentially
     harmful drugs to patients admitted to
     hospital after head injury. *J Neurol
     Neurosurg Psychiatry* 1995; 58:753–755

51. Tryba M, Cook D: Current guidelines on
     stress ulcer prophylaxis. *Drugs* 1997;
     54:581–596

52. Harrop JS, Sharan AD, Vaccaro AR, et al:
     The cause of neurologic deterioration after
     acute cervical spinal cord injury. *Spine*
     2001; 26:340-34

SHOCK

John P. Kress, MD, FCCP

SHOCK

Shock is a common condition necessitating admission to the ICU or occurring in the course of critical care. This chapter discusses the pathophysiology of various shock states, followed by recommendations for the diagnosis and treatment of each category of shock. Lastly a brief review of commonly used vasoactive agents is presented.

SHOCK DEFINED

Shock is defined by the presence of multisystem end-organ hypoperfusion. Clinical indicators include reduced mean blood pressure, tachycardia, tachypnea, cool skin and extremities, acute altered mental status, and oliguria. Hypotension is usually, though not always present. The end result of multiorgan hypoperfusion is tissue hypoxia, often clinically seen as lactic acidosis.

CLINICAL EVALUATION OF PATIENTS IN SHOCK

Most patients who present with shock are hypotensive. Since the mean blood pressure is the product of the cardiac output (CO) and the systemic vascular resistance (SVR), reductions in blood pressure can be categorized by decreased CO and/or decreased SVR. Accordingly, the initial evaluation of a hypotensive patient should evaluate the adequacy of the CO. Clinical evidence of diminished CO includes a narrow pulse pressure (a surrogate marker for stroke volume), and cool extremities with delayed capillary refill. Signs of increased CO include a widened pulse pressure (particularly with a reduced diastolic pressure), warm extremities with bounding pulses and rapid capillary refill. If a hypotensive patient has clinical signs of increased CO, one can infer that

the reduced blood pressure is a result of decreased SVR.

In hypotensive patients with clinical evidence of reduced CO, an assessment of intravascular and cardiac volume status is appropriate. A hypotensive patient with decreased intravascular and cardiac volume status may have a history suggesting hemorrhage or other volume losses (e.g., vomiting, diarrhea, polyuria). The jugular venous pulse is often reduced in such a patient. A hypotensive patient with an increased intravascular and cardiac volume status may have S3 and/or S4 gallops, increased jugular venous pressure (JVP), extremity edema, and crackles on lung auscultation. The chest X-ray may show cardiomegaly, congestion of the vascular pedicle (1), Kerley B lines and pulmonary edema. Chest pain and EKG changes consistent with ischemia may also be noted.

In hypotensive patients with clinical evidence of increased CO, a search for causes of decreased SVR is appropriate. The most common cause of high cardiac output hypotension is sepsis. Accordingly, one should search for signs of the systemic inflammatory response syndrome (SIRS), which include abnormalities in temperature ($\geq 38^\circ$ C or $\leq 36^\circ$ C), heart rate (≥ 90 beats/minute), respiratory rate (≥ 20 breaths/minute), and WBC count ($\geq 12,000/mm^3$ or $\leq 4,000/mm^3$ or ≥ 10 bands) (2). A person with SIRS and a presumed or confirmed infectious process fulfills criteria for sepsis. A person with sepsis and 1 or more organ failures fulfills criteria for severe sepsis. Other causes of high cardiac output hypotension include: liver failure, severe pancreatitis, burns and other trauma which elicit the systemic inflammatory response syndrome, anaphylaxis, thyrotoxicosis and peripheral arteriovenous shunts.

In summary, the 3 most common categories of shock include cardiogenic, hypovolemic and high CO with decreased SVR. Certainly these categories may overlap and occur simultaneously (e.g., hypovolemic and septic shock, septic and cardiogenic shock).

The initial assessment of a patient in shock as outlined above should take only a few minutes. It is important that aggressive, early resuscitation is instituted based on the initial assessment, particularly since there are data suggesting that early resuscitation of shock (both septic and cardiogenic) may improve survival (3, 4). If the initial bedside assessment yields equivocal or confounding data, more objective assessments such as echocardiography and/or central venous or pulmonary artery catheterization may be useful. The goal of early resuscitation is to reestablish adequate perfusion to prevent or minimize end organ injury.

During the initial resuscitation of patients in shock, principles of advanced cardiac life support should be followed. Since patients in shock may be obtunded and unable to protect the airway, an early assessment of the patient's airway is mandatory during resuscitation from shock. Early intubation and mechanical ventilation are often required. Reasons for institution of endotracheal intubation and mechanical ventilation include acute hypoxemic respiratory failure as well as ventilatory failure. Acute hypoxemic respiratory failure may occur in cardiogenic shock (pulmonary edema) as well as septic shock (pneumonia or ARDS). Ventilatory failure often occurs as a result of an increased load on the respiratory system. This load may present in the form of acute metabolic acidosis (often lactic acidosis) or decreased compliance of the lungs as a result of pulmonary edema. Inadequate perfusion to respiratory muscles in the setting of shock may be another reason for early intubation and mechanical ventilation. Normally, the respiratory muscles receive a very small percentage of the CO (5). However, in patients who are in shock with respiratory distress for the reasons listed above, the percentage of cardiac output dedicated to respiratory muscles may increase 10-fold or more (6, 7). Mechanical ventilation may relieve the patient of the work of breathing and permit redistribution of a limited cardiac output to other vital organs. Such patients often demonstrate signs of respiratory muscle fatigue including: inability to speak full sentences, accessory respiratory muscle use, paradoxical abdominal

muscle activity, extreme tachypnea (>40 breaths/minute), and decreasing respiratory rate despite an increasing drive to breathe.

Endotracheal intubation and mechanical ventilation with sedation and, if necessary, muscle paralysis will decrease oxygen demand of the respiratory muscles allowing improved oxygen delivery to other hypoperfused tissue beds (8). Patients in shock should be intubated before other procedures are performed, since attention to the airway and breathing may wane during such procedures.

Resuscitation

Resuscitation should focus on improving end organ perfusion, not simply raising the blood pressure. Accordingly, a patient with a reduced CO by clinical assessment with a decreased intravascular and cardiac volume status should receive aggressive intravenous resuscitation. The type of intravenous fluid is controversial, though recent data suggest that colloid (albumin) is not better than crystalloid and indeed may be associated with increased morbidity and mortality (9). Though 1 study reported improved outcomes in trauma patients whose volume resuscitation was delayed until definite surgical repair (average time to operation ~ 2 hours) (10), aggressive volume resuscitation in patients with reduced intravascular and cardiac volume status is merited in virtually all but perhaps torso trauma patients who can undergo surgical repair quickly. Early administration of vasoactive drugs in hypovolemic patients in order to increase the blood pressure is not recommended. This practice may impair the assessment of the patient's circulatory status and potentially delay definitive treatment. The transfusion of packed red blood cells to anemic patients in order to improve oxygen delivery is physiologically rational; however, recent data suggest that, as long as hemoglobin levels remain greater than 7 g/dL, this practice may not improve outcomes and perhaps even worsen outcomes in select subgroups of patients (11). Certainly, a conservative transfusion strategy does not apply to hemorrhaging, hypovolemic patients in shock. Blood products should be administered through a blood warmer, in order to minimize hypothermia and subsequent disturbances in coagulation. In summary, it is important to remember that oxygen delivery is the product of cardiac output, oxygen-carrying capacity of the blood, and arterial oxygen saturation. Each of these components must be considered and optimized when addressing resuscitation of patients in shock

Early reassessment after of the patient with purported hypovolemic shock after the initial resuscitation is extremely important. Concrete end points such as increased blood pressure and pulse pressure, improved capillary refill, urine output and mental status should be sought. The absence of a response suggests that the volume challenge may not be adequate. Careful and repeated searches for signs of volume overload (increased JVP, new gallop or extra heart sounds, pulmonary edema) should be done while the resuscitation is ongoing.

If the patient remains in shock despite adequate volume resuscitation, support with vasoactive drugs is appropriate. Occasionally, vasoactive drugs must be started "prematurely" when volume resuscitation needs are large. When severe hypotension and hypovolemia are present, this approach is occasionally needed to "buy time" while volume resuscitation is ongoing. This strategy is only rarely necessary and should only be instituted temporarily until volume resuscitation is accomplished. It is important to remember that vasoactive drugs may obscure hypovolemic shock by raising blood pressure in spite of a low cardiac output state.

Once intravascular volume has been restored, patients who remain in shock may benefit from vasoactive drugs. These drugs should be titrated to end-organ perfusion, rather than an arbitrary blood pressure value. Accordingly, mental status, urine output, lactic acidosis, capillary refill and skin temperature, and venous oxygen saturation are reasonable end points to target in these patients. If evidence of hypoperfusion persists, one should consider inadequate volume resuscitation, impaired cardiac output, inadequate hemoglobin, and/or inadequate oxygen saturation as a likely explanation. If objective information obtained by physical examination is unclear or ambiguous, additional information obtained via invasive monitoring (central venous pressure, pulmonary artery catheterization or echocardiography) may be useful. Echocardiography is a useful adjunct or even replacement to invasive pressure measurements and can be used to distinguish poor ventricular pumping function from hypovolemia; a good study can exclude or confirm tamponade, pulmonary hypertension, or significant valve dysfunction, all of which influence therapy and may supplement or replace the more invasive right heart catheterization. These topics are covered separately in another chapter in the syllabus.

CATEGORIZATION OF SHOCK

CARDIOGENIC SHOCK

The model of the heart as a pump is useful in considering cardiogenic shock. By definition, pump failure is seen when cardiac output is inappropriately low despite adequate input in the form of venous return (determined by right atrial pressure). The specific cause of decreased pump function must be considered. Left and/or right ventricular dysfunction may occur due to by decreased systolic contractility, impaired diastolic relaxation, increases in afterload, valvular dysfunction, or abnormal heart rate and rhythm.

Left Ventricular Failure

Systolic dysfunction. This is the classic example of cardiogenic shock. When left ventricular systolic function is impaired, the most common reason is acute coronary ischemia. The result is a reduction of cardiac output relative to increases in preload. Attempted compensation for this impaired pump function occurs via the Frank-Starling mechanism as well as by fluid retention by the kidneys and by increased venous tone mediated by the sympathetic nervous system. Patients present with reduced cardiac output and a resulting increased oxygen extraction ratio by the peripheral tissues. The low mixed venous oxygen saturation may exacerbate hypoxemia, especially in patients with pulmonary edema and intrapulmonary shunt physiology. As mentioned above, acute myocardial infarction or ischemia is the most common cause of left ventricular failure leading to shock. Cardiogenic shock is reported to complicate up to 10%of acute myocardial infarctions (12). Recent evidence supports the use of early aggressive revascularization using angioplasty or coronary artery bypass grafting in patients with cardiogenic shock (4). Survival benefit was seen in patients subjected to this strategy compared to medical management of cardiogenic shock, including those given thrombolytic therapy. Treatment of cardiogenic shock due to systolic dysfunction includes the judicious administration of volume if hypovolemia is present. A more precise characterization of the circulation can be obtained with the use of pulmonary artery catheterization and/or echocardiography—topics discussed in more detail in another chapter of the syllabus. Inotropic support includes the use of agents such as dobutamine or milrinone. Intra-aortic balloon counterpulsation may be used to support the circulation as a bridge to coronary artery revascularization.

Diastolic dysfunction. Increased left ventricular diastolic chamber stiffness and impaired left ventricular filling most commonly occur as a result of myocardial ischemia, though left ventricular hypertrophy and restrictive myocardial diseases may also contribute. Patients usually present with increased cardiac filling pressures despite a small left ventricular end diastolic volume as documented by echocardiography (usually best seen in the short axis view at the level of the papillary muscles). Aside from the management of acute ischemia, this condition may be difficult to treat. Volume administration can be tried, but many times only further increases diastolic pressure with little change in diastolic volume. Inotropic agents are usually ineffective. Aggressive management of tachycardia with volume adminstration and cautious use of negative chronotropic agents is a rational approach to therapy. Since very little ventricular filling occurs late in diastole in these patients, a very low heart rate (e.g., sinus bradycardia) may be detrimental. Often, careful titration of chronotropic agents to achieve the "optimal" heart rate that maximizes cardiac output is necessary. The maintenance of a normal sinus rhythm is important to maximize ventricular filling.

Valvular dysfunction. The management of valvular disease contributing to cardiogenic shock is guided by interventions to counter the specific pathophysiology. Accordingly, aortic stenosis is managed by efforts to decrease heart rate while maintaining sinus rhythm. Preload should be maintained and afterload must not be reduced, since there is a fixed afterload imposed by the aortic stenosis which may not tolerate further reductions in afterload via arteriolar dilation. Surgical evaluation or palliative valvuloplasty are other important considerations in cardiogenic shock complicated by aortic stenosis. Cardiogenic shock due to aortic insufficiency may present acutely and may require urgent surgical repair. Medical management includes the use of chronotropic agents to decrease regurgitant filling time and afterload reducing agents to facilitate forward flow. Mitral regurgitation may occur acutely as a result of ischemic injury to papillary muscles. Medical management includes attempts to establish and maintain sinus rhythm, as well as afterload reduction to decrease the percentage of regurgitant blood flow. This may be accomplished with medications such as nitroprusside or intra-aortic balloon counterpulsation as a bridge to mitral valve repair or replacement. Mitral stenosis contributing to cardiogenic shock is managed by negative chronotropic agents, which seek to maximize diastolic filling time across the stenotic valve. Lastly, hypertrophic cardiomyopathy may contribute to cardiogenic shock. This lesion is managed by maintenance of preload with volume administration and negative inotropic and chronotropic agents that serve to decrease the obstruction of the left ventricular outflow tract during systole. Rarely, acute obstruction of the mitral valve by left atrial thrombus or myxoma may also result in cardiogenic shock. These conditions generally require acute surgical interventions.

Cardiac arrhythmias. Dysrhythmias may exacerbate shock in critically ill patients. Details on the management of dysrhythmias are beyond the scope of this chapter and the reader is referred to other sections of the syllabus for further discussion of this topic.

Right Ventricular (RV) Failure. Right ventricular failure resulting in cardiogenic shock is typically associated with increased right atrial pressure and reduced cardiac output. Though the most common reason for RV failure is concomitant left ventricular failure, this section will discuss management of isolated RV failure. Right ventricular infarction may result in RV failure, usually accompanied by inferior myocardial infarction. Elevated JVP in the presence of clear lungs are the classic physical findings seen in acute RV infarction. It is important to distinguish RV infarction from cardiac tamponade. Echocardiography may be helpful in making this distinction. Therapy includes volume administration, dobutamine to increase RV inotropy (13) and norepinephrine, which may improve RV endocardial perfusion.

Right ventricular failure as a result of increases in right heart afterload may be due to pulmonary embolism, ARDS and other causes of alveolar hypoxia, hypercapnia and metabolic acidosis. Management is focused at treating the underlying physiologic derangement, with circulatory support again centered on inotropic agents as well as norepinephrine (14, 15). Treatment of RV failure is complicated, since volume administration may result in worsening RV function by causing mechanical overstretch and/or by reflex mechanisms that depress contractility (16). However, some investigators have found volume administration to result in favorable hemodynamics in acute RV failure due to increased RV afterload (17). Optimal management is often facilitated by echocardiographic or pulmonary artery catheter directed therapy. Thrombolytic therapy for acute pulmonary embolism complicated by cardiogenic shock has been shown to improve survival (18) and is currently accepted as a recommended strategy (19). Hypoxic pulmonary vasoconstriction may be reduced by improving alveolar and mixed venous oxygenation by administering supplemental oxygen. More aggressive correction of hypercapnia and acidemia may be necessary in patients with acute right heart syndromes. Pulmonary vasodilator therapy (e.g., inhaled nitric oxide and prostaglandin E_1) may be considered, though outcome benefits in the acute setting are largely lacking.

Pericardial Tamponade and other Syndromes Causing External Compression of the Heart. Cardiac tamponade impairs diastolic filling, resulting in shock. The diagnosis is established by the presence of elevated jugular venous pulse with Kussmaul's sign and pulsus paradoxus. Pulmonary artery catheterization may reveal a decreased cardiac output with equalization of right atrial, left atrial (PCWP) and RV diastolic pressures. Echocardiography reveals pericardial fluid with diastolic collapse of the atria and right ventricle, and right-to-left septal shift during inspiration. Other causes of external cardiac compression include tension pneumothorax, elevated intra-abdominal pressure (e.g., tense ascites)—so called abdominal tamponade, large pleural effusions and pneumopericardium. Treatment is focused at the underlying cause and includes pericardial drainage with a catheter or surgical "window" in the case of pericardial tamponade. In unstable patients, blind drainage of the pericardial sac with a needle may be necessary. Medical management of the circulatory pathophysiology of tamponade includes the use of aggressive volume administration as well as inotropic and chronotropic support to increase heart rate and thus maintain forward flow.

DECREASED VENOUS RETURN

Hypovolemia is the most common cause of shock due to decreased venous return. The venous circuit has tremendous capacitance potential and venoconstriction in response to hypovolemia can compensate for initial decreases in intravascular volume. Orthostatic changes in blood pressure and heart rate may be seen early in hypovolemic shock (20). At a level of approximately 40% loss of intravascular volume, venoconstriction driven by the sympathetic nervous system can no longer maintain mean arterial blood pressure.

In hypovolemic shock, tissue injury (especially gut ischemia) and resulting systemic inflammation may lead to ongoing shock despite replacement of volume losses (21). This is particularly relevant if resuscitation is delayed and underscores the importance of early aggressive resuscitation of hypovolemic shock. The phenomenon of systemic inflammation as it pertains to shock will be discussed in more detail in the section on septic shock.

Other causes of shock due to decreased venous return include severe neurologic damage or drug exposure resulting in hypotension due to loss of venous tone. The prototypical example of loss of venous tone due to drug exposure is anaphylaxis. This unregulated immunologically-mediated release of histamine can result in profound shock requiring aggressive catecholamine support (epinephrine is the drug of choice). Septic shock is a common cause of shock due to decreased venous tone and is discussed separately in the following section. All of these processes result in decreased venous tone and impaired venous return resulting in decreased cardiac output and blood pressure. Obstruction of veins due to compression (e.g., pregnancy, intra-abdominal tumor), thrombus formation, or tumor invasion increases the resistance to venous return and may occasionally result in shock.

The principal therapy of hypovolemic shock and other forms of shock due to decreased venous return is aggressive volume resuscitation while attempting to reverse the underlying problem driving the pathophysiology. This has been described in more detail above. In hemorrhagic shock, resuscitation with packed red blood cells should be done through a blood warmer. The optimal hemoglobin concentration is controversial and transfusion should be paced by the extent of ongoing blood loss. After large volume red blood cell transfusions, dilutional thrombocytopenia and reduction in clotting factors should be anticipated, sought and corrected with platelet and plasma product transfusions as directed by platelet count and coagulation assays.

HIGH CARDIAC OUTPUT HYPOTENSION

Septic Shock

Septic shock is the most extreme presentation of a spectrum of pathophysiologic responses to an infectious insult. Sepsis is defined by the presence of the systemic inflammatory response syndrome in the presence of known or suspected infection (2). Severe sepsis occurs when patients with sepsis accrue 1 or more organ failure(s). Septic shock is seen in patients with severe sepsis who manifest shock as described above. Any infectious organism may result in sepsis and septic shock, including all bacteria, fungi, viruses and parasites. As noted above, patients typically present with evidence of high cardiac output (assuming hypovolemia has been resuscitated). These patients have a widened pulse pressure, warm extremities, brisk capillary refill, and a reduced diastolic and mean blood pressure. A subgroup of patients with septic shock may present with depressed cardiac function. Circulating myocardial depressant factors have been identified in some septic patients (22-24), but the reason only a small subgroup of patients manifest cardiac depression is not well understood.

Sepsis is a significant problem in the care of critically ill patients. It is the leading cause of death in noncoronary ICUs in the United States (25). Current estimates suggest that more than 750,000 patients are affected each year (26) and these numbers are expected to increase in the coming years as the population continues to age and a greater percentage of people vulnerable to infection will likely seek medical care.

Decades of research have focused on modifying the pathophysiologic responses of the body to severe infection. For many years, an unregulated proinflammatory state was thought to be the driving force behind severe sepsis and septic shock. Numerous trials attempting to block a particular inflammatory pathway were conducted without any survival benefits noted (27). More recently, the pathophysiology behind severe sepsis has become better understood. Currently, the pathophysiology of severe sepsis is thought to be driven by unregulated inflammation (via cytokines such as interleukin 6 and tumor necrosis factor), coupled to a hypercoagulable state favoring microvascular coagulation and impaired fibinolysis. Such unregulated microvascular coagulation is thought to lead to impaired tissue perfusion and predispose patients to the multiple organ dysfunction syndrome that is commonly observed in severe sepsis (28). Activated protein C has a salutary impact on all 3 pathophysiologic derangements noted in severe sepsis. Recently, a survival benefit was reported in patients with severe sepsis treated with recombinant activated protein C (29). This study was the first to ever demonstrate a survival benefit from a therapy directed at modifying the underlying pathophysiology of severe sepsis. Because of its anticoagulant properties, there was a small but significant increase in bleeding complications associated with activated protein C.

The mainstay of therapy for septic shock is aggressive supportive care. This includes early identification of the source of infection with eradication by surgical or percutaneous drainage, if possible. Over 80% of patients with severe sepsis will require ventilatory support for respiratory failure, which should be instituted early for reasons outlined earlier in this chapter. Circulatory failure is supported with aggressive volume administration to correct any component of hypovolemia. Objective monitoring using CVP, pulmonary artery catheterization and echocardiography should be used early to guide therapy. Vasoactive support is directed by the underlying circulatory derangement. The optimal extent of volume resuscitation is controversial. Some clinicians favor aggressive volume administration, while others favor earlier use of vasoactive drugs (keeping patients "dry"). Trials are ongoing to attempt to better answer this difficult question. Early institution of broad spectrum antibiotic therapy focused on potential pathogens has been shown to improve survival (30, 31). Acute renal failure in septic shock carries a poor prognosis. Recent literature supports the use of an aggressive approach to renal replacement therapy, with a survival benefit demonstrated with daily hemodialyis compared to alternate day hemodialysis (32). The use of low dose dopamine as a renal protective strategy was recently found to be of no benefit in preventing acute tubular necrosis in patients with SIRS and acute renal insufficiency (33). Other therapeutic interventions in severe sepsis await further evaluation. Early trials evaluating the utility of high dose corticosteroids

in septic shock failed to demonstrate a survival benefit (34, 35). Corticosteroid therapy remains controversial and further studies are needed before it can be recommended for widespread use. Recent data suggest that the response to an ACTH stimulation test may have important prognostic implications (36). Whether lower doses of corticosteroids provide survival benefit in severe sepsis remains to be determined.

Other Types of Shock

Adrenal insufficiency. Adrenal insufficiency is often viewed as a rare occurrence in critically patients. However, a recent study reported a 54% incidence of blunted adrenal response to ACTH in patients with septic shock (36). This number may be a generous estimate since the parameters for defining adrenal insufficiency are not universally agreed upon (37); nevertheless, adrenal insufficiency may not be as rare as previously thought. It is reasonable to consider testing all patients who present with septic or other occult reasons for shock with an ACTH stimulation test. Conventionally, this test is performed in the morning with a baseline cortisol level drawn and then 250 mcg of ACTH administered intravenously. Thirty and 60-minute cortisol levels are then drawn. A level greater than 20 mcg/dL is viewed as an appropriate response. If adrenal insufficiency is suspected, dexamethasone (does not cross react with the cortisol laboratory assay) should be administered while the ACTH stimulation test is performed.

Neurogenic shock typically occurs as a result of severe injury to the central nervous system. The loss of sympathetic tone results in venodilation and with venous blood pooling. Mainstays of therapy include volume repletion and vasoactive support with drugs that have venoconstricting properties

Severe hypothyroidism or hyperthyroidism may result in shock. Myxedema presenting as shock should be treated with administration of intravenous thyroid hormone. One should watch carefully for myocardial ischemia and/or infarction, which may complicate aggressive thyroid replacement. Thyroid storm requires urgent therapy with

Lugol's solution, propylthiouracil, steroids, propranolol, fluid resuscitation, and identification of the precipitating cause. Pheochromocytoma often present with a paradoxical hypertension despite a state of shock and impaired tissue perfusion. Intravascular volume depletion is masked by extreme venoconstriction from endogenous catecholamines in pheochromocytoma. The increase in afterload caused by endogenous catecholamines may also precipitate a shock-like state. Treatment includes aggressive volume replacement as well as β and α adrenergic blockade. A search for the location of the pheochromocytoma with subsequent surgical removal is indicated.

Vasoactive Agents

The choice of vasoactive medications should be based upon the underlying pathophysiology of the circulation as gleaned by the physical examination and supplemented by more sophisticated measurements. It is sobering to realize that despite widespread use of these agents for many decades, there are no outcomes studies to guide clinicians with regard to a particular agent in the management of shock.

Dobutamine. Dobutamine is a powerful inotrope that stimulates both β-1 and β-2 receptors. The end result is typically an increase in cardiac output with diminished systemic vascular resistance. This reduction in afterload may benefit patients with left ventricular systolic dysfunction.

Milrinone. Milrinone is an inotropic agent that induces a positive inotropic state via phosphodiesterase inhibition. It has potent vasodilating properties that decrease both systemic and pulmonary vascular resistance. A recent study of patients with acute exacerbations of congestive heart failure did not demonstrate a benefit with regard to days hospitalized for cardiovascular causes, in-hospital mortality, 60-day mortality, or the composite incidence of death or hospital readmission. Rather, hypotension and new atrial arrhythmias were found to occur more frequently in patients who received milrinone compared to placebo (38).

Dopamine. Dopamine is purported to have varying physiologic effects at different doses. Classically, "low-dose" dopamine (1-3 mcg/kg/minute is thought to stimulate dopaminergic receptors and increase renal and mesenteric blood flow. This notion has recently been disproven, however (33, 39). Indeed there is evidence that dopamine may impair mesenteric perfusion to a greater degree than norepinephrine (40). As data are accumulating reporting the ill effects of dopamine in shock, this agent has recently fallen out of favor in the view of many clinicians, with other agents such as norepinephrine being more widely used (see below) (41).

Norepinephrine. Norepinephrine stimulates α-1 as well as β receptors. Data are now accumulating suggesting norepinephrine may be a preferred drug in septic and other vasodilatory types of shock. It appears to have a lesser propensity to cause renal injury (42) and provides a more reliable increase in blood pressure compared to dopamine (43). A recent prospective observational cohort study found a significant reduction in mortality when compared to dopamine and/or epinephrine in patients with septic shock (44).

Phenylephrine. Phenylephrine is a pure α–1 agonist, which results in veno- and arteriolar constriction. It often elicits a reflex bradycardia mediated via baroreceptors. This may prove useful in patients with tachydysrhythmias accompanied by hypotension. In a prospective observational study of patients with septic shock, phenylephrine was found to increase blood pressure, SVR and cardiac index when added to low dose dopamine or dobutamine after volume resuscitation (45). There is a theoretical concern that alpha agonism may precipitate myocardial ischemia, though are few objective data to support or refute this concern.

Epinephrine. Epinephrine has both α as well as β agonist properties. It has potent inotropic as well as vasoconstricting properties. It appears to have a higher propensity toward precipitating mesenteric ischemia (46), a property that limits its utility as a first line agent for the management of shock, regardless of the underlying etiology.

Vasopressin. The use of vasopressin as a vasoactive agent has increased tremendously in the last few years. Patients who present with septic shock or late phase hemorrhagic shock have been shown to have a relative deficiency of vasopressin. A recent study found patients with septic shock to demonstrate an increase in blood pressure and urine output without evidence of impaired cardiac, mesenteric or skin perfusion when treated with "low dose" (40 milliunits per minute) vasopressin (47). The exact role of vasopressin in various shock states requires further investigation.

REFERENCES

1. Ely EW, Smith AC, Chiles C, et al: Radiologic determination of intravascular volume status using portable, digital chest radiography: a prospective investigation in 100 patients. *Crit Care Med* 2001; 29:1502

2. Bone RC, Balk RA, Cerra FB, et al: Definitions for sepsis and organ failure and guidelines for the use of innovative therapies in sepsis. The ACCP/SCCM Consensus Conference Committee. American College of Chest Physicians/Society of Critical Care Medicine. *Chest* 1992; 101:1644

3. Rivers E, Nguyen B, Havstad S, et al: Early goal directed therapy in the treatment of severe sepsis and septic shock. *N Engl J Med* 2001; 345:1368

4. Hochman JS, Sleeper LA, Webb JG, et al: Early revascularization in acute myocardial infarction complicated by cardiogenic shock. Shock Investigators. Should we emergently revascularize occluded coronaries for cardiogenic shock? *N Engl J Med* 1999; 341:625

5. Rochester DF, Pradel-Guena M. Measurement of diaphragmatic blood flow in dogs from xenon 133 clearance. *J Appl Physiol* 1973; 34:68

6. Hussain SNA, Roussos C: Distribution of respiratory muscle and organ blood flow during endotoxic shock in dogs. *J Appl Physiol* 1985: 59:1802

7. Robertson CH Jr., Foster GH, Johnson RL Jr.: The relationship of respiratory failure to the oxygen consumption of, lactate production by, and distribution of blood flow among respiratory muscles during increasing inspiratory resistance. *J Clin Invest* 1977; 59:31

8. Hall JB, Wood LDH. Liberation of the patient from mechanical ventilation. *JAMA* 1987; 257:1621

9. Cochrane Injuries Group Albumin Reviewers Human albumin administration in critically ill patients: systematic review of randomised controlled trials. *BMJ* 1998; 317:235

10. Bickell WH, Wall MJ Jr, Pepe PE, et al" Immediate versus delayed fluid resuscitation for hypotensive patients with penetrating torso injuries. *N Engl J Med* 1994; 331:1105

11. Hebert PC, Wells G, Blajchman MA, et al: A multicenter, randomized, controlled clinical trial of transfusion requirements in critical care. Transfusion Requirements in Critical Care Investigators, Canadian Critical Care Trials Group. *N Engl J Med* 1999; 340:409

12. Goldberg RJ, Gore JM, Alpert JS, et al: Cardiogenic shock after acute myocardial infarction: incidence and mortality from a community-wide perspective, 1975 to 1988. *N Engl J Med* 1991; 325:1117

13. Dell'Italia LJ, Starling MR, Blumhardt R, et al: Comparative effects of volume loading, dobutamine and nitroprusside in patients with predominant right ventricular infarction. *Circulation* 1985; 72:1327

14. Hirsch LJ, Rooney MW, Wat SS, et al: Norepinephrine and phenylephrine effects on right ventricular function in experimental canine pulmonary embolism. *Chest* 1991; 100:796

15. Layish DT, Tapson VF: Pharmacologic hemodynamic support in massive pulmonary embolism. *Chest* 1997; 111:218

16. Ghignone M, Girling L, Prewitt RM: Volume expansion versus norepinephrine in treatment of a low cardiac output complicating an acute increase in right ventricular afterload in dogs. *Anesthesiology* 1984; 60:132

17. Mathru M, Venus B, Smith R, et al: Treatment of low cardiac output complicating acute pulmonary hypertension in normovolemic goats. *Crit Care Med* 1986; 14:120

18. Jerjes-Sanchez C, Ramirez-Rivera A, Gareia M de L, et al: Streptokinase and heparin versus heparin alone in massive pulmonary

embolism: a randomized controlled trial. *J Thromb Thrombolysis* 1995; 2:227

19. Arcasoy SM, Kreit JW: Thrombolytic therapy of pulmonary embolism: a comprehensive review of current evidence. *Chest* 1999; 115:1695

20. Knopp R, Claypool R, Leonardt D: Use of the tilt test in measuring acute blood loss. *Ann Emerg Med* 1980; 9:72

21. Barroso-Aranda J, Schmid-Schonbein GW, Zweifach BW, et al: Granulocytes and no-reflow phenomenon in irreversible hemorrhagic shock. *Circ Res* 1988; 63:437

22. Parker MM, Shelhamer JH, Bacharach SL, et al: Profound but reversible myocardial depression in patients with septic shock. *Ann Intern Med* 1984; 100:483

23. Schremmer B, Dhainault J: Heart failure in septic shock: Effects of inotropic support. *Crit Care Med* 1990; 18:549

24. Parrillo JE, Burch C, Shelhamer JH, et al: A circulating myocardial depressant substance in humans with septic shock. *J Clin Invest* 1985; 76:1539

25. Sands KE, Bates DW, Lanken PN, et al: Epidemiology of Sepsis Syndrome in Eight Academic Medical Centers. *JAMA* 1997; 278:234

26. Angus DC, Linde-Zwirble WT, Lidicker J, et al: Epidemiology of severe sepsis in the United States: analysis of incidence, outcome, and associated costs of care. *Crit Care Med* 2001; 29:1303

27. Bone RC: Why sepsis trials fail. *JAMA* 1996; 276:565

28. Kidokoro A, Iba T, Fukunaga M, et al: Alterations in coagulation and fibrinolysis during sepsis. *Shock* 1996; 5:223

29. Bernard GR, Vincent JL, Laterre PF: Recombinant human protein C Worldwide Evaluation in Severe Sepsis (PROWESS) study group. Efficacy and safety of recombinant human activated protein C for severe sepsis. *N Engl J Med* 2001; 344:699

30. Ibrahim EH, Sherman G, Ward S, et al: The influence of inadequate antimicrobial treatment of bloodstream infections on patient outcomes in the ICU setting. *Chest* 2000; 118:146

31. Kollef MH, Sherman G, Ward S, et al: Inadequate antimicrobial treatment of infections: a risk factor for hospital mortality among critically ill patients. *Chest* 1999; 115:462

32. Schiffl H, Lang SM, Fischer R: Daily hemodialysis and the outcome of acute renal failure. *N Engl J Med* 2002; 346:305

33. Bellomo R, Chapman M, Finfer S, et al: Low-dose dopamine in patients with early renal dysfunction: a placebo-controlled randomised trial. Australian and New Zealand Intensive Care Society (ANZICS) Clinical Trials Group. *Lancet* 2000; 356:2139

34. Bone RC, Fisher CJ, Clemmer TP, et al: A controlled clinical trial of high-dose methylprednisolone in the treatment of severe sepsis and septic shock. *N Engl J Med* 1987; 317:653

35. The Veterans Administration Systemic Sepsis Cooperative Study Group. Effect of high-dose glucocorticoid therapy on mortality in patients with clinical signs of systemic sepsis. *N Engl J Med* 1987; 317:659

36. Annane D, Sebille V, Troche G, et al: A 3-level prognostic classification in septic shock based on cortisol levels and cortisol response to corticotropin. *JAMA* 2000; 283:1038

37. Zaloga GP: Sepsis induced adrenal deficiency syndrome. *Crit Care Med* 2001; 29:688

38. Cuffe MS, Califf RM, Adams KF, et al: The Outcomes of a Prospective Trial of Intravenous Milrinone for Exacerbations of Chronic Heart Failure (OPTIME-CHF) Investigators. Short-term intravenous milrinone for acute exacerbation of chronic heart failure: a randomized controlled trial. *JAMA* 2002; 287:1541

39. Hannemann L, Reinhart K, Grenzer O, et al: Comparison of dopamine to dobutamine and norepinephrine for oxygen delivery and uptake in septic shock. *Crit Care Med* 1995; 23:1962

40. Marik PE, Mohedin M: The contrasting effects of dopamine and norepinephrine on systemic and splanchnic oxygen utilization in hyperdynamic sepsis. *JAMA* 1994; 272:1354

41. Nasraway SA: Norepinephrine: No more "leave 'em dead"? *Crit Care Med* 2000; 28:3096

42. Desjars P, Pinaud M, Bugnon D, et al: Norepinephrine therapy has no deleterious renal effects in human septic shock. *Crit Care Med* 1989; 17:426

43. Martin C, Papazian L, Perrin G, et al: Norepinephrine or dopamine for the treatment of hyperdynamic septic shock? *Chest* 1993; 103:1826

44. Martin C. Viviand X. Leone M. Thirion X: Effect of norepinephrine on the outcome of septic shock. *Crit Care Med* 2000; 28:2758

45. Gregory JS, Bonfiglio MF, Dasta JF, et al: Experience with phenylephrine as a component of the pharmacologic support of septic shock. *Crit Care Med* 1991; 19:1395

46. Levy B, Bollaert PE, Charpentier C, et al: Comparison of norepinephrine and dobutamine to epinephrine for hemodynamics, lactate metabolism, and gastric tonometric variables in septic shock: a prospective, randomized study. *Intensive Care Med* 1997; 23:282

47. Tsuneyoshi I, Yamada H, Kakihana Y, et al: Hemodynamic and metabolic effects of low-dose vasopressin infusions in vasodilatory septic shock. *Crit Care Med* 2001; 29:487

SEVERE PNEUMONIA

Michael S. Niederman, MD

Objectives

- Define the epidemiology of community-acquired pneumonia and risk factors for mortality
- Discuss the common etiologic pathogens of severe CAP
- Review current treatment strategies for severe CAP
- Discuss the clinical relevance of atypical pathogens and penicillin-resistant pneumococci
- Describe the pathogenesis of VAP
- Discuss the organisms that cause VAP
- Outline therapies for VAP

COMMUNITY-ACQUIRED PNEUMONIA

Pneumonia and influenza together are the sixth leading cause of death in the United States and the number one cause of mortality from infectious diseases. Community-acquired pneumonia (CAP) occurs in approximately 6 million people annually, with 20-30% requiring hospital admission.

Epidemiology and Risk Factors for Mortality

In a recent meta-analysis, the overall mortality for 33,148 patients reported in 127 studies was 13.7%, ranging from 5.1% in a population that was both hospitalized and ambulatory to 13.6% for hospitalized patients. In the elderly, mortality was 17.6%, while among nursing home patients it was 30.8%, and among those admitted to the ICU it was 36.5%. When pneumococcus was responsible, the mortality rate was 12.3%, a rate similar to that seen when no pathogen could be identified (12.8%). Certain pathogens such as *P. aeruginosa*, other gram-negatives (such as *K. pneumoniae*), and *S. aureus* had higher associated mortality rates.

A number of prognostic factors for mortality were identified, the most important being underlying neurologic disease, BUN > 20 mg/dl, respiratory rate > 20/min, systolic hypotension, hypothermia, bacteremia, multilobar disease, coexisting malignancy, and underlying congestive heart failure. The presence of a comorbid illness, more than specific bacteriology or patient age, is the major determinant of early and late mortality in CAP patients. In 1 study, 16% of all hospitalized CAP patients died, but an additional 32% of discharged patients died from all causes in the subsequent 2 years. Patients with CAP are at risk for recurrent infection indicating the need to vaccinate all pneumonia patients prior to discharge in an effort to avoid this complication, which has a very high mortality rate.

The British Thoracic Society rule uses certain clinical and laboratory features to identify certain high-risk patients who might have been unrecognized otherwise, and should be assessed on initial evaluation. It uses only 3 variables: respiratory rate ≥ 30/min, BUN > 19.6 mg/dl, and diastolic blood pressure ≤ 60 mm Hg. The presence of 2 of these 3 variables increases mortality 9- to 21-fold. More recently, confusion has been added as a fourth variable and, if 2 of 4 variables are present, there is a similar increase risk for death and need for ICU admission. Other factors that are associated with a poor outcome in CAP include: age > 65 years, the presence of comorbid illness, altered mental status, temperature > 38.3°C, extrapulmonary sites of infection, extremes of white blood cell count, multilobar radiographic abnormalities, evidence of sepsis, respiratory failure, the presence of end organ dysfunction secondary to severe infection, delays in the initiation of appropriate antibiotic therapy, prolonged illness prior to therapy, and indistinct clinical features on presentation (i.e., afebrile, absence of pleuritic chest pain). When multiple factors predicting a complicated course are present, hospitalization is indicated.

The pneumonia PORT study has led to the development of a prediction rule for deciding who should be admitted to the hospital with CAP. This rule divides patients into 5 groups with different risk of death, and suggests that outpatient care be given for classes I and II, admission for classes IV and V, and individualized decision for class III. The system heavily weighs age and comorbid illness. In a large prospective study, the rule was successful in increasing the number of low-risk patients who were discharged, compared to situations when the rule was not used, but even at sites that used the rule, 31% of low risk patients were still admitted, emphasizing the fact that the admission decision remains an "art of medicine" decision which cannot be easily determined by a rule.

Pathogenesis

Most of the pathogens responsible for CAP reach the lung after first colonizing the oropharynx. Since patients with serious comorbidity have an increased risk of gram-negative colonization of the oropharynx, those same patients appear to have an increased risk of pneumonia due to these types of pathogens. Community respiratory pathogens that can enter via inhalation, without preceding oropharyngeal colonization, include certain viruses, *M. tuberculosis* and Legionella.

One of the serious but infrequent complications of CAP is acute lung injury, presumably due to activation of inflammatory mediators in the lung. Investigators have evaluated the normal host response to pneumonia in order to determine if the inflammatory response remains localized to the lung or if it enters into the systemic circulation, thereby creating the conditions that lead to lung injury and ARDS. In studies of unilateral pneumonia, the infected lung had enhanced production of TNF-alpha, IL-1 beta, IL-6, and IL-8 with little effect on the contralateral lung or systemic circulation. IL-8 may be a key mediator since it can recruit neutrophils to sites of infection, and alveolar levels of this cytokine correlate with the number of neutrophils in the alveolar space. The fact that the cytokine response to pneumonia is usually localized may explain why ARDS is an infrequent complication of CAP.

Pathogens

Bacteria, viruses, and "atypical pathogens" (*Mycoplasma pneumoniae* and *Chlamydia pneumoniae*) account for most cases of CAP, but in some 50% of patients a microbiologic diagnosis is not established, reflecting the limitations of current diagnostic testing, particularly in those patients who have received prior antibiotic therapy. In 1 recent study, a transthoracic needle aspirate was used in patients without a known diagnosis, and many of these patients were shown to have pneumococcal infection. While this organism can account for many undiagnosed patients, it is also possible that not all pathogens causing CAP have been identified and studied, and new pathogens are commonly being described. The distribution of individual pathogens has also varied in studies, depending on the location of the study and the types of patients evaluated. For example, in a study of 385 patients at an inner city U.S. hospital, 205 of whom were HIV-negative, pneumococcus was found in 15%, *H. influenzae* in 7.3%, atypical pathogens in 8%, and in 37% no agent was identified. Most of these patients were older, and 65% had a smoking history and 30% were classified as alcoholic. This distribution of etiologic agents contrasts with the results of a study done in Israel. Here 346 patients were evaluated and a diagnosis was established in 81%. Pneumococcus was found in 43%, *M. pneumoniae* in 29%, *C. pneumoniae* in 18%, Legionella in 16%, and viruses in 10%. Interestingly, 38% of the patients had multiple organisms present simultaneously. In a recent U.S. study, 2,776 patients were studied and a possible etiologic diagnosis was made in 44.3%. In this group, *M. pneumoniae* was most common (32.5%), followed by pneumococcus (12.6%), *C. pneumoniae* (8.9%), influenza (7.4%), *H. influenzae* (6.6%) and then gram-negative bacilli and Legionella. In many of the more recent studies, atypical pathogen infections are common, often as coinfection with bacterial pathogens. In addition, the atypical organisms are not seen only in young and healthy adults, but also in older patients, particularly *C. pneumoniae* and Legionella. When atypical pathogens occur as part of a mixed infection, the

Table 1. Modifying factors that increase the risk of infection with specific pathogens

Penicillin-resistant and drug-resistant pneumococci:
>   Age > 65 years
>   Beta-lactam therapy within the past 3 months
>   Alcoholism
>   Immune suppressive illness (including therapy w/corticosteroids)
>   Multiple medical comorbidities
>   Exposure to a child in a day care center

Enteric gram-negatives:
>   Residence in a nursing home
>   Underlying cardiopulmonary disease
>   Multiple medical comorbidities
>   Recent antibiotic therapy

Pseudomonas aeruginosa:
>   Structural lung disease (bronchiectasis)
>   Corticosteroid therapy (> 10 mg prednisone/day)
>   Broad spectrum antibiotic therapy for > 7 days in the past month
>   Malnutrition

outcome may be more complex and length of stay longer than if a single organism is causing infection. The elderly may have different pathogens than younger patients, with a higher incidence of infection with *H. influenzae* and enteric gram-negatives.

In general, the pathogens causing CAP vary in relation to specific patient factors. The American Thoracic Society has categorized patients into 4 groups, each with its own list of likely pathogens (Figure and Tables 1-3), by assessing: illness severity (mild, moderate, or severe); the place of therapy (inpatient or outpatient); and the presence of cardiopulmonary disease and or modifying factors. Modifying factors (Table 1) are clinical conditions that put the patient at risk for infection with specific pathogens such as drug-resistant pneumococci, enteric gram negatives, and *Pseudomonas aeruginosa*. For all groups, the most common pathogen is pneumococcus, and therapy for CAP should always provide adequate coverage for this organism. In the elderly and chronically ill, *H. influenzae* (10-20

% of cases) and enteric gram-negative bacteria (20-40% of cases) are common organisms, but anaerobes must also be considered in those at risk for aspiration due to impaired consciousness or altered swallowing reflexes. In severe CAP, pneumococcus is the most common organism but studies have also found Legionella, *H. influenzae*, and enteric gram-negatives as important organisms. *P. aeruginosa* has been identified from the

Table 2.

Hospitalized Patients with Community-Acquired Pneumonia With Cardiopulmonary Disease +/or Modifying Factors

Probable organisms

       <u>*Streptococcus pneumoniae*</u> (including DRSP)
       <u>*Hemophilus influenzae*</u>
       Atypical pathogens such as <u>*M. pneumoniae*</u> or <u>*C. pneumoniae*</u>, alone or as mixed infection
       Aerobic gram-negative bacilli
       Legionella species
       Respiratory viruses
       Miscellaneous
              <u>*S. aureus, Moraxella catarrhalis*</u>,
              <u>Mycobacterium tuberculosis</u>, endemic fungi

Therapy

       Selected beta-lactam with antipneumococcal activity (ceftriaxone, cefotaxime, ampicillin/sulbactam, high dose ampicillin) (intravenous)
              PLUS
       Macrolide (decide oral or intravenous) OR doxycycline (decide oral or intravenous)
              OR

Hospitalized Patient with No Cardiopulmonary Disease and No Modifying Factors

Probable Organisms

       S. pneumoniae
       H. influenzae
       M. pneumoniae
       C. pneumoniae
       Mixed infection (bacteria plus atypical pathogen)
       Viruses
       Legionella sp.
       Miscellaneous : M. tuberculosis, endemic fungi, P. carinii

Therapy

       Intravenous azithromycin alone
            If macrolide allergic or intolerant: doxycycline and a beta-lactam, OR monotherapy with an antipneumococcal fluoroquinolone

respiratory tract cultures of 5-15% of all patients with severe CAP.

While this categorization is useful in suspecting certain pathogens when other specific clues are absent, there are some epidemiologic findings which point to the presence of specific pathogens. *Legionella pneumophila* should be considered in the late summer and with exposure to contaminated water sources (cooling towers, air conditioning, saunas); *C. burnetii* (Q fever) can follow exposure to infected cats,

cattle, sheep, and goats. Exposure to turkeys, chicken, and psittacine birds can lead to infection with *Chlamydia psittaci*, while contaminated bat caves may lead to Histoplasmosis. Immigrants from Asia, India, or Central America should always be evaluated for tuberculosis, and meliodosis should be considered in patients who have traveled to Southeast Asia. Other epidemiologic associations with specific pathogens are listed in Table 4.

Table 3.

Hospitalized Patients with Severe Community-Acquired Pneumonia

No Pseudomonal Risk Factors
  <u>Streptococcus pneumoniae</u> (ncluding DRSP)
    Legionella species
    <u>H. influenzae</u>
    Enteric gram-negatives
    <u>S. aureus</u>
    <u>M. pneumoniae</u> or <u>C. pneumoniae</u>
      Respiratory viruses
      Miscellaneous: <u>M. tuberculosis</u>, Endemic fungi
Therapy
      Macrolide OR Antipneumococcal quinolone
            PLUS

Hospitalized Patients with Severe Community-Acquired Pneumonia

Pseudomonal risks
  <u>Streptococcus pneumoniae</u> (including DRSP)
    Legionella species
    <u>H. influenzae</u>
    Enteric gram-negatives (including *P. aeruginosa*)
    <u>S. aureus</u>
    <u>M. pneumoniae</u> or <u>C. pneumoniae</u>
      Respiratory viruses
      Miscellaneous: <u>M. tuberculosis</u>, Endemic fungi
Therapy
      Ciprofloxacin PLUS antiPseudomonal, antipneumococcal beta lactam (imipenem,
meropenem, cefepime, piperacillin/tazobactam)
                  OR
      Nonpseudomonal quinolone (levofloxacin, gatifloxacin, moxifloxacin) or macrolide
      PLUS antiPseudomonal, antipneumococcal beta lactam (imipenem, meropenem, cefepime,
piperacillin/tazobactam) PLUS aminoglycoside

COMMENTS ABOUT SPECIFIC PATHOGENS

<u>Pneumococcus</u>: A gram-positive diplococcus, with 85% of cases caused by 23 of the 84 serotypes. Commonly preceded by viral illness, this may cause lobar or bronchopneumonia. It is a common infection in those with asplenia, multiple myeloma, heart failure, alcoholism. The current vaccine includes 23 serotypes. Controversy about vaccine efficacy shows that it is safe, but it may not be effective in the chronically ill. Case-control methodology has been used to show efficacy.

Penicillin-resistant Streptococcus pneumoniae (PRSP) is becoming a problem in some areas. In the United States, over 40% of pneumococci are penicillin-resistant, with rates varying widely from region to region. Most have intermediate (penicillin MIC ≥ 0.12 mg/ml but < 2.0 mg/L) rather than high-level resistance (penicillin MIC ≥ 2 mg/L). The clinical relevance of *in vitro* resistance is debated, but there are data to show an increased risk of death if patients have organisms with a penicillin MIC of at least 4 mg/L, which is currently an uncommon occurrence. Resistance is rarely a *de novo* event and is uncommon in low-risk patients, but rather is seen in immunosuppressed and chronically ill

Table 4. EPIDEMIOLOGIC CONDITIONS RELATED TO SPECIFIC PATHOGENS IN PATIENTS WITH COMMUNITY-ACQUIRED PNEUMONIA

CONDITION	COMMONLY ENCOUNTERED PATHOGENS
Alcoholism	*Streptococcus pneumoniae* (including PRSP), anaerobes, gram-negative bacilli
COPD/smoker	*S. pneumoniae, H. influenzae, Moraxella catarrhalis, Legionella*
Nursing home residency	*S. pneumoniae*, gram-negative bacilli, *H. influenzae, S. aureus*, anaerobes, *C. pneumoniae*
Poor dental hygiene	Anaerobes
Epidemic Legionnaire's disease	*Legionella* species
Exposure to bats	Histoplasma capsulatum
Exposure to birds	Chlamydia psittaci, Cryptococcus neoformans, *H. capsulatum*
Exposure to rabbits	Francisella tularensis
Travel to SW USA	Coccidioidomycosis
Exposure to farm animals or parturient cats	Coxiella burnetii (Q fever)
Influenza active in community	Influenza, *S. pneumoniae, S. aureus, H. influenzae*
Suspected large volume aspiration	Anaerobes, chemical pneumonitis, or obstruction
Structural disease of lung (bronchiectasis, cystic fibrosis, etc.)	*P. aeruginosa, P. cepacia* or *S. aureus*
Injection drug use	*S. aureus*, anaerobe, tuberculosis
Endobronchial obstruction	Anaerobes
Recent antibiotic therapy	Drug-resistant pneumococci, *P. aeruginosa*

patients, especially if they have received a beta-lactam antibiotic in the preceding 3 months, although cases of epidemic transmission of resistant organisms have been reported. Other risk factors for PRSP include age > 60, alcoholism, and multiple medical comorbidity.

The mortality rate of hospitalized patients with pneumococcal CAP exceeds 20%, but is related to the status of the patient's immune defenses and overall health and not whether the organism is penicillin-resistant. Although most studies have shown that patients with penicillin-resistant organisms have the same mortality rate as patients who are infected with penicillin-sensitive organisms, those with very high levels of resistance may have an increased risk of death. Penicillin resistance may mean multidrug resistance, and there is a high coincidence of macrolide and trimethoprim-sulfa resistance among penicillin-resistant pneumococci. Although quinolone resistance is uncommon for pneumococci, the less-active agents ciprfloxacin and levofloxacin have been associated with failures of therapy due to resistance, especially if patients have received recent therapy with a quinolone.

Risk factors for mortality include the presence of bacteremia, the finding of bronchopneumonia rather than lobar consolidation, and the presence of multiple comorbid illnesses. Regardless of resistance pattern, therapy for pneumococcus with high-dose penicillin (2 million units every 4 hours) or a third-generation cephalosporin (cefotaxime or ceftriaxone) is adequate for invasive pulmonary disease, provided that central nervous system involvement is not present. The incidence of penicillin resistance is rising in certain communities, and a knowledge of the frequency of the problem and of local antimicrobial susceptibilities is necessary to assure adequate initial antibiotic therapy because some agents, such as trimethoprim-sulfamethoxizole, are increasingly ineffective against pneumococci. The new fluoroquinolones may represent appropriate empiric therapy for patients with suspected resistance. If they are used, there are differences in activity against pneumococci, with the least to most active agents being, in order: levofloxacin less active than gatifloxacin or moxifloxacin.

Legionella pneumophila is a weakly staining gram-negative organism. Legionella is a water-borne organism, and should be suspected in all patients with severe CAP, and in other patients based on a careful epidemiologic evaluation. Increased risk is present in those who are immune compromised, have malignancy, are a smoker, or who have chronic lung disease, or age > 50. There is no constellation of clinical signs that is specific for Legionella infection. In addition to respiratory symptoms, may have confusion, diarrhea, elevated liver function tests, hyponatremia, and relative bradycardia.

Legionella is a commonly identified pathogen in patients with severe CAP, but its overall incidence is uncertain. Unless careful diagnostic testing is done, underestimation of its frequency is likely. Sputum samples that grow Legionella often have few polymorphonuclear cells and may be discarded by microbiology labs. Most cases cannot be diagnosed by a single immunofluorescent antibody titer (often negative at the time of the acute illness), and are only recognized if acute and convalescent serum titers are examined for a fourfold rise. The urinary antigen is a more sensitive single test, but is specific only for infection with *L. pneumophila* serogroup I.

Mycoplasma pneumoniae: Usually a mild illness, but it can be severe with complications of hemolytic anemia, myocarditis, hepatitis, cold agglutinins, meningoencephalitis. Serologic diagnosis.

S. aureus can cause CAP, particularly when bacterial pneumonia complicates influenza, or when right-sided endocarditis or cavitary lung lesions are present. *S. aureus* is also seen after influenza, with chronic lung disease. May lead to cavities (pneumatoceles). Empyema is common.

Chlamydia pneumoniae (the TWAR agent) is a common pathogen in young adults with tracheobronchitis and/or pneumonia, and often leads to a syndrome of "adult croup." The role of *C. pneumoniae* as a respiratory pathogen is uncertain, with some studies suggesting that it functions as a copathogen more often than as a single agent. Confusion results because the organism can be isolated along with other pathogens, its clinical features cannot be differentiated from those of pneumonia caused by other organisms, and patients can recover without specific therapy. One recent study has shown that it can occur in the elderly, including those who reside in nursing homes, and it may spread person-to-person. The mortality rate can be high in certain populations, and it may lead to severe forms of CAP.

Aspiration/Lung abscess: Aspiration may involve acid (chemical pneumonitis), inert liquids, or particulate matter (suffocation or postobstructive pneumonia), or oropharyngeal bacteria (aspiration pneumonia or lung abscess). Aspiration pneumonia often is polymicrobial, involving anaerobes, and may cavitiate, and can be an indolent infection that is confused with malignancy. If lung abscess is seen in an edentulous patient (no mouth anaerobes), consider lung malignancy, foreign body, or GI source of chronic aspiration (esophageal diverticulum). The cavity usually has an air fluid level and is > 2 cm. Cavities from bacterial infection tend to be thick-walled with a ragged inner lining. Lung abscess cavities usually have an air-fluid level. TB cavities, by contrast, tend to be thin-walled, air-filled (without an air-fluid level), and the inner wall is smooth. Aspiration pneumonia occurs in the superior segment of the lower lobe or the posterior segments of the upper lobe if aspiration occurs when supine, and in the lower lobe if aspiration occurs when upright. Patients with aspiration risks and also with poor dentition, a lower lobe infiltrate and pleural or chest wall involvement should be considered as possibly having *actinomycosis*.

Influenza: Can be complicated by pneumonia. RNA virus, with types A and B. Type A infection is generally more severe. Vaccine is trivalent and directed at both types of influenza and reduces mortality from respiratory illness. Amantidine and rimantadine are active only against type A. The new antivirals osteltamivir and zanamivir are active against both influenza A and B. Fall and early spring are most common for epidemics. Attack rates are not increased in the elderly, but mortality is. Pneumonia may be viral or secondary bacterial. The latter occurs as the patient is improving from his initial infection and is most commonly due to pneumococcus, *S. aureus*, *H. influenzae,* or gram-negative. New interest in diagnosing influenza has come with the advent of the neuraminidase inhibitors zanamivir and oseltamivir. The former is given as a dry powder inhaler, and the latter as a pill.

In HIV-positive patients, pneumococcus and *H. influenzae* are common, but CAP with *P. aeruginosa* has been reported, and infection with *Pneumocystis carinii* and *M. tuberculosis* must always be considered.

A newly described pathogen is the hantavirus, carried by rodents and first identified in the Four Corners area of New Mexico in May 1993. The hantavirus pulmonary syndrome is life-threatening and characterized by fulminant respiratory failure after a brief prodromal illness with symptoms of fever, myalgia, cough, dyspnea, gastrointestinal symptoms, and headache. Patients are generally tachypneic and hypotensive with rapidly progressive pulmonary edema. Mortality is high, with only nonspecific and supportive therapy available.

DIAGNOSTIC EVALUATION

Because of limited yield, extensive diagnostic testing is not indicated for most CAP patients. However, certain tests can help to determine the severity of illness and presence of extrapulmonary complications. Blood cultures are positive in only 15% of patients, but provide both therapeutic and prognostic information. Controversy about the value of sputum's stain and culture continues, but a sputum culture alone is not a reliable way to identify the etiologic pathogen for CAP. It is clear that if diagnostic testing is done, it should be done promptly, as delays in the administration of antibiotics more than 8 hours after coming to the hospital are associated with increased mortality. Sputum culture should be reserved for situations when an unusual or drug-resistant pathogen is suspected, particularly if the patient has not responded to initial empiric therapy. Limitations to the use of stain include: not all patients are able to produce an adequate specimen (> 25 polys/LPF, < 10 squames/LPF), the stain is often interpreted by technicians who are unfamiliar with the clinical circumstances, results are often negative if the patient has taken antibiotics. In addition, a stain can be either sensitive or specific, but not both, and probably if used should be used for its specificity. The finding of any gram-positive diplococcus is very sensitive for finding samples that will grow pneumococcus, but the finding is not very specific. On the other hand, the finding of a predominance of gram-positive diplococci, is more specific, but of course less sensitive.

An extensive diagnostic evaluation can also be useful when an unusual pathogen (e.g., an endemic fungus, *C. psittaci*) is suspected. Serologic testing is not routinely indicated, and should be reserved for nonresponding patients and for epidemiologic studies. Most serologic tests are positive when there is a 4-fold rise in titer, and this necessitates the collection of convalescent titers, as acute testing is rarely positive. Bronchoscopy and transtracheal aspirates are not usually indicated for CAP patients, but are of value in HIV-positive or other immunosuppressed patients. Patients with severe CAP often undergo an extensive diagnostic evaluation, but studies have not shown a benefit from having a specific etiologic diagnosis. When a patient with CAP is not responding to initial empiric therapy, a reevaluation is needed, which is directed at identifying noninfectious processes that mimic pneumonia, unusual or drug-resistant organisms, as well as both infectious and noninfectious complications of pneumonia. Diagnostic studies in this setting may include bronchoscopy with cultures, CT scanning of the chest, and possibly open lung biopsy, but the latter has its greatest value if a noninfectious process is suspected (bronchiolitis obliterans with organizing pneumonia, pulmonary vasculitis, etc.).

The classification of the clinical presentation into "typical " and "atypical" patterns is generally of little use for predicting the microbial etiology. Not only are the clinical features caused by specific organisms not diagnostic, but some organisms, such as Legionella, lead to a clinical picture that overlaps both patterns. Clinical features usually do not accurately predict etiology because certain patient populations, particularly the elderly and chronically ill, often have an inadequate response to infection. An elderly patient with a virulent bacterial CAP may present with confusion, incontinence, falling, or worsening of a comorbid illness, rather than with fever, respiratory symptoms, and other features of the "typical" pneumonia syndrome.

THERAPY

Based on the likely organisms, therapy will differ for each of the 4 patient subsets with CAP. Recent data show that atypical pathogen coinfection is common enough that all patients should be treated for these organisms, using either a quinolone alone, or a macrolide added to a beta-lactam. In general, trimethoprim-sulfamethoxizole is no longer a useful therapy because of the increased incidence of pneumococcal resistance to this agent. The new fluoroquinolones (levofloxacin, gatifloxacin, and moxifloxacin) are monotherapy options for complicated outpatients, and cover gram positives, gram-negatives, and atypical pathogens, and are active against penicillin-resistant or sensitive pneumococci.

For hospitalized patients with nonsevere CAP, in the absence of cardiopulmonary disease and modifying factors (these patients are rarely admitted), therapy should be with an intravenous macrolide alone (such as azithromycin) (Table 2). For the hospitalized patient with cardiopulmonary disease and/or modifying factors, therapy should be with a third-generation cephalsporin (cefotaxime, ceftriaxone, ampicillin/sulbactam, high-dose ampicillin), combined with an oral or intravenous macrolide (or tetracycline), or alternatively, with a new antipneumococcal quinolone alone (levofloxacin, gatifloxacin, moxifloxacin).

Patients with severe CAP (Table 3) should be considered for admission to an intensive care unit and require a more aggressive therapeutic approach. Severe CAP has no uniform definition, but it is characterized by the presence of septic shock, or the need for mechanical ventilation; or alternatively, by at least 2 of the following 3: systolic BP < 90 mm Hg, PaO_2/FiO_2 ratio < 250, or multilobar pneumonia. Other criteria that suggest severe infection include: respiratory rate > 35/min; increase in the size of lung infiltrates by > 50% in 48 hours; oliguria; or acute renal failure. The role of the ICU in severe illness has been debated, but the ICU probably has its greatest value if used early in the course of severe disease.

Pathogens which lead to severe CAP are distinct and slightly different from those seen in other populations, and include pneumococcus, Legionella, and enteric gram-negative bacilli. Several studies have demonstrated that when initial empiric therapy was directed at these organisms and accompanied by a prompt clinical response, outcome was better than if ineffective therapy was used. In these studies, identification of the pathogen has not led to an improved outcome, raising questions about the value of extensive diagnostic testing even in these critically ill patients. For patients with severe CAP, an intravenous macrolide or quinolone should be combined with additional agents, the type and number being dictated by the presence of Pseudomonal risk factors (Table 3).

For hospitalized patients who improve with initial therapy, an early switch to oral antibiotics is appropriate and may not only shorten length of stay, but may also improve overall outcome. Criteria for early oral therapy include the absence of fever on at least 2 consecutive determinations, the absence of an unstable medical illness, a declining white blood cell count, improvement in cough and dyspnea, and the ability to take oral medications. In general, patients who receive effective therapy will improve in 48-72 hours, but the nonresponding patient should have an extensive diagnostic evaluation to identify unusual or drug-resistant pathogens, noninfectious mimics of pneumonia (vasculitis, bronchiolitis obliterans with organizing pneumonia), and complications of pneumonia. In the patient responding to therapy, radiographic resolution can be slow, with only 50% of a young, healthy population having radiographic clearing by 2 weeks. Slower resolution is seen in those with bacteremia, advanced age, multilobar involvement, or underlying chronic obstructive lung disease.

Vaccination. The mainstay of CAP prevention is vaccination with both the pneumococcal and influenza vaccines. Pneumococcal vaccine should be given to all patients over age 65, and to patients, regardless of age, who have chronic heart, lung, and other medical illnesses. Patients who are asplenic, or those with hematologic malignancy or HIV infection should also be vaccinated. Hospital-based immunization with pneumococcal vaccine has been suggested for the majority of patients admitted for any diagnosis, because as many as 60% of all patients with CAP have been hospitalized for some reason in the preceding 4 years. The current ACIP recommendation is to repeat pneumococcal vaccination after 5 years in patients who are likely to have had a rapid decline in antibody concentrations. These include patients with chronic renal failure, organ or bone marrow transplantation, and patients at risk for fatal infection, particularly those who are asplenic.

Influenza vaccination reduces hospital admissions and mortality rates if administered before an outbreak. Repeated influenza vaccination in elderly patients is both safe and effective in preventing influenza illness and its complications. In healthy adults, the influenza vaccine can reduce the incidence of upper respiratory illness, while in a nursing home population it can reduce hospitalization rates, pneumonia rates and mortality. Antiviral therapy with amantadine or rimantidine, which are active only against influenza A virus, or oseltamivir or zanamivir (active against influenza A and B) is used to supplement vaccination in immune deficient patients. Antiviral therapy is indicated during an influenza outbreak in a closed environment (such as a nursing home) for all unvaccinated high-risk persons for least 2 weeks following the late administration of vaccine. New studies with topical antiviral agents are promising, and these agents may have a role in the future.

NOSOCOMIAL PNEUMONIA

The incidence of nosocomial, or hospital-acquired pneumonia (HAP) varies in relation to the concomitant comorbidity in a given patient population. While 10% of patients requiring ICU care after general surgery develop this infection, 20% of those intubated and up to 70% of those with ARDS will develop HAP. In critically ill, mechanically ventilated patients, the incidence of HAP is 1% per day during the first month of ventilation. However, since most patients are ventilated for short periods, up to half of all episodes of VAP occur within the first 4 days of ventilation (early onset VAP). Recent data show that the risk of pneumonia is 3% per day in the first 5 days, 2% per day on days 5-10, and then 1% per day on days 10-15. The mortality rate of HAP can exceed 50% in mechanically ventilated patients, especially if the infection involves potentially resistant enteric gram-negatives such as *P. aeruginosa* and *Acinetobacter* organisms that are particularly common in patients who have received prior antibiotic therapy. Case-control studies in mechanically ventilated patients indicate that 50% of HAP patients die as a direct result of this infection and not as a consequence of their underlying serious illness. One of the factors that adds to attributable mortality is the use of inadequate therapy, and this is more likely if patients are infected with antibiotic resistant organisms.

Using the National Nosocomial Infections Surveillance (NNIS) system, the CDC regularly collects data about nosocomial infections, and has reported the data collected between 1992 and 1997 in medical ICUs throughout the United States, involving 181,993 patients. The data come from 112 medical ICUs in 97 hospitals, and the most common infections by site were: urinary tract (31%), pneumonia (27%), primary bacteremia (19%), followed by all other infections. The common sites of infection were often device-related, with 87% of bacteremias associated with central lines, 86% of pneumonias with mechanical ventilation, and 95% of UTIs with urinary catheters. The most common pathogens for primary bacteremia were coagulase negative staphylococci (36%), followed by enterococci (16%) and *S. aureus* (13%). Central line infections were especially associated with coagulase negative staphylococci. With nosocomial pneumonia, gram–negatives predominated (64%), with *P. aeruginosa* being most common (21%), followed by Enterobacter (9%), *Klebsiella pneumoniae* (8%), and Acinetobacter (6%). *Staphylococcus aureus* was present in 20% of nosocomial pneumonia episodes. In ventilator-associated pneumonia, Pseudomonas and Acinetobacter were most common, while *E. coli* was more common in nonventilated patients. Not surprisingly, overall nosocomial infection rate correlated with average length of stay and device use. The pooled mean rate of ventilator-associated pneumonia was 6.5 per 1,000 ventilator days. There was no association between device-associated infection rates and number of hospital beds, number of ICU beds, and length of stay.

Pathogenesis and risk factors. Patients usually develop HAP because of impaired host defenses and the consequent inability to contain encountered bacteria. In other patients, HAP develops because bacteria in the ICU environment are sufficiently numerous or virulent to overcome either normal or impaired host defenses. Recognized risk factors for HAP include patient-related conditions, therapeutic interventions, and infection-control-related factors. Patient factors predisposing to HAP include the primary critical illness (shock, sepsis, extrapulmonary infection, respiratory failure) and underlying comorbid illness (diabetes, azotemia, COPD, central nervous system dysfunction, recent surgery).

Therapeutic interventions that increase HAP risk include sedatives, corticosteroids, cytotoxic agents, antacids, antibiotic therapy, enteral feeding, and especially endotracheal intubation. Patients can be exposed to large numbers of bacteria via the endotracheal tube, which itself can harbor a bacterial biofilm or serve as a conduit from a colonized oropharynx. In addition, secretions pooling above the endotracheal tube cuff often contain bacteria that can be aspirated into the lung. Proper attention to cuff pressure can minimize the leaking of secretions around the endotracheal tube cuff. Even though endotracheal tubes are often contaminated with organisms, they should not be routinely changed, as reintubation itself serves as a pneumonia risk. An exception may be replacement of a nasotracheal tube with an orotracheal tube; nasal tubes promote nosocomial sinusitis, a source of pathogens for HAP. With the advent of noninvasive ventilation to manage respiratory failure, pneumonia has been less common in patients managed with this modality, compared to mechanical ventilation and endotracheal intubation.

Nosocomial sinusitis has been identified in the past as a risk factor for nosocomial pneumonia, and now an intervention study demonstrates that aggressive diagnosis and treatment of sinusitis can prevent pneumonia and mortality. In a study, 399 intubated patients, expected to be ventilated for > 7 days, were enrolled and randomized to a group that had a systematic search for sinusitis when fever was present, and a control group that did not. Surprisingly, ALL patients were nasotracheally intubated, and all gastric tubes were nasally inserted, a practice that should be questioned given the data in this study and the other before it. A total of 199 patients were in the intervention group, and whenever fever was present, the protocol required sinus CT scans at days 4 and 8 after intubation and then every 7 days. If radiographic sinusitis was present, a transnasal culture was obtained and sinusitis diagnosed if cultures showed > 1,000 organisms/ml. Patients with sinusitis were treated with antibiotics and sinus lavage every 8 hours. Nosocomial pneumonia was diagnosed in all patients by the finding of a new infiltrate and a positive PSB culture. The authors found that 110 of the 199 study patients had radiographic sinusitis, and a total of 80 fulfilled microbiologic criteria and clinical criteria for sinusitis. Ventilator-associated pneumonia (VAP) occurred in 37/199 of the intervention patients (23 with sinusitis, 14 without) and 51/200 of the controls (p = 0.02). For the 23 patients with both VAP and sinusitis, the pneumonia occurred at the same time of sinusitis or later in 16/23, and with the same organism in 43%. Interestingly, the mortality rate of the intervention group (36%) was significantly lower than the mortality of the control group (46%), suggesting that aggressive diagnosis and therapy of sinusitis can have a favorable impact on patient outcome. When the data are examined for the relationship of VAP and sinusitis, the finding was that VAP occurred in 29% of those with sinusitis (23/80) and in only 12% without sinusitis (14/119). Methodologic issues with the study include that nasal tubes were used, and if sinusitis was diagnosed, they were not removed. It therefore is unclear how valuable this protocol is for an ICU that does not use nasotracheal tubes.

The stomach's role in HAP pathogenesis is uncertain. Elevation of gastric pH by antacids, H2 antagonists, or enteral feeding can lead to gastric overgrowth by enteric gram-negative bacteria. However, the frequency with which these organisms lead to pneumonia is uncertain. Some, but not all, studies in critically ill patients show reduced HAP rates when sucralfate is used for intestinal bleeding prophylaxis instead of antacids or H2 antagonists. Many factors influence whether gastric contents reach the lung, including increased reflux in the supine position or with enteral feeding tube placement in the stomach rather than the

Table 5. GROUP 1: NO UNUSUAL RISK FACTORS; MILD-MODERATE HAP; ONSET ANY TIME; OR SEVERE HAP WITH EARLY ONSET

CORE PATHOGENS:	CORE ANTIBIOTICS:
Enteric Gram-negative organisms (Nonpseudomonal)	Cephalosporin: Second generation, Nonpseudomonal third-generation, or fourth-generation
Enterobacter spp.	OR
E. coli	Beta-lactam/Beta-lactamase inhibitor
Klebsiella spp.	
Proteus spp.	Penicillin Allergic
S. marcescens	
	Fluoroquinolone
H. influenzae	or Clindamycin + Aztreonam
Methicillin-sensitive *S. aureus*	
S. pneumoniae	

small bowel, gastric volume, and nasogastric tube diameter.

Infection-control risk factors for HAP include the failure to routinely use hand washing or isolation of resistant pathogens and the use of contaminatedrespiratory therapy equipment. Respiratory therapy equipment does not commonly bring bacteria to the lung. Even if ventilator circuits are changed as infrequently as once a week or are never changed, HAP risk is not increased.

Bacteriology. All HAP patients are at risk for infection with a "core" group of organisms, which include nonresistant enteric gram negatives (*Enterobacter, E. coli, Klebsiella, Proteus,* and *S. marcescens*), *H. influenzae,* methicillin-sensitive *S. aureus,* and *S. pneumoniae.* These organisms are particularly likely if no unusual risk factors are present, and if the pneumonia begins within the first 5 days of hospitalization (early onset HAP) (Table 5). When risk factors are present, or if the pneumonia begins on day 5 or later (late onset HAP), then the likely pathogens change. In addition to the core organisms, patients with witnessed aspiration are also at risk for anaerobes; those with coma, head injury, and diabetes are especially at risk for *S. aureus* infection; those with a prolonged ICU stay, prior antibiotics, corticosteroids, malnutrition, or structural lung disease are at risk for *P. aeruginosa* and *Acinetobacter;* and those who have had a prolonged ICU stay and prior antibiotics are also at risk for methicillin-resistant *S. aureus* (MRSA) (Table 6). When HAP is severe, in the presence of risk factors, or if it is of late onset, resistant gram-negatives and MRSA are particularly likely (Table 7).

In the setting of severe pneumonia, drug resistant organisms are likely, particularly if the patient has been treated with antibiotics, corticosteroids, and prolonged ventilation. These resistant organisms include gram-negatives as well as MRSA. MRSA is an increasingly common pathogen causing VAP, and is more likely in patients who have received prolonged ventilation and prior antibiotics.

One group of organisms that is of unclear significance in VAP is anaerobes, and now a careful bronchoscopic study has found that these organisms almost never are involved in this infection. In this study, PSB and BAL were done in 143 patients with 185 episodes of suspected VAP, and in 25 patients with aspiration pneumonia who were ventilated. A total of 63 of 185 suspected episodes and 12/25 aspiration patients met microbiologic criteria for pneumonia. The organisms included common gram-negative and gram-positive

Table 6. GROUP 2: MILD-MODERATE HAP; WITH RISK FACTORS; ONSET ANY TIME

CORE PATHOGENS PLUS:

CORE ANTIBIOTICS PLUS:

Anaerobes (Witnessed aspiration, recent thoraco-abdominal surgery)

Clindamycin
or Beta-lactam/Beta-lactmase
   inhibitor (alone)

S. aureus (Coma, head trauma, diabetes, renal failure)

+/- Vancomycin (until MRSA is ruled out)

Legionella (High dose corticosteroids)

Erythromycin +/- Rifampin

Prolonged ICU stay, prior antibiotics, corticosteroid therapy, structural lung disease

Treat as severe pneumonia (Group 3)

organisms, but only 1 patient from the entire group had an anaerobic organism isolated.

The authors conclude from these findings that routine anaerobic therapy is not needed in ventilated patients with VAP or aspiration pneumonia.

<u>Diagnosis and treatment</u>. The clinical diagnosis of HAP is made when a patient has a new or progressive lung infiltrate plus at least 2 of the following: fever, purulent sputum, or leukocytosis. This clinical definition is sensitive, but patients with other disease processes may be misdiagnosed as having HAP. The differential diagnosis includes congestive heart failure, atelectasis, pulmonary infarction, and inflammatory diseases (such as acute lung injury). In addition, many patients who have VAP can have coexisting infections including sinusitis, intraabdominal infection, and central line infections.

The overdiagnosis of HAP is a particular concern in mechanically ventilated patients. Quantitative cultures of respiratory secretions, obtained bronchoscopically or with a blind catheter or brush insertion, have been used to define whether pneumonia is present. This approach is controversial because it relies on defining a microbiologic "threshold concentration" in respiratory secretions above which pneumonia is diagnosed. Early forms of pneumonia may go undiagnosed with this approach, and there are technical problems involved in collecting samples and

interpreting results, especially in patients who are concurrently receiving antibiotics. The impact of these procedures on the outcome of patients with VAP has been addressed by a number of studies. In these studies, bronchoscopy has not always had a benefit, but if a benefit was present, it was seen in populations that often received inadequate antibiotic therapy, due to a high frequency of drug-resistant organisms. Although bronchoscopy has been reported to lead to fewer patients getting antibiotics and to less antibiotic resistance than management by clinical tools, not all studies have found this. In fact, in 1 study, similar benefits were seen when the clinical pulmonary infection score (CPIS) was used to decide whether to continue empiric antibiotic therapy, after observing the patient's clinical course for 3 days during therapy. If quantitative cultures are not collected, the etiologic pathogen can still be identified in intubated patients (along with other colonizing but not infecting organisms), by collecting tracheal aspirates for culture. The role of expectorated or suctioned sputum cultures in nonintubated patients is controversial.

One thing that has become clear in studies of VAP is that initial antibiotic therapy must be accurate in order to assure the best possible outcome. If therapy is not accurate (and invasive methods may delay the initiation of therapy, and maybe even appropriate therapy), then outcome is poor,

Table 7. GROUP 3: SEVERE HAP, EARLY ONSET WITH RISK FACTORS OR LATE ONSET

CORE PATHOGENS PLUS:	AMINOGLYCOSIDE OR CIPROFLOXACIN PLUS ONE OF THE FOLLOWING:
P. aeruginosa *Acinetobacter spp.*	Antipseudomonal penicillin Beta-lactam/Beta-lactamase inhibitor Ceftazidime or cefoperazone Fourth-generation Cephalosporin (cefepime) Imipenem, Meropenem Azotreonam
Consider MRSA	+/- Vancomycin

even if microbiologic data become available and explain why the initial therapy was incorrect. Thus, initial therapy is usually empiric and based upon the suspected etiologic pathogens (Tables 5-7). Many patients without special risk factors, and can be used in the ICU patient with early onset infection and no special risk factors. Combination therapy is superior to monotherapy for bacteremic *P. aeruginosa* infection and should be used in this setting. For non-bacteremic *P. aeruginosa* infection, combination therapy is often used to prevent the emergence of resistance during therapy, but the optimal combination regimen is not defined, and the addition of an aminoglycoside to a beta lactam agent may have little benefit. However, current practice is to use combination therapy for severe, late-onset HAP, or for patients with severe early-onset HAP in the presence of certain risk factors, in an effort to prevent resistance, but more data supporting the efficacy of this approach are needed. Combination can involve an anti-Pseudomonal beta lactam, with either an aminoglycoside or ciprofloxacin, but the latter may be preferable because of its excellent penetration into respiratory secretions and because of the limited efficacy and enhanced renal toxicity associated with aminoglycosides. Stepdown to monotherapy may be appropriate if *P. aeruginosa* or another highly resistant pathogen is not isolated from the tracheal aspirate of an intubated patient. Agents that can be used as monotherapy for severe pneumonia, not due to a drug-resistant organism, include: ciprofloxacin (dosed 400

patients can be treated with a single broad-spectrum agent, but certain resistant organisms require combination therapy. Monotherapy can be used for non-ICU HAP

mg every 8 hours), imipenem (1 gram every 8 hours), meropenem, cefepime, and piperacillin/tazobactam. If patients have risk factors for MRSA (above), it may be necessary to add coverage for this organism, pending the results of tracheal aspirate cultures. This is especially the case if the tracheal aspirate gram stain shows gram-positive organisms. Therapy of MRSA can be with vancomycin or one of its alternatives, such as linezolid or quinupristin/dalfopristin.

In 2 recent studies, piperacillin/tazobactam was an effective monotherapy for HAP. In the first study piperacillin/tazobactam (P/T) (3g/375mg every 4 hours) was compared to ceftazadime with each arm being given tobramycin, which could be discontinued after respiratory culture results were known. A total of 300 patients were enrolled, with 136 clinically evaluable. The P/T group had a significantly higher clinical success rate (74% versus 50%), higher frequency of eradication of baseline pathogens (66% versus 38%), and lower mortality (7.7% versus 17%) than the ceftazadime group. The patients generally did not have severe illness (only 20% had severe illness), and the need to use antibiotics every 4 hours is somewhat limiting. However, in a second study, a dose of 4.5 grams P/T 3 times daily was used , and approximately 50% of the study group were mechanically ventilated patients. The mean APACHE II score in this study was 14.7. P/T was compared to imipenem, and it was associated with significantly more success and less failures, greater success against *P. aeruginosa* (90% versus 50%), and with fewer episodes of *P. aeruginosa* resistance during therapy, even when used as a monotherapy regimen. These data suggest that piperacillin/tazobactam can be used in mechanically ventilated patients as monotherapy for severe HAP, adding it to a list that includes a number of other agents.

Prevention. Attention to pneumonia risk factors and infection control efforts are the most effective preventive strategies. Recently, a specially adapted endotracheal tube that allows for the suction of subglottic secretions pooled above the endotracheal tube cuff, has been shown to prevent some episodes of HAP. Prophylactic antibiotics, either as an aerosol or as part of a selective digestive decontamination strategy, do not lead to a reduction in mortality and raise concerns about the emergence of resistant pathogens. Such uses of antibiotics are experimental and should not be used in routine clinical practice.

REFERENCES

REFERENCES FOR CAP

1. Niederman MS, Mandell LA, Anzueto A, et al: Guidelines for the management of adults with community-acquired lower respiratory tract infections: Diagnosis, assessment of severity, antimicrobial therapy and prevention. *Am J Respir Crit Care Med* 2001; 163, 1730-1754
    This document reviews the literature relevant to the management of community-acquired pneumonia and presents an empiric approach to management based on an assessment of severity of illness, place of therapy (inpatient or outpatient), and the presence of cardiopulmonary disease and/or modifying factors. There is also a discussion of the bacteriology of community-acquired pneumonia, the recommended approach to diagnostic testing, criteria for hospitalization and for admission to the intensive care unit, and an approach to evaluating the patient who has not responded to initial empiric therapy.

2. Pallares R, Linares J, Vadillo M, Cabellos C, Manresa F, Viladrich PF, et al: Resistance to penicillin and cephalosporin and mortality from severe pneumococcal pneumonia in Barcelona, Spain. *N Engl J Med* 1995; 333: 474-480
    Results of a 10-year prospective study of 504 adults with invasive pneumococcal disease in Spain are presented, reporting an incidence of penicillin resistance approaching 30%. Factors associated with mortality were examined, and the authors found that penicillin resistance per se was not associated with an enhanced risk of dying. Adequate outcome was achieved, even for resistant strains, with the use of high-dose penicillin or with the use of cefotaxime or ceftriaxone.

3. Lieberman D, Schlaeffer F, Boldur I, Lieberman D, Howrowitz S, Friedman MG, et al: Multiple pathogens in adult patients admitted with community-acquired pneumonia: A 1-year prospective study of 346 consecutive patients. *Thorax* 1996; 51:179-184
    This prospective study of 346 hospitalized patients with community-acquired pneumonia conducted in Israel, found a surprisingly high incidence of atypical pathogen infection in the context of identifying an etiologic diagnosis in 80.6% of all patients, a far greater number than in many similar studies. The most commonly identified pathogen was pneumococcus, but M. pneumoniae was found in 29.2%, C. pneumoniae in 17.9%, and Legionella in 16.2%. The high frequency of atypical pathogens can be explained by the careful serologic testing done and by the fact that 38.4% of all patients had more than 1 pathogen identified. Atypical

pathogens were seen in patients of all ages, and *C. pneumoniae* was found more in older patients than in those less than age 55. The implications of these findings for therapy are uncertain since only about half of the patients with atypical pathogens received specific therapy. One possible role of atypical pathogens that is discussed is as agents that potentiate the role of bacterial organisms.

4. Duchin JS, Koster FT, Peters CJ, Simpson GL, Tempest B, Zaki SR, et al: Hantavirus pulmonary syndrome: A clinical description of 17 patients with a newly recognized disease. *N Engl J Med* 1994; 330:949-955
This report describes the clinical and pathologic findings of the first 17 patients with the hantavirus pulmonary syndrome. The mean age of patients was 32.2 years, and the case fatality rate was 76%, with 88% developing rapidly progressive noncardiogenic pulmonary edema. Most patients had fever, myalgias, cough, or dyspnea, along with gastrointestinal symptoms and headache. Although hantavirus is not a new organism, this is the first description of a pulmonary syndrome resulting from this agent.

5. Mundy LM, Auwaerter PG, Oldach D, Warner ML, Burton A, Vance E, et al: Community-acquired pneumonia: Impact of immune status. *Am J Respir Crit Care Med* 1995; 152:1309-1315
In a 1-year prospective study, 385 patients with CAP at an inner-city hospital were evaluated. The study is unique because both HIV infected and nonimmune-suppressed patients were evaluated, and the impact of immune status on bacteriology was examined. In the 205 non-HIV-infected patients, pneumococcus was the most common pathogen, while H. influenzae, gram-negative bacilli, and atypical pathogens were the next most frequently identified causes of CAP, but no diagnosis was found in 37%. The distribution of pathogens was such that the authors

concluded that the ATS guidelines for CAP were appropriate for the population that they treated, and they endorsed the selective (rather than routine) use of macrolide therapy for hospitalized patients with CAP.

6. Plouffe JF, Breiman RF, Facklam RR, et al: Bacteremia with Streptococcus pneumoniae: Implications for therapy and prevention. *JAMA* 1996; 275:194-198

7. Bartlett JG, Breiman RF, Mandell LA, File TM: Community-acquired pneumonia in adults: Guidelines for management. *Clin Infect Dis* 1998; 26:811-838
New and comprehensive guidelines for CAP from the IDSA, that differ in several ways from the ATS guidelines.

8. Fine MJ, Smith MA, Carson CA, Mutha SS, Sankey SS, Weissfeld LA, Kapoor WN: Prognosis and outcomes of patients with community-acquired pneumonia: A meta-analysis. *JAMA* 1996; 275:134-141
Using 137 references, a meta-analysis of factors predicting mortality in CAP was conducted, examining 33,148 patients in 127 study cohorts. The data provide an excellent view of the epidemiology of CAP, broken down into relevant outpatient and inpatient subsets. The predictors of mortality are identified, and the impact of bacteriology on outcome is reported. By virtue of the number of patients examined, this report is a state of the art summary of the mortality impact of CAP and its determinants.

9. Ewig S, Ruiz M, Mensa J, Marcos MA, Martinez JA, Arancibia F, Niederman MS, Torres A: Severe community-acquired pneumonia: Assessment of severity criteria. *Am J Respir Crit Care Med* 1998; 158:1102-1108
Although the original ATS guidelines for CAP defined an entity termed "severe CAP," recent observations have suggested that this definition was overly inclusive, and that many patients who fit the definition did not actually need

intensive care admission. In this study of 395 patients, a modified rule for severe illness was derived from the ATS definition, because that definition (using only a single criteria for severe illness) had a specificity of only 32%. The modified rule defined the need for ICU admission as the presence of 2 of 3 "minor" criteria (systolic BP < 90 mm Hg, multilobar infiltrates, PaO2/FiO2 ratio < 250) or 1 of 2 "major" criteria (need for mechanical ventilation or septic shock). This modified definition had a sensitivity of 78% and a specificity of 94%, and a negative predictive value of 95%.

Other references

1. Marston BJ, Plouffe JF, File TM Jr, et al: Incidence of community-acquired pneumonia requiring hospitalization. Results of a population-based active surveillance Study in Ohio. The Community-Based Pneumonia Incidence Study Group. *Arch Int Med* 1997; 157:1709-1718

2. Metaly JP, Schulz R, Li Y-H, Singer DE, Marrie TJ, Coley CM, et al: Influence of age on symptoms at presentation in patients with community-acquired pneumonia. *Arch Intern Med* 1997; 157:1453-1459

3. Kauppinen MT, Saikku P, Kujala P, Herva E, Syrjala H: Clinical picture of *Chlamydia pneumoniae* requiring hospital treatment: A comparison between chlamydial and pneumococcal pneumonia. *Thorax* 1996; 51:185-189

4. Fine MJ, Auble TE, Yealy DM, et al: A prediction rule to identify low-risk patients with community-acquired pneumonia. *N Engl J Med* 1997; 336:243-250

5. Ruiz M, Ewig S, Torres A, Arancibia F, Marco F, Mensa J, Sanchez M, Martinez JA: Severe community-acquired pneumonia: Risk factors and follow-up epidemiology. *Am J Respir Crit Care Med* 1999; 160:923-929

6. Leroy O, Santre C, Beuscart C: A 5-year study of severe community-acquired pneumonia with emphasis on prognosis in patients admitted to an ICU. *Intensive Care Med* 1995; 21:24-31

7. Neill AM, Martin IR, Weir R, et al: Community-acquired pneumonia: Etiology and usefulness of severity criteria on admission. *Thorax* 1996; 51:1010-1016

REFERENCES NOSOCOMIAL PNEUMONIA

1. Campbell GD, Niederman MS, Broughton WA, Craven DE, Fein AM, Fink MP, et al: Hospital-acquired pneumonia in adults: Diagnosis, assessment of severity, initial antimicrobial therapy, and preventative strategies: A consensus statement. *Am J Respir Crit Care Med* 1996; 153:1711-1725

2. Kollef M, Shapiro SD, Fraser VJ, Silver P, Murphy DM, Trovillion E, et al: Mechanical ventilation with or without 7-day circuit changes: A randomized controlled trial. *Ann Intern Med* 1995; 123:168-174
A randomized controlled trial of 300 mechanically-ventilated patients admitted to an ICU for more than 5 days evaluated the routine changing of ventilator circuits every 7 days versus no routine changes. Ventilator-associated pneumonia was diagnosed using clinical criteria and occurred in 24.5% of patients receiving no routine changes and in 28.8% of patients receiving routine changes. Mortality rates were comparable in both groups, but the failure to routinely change tubing was associated with substantial cost savings.

3. Rouby JJ, Laurent P, Gosnach M, Cambau E, Lamas G, Zouaqui A, et al: Risk factors and clinical relevance of nosocomial maxillary sinusitis in the critically ill. *Am J Respir Crit Care Med* 1994; 150:776-783

A prospective study of 162 patients mechanically ventilated for more than 7 days evaluated the incidence of nosocomial sinsusitis and the influence of inserting tracheal and gastric tubes through the nose rather than through the mouth. In patients who did not start with radiographic maxillary sinusitis, the use of oral or nasal tubes was selected randomly. Those who had nasal tubes inserted had a 95.5% incidence of sinusitis, while those who had oral tubes had a 22.5% incidence of radiographic sinusitis. The relevance of sinusitis was shown by the finding that 67% of patients with bacteriologically-confirmed infectious sinusitis also developed nosocomial pneumonia.

4. Vallés J, Artigas A, Rello J, Bonsoms N, Fantanals D, Blanch L, et al: Continuous aspiration of subglottic secretions in preventing ventilator-associated pneumonia. *Ann Intern Med* 1995; 122:179-186

In a randomized, controlled, and blinded study, 76 patients were managed with an endotracheal tube that allowed for the continuous aspiration of subglottic secretions (CASS), while 77 were managed with conventional endotracheal tubes. The use of CASS was associated with a significant (p < 0.03) reduction in the incidence of nosocomial pneumonia and a reduction in the number of infections due to gram-positive cocci and H. influenzae, but no difference in the number of infections caused by P. aeruginosa or other resistant gram-negatives. When pneumonia developed, it occurred later in CASS patients than in control patients. The simplicity of this method for pneumonia prevention is very appealing, and contrasts with other more complex and less effective methods, as pointed out in the accompanying editorial.

5. Prod'hom G, Leuenberger P, Koerfer J, Blum A, Chiolero R, Schaller MD, et al: Nosocomial pneumonia in mechanically ventilated patients receiving antiacid, ranitidine, or sucralfate as prophylaxis for stress ulcer: A randomized controlled trial. *Ann Intern Med* 1994; 120:653-662

In a randomized controlled trial, intubated ICU patients were given intestinal bleeding prophylaxis with antacids (n = 81), a continuous infusion of ranitidine (n = 80) or sucralfate (n = 83). Bleeding rates were identical with each regimen (p > 0.2), and the rates of early-onset nosocomial pneumonia were also similar. However, patients who received sucralfate had a markedly reduced incidence (5%) of late-onset pneumonia compared to patients who received other regimens (P = 0.022). The distinction between early- and late-onset pneumonia that was made in this study had implications for prevention strategies and also had relevance to bacteriology, with the pathogens responsible for each type of pneumonia being dramatically different.

6. Niederman MS, Torres A, Summer W: Invasive diagnostic testing is not needed routinely to manage suspected ventilator-associated pneumonia. *Am J Respir Crit Care Med* 1994; 150:565-569

This editorial critically reviews the literature relevant to the use of invasive methods (bronchoscopic lavage and brushing) for the diagnosis of ventilator-associated pneumonia. The authors conclude that invasive methods should not replace clinical judgment in deciding when to use antibiotics for suspected nosocomial pneumonia. Problems with invasive methods include the possibility of overlooking early forms of infection and the inaccuracy of the methods in patients who are already receiving antibiotics. An opposing editorial opinion accompanies this article and argues in favor of invasive methods.

7. Hatala R, Dinh T, Cook DJ: Once-daily aminoglycoside dosing in immunocompetent adults: A meta-

analysis. *Ann Intern Med* 1996; 124:717-725

8. Cometta A, Baumgartner JD, Lew D, et al: Prosptective randomized comparison of imipenem monotherapy with imipenem plus netilmicin for treatment of severe infections in nonneutropenic patients. *Antimicrobial Agents and Chemotherapy* 1994; 38:1309-1313

9. Lowenkron SE, Niederman MS: Definition and evaluation of the resolution of nosocomial pneumonia. Seminars in Respiratory Infections. 1992; 7:271-281

10. Hilf M, Yu VL, Sharp J, Zuravleff JJ, Korvick JA, Muder RR: Antibiotic therapy for *Pseudomonas aeruginosa* bacteremia: Outcome correlations in a prospective study of 200 patients. *Am J Med* 1989; 87:540-546

11. Kollef MH, Silver P, Murphy DM, Trovillion E: The effect of late-onset ventilator-associated pneumonia in determining patient mortality. *Chest* 1995; 108:1655-1662

12. Fagon JY, Chastre J, Vaugnat A, Trouillet JL, Novara A, Gibert C: Nosocomial pneumonia and mortality among patients in intensive care units. *JAMA* 1996; 275:866-869
The 1,978 consecutive patients admitted to the ICU were evaluated to define the incidence of nosocomial pneumonia and its impact on mortality by using a logistic regression model. Among the 16.6% who developed pneumonia, mortality was 52.4%, compared to a mortality of 22.4% in patients without pneumonia. These data led the authors to conclude that pneumonia does lead to the death of critically ill patients having an "attributable mortality," but the findings are not in agreement with the conclusions of other investigators, and the controversy associated with this issue is discussed.

Other references

1. Richards MJ, Edwards JR, Culver DH, Gaynes RP, et al: Nosocomial infections

in medical intensive care units in the United States. *Crit Care Med* 1999; 27:887-892

2. Holzapfel L, Chastang C, Demingeon G, Bohe J, Pirilla B, Courpry A: A randomized study assessing the systematic search for maxillary sinusitis in nasotracheally mechanically-ventilated patients: Influence of nosocomial maxillary sinusitis on the occurrence of ventilator-associated pneumonia. *Am J Respir Crit Care Med* 1999; 159:695-701

3. Marik PE, Careau P: The role of anaerobes in patients with ventilator–associated pneumonia and aspiration pneumonia: A prospective study. *Chest* 1999; 115:178-183

4. Joshi M, Bernstein J, Solomkin J, Wester BA, Kuye O, et al: Piperacillin/tazobactam plus tobramycin versus ceftazadime plus tobramycin for the treatment of patients with nosocomial lower respiratory tract infections. *J Antimicrob Chemother* 1999; 43:389-397

5. Jaccard C, Troillet N, Harbarth S, Zanetti G, Aymon D, Schneider R, et al: Prospective randomized comparison of imipenem-cilastatin and piperacillin-tazobactam in nosocomial pneumonia or peritonitis. *Antimicrobial Agents and Chemotherapy* 1998; 42:2966-2972

6. Kollef M: Inadequate antimicrobial treatment: An important determinant of outcome for hospitalized patients. *Clin Infect Dis* 2000; 31(Suppl 4):S131-S138

7. Sachez-Nieto JM, Torres A, Garcia-Cordoba F, El-Ebiary M, Carrillo A, Ruiz J, Nunez ML, Niederman M: Impact of invasive and noninvasive quantitative culture sampling on outcome of ventilator-associated pneumonia. *Am J Crit Care Med* 1998; 157:371-376

8. Fagon JY, Chastre J, Wolff M, Gervais C, Parer-Aubas S, Stephan F, Similowski T, et al: Invasive and noninvasive strategies for management of suspected ventilator-associated

pneumonia: A randomized trial. *Ann Intern Med* 2000; 132:621-630

9. Luna CM, Vujacich P, Niederman MS, et al: Impact of BAL data on the therapy and outcome of ventilator associated pneumonia. *Chest* 1997; 111:676-685

10. Kollef MH, Sherman G, Ward S, Fraser VJ: Inadequate antimicrobial treatment of infections: A risk factor for hospital mortality among critically ill patients. *Chest* 1999; 115:462-474

11. Rello J, Sa-Borges M, Correa H, Leal SR, Baraibar J: Variations in etiology of ventilator-associated pneumonia across 4 treatment sites: Implications for antimicrobial prescribing practices. *Am J Respir Crit Care Med* 1999; 160:608-613

12. Singh N, Rogers P, Atwood CW, Wagener MM, Yu VL: Short–course empiric antibiotic therapy for patients with pulmonary infiltrates in the intensive care unit: A proposed solution for indiscriminate antibiotic prescription. *Am J Respir Crit Care Med* 2000; 162:505-511

INFECTIONS IN AIDS PATIENTS AND OTHER IMMUNOCOMPROMISED HOSTS

George H. Karam, MD, FCCP

Objectives

- To propose an approach to the immunocompromised patient based on identification of defects in 3 major host defense systems
- To review the likely pathogens, their clinical presentations, and therapeutic options in patients with neutropenia
- To summarize the various limbs in humoral immunity, with particular attention to the clinical situations of asplenia and splenic dysfunction
- To outline the categories and clinical presentations of pathogens likely to be encountered with deficits of cell-mediated immunity
- To focus on the broadening number of clinical issues in patients whose cell-mediated immunity defect is on the basis of HIV infection

Key Words: neutropenia; humoral immunity; asplenia; cell-mediated immunity; human immunodeficiency virus

TABLE OF ABBREVIATIONS

CMV	cytomegalovirus
CSF	colony-stimulating factor
CVI	common variable immunodeficiency
ESBL	extended-spectrum β-lactamases
HIV	human immunodeficiency virus
IDSA	Infectious Diseases Society of America
IL	interleukin
MAC	*Mycobacterium avium* Complex
MRSA	methicillin-resistant *Staphylococcus aureus*
NEC	neutropenic enterocolitis

INTRODUCTION

In the clinical approach to patients with fever presumed to be infectious in etiology, a basic consideration is whether the patient is a normal host or one who is immunocompromised. A traditional method has been to consider host defense in immunocompromised patients as being in 1 of 2 categories: a) mechanical factors, including barrier systems such as skin and mucous membranes (which are protective against infection) or foreign bodies such as intravascular and urinary catheters (which predispose to infection); and b) cellular host defense, which includes the 3 major categories of primary neutrophil defense, humoral immunity, and cell-mediated immunity. Use of an approach that identifies the defective limb of host defense allows for directed therapeutic decisions that are based on likely pathogens for the involved site.

Recent attention has been focused on the concept of type 1 and type 2 immunity as they interrelate with humoral and cell-mediated immunity (*Clin Infect Dis* 2001; 32:76-102). Subpopulations of CD4$^+$ lymphocytes are important in both humoral immunity and cell-mediated immunity, with T helper type 1 (Th1) and T helper type 2 (Th2) cells being the most relevant. All T helper lymphocytes start out as naive Th0 cells, which, after being activated, are capable of "polarizing" or differentiating into either Th1 or Th2 effector cells. Although multiple factors are involved, the key to polarization of Th0 cells into the Th1 phenotype is interleukin-12 (IL-12), whereas interleukin-4 (IL-4) is needed for Th2 polarization. These events may not occur until an activated T cell arrives at the site of danger and samples the local cytokine milieu to determine if an inflammatory or antibody response is appropriate. In questionable circumstances, the Th2 outcome is favored over the Th1 differentiation since IL-4 dominates IL-12. Th1 cells, which are involved with type 1 immunity, secrete interferon-gamma (IFN-γ), IL-2, and lymphotoxin-α as the cytokines chiefly responsible for their proinflammatory effect. The Th1 cell is associated with strong cell-mediated immunity and weak humoral immunity. Th2 cells are involved with type 2 immunity, are influenced by IL-4, IL-10, and IL-13, stimulate high titers of antibody production, and are associated with suppression of cell-mediated immunity and with strong humoral immunity. When integrated into the traditional approach of cell-mediated immunity and humoral immunity, type 1 and type 2 immunity have important therapeutic implications in the care provided for immunocompromised patients.

PRIMARY NEUTROPHIL FUNCTION

The polymorphonuclear leukocyte is the major phagocyte for both primary neutrophil defense and humoral immunity. Once a pathogen is ingested by these cells and is intracellular, killing is generally an easy process. Pathogens that classically infect patients with primary neutrophil problems are those that may be ingested without opsonization. The system of neutrophil defense has been described as being responsible for defending against organisms that are easy to eat and easy to kill.

An important pathophysiologic consideration is that polymorphonuclear leukocytes may have either an extravascular or intravascular location. After leaving the bloodstream, these phagocytes go to 2 major sites: the subepithelial area of skin and the submucosal area of the gastrointestinal tract. Recognition of this fact allows for an understanding of the organisms that classically infect neutropenic patients.

As represented in Table 1, neutrophil dysfunction may occur on either a qualitative or quantitative basis. Qualitative defects characteristically occur in children and are associated with polymorphonuclear leukocytes that are normal in number but abnormal in function. Classic qualitative defects of polymorphonuclear leukocytes are related to dysfunction in one of the following processes: a) diapedesis (the ability to leave the intravascular space via endothelial channels); b) chemotaxis (movement to the site of infection); c) ingestion (the process of attaching to the pathogen and then getting that pathogen within the cell, where killing takes place); and d) intracellular killing (which may occur via either oxygen-dependent or oxygen-independent mechanisms).

Quantitative defects, which are the more characteristic neutrophil problems in adults, clinically present as the entity interchangeably referred to as either granulocytopenia or neutropenia. Characteristic conditions that may lead to neutropenia are listed in Table 1. Although eosinophils are classified as granulocytes, for most clinical purposes the granulocyte count is calculated by added the percentage of polymorphonuclear leukocytes and band forms, and then multiplying the total white blood cell count by that percentage. In the guidelines of the Infectious Diseases Society of America (IDSA) for management of febrile, neutropenic patients, a calculated granulocyte count of <500/mm^3 indicates absolute neutropenia; a granulocyte count <1,000 cells/mm^3 with a predicted decline to <500/mm^3 should be considered neutropenia (*Clin Infect Dis* 2002; 34:730-751). In the setting of neutropenia and fever, the clinician must assume that the patient has impaired natural defense against the pathogens defended against by this limb of host defense.

The clinical course of patients with neutropenia is variable and may be explained in part by the integrity of the gut mucosa. In conditions such as aplastic anemia or HIV-associated neutropenia, the gut mucosa is usually intact, and those patients have a lower incidence of bacteremia. In contrast, patients who receive chemotherapeutic agents that cause mucositis have loss both of the mechanical barrier of gut mucosa and of submucosal polymorphonuclear leukocytes. These patients are more likely to experience Gram-negative bacteremia and fungemia.

Infections due to bacteria are classically encountered when the neutropenia is either rapid in development or profound (especially with counts <100 cells/mm^3). The pathogens most likely to infect neutropenic patients are listed in Table 2. The bacteria characteristically involved are skin and gut flora, as might be predicted

Table 1. Conditions causing neutrophil dysfunction

Qualitative Defects	Quantitative Defects (Neutropenia)
Impaired diapedesis	Acute leukemia
Impaired chemotaxis	Invasion of bone marrow by neoplasms
Impaired ingestion	Treatment with agents toxic to marrow
Impaired intracellular killing	Drug idiosyncracy
	Splenic sequestration syndromes
	HIV-associated neutropenia
	Idiopathic chronic neutropenia

from the loss of subepithelial and submucosal polymorphonuclear leukocytes. Although any of the enterobacteriaceae (e.g., *Escherichia coli* or *Klebsiella*) may cause infection in this setting, the most life-threatening pathogen is *Pseudomonas aeruginosa*. Because of this (and despite the relative decline in the incidence of infection caused by this pathogen in neutropenic patients), a basic principle in empiric therapy of febrile neutropenic patients is coverage of *P. aeruginosa*. The classic skin lesion that suggests such an infection is ecthyma gangrenosum. These lesions have a central area of hemorrhage surrounded by a halo of uninvolved skin with a narrow pink or purple rim. Histologically, the infection involves dermal veins, and clinically it may progress to bullae formation. Although other Gram-negative pathogens have been reported to cause such a process, the clinician should assume that ecthyma gangrenosum is caused by *P. aeruginosa* until this pathogen has been excluded.

In recent years, infections caused by Gram-positive organisms have significantly increased in neutropenic patients. These pathogens, which are listed in Table 2, have increased in part because of the expanded use of invasive devices like intravascular catheters, which breach the mechanical barrier of the skin. The important clinical finding of cavitary pulmonary infiltrates may be a clue to infection by either *Staphylococcus aureus* or *Corynebacterium jeikeium*. Notable among the Gram-positive pathogens is infection caused by viridans streptococci (e.g., *Streptococcus mitis*), which may result in the viridans streptococcal shock syndrome. In a recent prospective study of

485 episodes of bacteremia in neutropenic patients with cancer (*Clin Infect Dis* 2000; 31:1126-1130), viridans streptococci caused a total of 88 episodes (18%). Ten (11%) of these 88 cases were associated with serious complications, including acute respiratory distress syndrome (ARDS) plus septic shock (5 cases), ARDS (3 cases), and septic shock (2 cases). Of the patients with serious complications of their streptococcal bacteremia, 3 (30%) had a cutaneous rash, which in other reports has been associated on occasion with desquamation. Severe oral mucositis, high-dose chemotherapy with cyclophosphamide, and allogeneic bone marrow transplantation were the only variables found to be significantly associated with the development of complications. Of the patients with complications, 36% showed diminished susceptibility to penicillin, and approximately one-half were resistant to ceftazidime. Because of less predictable coverage against Gram-positive organisms, this process has been described in other reports to occur with an increased incidence in neutropenic patients who have received the prophylactic administration of trimethoprim/sulfamethoxazole or a fluoroquinolone.

A life-threatening complication that may occur in patients who have received chemotherapy is neutropenic enterocolitis (NEC). Previously referred to as typhlitis because of the cecum as the predominant site in many cases, NEC may involve the terminal ileum, the cecum, and the colon (with the ascending portion the most frequently involved). Pathogenetically, the process may occur on

Table 2. Important pathogens causing infection in neutropenic patients

---

Gram-positive organisms
        Staphylococcus aureus
        Coagulase-negative staphylococci
        Enterococci
        Viridans streptococci
        Corynebacterium jeikeium

Enterobacteriaceae

Pseudomonas aeruginosa

Anaerobes, including *Bacteroides fragilis*

Fungi
        Yeasts, most notably *Candida* species
        Filamentous fungi, most notably
        Aspergillus

---

several bases including destruction of gastrointestinal mucosa by chemotherapy, intramural hemorrhage due to severe thrombocytopenia, and alterations in gastrointestinal tract flora. Patients characteristically present with the triad of fever, abdominal pain, and diarrhea, but these findings may be seen with other conditions including *Clostridium difficile* toxin-induced colitis and ischemic colitis. Ultrasound findings include echogenic thickening of the mucosa and bowel wall. Although isodense cecal wall thickening is the most notable computer tomographic finding, the distal ileum and remaining colon are also frequently involved. Although optimal therapy has not been definitively established, conservative medical management appears to be effective for most patients (*Clin Infect Dis* 1998; 27:695-699).

Although the level of temperature elevation which mandates antimicrobial therapy in neutropenic patients may be influenced by the degree of neutropenia, fever in neutropenic patients has been defined as a single oral temperature of >38.5°C (101°F) or as a temperature of ≥38.0°C (100.4°F) over at least 1 hour. In such patients, empiric antibiotics should be started after appropriate cultures are obtained. Because the patients do not have adequate neutrophils to provide natural host defense, all antimicrobial agents administered should be bactericidal. The classic regimen has been an antipseudomonal β-lactam antibiotic (e.g., piperacillin or ceftazidime) in combination with an aminoglycoside. Although some centers acknowledge a decreasing prevalence of infection caused by *Pseudomonas aeruginosa*, the recommendation for coverage against this pathogen in febrile neutropenic patients is prompted by the higher rates of mortality that may occur when this pathogen infects neutropenic patients. A review of 410 episodes of *Pseudomonas* bacteremia in patients with cancer identified that outcome was related to the interval between the onset of the bacteremia and the institution of appropriate therapy (*Arch Intern Med* 1985; 145:1621-1629). In neutropenic patients in this study who had *P. aeruginosa* bacteremia and in whom therapy was delayed, 26% died within 24 hours and 70% died within 48 hours.

Influenced by multiple factors, including the potential for acute mortality in neutropenic patients who are bacteremic with *P. aeruginosa*, the IDSA has in its most recent recommendations for management of febrile neutropenic patients (*Clin Infect Dis* 2002; 34:730-751) offered suggestions for empiric antimicrobial therapy. In these recommendations, it was noted that the initial evaluation should determine 1) whether the patient is at low risk for complications (with the specifics defined in these guidelines), and 2) whether vancomycin therapy is needed. For low-risk adults only, an oral regimen using ciprofloxacin plus amoxicillin-clavunate was suggested. Options in patients for monotherapy with vancomycin not being needed include 1 of the following agents: cefepime or ceftazidime; or imipenem or meropenem. Options for combination therapy were an aminoglycoside plus an antipseudomonal penicillin, cephalosporin (cefepime or ceftazidime), or carbapenem. In those patients in whom vancomycin is indicated (discussed in the following paragraph), 3 options were presented: cefepime or ceftazidime plus vancomycin, with or without an aminoglycoside; carbapenem plus vancomycin, with or without an aminoglycoside; or an antipseudomonal penicillin plus an aminoglycoside and vancomycin. Prior to the publication of the 2002 IDSA guidelines, a prospective, multicenter, double-blind, randomized clinical trial has shown that piperacillin-tazobactam given as monotherapy was as effective as the combination of piperacillin-tazobactam plus amikacin for the treatment for adults who were febrile and neutropenic (*Clin Infect Dis* 2001; 33:1445-1452). Even though an antipseudomonal penicillin was offered as an option in the 2002 IDSA guidelines for combination therapy without vancomycin and for therapy in which vancomycin was indicated, it was not presented as an option for monotherapy when vancomycin was not indicated.

Two recent patterns of resistance may influence the choice of therapy for febrile neutropenic patients. An ongoing controversy remains regarding whether an agent like vancomycin, which would cover such pathogens as methicillin-resistant *Staphylococcus aureus* (MRSA), penicillin- and cephalosporin-resistant *Streptococcus pneumoniae*, and *Corynebacterium jeikeium*, should be included in the initial regimen. Because of the risk of selecting vancomycin-resistant enterococci or vancomycin-resistant staphylococci with injudicious use of vancomycin, the IDSA guidelines for management of febrile neutropenic patients discouraged vancomycin use in routine empiric therapy for a febrile neutropenic patient and has recommended that this agent be used in the following settings: a): clinically suspected serious catheter-related infections (e.g., bacteremia, cellulitis); b) known colonization with methicillin-resistant *S. aureus* or penicillin- and cephalosporin-resistant *Streptococcus pneumoniae*; c) positive results of blood cultures for gram-positive bacteria before final identification and susceptibility testing; and d) hypotension or other evidence of cardiovascular impairment.

Published in the *Journal of Clinical Oncology* (2000; 18:3558-3585) are the most recent guidelines of the American Society of Clinical Oncology (SGO) for colony-stimulating factors (CSFs). Clinical situations for which recommendations were made in adults include the following: a) when the expected incidence of neutropenia is ≥40% (although there are some special circumstances detailed in the SGO

guidelines that might be a valid exception); b) as adjuncts to progenitor-cell transplantation; c) after completion of induction chemotherapy in patients ≥55 years of age who have acute myeloid leukemia (AML); and d) after completion of the first few days of chemotherapy of the initial induction or first postremission course in patients with acute lymphoblastic leukemia (ALL). In the 1996 guidelines of the SGO, CSFs were recommended after documented febrile neutropenia in a prior chemotherapy cycle to avoid infectious complications and maintain dose-intensity in subsequent treatment cycles when chemotherapy dose-reduction is not appropriate (*J Clin Oncol* 1996; 14:1957-1960). This was modified in the 2000 guidelines since there are no published regimens that have demonstrated disease-free or overall survival benefits when the dose of chemotherapy was maintained and secondary prophylaxis was instituted. Based on these data, it was recommended in the setting of many tumors exclusive of curable tumors (e.g., germ cell tumors) that dose reduction after an episode of severe neutropenia should be considered as a primary therapeutic option. CSFs should be avoided in patients receiving concomitant chemotherapy and radiation therapy, particularly involving the mediastinum. Since no large-scale prospective, comparative trials evaluating the relative efficacy of G-CSF versus GM-CSF are available, guidelines about equivalency of these preparations were not proposed. Certain patients with fever and neutropenia are at higher risk for infection-associated complications and have prognostic factors that are predictive of poor clinical outcome. The use of a CSF for such high-risk patients may be considered, but the benefits of a CSF in these circumstances have not been proven. Potential clinical factors mentioned in the 2000 guidelines include profound (ANC<100/μL) neutropenia, uncontrolled primary disease, pneumonia, hypotension, multiorgan dysfunction (sepsis syndrome), and invasive fungal infection. Age greater than 65 years and posttreatment lymphopenia were mentioned as potentially being other high-risk factors, but it was acknowledged that these have not been consistently confirmed by multicenter trials.

A major predisposition to fungal infection is prolonged neutropenia. Although the list of fungal organisms identified in neutropenic patients has increased significantly in recent years, the most important pathogens to consider are *Candida* species and *Aspergillus* species. On the basis of neutropenia, indwelling catheters, broad-spectrum antibiotics, and mucositis, neutropenic patients are at risk for candidemia. The clinical presentation may range from unexplained fever to a septic appearance. Autopsy series have suggested that as many as 50% of patients with evidence of metastatic candidal infections in visceral organs may have had negative antemortem blood cultures for *Candida*. The characteristic clinical infection in this setting is chronic disseminated candidiasis, which has also been referred to as hepatosplenic candidiasis. This illness may present as unexplained fever, right upper quadrant tenderness, and elevated alkaline phosphatase. During the period of neutropenia, imaging studies may be negative, but as the granulocyte count improves, patients may demonstrate bull's-eye liver lesions on ultrasound and hypodense liver defects on abdominal CT scan.

Aspergillus is a nosocomial pathogen, which may be associated with vascular invasion and extensive tissue necrosis. The lungs are a prime site of infection, with a spectrum of disease that includes pulmonary infiltrates or cavitary lung lesions. Infection of the paranasal sinuses and central nervous system may also occur (*Medicine* 2000; 79:250-260). Because of the nosocomial nature of this organism, it may be introduced into the skin with catheter insertion. With the lack of both intravascular and subepithelial polymorphonuclear leukocytes, and because of the vascular invasion, the skin lesions may be concentrically enlarging and necrotic. Blood cultures are not likely to reveal this pathogen.

There is not a consensus recommendation about when empirical antifungal therapy should be started for neutropenic patients who have persistent fever. The clinical guidelines of the IDSA for treatment of infections caused by *Candida* suggest using persistent unexplained fever despite 4-6 days of appropriate antibacterial therapy *(Clin Infect Dis* 2000; 30:662-678), but

the IDSA guidelines for therapy in febrile neutropenic patients suggest beginning empirical antifungal treatment when there is persistent fever for >3 days after antibacterial therapy is instituted in patients expected to have neutropenia for longer than 5-7 more days (*Clin Infect Dis* 2002; 34:730-751). Since amphotericin B has activity against most *Candida* species as well as *Aspergillus*, it has been the agent most often used. Liposomal amphotericin B has been shown to be as effective as conventional amphotericin B for empirical antifungal therapy in patients with fever and neutropenia, and it is associated with fewer breakthrough fungal infections, less infusion-related toxicity, and less nephrotoxicity (*N Engl J Med* 1999; 340:764-771). More recently, a randomized, international, multicenter trial found that voriconazole (a new second-generation triazole with both *Aspergillus* and *Candida* activity) was comparable to liposomal amphotericin B for empirical antifungal therapy and was noted to be a suitable alternative (*N Engl J Med* 2002; 346:225-234). A statistically significant noteworthy observation in this report was that patients receiving voriconazole had more episodes of transient visual changes (22%) than did those receiving liposomal amphotericin B (1%).

Table 3. Major clinical situations resulting in disorder of immunoglobulin production

---

Congenital agammaglobulinemias
Common variable immunodeficiency (acquired hypogammaglobulinemia)
Multiple myeloma
Waldenstrom's macroglobulinemia
Heavy chain disease
B-cell lymphomas
Chronic lymphocytic leukemia
T-cell deficiency states
Hyposplenic states

HUMORAL IMMUNITY

For certain organisms to be ingested by polymorphonuclear leukocytes, there is a requirement that those organisms undergo opsonization, a process in which organisms are encased by a factor which then allows the phagocyte to attach. Once intracellular, these organisms are readily killed by the phagocyte. The humoral immune system provides for such opsonization through its major components of antibody and complement and may be summarized as providing protection against pathogens that are hard to eat but easy to kill.

The antibody component of humoral immunity is dependent on the transformation of B lymphocytes into plasma cells, which produce as major opsonins IgG and IgM. A structural part of these antibodies is a component referred to as the Fc segment. Polymorphonuclear leukocytes have a receptor for this Fc segment. These Fc segments attach to the Fc receptor on the phagocyte, allowing the polymorphonuclear leukocyte to ingest the organism in a process that has been referred to as the "zipper" phenomenon of phagocytosis.

In addition to antibody, complement may serve as an opsonizer. Of the various complement components, the one most important for opsonization is C3b, which may be generated through 2 different pathways. In the classic complement pathway, the formation of antigen-antibody complexes turns on the complement cascade. Once C3 is activated, it is cleaved by C3 esterase to yield C3b. A limitation of the classic complement pathway is the requirement for antibody production, which may take hours to develop. In situations such as the acute development of pneumococcal infection, there is an immediate need for host defense that cannot wait for antibody production. It is in this setting that the alternative complement pathway (also known as the properdin system) becomes important. Instead of requiring an antigen-antibody complex to turn on the cascade, the alternative pathway is dependent on cell wall components such as teichoic acid and peptidoglycans found in Gram-positive organisms and lipopolysaccharides found in Gram-negative organisms. These lead to proteolytic cleavage of C3 to generate C3b, and this mechanism can lead to immediate opsonization. Clinically important is the fact that this alternative complement pathway is housed in the spleen and will therefore be deficient or absent in patients with splenic absence or hypofunction.

Within the category of defective humoral immunity are 4 clinically relevant situations: a) disorders of immunoglobulin production; b) asplenia or hyposplenic states; c) hypocomplementemia; and d) impaired neutralization of toxins.

The major clinical situations that result in disorders of immunoglobulin production are summarized in Table 3. Included in these processes is the lack of B cell regulation, with its resultant production of abnormal immunoglobulins, which occurs on the basis of T-cell deficiency states in conditions such as HIV infection.

The characteristic pathogens infecting patients with impairment of immunoglobulin production are included in Table 4. Of the bacteria, the common feature is encapsulation, with the capsule essentially making them slippery and therefore dependent on opsonization for phagocyte attachment. Of the pathogens defended against by humoral immunity, the 1 that most frequently causes an acute life-threatening infection is *Streptococcus pneumoniae*. In recent years, it has been noted that the severity of infection with *Str. pneumoniae* may be accentuated in patients with alcoholism or in those who are HIV-infected. In both patient groups, this pathogen may initially present as the etiologic agent of community-acquired pneumonia, which may be multilobar, with a high incidence of bacteremia and an increased risk of acute respiratory distress syndrome. An important consideration regarding infection with this pathogen is the increasing prevalence of penicillin resistance. Despite appropriate antibiotics and supportive care, the mortality in this setting remains high.

Also included among the pathogens that infect patients with defects in immunoglobulin production are certain viruses, including enteroviruses, influenza viruses, and arboviruses. Enteroviruses, particularly echovirus 24, have been associated with a clinical complex consisting of dermatomyositis-like skin lesions, edema, and neurologic problems. This has been referred to as chronic enteroviral meningoencephalitis.

Table 4. Pathogens in patients with defective humoral immunity

Disorders of Immunoglobulin Production	Asplenic State or Splenic Dysfunction
Streptococcus pneumoniae	*Streptococcus pneumoniae*
Haemophilus influenzae	*Capnocytophaga canimorsus*
Encapsulated strains of gram-negative bacilli	(DF-2; Dysgonic Fermenter-2)
Enteroviruses, particularly echovirus 24	*Babesia microti*
Influenza viruses	*Plasmodium species*
Arboviruses	*Haemophilus influenzae*
Pneumocystis carinii	*Neisseria* species
Giardia lamblia	

Common variable immunodeficiency (CVI) is associated with functional abnormalities of both B and T cells, but is usually classified as a primary antibody deficiency syndrome. Characterized by hypogammaglobulinemia and recurrent bacterial infections, CVI usually does not become clinically apparent until the second or third decade of life. Affected patients have an increased risk of autoimmune, granulomatous, and lymphoproliferative diseases. Even though recurrent bacterial infections of the respiratory tract are the most common, diarrhea due to *Giardia lamblia* is frequently encountered. This reflects the importance of local immunoglobulin production in the gastrointestinal tract as a component of defense against *Giardia lamblia*. Since some of the common pathogens infecting the respiratory or gastrointestinal tracts are dependent on antibody production for host defense, concomitant infection of these 2 body sites should raise the suspicion of immunoglobulin deficiency states such as CVI. Intravenous immunoglobulin may be efficacious in patients with this clinical entity, but anaphylaxis with such therapy has been reported. Anatomic asplenia, as well as the hyposplenic states which occur in persons with sickle cell disease (due to autoinfarction of the spleen) and in patients with Hodgkin's disease (especially after therapy), are also important predispositions to infection. The propensity for infection in these patients occurs on the basis of impairment of several immunologic functions: a) Relative to other lymphoid organs, the spleen

has a greater percentage of B lymphocytes and is therefore involved in the production of antibody to polysaccharide antigens, b) The spleen participates as a phagocytic organ, removing opsonin-coated organisms or damaged cells from the circulation, and c) Alternative complement pathway components are provided by the spleen. An important clinical clue to heighten awareness of both functional and anatomic asplenia is the presence of Howell-Jolly bodies on the peripheral blood smear.

The important pathogens involved in infections in patients without a spleen or with splenic dysfunction are summarized in Table 4. Responsible for about 80% of overwhelming infections in asplenic patients (*Infect Med* 1996; 13:779-783), *Streptococcus pneumoniae* should be given a particularly high index of suspicion since the clinical entity of post-splenectomy pneumococcal sepsis may initially present as only a flu-like illness with fever and myalgias. Within the course of a few hours, untreated patients may develop a fulminant course that includes disseminated intravascular coagulation, purpura fulminans, symmetrical peripheral gangrene, shock, and ultimately death. Although *Streptococcus pneumoniae* and *Haemophilus influenzae* are pathogens encountered in patients with either disorders of immunoglobulin production or splenic dysfunction, the pathogens infecting the asplenic or hyposplenic patient are otherwise different. Included are 2 pathogens, *Babesia microti* and *Plasmodium* species, which infect erythrocytes to cause hemolytic states and which require removal of parasitized red blood

Table 5. Important clinical situations associated with defects in cell-mediated immunity

Aging
During and following certain viral illnesses
Thymic dysplasia
Sarcoidosis
Congenital situations associated with defects in cell-mediated immunity
Third-trimester pregnancy
Lymphatic malignancies of T-cell origin
Immunosuppressive therapy, especially corticosteroids and cyclosporine
AIDS and HIV-related disorders

cells by the spleen as a protective defense. *Capnocytophaga canimorsus* (formerly Dysgonic Fermenter-2, or DF-2) produces an acute illness with eschar formation following dog bites to asplenic individuals.

Patients with deficiencies in the late complement components (C5 through C8) may present with recurrent *Neisseria* species infections. The total hemolytic complement (CH_{50}) is the best screening test for this population. If the assay is normal, one can essentially exclude complement deficiency. In addition, an X-linked properdin deficiency associated with absence of the alternative complement pathway may produce a similar picture of severe meningococcal disease.

Completing the spectrum of clinical problems that may occur on the basis of defective humoral immunity is less-than-optimal neutralization of toxins produced in diphtheria, tetanus, and botulism.

Intravenous gammaglobulin is a polyvalent antibody product that contains the IgG antibodies which regularly occur in the donor population as well as traces of IgA and IgM and immunoglobulin fragments. Its half-life of 3 weeks allows for once-monthly dosing for prophylaxis in patients with primary humoral immunodeficiency. For bone marrow transplant patients ≥20 years of age, it has been shown to decrease the risk of septicemia and certain other infections, including interstitial pneumonia, in the first 100 days posttransplant. In this patient population, dosing is more frequent than in prophylaxis for primary humoral immunodeficiency. Contraindications to its use

include selective IgA deficiency and severe systemic reactions to human immune globulin.

Prevention of disease with vaccine is important in patients with defects in humoral immunity, although responses to vaccine may be attenuated. Included among those adults for whom the 23-valent pneumococcal vaccine is recommended are persons with functional or anatomic asplenia, chronic cardiovascular disease, chronic pulmonary disease, diabetes mellitus, alcoholism, chronic liver disease, cerebrospinal fluid leaks, and immunocompromised states including malignancy and HIV infection. In a recent review by the Centers for Disease Control and Prevention (*MMWR* 1997; 46[RR-8]:1-24), revaccination once was recommended for 2 groups: a) persons age ≥2 years who are at highest risk for serious pneumococcal infection and those who are likely to have a rapid decline in pneumococcal antibody levels (e.g., functional or anatomic asplenia, HIV infection, leukemia, lymphoma, Hodgkins disease, multiple myeloma, generalized malignancy, chronic renal failure, nephrotic syndrome, other conditions associated with immunosuppression [including transplantation], and those receiving immunosuppresive chemotherapy [including steroids]), provided that 5 years have elapsed since receipt of the first dose of pneumococcal vaccine; and b) persons aged ≥65 years if they received the vaccine 5 years previously and were <65 years old at the time of the primary vaccination. Routine vaccination with the quadravalent *Neisseria meningitidis* vaccine is recommended for certain high-risk groups, including persons who have terminal complement component deficiencies and those who have anatomic or functional asplenia (*MMWR* 2000; 49[RR-7]:1-20). Although the need for revaccination of adults has not been determined, antibody levels to *N. meningitidis* rapidly decline over 2-3 years, and revaccination may be considered 3-5 years after receipt of the initial dose. Prophylaxis against meningococcal infection may be with rifampin (600 mg orally every 12 hours for 2 days), ciprofloxacin (500 mg orally as single dose), or ceftriaxone (250 mg intramuscularly as a single dose). *Haemophilus influenzae* B (Hib) vaccines are immunogenic in splenectomized adults and may be considered for this group (*MMWR* 1993; 42([R-4]:1-12). When elective splenectomy is planned, pneumococcal, meningococcal, and Hib vaccination should precede surgery by at least 2 weeks, if possible.

CELL-MEDIATED IMMUNITY

The cell-mediated immune system is dependent on the interrelationship of T lymphocytes with macrophages. In contrast to primary neutrophil defense and humoral immunity, in which the polymorphonuclear leukocyte is the major phagocyte, the predominant phagocytic cell in cell-mediated immunity is the macrophage. On initial exposure to an antigen, T lymphocytes become sensitized. When restimulated these sensitized T lymphocytes produce a group of lymphokines,

including macrophage activation factor. It is this substance that stimulates macrophages to better ingest and kill pathogens. In contrast to polymorphonuclear leukocytes, macrophages can readily ingest microorganisms but have a difficult time with intracellular killing. This system may be summarized as providing protection against pathogens that are easy to eat but hard to kill.

Some of the disorders and clinical situations associated with defects in cell-mediated immunity are listed in Table 5. With aging alone, patients have a decrease in cell-mediated immunity. Pregnant women in their third trimester have a transient loss of cell-mediated immunity, which spontaneously reconstitutes itself within about 3 months of delivery. Immunosuppressive drugs (including corticosteroids and cyclosporine) and HIV infection are associated with defects in this limb of host defense. Both steroids and HIV infection decrease total T lymphocyte numbers, resulting in production of abnormal amounts of lymphokines like macrophage activation factor. In contrast, cyclosporine does not decrease lymphocyte numbers but decreases the functional capacity of lymphocytes to produce lymphokines. Irrespective of the mechanism, a decrease in the production of macrophage activation factor decreases the stimulus for macrophages to optimally serve as the primary phagocytic cell in this host defense system.

The pathogens infecting patients with defects in cell-mediated immunity are

Table 6. Pathogens in disorders of cell-mediated immunity

Bacteria	Fungi	Viruses	Parasites/Protozoa	Others
Mycobacteria	*Cryptococcus*	Herpes simplex	*Pneumoncystis*	*Treponema*
Listeria	*Histoplasma*	Varicella-zoster	*Toxoplasma*	*pallidum*
Nocardia	*Coccidioides*	Cytomegalovirus	*Strongyloides*	Chlamydiae
Rhodococcus	*Blastomyces*	Epstein-Barr virus	*Giardia*	Rickettsiae
Salmonella	*Candida*	Polyoma viruses	*Cryptosporidium*	
Legionella	*Aspergillus*	Adenoviruses	*Isospora*	
Brucella		Measles virus	*Microsporidia*	
Bartonella			Amebae	
(formerly			*Leishmania*	
Rochalimaea)			*Trypanosoma*	

summarized in Table 6 and can be divided into 5 categories: a) bacteria (which have as a common characteristic an intracellular location); b) fungi (which often become clinically manifested in the setting of previous epidemiologic exposure); c) viruses (most characteristically, DNA viruses); d) parasites and protozoa; and e) a miscellaneous group (into which some include spirochetes).

Intracellular Bacteria

Mycobacterium tuberculosis

Although tuberculosis can be a problem in any patient with defective cell-mediated immunity, it has attracted recent attention because of the copathogenesis that may occur in individuals who are dually infected with the intracellular pathogens *M. tuberculosis* and HIV-1. It has been suggested by some that mycobacteria and their products may enhance viral replication by inducing nuclear factor kappa-B, the cellular factor that binds to promoter regions of HIV. The presentation of tuberculosis in HIV-infected persons is variable and is influenced by the level of immunosuppression. With CD4 counts >300 cells/mm^3, the pattern of typical reactivation tuberculosis with cavitary disease or upper lobe infiltrates is more common. When CD4 cells fall to <200/mm^3, the pattern of disease is more typically middle to lower lobe disease with or without intrathoracic lymphadenopathy. In patients with CD4 counts at this level, extrapulmonary tuberculosis has been reported in at least 50%. Persons with serologic evidence of HIV infection and pulmonary tuberculosis fulfill the case definition for AIDS. These individuals with drug-susceptible strains tend to respond well to standard antituberculous therapy given as a short-course regimen for 6 months (*MMWR* 1998; 47[RR-20]:1-58). After initiation of antituberculosis therapy, some patients experience a paradoxical reaction, which is the temporary exacerbation of tuberculosis symptoms in the form of hectic fevers, lymphadenopathy, worsening of chest radiographic findings, and worsening of extrapulmonary lesions. These reactions are not associated with changes in *M. tuberculosis* bacteriology, and patients generally feel well

with no signs of toxicity. Such reactions have been attributed to recovery of delayed hypersensitivity response and an increase in exposure and reaction to mycobacterial antigens after bactericidal antituberculosis therapy is initiated. These reactions have been especially notable in individuals concurrently treated with antituberculosis and antiretroviral therapy. A noteworthy issue in HIV-infected patients is the interaction between antituberculosis drugs and antiretroviral therapy, including that with protease inhibitors. The rifamycins (e.g., rifampin and rifabutin) accelerate the metabolism of protease inhibitors through induction of hepatic P$_{450}$ cytochrome oxidases. Rifabutin has comparable antituberculous activity but with less hepatic P$_{450}$ cytochrome enzyme-inducing effect than rifampin. Based on these facts, CDC recommendations in 1998 for the therapy of tuberculosis in HIV-infected patients stated that "Because rifampin markedly lowers the blood levels of these (nonnucleoside reverse transcriptase inhibitors [NNRTI] and protease inhibitors) and is likely to result in suboptimal antiretroviral therapy, the use of rifampin to treat active TB in a patient who is taking a protease inhibitor or an NNRTI is always contraindicated." (*MMWR* 1998; 47[RR-20]:12). In 2000, the CDC issued updated guidelines which altered some of these contraindications (*MMWR* 2000; 49:185-189). These new data suggest that rifampin can be used for the treatment of active tuberculosis in 3 situations: 1) in a patient whose antiretroviral regimen includes the NNRTI efavirenz and 2 other nucleoside reverse transcriptase inhibitors (NRTIs); 2) in a patient whose antiretroviral regimen includes the protease inhibitor ritonavir and 1 or more NRTIs; or 3) in a patient whose antiretroviral regimen includes the combination of 2 protease inhibitors (ritonavir and either saquinavir hard-gel capsule [HGC] or saquinavir soft-gel capsule [SGC]). In addition, the updated guidelines recommend substantially reducing the dose of rifabutin (150 mg 2 or 3 times per week) when it is administered to patients taking ritonavir (with or without saquinavir HGC or saquinavir SGC) and increasing the dose of rifabutin (either 450 mg or 600 mg daily or 600 mg 2 or 3 times per week) when rifabutin is used concurrently with efavirenz.

Two clinically-relevant trends related to tuberculosis deserve comment. One is an apparent increase in tuberculosis reactivation associated with TNF-alpha inhibitors (e.g., infliximab) used to treat rheumatoid arthritis and Crohn's disease, with extrapulmonary tuberculosis being especially noted (*N Engl J Med* 2001; 345:1098-1104). The other relates to the reports of liver failure and death after 2-month therapy with rifampin and PZA (*MMWR* 2001; 50:733-735).

Some recent attention has been focused on measures that foster Type 1 immunity as a means of treating patients with tuberculosis who do not respond to standard therapy. Low-dose adjuvant IL-2 was added to the regimen of patients with multidrug-resistant tuberculosis who responded poorly to antituberculous therapy (*Novartis Found Symp* 1998; 217:99-106). This resulted in reduction or clearance of acid-fast bacilli from sputum as well as with enhanced activation of the immune system. This supports the concept that Type 1 immunity may be a form of adaptive host defense.

A significant change has recently occurred regarding tuberculosis infection. For many decades, the terms "preventive therapy" and "chemoprophylaxis" were used to describe persons with a positive tuberculin test but no symptoms or signs of active tuberculosis. The terminology "preventive" was inaccurate in that it referred to use of an agent like isoniazid to prevent development of active tuberculosis in persons known or likely to be infected with *M. tuberculosis*; it was not intended to imply prevention of true primary infection. To provide a more accurate descriptor for such therapy, the American Thoracic Society in a 2000 official statement introduced the terminology "latent tuberculosis infection" (LTBI) as a substitute for "preventive therapy" and "chemoprophylaxis." (*Am J Respir Crit Care Med* 2000; 161:S221-S247). It acknowledged the role of LTBI as an important element in control of tuberculosis. It has been stated that HIV-infected persons with a positive tuberculin skin test have about a 7% chance per year of developing tuberculous disease. In a prospective cohort study of persons with HIV infection in the United States, the annual risk of active TB among HIV-infected persons with a positive tuberculin test was 4.5

cases per 100 person years. Based on reports such as these, it is recommended that HIV-infected persons with a tuberculin skin test with ≥5-mm induration be given treatment for latent tuberculosis. In the 2000 guidelines for treatment of LTBI, tuberculin positivity was also set at ≥5-mm induration for patients with organ transplants and other immunosuppressed patients receiving the equivalent of ≥15 mg/day of prednisone for 1 month or more. It was noted that the risk of tuberculosis in patients treated with corticosteroids increases with higher dose and longer duration. Data summarized by the Centers for Disease Control and Prevention (*MMWR* 1998; 47[RR-20]:20) suggested that a) the optimal duration of isoniazid preventive therapy should be >6 months, b) therapy for 9 months appeared to be sufficient; and c) therapy for >12 months did not appear to provide additional protection.

Mycobacterium avium Complex (MAC)

Among individuals with defective cell-mediated immunity, MAC classically infects HIV-infected persons when their CD4 cells are <50/mm^3. In patients with AIDS, there are several lines of evidence suggesting that most patients with disseminated MAC have recently acquired the organisms, in contrast to the reactivation that is common with tuberculosis (*J Infect Dis* 1999; 179[Suppl 3]:S461-465) Adherence of the organisms to the gut wall is the initial event in invasion, followed by entry into the lamina propria and then phagocytosis by macrophages. Local replication of organisms leads to the endoscopically visable 2-4 mm punctate lesions that are the hallmark of MAC disease in the gut. The clinical presentation is that of a wasting syndrome marked by fever, night sweats, weight loss, diarrhea, anorexia, and malaise. Despite positive sputum cultures, serious pulmonary infection is not common in HIV-infected patients. The organism is most characteristically isolated from blood, stool, respiratory secretions, bone marrow, gastrointestinal tract mucosa, and lymph nodes (although granuloma formation is minimal or absent). A unique pathophysiologic abnormality seen in about 5% of AIDS patients with MAC disease is marked (20-40 times normal) elevations in serum alkaline phosphatase with little elevation of transaminases, bilirubin, or other parameters of hepatic function. This is felt to occur on the basis on interference with enzyme metabolism rather than on hepatic tissue destruction. In those patients with symptomatic disease, a multidrug regimen is recommended that should include either azithromycin or clarithromycin in combination with ethambutol. Additional drugs that may be added to this regimen include clofazimine, ciprofloxacin, rifabutin, and amikacin. The response to therapy is variable among patients, and the acquisition of drug resistance is common, especially with monotherapy. Although rifabutin was the initial agent approved for prophylaxis against MAC infection, recent recommendations for the prevention of opportunistic infections in HIV-infected persons have listed clarithromycin or azithromycin as the agent of choice (http://www.hivatis.org). This recommendation may have been influenced by the fact that macrolides should result in less interaction with the cytochrome P_{450} system than occurs with rifabutin.

Listeria monocytogenes

This intracellular Gram-positive rod characteristically infects persons with malignancy, diabetes mellitus, or renal transplantation on immunosuppressive therapy. Neonates and pregnant women are also at risk, and the infection occurs with increased frequency with cirrhosis. About one-third of patients in some series have no known risk factor, and it has only recently been considered a cause of febrile gastrointestinal illness in immunocompetent persons (*N Engl J Med* 2000; 342:1236-1241). *Listeria* may be acquired via consumption of certain contaminated raw vegetables (with cole slaw as a source in some outbreaks), certain contaminated canned products (with sterile canned corn kernels as the source in 1 outbreak), raw food from animal sources (e.g., beef, pork, or poultry), unpasteurized milk, or foods made from raw milk (notably, certain soft cheeses). The most common clinical presentations are of CNS infection, sepsis, or a flu-like illness. When it causes acute meningitis, *Listeria* may be

associated with a variable glucose level or with a cerebrospinal fluid lymphocytosis or monocytosis. Gram's stain of the cerebrospinal fluid is positive in only about one-fourth of patients. The infection has a predilection for the base of the brain with resultant focal neurologic signs, particularly cranial nerve involvement, in up to 40% of patients. Hydrocephalus may be a complication of this localization. Bacteremia is another common presentation, with cerebritis or brain abscess being less frequent. Therapy is with high-dose ampicillin or penicillin intravenously. Some favor the addition of a parenteral aminoglycoside with these agents even for treatment of meningitis, recognizing that the aminoglycosides administered parenterally in adults will not cross the blood-brain barrier but may help eradicate infectious sites outside the central nervous system. For penicillin-allergic patients, trimethoprim-sulfamethoxazole is possibly effective. Extremely noteworthy is that there is no role for cephalosporin therapy in treating infection caused by *Listeria*. Because of the intracellular location of the organisms, 3 weeks of therapy are recommended for serious infections.

Nocardia asteroides

These filamentous aerobic Gram-positive rods are weakly acid-fast and characteristically produce disease in patients with lymphoreticular neoplasms or who have received long-term corticosteroid therapy. Because the organism most commonly infects humans through the respiratory tract, the classic pattern of infection is pulmonary disease, which may take the form of nodular infiltrates, cavitary lesions, or diffuse infiltrates with or without consolidation. Pustular skin lesions and neurologic disease in the form of encephalitis or brain abscess complete the triad of the most common presentations by this pathogen. Less likely organs to be involved are liver and kidney. In the report from The Johns Hopkins Hospital of 59 patients diagnosed with nocardiosis over an 11-year time span, *Nocardia* was isolated most commonly from the respiratory tract (76%), followed by soft tissue (13%), blood (7%), and central nervous system (5%) (*Infect Dis Clin Pract* 2001; 10:249-254). In this series, the infection was common in AIDS patients as well as in transplant recipients. In both groups of patients, disease developed in some despite prophylactic therapy against other pathogens with trimethoprim/sulfamethoxazole. Standard therapy is with sulfonamides. Trimethoprim-sulfamethoxazole is often used because of its convenient intravenous dosing; however, it has not been definitively proven that the combination is synergistic at the drug ratios that usually are achieved in serum or cerebrospinal fluid.

Rhodococcus equi

Formerly called *Corynebacterium equi*, this partially acid-fast, aerobic, intracellular Gram-positive rod-coccus has been the cause of more than 100 reported cases of infection since the organism was described in 1967 as the cause of disease in humans (*Clin Infect Dis* 2002; 34:1379-1385). Even though the organism has been rarely reported to cause infection in immunocompetent patients, immunocompromised patients, especially those with HIV infection, are the ones most likely to develop clinical disease due to this pathogen. The most characteristic pattern of infection is described as a progressive pneumonia that may cavitate. Bacteremia is common in immunocompromised patients. Like *Nocardia*, it has also been associated with neurologic and skin lesions. The intracellular location has made the organism difficult to treat, and principles of therapy include a prolonged duration of antibiotics often in association with drainage. In vitro, *R. equi* is usually susceptible to erythromycin, rifampin, fluoroquinolones, aminoglycosides, glycopeptides (e.g., vancomycin), and imipenem, and it has been suggested that immunocompromised patients and patients with serious infections receive intravenous therapy with 2-drug or 3-drug regimens that include vancomycin, imipenem, aminoglycosides, ciprofloxacin, rifampin, and/or erythromycin (*Clin Infect Dis* 2002; 34:1379-1385). The choice of agents used and the duration of therapy are dependent on both the patient's host defense status and the site of infection. Oral antibiotics may be an option in certain immunocompetent patients with localized infection.

Salmonella Species

Patient populations with defective cell-mediated immunity that develop bacteremia with this intracellular Gram-negative rod include those with hematologic malignancies, systemic lupus erythematosus, and HIV infection. In those persons with HIV infection, a febrile typhoidal illness without diarrhea accounts for about 45% of the disease caused by this pathogen. More common is an illness associated with fever, severe diarrhea, and crampy abdominal pain. Compared to *Shigella* and *Campylobacter*, there is a lower incidence of bloody diarrhea and fecal leukocytes with *Salmonella* infection. Since HIV-infected persons do not reconstitute their cell-mediated immunity, recurrent nontyphoidal bacteremia is considered an indication for secondary antibacterial prophylaxis.

Legionella Species

Legionella causes more severe disease in transplant recipients, patients who receive corticosteroids, and HIV-infected persons. Immunocompromised patients with legionellosis may present with variable patterns of multisystem disease. Of these, fever with a scanty productive cough is often described. In individuals receiving corticosteroids, cavitary lung lesions with abscess formation may occur. Dissemination seems to occur via bacteremic spread of the organism. In a review of legionnaires' disease, the most common extrapulmonary site was reported to be the heart (including myocarditis and pericarditis), and one would need to assume that such organ system involvement might be possible in immunocompromised patients (*N Engl J Med* 1997; 337:682-687). Other patterns of extrapulmonary involvement by *Legionella* may take the form of sinusitis, cellulitis, pyelonephritis, and pancreatitis. Patients with hairy-cell leukemia, a disorder of monocyte deficiency and dysfunction, have an increased incidence of *Legionella* pneumonia. *Legionella* infection should be suspected in those individuals who do not respond to therapy with a β-lactam antibiotic. Useful in the acute diagnosis is the *Legionella* urinary antigen assay, which has been stated to be 70% sensitive and 100% specific in diagnosing infection caused by *L. pneumophila* serogroup I. Erythromycin has traditionally been considered the agent of choice for treatment of this infection, but recent reviews have suggested that the fluoroquinolones may be more efficacious *(N Engl J Med* 1997; 337:682-687). Because of increased efficacy and the fact that macrolides like erythromycin may have pharmacologic interactions with immunosuppressive agents used in transplant patients, some investigators feel that a fluoroquinolone should be added to the standard regimen for treating Legionnaires' disease in transplant recipients with nosocomial pneumonia if the causative agent has not been identified. Some have suggested that rifampin be used as adjunctive therapy for severe *Legionella* infections, but this must be taken in context of the facts that (1) no prospective studies have evaluated such therapy, and (2) rifampin has the potential to induce the cytochrome P_{450} system and therefore cause a significant interaction with immunosuppressive therapy.

Brucella Species

Even though intracellular brucellae require cell-mediated immunity for eradication, the spectrum of brucellosis in immunocompromised hosts has not been frequently described. Because of the ability for splenic localization with the formation of suppurative lesions which might require splenectomy, this organism may cause further impairment of an otherwise compromised immune system.

Bartonella (Formerly *Rochalimaea*) Species

The small Gram-negative organisms in this genus may be demonstrated with Warthin-Starry staining or by electron microscopy. The patterns of infection in HIV-infected persons include the following: a) bacteremia (in the absence of focal vascular proliferative response in tissue); b) bacillary angiomatosis (BA); and c) peliosis hepatitis (PH). BA presents in the later

phases of HIV infection, usually with CD4 counts <100 cells/mm³. The condition is associated with a unique vascular lesion that may involve virtually every organ system either alone or in association with other sites of involvement. Of these, skin lesions are the most commonly recognized, with characteristic lesions being red and papular and therefore resembling Kaposi's sarcoma. Characteristic of the lesions is a long duration of symptoms or physical findings prior to diagnosis. Species causing such a process include *B. henselae* and *B. quintana*. PH refers to the blood-filled peliotic changes in the parenchyma of the liver or spleen that occur because of infection with these 2 species. Since these organisms are at present difficult to culture from blood or tissue, histopathology may be the study that directs further diagnostic evaluation. Erythromycin is considered the drug of choice with tetracycline being an alternative agent.

Fungi

Cryptococcus neoformans

Cryptococcal meningitis is an important infection in HIV-infected persons, particularly when CD4 counts are <100 cells/mm³, but may also occur in other populations, including elderly persons. The organism enters the body through the lung, and the associated finding of pulmonary infiltrates in an HIV-infected person with meningitis should raise the suspicion of this diagnosis. The organism has a propensity to enter the bloodstream and may be detected in routine blood cultures. The resulting fungemia is often associated with multisegment pulmonary infiltrates and with skin lesions. Infection in the HIV population may present as a noninflammatory infection of the central nervous system, and the clinical features are therefore different than one might expect in classic forms of meningitis caused by other pathogens. The history is frequently of a subacute or chronic illness associated mainly with headache. Physical exam may not reveal classic findings such as nuchal rigidity. Because of the lack of inflammation in the central nervous system, the cerebrospinal fluid formula may include <20 white blood cells/mm³, normal glucose, and normal protein. These findings make cerebrospinal fluid studies such as India ink, cryptococcal antigen, and fungal culture mainstays in the diagnosis. The National Institute of Allergy and Infectious Diseases Mycoses Study Group and AIDS Clinical Trials Group reported the findings on 381 patients with cryptococcal meningitis treated in their double-blind multicenter trial (*N Engl J Med* 1997; 337:15-21). Conclusions from this trial of AIDS-associated cryptococcal meningitis were that induction treatment for 2 weeks with the combination of amphotericin B (0.7 mg/kg/day) plus flucytosine (100 mg/kg/day in patients who were tolerant of this agent), followed by therapy with fluconazole (400 mg orally per day for 8 weeks) is safe and effective and should be considered the treatment of choice. Noted in this report was the observation that high intracranial pressures have been associated with catastrophic neurologic deterioration and death in the absence of hydrocephalus. Of the patients in this study, 13 of 14 early deaths and 40% of deaths during weeks 3 through 10 were associated with elevated intracranial pressure. Based on the association of elevated intracranial pressure and mortality in patients with cryptococcal meningitis, it was suggested that measurement of intracranial pressure be included in the management of such patients. Included in the recommendations were daily lumbar punctures, use of acetazolamide, and ventriculoperitoneal shunts for asymptomatic patients with intracranial CSF pressure >320 mm and for symptomatic patients with pressures >180 mm. More recently (*Clin Infect Dis* 2000; 30:47-54), it was recommended in the absence of focal lesions that opening pressures ≥250 mm H_2O be treated with large-volume CSF drainage (which was defined in this report as allowing CSF to drain until a satisfactory closing pressure had been achieved, commonly <200 mm H_2O). IDSA guidelines for the management of cryptococcal meningitis in HIV-infected persons with opening CSF pressure of >250 mm H_2O recommended lumbar drainage sufficient to achieve closing pressure ≤200 mm H_2O or 50% of initial opening pressure (*Clin Infect Dis* 2000; 30:710-718). Maintenance therapy is required following completion of primary therapy, and

recent studies have defined fluconazole as the agent of choice.

Histoplasma capsulatum

The clinical entity of progressive disseminated histoplasmosis has become increasingly recognized because of HIV infection. The illness may occur on the basis of either reactivation or primary disease, making the epidemiologic history of travel to or residence in endemic areas crucial. Although patients may present with such nonspecific findings as fever, fatigue, weakness, and weight loss, a characteristic presentation in about half of patients is diffuse interstitial or miliary pulmonary infiltrates associated with hypoxemia and mimicking *Pneumocystis carinii* pneumonia. These patients may concomitantly demonstrate reticuloendothelial involvement in the forms of hepatosplenomegaly, lymphadenopathy, and bone marrow involvement. A subgroup may present with a septic syndrome that can include disseminated intravascular coagulation. Small intracellular periodic acid-Schiff (PAS) positive, yeast-like organisms are the characteristic morphologic form of the organism. Although the organism may be isolated from sputum, tissue, or blood, the *H. capsulatum* polysaccharide antigen (HPA) from blood, urine, or cerebrospinal fluid may serve as a more rapid diagnostic study. In the guidelines of the IDSA for treating disseminated histoplasmosis, immunocompromised patients were divided into those with AIDS and those without AIDS (*Clin Infect Dis* 2000; 30:688-695). In those without AIDS who were sufficiently ill to require hospitalization, amphotericin B, 0.7-1.0 mg/kg/day was recommended. It was noted that most patients respond quickly to amphotericin B and can then be treated with itraconazole, 200 mg once or twice daily for 6-18 months. For patients with AIDS, it was recommended that therapy be divided into an initial 12-week intensive phase to induce a remission in the clinical illness and then followed by a chronic maintenance phase to prevent relapse. Amphotericin B was recommended for patients sufficiently ill to require hospitalization, with replacement by itraconazole, 200 mg twice daily (when the patient no longer requires hospitalization of intravenous therapy), to complete a 12-week total course of induction therapy. Itraconazole, 200 mg 3 times daily for 3 days and then twice daily for 12 weeks, was recommended for patients who have mild or moderately severe symptoms who do not require hospitalization. Maintenance therapy with itraconazole for life was included in the recommendations.

Coccidioides immitis

In HIV-infected persons as well as in transplant recipients, this fungal pathogen occurs most commonly in those individuals from endemic areas. The illness may resemble *P. carinii* pneumonia with diffuse reticulonodular infiltrates. The classic clinical pattern of disease, manifested as dissemination to sites such as meninges, skin, and joints, is not altered by HIV infection. In the IDSA guidelines for the treatment of coccidioidomycosis, it was noted that bilateral reticulonodular or miliary infiltrates produced by *C. immitis* usually implies an underlying immunodeficiency state (*Clin Infect Dis* 2000; 30:658-661). In such circumstances, therapy usually starts with amphotericin B. Several weeks of therapy are often required for improvement, at which point an oral azole may replace amphotericin. Included in the IDSA guidelines for treatment of coccidioiomycosis are recommendations for the management of meningitis, which includes a role for oral fluconazole in certain patients.

Candida Species

Host defense against *Candida* is provided by both neutrophils and cell-mediated immunity. In addition, the immunocompetent host may develop blood-borne infection with this pathogen, and notable risk factors for this include surgery (particularly of the gastrointestinal tract), broad-spectrum antibiotics, hyperalimentation, and intravascular catheters. With HIV infection, *Candida* may present in a hierarchal pattern. With CD4 counts in the 400 to 600 cells/mm^3 range, women may develop recurrent vulvovaginal candidiasis (RVVC). At CD4 levels of ~250 cells/mm^3, oral candidiasis is the expected clinical entity. The

clinical presentation of odynophagia in a patient with oral candidiasis and a CD4 count of <100 cells/mm^3 strongly raises the diagnosis of *Candida* esophagitis. These candidal infections generally respond well to therapy, and because of this, primary prophylaxis is not generally recommended. A recent trend has been toward non-*albicans* strains of *Candida* and toward strains of *Candida albicans* that are fluconazole-resistant. Patterns of azole use have probably contributed to such problems. Recurrent use of fluconazole in HIV-infected patients has been associated with an increasing number of reports of *Candida* species resistant to this agent. In a bone marrow transplant unit in which patients were given fluconazole (400 mg daily, oral or iv) for the first 75 days after transplantation, 5% of patients became colonized with fluconazole-resistant strains of *C. albicans*, and 53% of patients had at least 1 mouthwashing sample that yielded non-*albicans* species of *Candida* during the course of their bone marrow transplantation (*Clin Infect Dis* 2000; 181:309-316).

Aspergillus Species

As is the case with *Candida*, *Aspergillus* may cause infection in patients with defects in either neutrophil function or cell-mediated immunity. In addition to being a nosocomial pathogen, infection with this agent may represent reactivation disease. This may be especially notable in patients who have received a bone marrow transplant or in those after solid organ transplantation. In AIDS patients with the concomitant problems of neutropenia, corticosteroid therapy, or ethanol use, invasive pulmonary or disseminated aspergillosis may occur. This tends to present in the later stages of HIV infection, especially when CD4 cells are <50/mm^3.

Infection with, and treatment of, *Aspergillus* provide some important insights into the evolving clinical importance of type 1 immunity. Patients with chronic granulomatous disease have an increased incidence of infection with *Aspergillus*. Treatment of these patients with recombinant interferon-γ stimulates killing of this pathogen and reduces the frequency and severity of clinically apparent fungal infection (*Clin Infect Dis* 2001; 32:76-102). This observation is important in that it conveys a treatment option for INF-γ based on an understanding of the role of type 1 immunity in defending against certain fungal pathogens. The traditional treatment for *Aspergillus* has been amphotericin B given at maximum tolerated doses (e.g., 1-1.5 mg/kg/day) and continued despite modest increases in serum creatinine (*Clin Infect Dis* 2000; 30:696-709). Lipid formulations of amphotericin are indicated in 2 circumstances: for the patient who has impaired renal function or develops nephrotoxicity while receiving amphotericin B deoxycholate (*Clin Infect Dis* 2000; 30:696-709) and for patients who have undergone a bone marrow transplant (*Clin Infect Dis* 1999; 29:1402-1407). Oral itraconazole may be an alternative in certain settings. The echinocandin caspofungin has been recently approved for patients who fail amphotericin. Evolving data now suggest the potential for a clinically important role for voriconazole in the treatment of *Aspergillus* infections.

Viruses

Herpes simplex Virus (HSV)

The patterns of HSV infection vary according to the underlying immunosuppression status. Patients with hematologic or lymphoreticular neoplasms may develop disseminated mucocutaneous HSV lesions. In transplant patients, esophagitis, tracheobronchitis, pneumonitis, or hepatitis are characteristic presentations. HIV-infected persons can have a vast array of clinical conditions caused by HSV, including esophagitis, colitis, perianal ulcers (often associated with urinary retention), pneumonitis, and a spectrum of neurologic diseases. Acyclovir remains the drug of choice for these infections. However, acyclovir-resistant strains have emerged for which foscarnet may be the alternative therapy.

Varicella-zoster Virus (VZV)

As is the case with HSV infection, VZV may present differently according to the underlying type of immunosuppression. With both chickenpox and shingles in patients with solid and hematologic malignancies, cutaneous dissemination may occur and may be associated with such visceral involvement as pneumonitis, hepatitis, and meningoencephalitis. Herpes zoster may be multidermatomal in HIV-infected persons, and this may be the initial clue to the diagnosis of HIV infection. Treatment options for both varicella and zoster have been summarized (*Ann Intern Med* 1999; 130:922-932). Acyclovir, famciclovir, and valacyclovir are presented according to the disease, the pattern of immunosuppression, and the requirement for intravenous versus oral therapy. With the depression of cell-mediated immunity that occurs during the third trimester of pregnancy (*Rev Infect Dis* 1984; 6:814-831), there is increased risk of dissemination of VZV to the lungs during pregnancy. A recently published case-control analysis of 18 pregnant women with VZV pneumonia compared with 72 matched control subjects identified cigarette smoking and >100 skin lesions as markers for developing varciella pneumonia in pregnancy (*J Infect Dis* 2002; 185:422-427). In immunocompromised patients and pregnant women who are exposed to chickenpox and in whom there is no clinical or serologic evidence of immunity to VZV, administration of VZ immune globulin (VZIG) may prevent or significantly modify VZV infection (*Ann Intern Med* 1999; 130:922-932).

Cytomegalovirus (CMV)

For perspective, it is important to recognize the 3 major consequences of CMV infection in solid-organ transplantation recipients: (1) CMV disease, including a wide-range of clinical illnesses; (2) superinfection with opportunistic pathogens; and (3) injury to the transplanted organ, possibly enhancing chronic rejection (*Clin Infect Dis* 2001; 33[Suppl 1]:S33-S37). The virus may be present in the forms of latency (infection without signs of active viral replication), active infection (viral replication in blood or organs), and primary infection (active infection in a previously nonimmune seronegative person). A recent study addressed the impact of primary infection in bone marrow recipients who were CMV-seronegative and who received stem cells from CMV-seropositive recipients (*Clin Infect Dis* 2002; 185:273-282). These patients died of invasive bacterial and fungal infections at a rate greater than that of patients who did not have primary infection, and it was hypothesized that primary CMV infection has immunomodulatory effects that predispose to such secondary infections.

The spectrum of clinically-active CMV infection in immunocompromised patients is broad and may vary according to the immunosuppressive condition. In HIV-infected patients, the classic presentation has been chorioretinitis but may also include gastrointestinal ulcerations, pneumonitis, hepatitis, encephalopathy, adrenalitis, and a painful myeloradiculopathy. Some immunosuppressed patients present with only a mononucleosis-like syndrome consisting of fever and lymphadenopathy.

New approaches in both hematopoietic stem cell or solid organ transplant recipients emphasize the use of prophylactic or preemptive therapy based on CMV monitoring. Although serologic tests have previously been suggested to have a potential role in directing CMV therapy in bone marrow transplant patients and heart transplant patients, serologies are not the most reliable studies in predicting the presence of CMV infection or clinical disease. The appearance of CMV protein pp65 (CMV-pp65) in peripheral blood leukocytes has proved to be superior to tests based on virus isolation (*Clin Infect Dis* 2001; 33[Suppl 1]:S33-S37) and has correlated with subsequent development of CMV disease. In addition to CMV antigenemia, DNA/RNAemia (especially quantitative PCR) is clinically useful, and detection tests for both are methods of choice for diagnosis and monitoring of active CMV infection after organ transplantation.

For the purpose of developing consistent reporting of CMV in clinical trials, definitions of CMV infection and disease were developed and published (*Clin Infect Dis* 2002; 34:1094-1097). In addition, an approach to the management of CMV infection after solid-organ transplantation has been recently published, and several clinically relevant messages are provided in it (*Clin Infect Dis* 2001; 33[Suppl 1]:S33-S37). In managing CMV infection, the clinician needs to

be aware of 4 types of treatment options: (1) therapeutic use (treatment based on the presence of established infection); (2) prophylactic use (use of antimicrobial therapy from the earliest possible moment); (3) preemptive use (antimicrobial therapy before clinical signs of infection); and (4) deferred therapy (initiation of therapy after onset of disease). In the therapeutic setting of CMV disease after solid organ transplantation, intravenous ganciclovir is the drug of choice, with anti-CMV hyperimmunoglobuilin preparations being useful adjuncts in seronegative recipients of seropositive organs and with foscarnet (because of its inherent toxicity) being considered as rescue therapy. Although ganciclovir has for years been the mainstay of therapy for CMV retinitis in AIDS patients, valganciclovir (an oral prodrug of ganciclovir) has been approved as an effective treatment option. In addition, studies are ongoing using valgancivlovir as both preemptive and definitive therapy of CMV infections in transplant patients. An immune reconstitution syndrome including visual blurring months after successful therapy of CMV retinitis has been described in AIDS patients who have been started on highly active antiretroviral therapy (HAART) (*Retina* 2001; 12:1-9). The role for prophylaxis against CMV was summarized based on the type of organ transplanted (*Clin Infect Dis* 2002; 34:1094-1097). With detection of CMV antigenemia at a predefined level, intravenous ganciclovir may have a role in preventing CMV disease in certain patient populations. Maintenance therapy is required for life in AIDS patients after completion of primary therapy for CMV retinitis.

Epstein-Barr Virus (EBV)

The pathobiology of EBV is important in understanding the evolution of EBV-associated disease in immunocompromised patients. Although early studies indicated that EBV replicated in epithelial cells in the oropharynx, more recent studies suggest that B cells in the oropharynx may be the primary site of infection (*N Engl J Med* 2000; 343:481-492). This has led to the thought that resting memory B cells are the site of persistence of EBV within the body, with the number of latently infected cells remaining stable over years (*Immunity* 1998; 9:395-404). What has not been definitively elucidated at the present time is the role of oral epithelial cells in the transmission and latency of EBV. Even though the finding of antibodies against EBV viral proteins and antigens is consistent with the fact that there is some degree of humoral immunity to the virus, it is the cellular immune response that is the more important for controlling EBV infection. Important among the proteins produced by EBV is latent membrane protein 1 (LMP-1), which acts as an oncogene and whose expression in an animal model has resulted in B-cell lymphomas. In patients with AIDS or who have received organ or bone marrow transplants, an inability to control proliferation of latently EBV-infected cells may lead to EBV lymphoproliferative disease, which in tissue may take the form of plasmacytic hyperplasia, B-cell hyperplasia, B-cell lymphoma, or immunoblastic lymphoma (*N Engl J Med* 2000; 343:481-492). It has been suggested that therapy for EBV lymphoproliferative disease include reduction in the dose of immunosuppressive medication when possible. More specific, definitive recommendations for therapy are not available, but potential options have been reviewed (*N Engl J Med* 2000; 343:481-492).

Completing the spectrum of EBV disease in immunocompromised patients is oral hairy leukoplakia, a common, nonmalignant hyperplastic lesion of epithelial cells seen most characteristically in HIV-infected patients. In its classic presentation, hairy leukoplakia presents as raised white lesions of the oral mucosa, especially on the lateral aspect of the tongue. Contributing to the ongoing attempts to elucidate the pathobiology of EBV, a study of serial tongue biopsy specimens from HIV-infected patients demonstrated EBV replication in normal tongue epithelial cells (in contrast to the lack of active viral replication in certain EBV-associated malignancies) and suggested that the tongue may be a source of EBV secretion into saliva (*Clin Infect Dis* 2001; 184:1499-1507). In this clinical trial, valacyclovir treatment completely abrogated EBV replication, resulting in resolution of hairy leukoplakia when it was present, but EBV replication returned in normal tongue epithelial cells after valacyclovir treatment. These findings are consistent with clinical experience that the lesions of hairy leukoplakia respond to antiviral therapy but recur once therapy is stopped. Topics not evaluated in this study, but important in the understanding of EBV, are whether other oral epithelial cells support viral replication and whether oral epithelial cells participate with B cells in viral latency.

Polyoma Viruses (Including JC Virus and BK Virus)

Clinically important members of this class of double-stranded DNA viruses include BK virus and JC virus. Primary infection with BK virus is generally asymptomatic and occurs in childhood. Following primary infection, the virus can remain latent in many sites, with the most notable being the kidney. With cellular immunodeficiency, the virus can reactivate and cause clinical disease. Although the kidney, lung, eye, liver, and brain are sites of both primary and reactivated BK virus-associated disease, the most characteristic disease entities are hemorrhagic and nonhemorrhagic cystitis, ureteric stenosis, and nephritis, and these occur most often in recipients of solid organ or bone marrow transplants (*Clin Infect Dis* 2001; 33:191-202). JC virus is the etiologic agent in progressive multifocal leukoencephalopathy (PML). In this primary demyelinating process involving white matter of cerebral hemispheres, patients present subacutely with confusion, disorientation, and visual disturbances, which may progress to cortical blindness or ataxia. Cerebrospinal fluid is characteristically acellular. A feature on neuroradiology imaging studies is lack of mass effect. No definitive therapy is presently available for this infection, and clinical efforts have recently focused on the role of immune reconstitution in modifying the clinical course of the illness. In a multicenter analysis of 57 consecutive HIV-positive patients with PML, neurologic improvement or stability at 2 months after therapy was demonstrated in 26% of patients who received highly active antiretroviral therapy (HAART) in contrast to improvement in only 4% of patients who did not receive HAART (*P*=0.03) (*J Infect Dis* 2000;

182:1077-1083). In this study, decreases in JC virus DNA to undetectable levels predicted a longer survival. In the context that untreated PML may be fatal within 3 to 6 months, such potential for preventing neurologic progression and improving survival by controlling JC virus replication becomes clinically relevant.

Adenoviruses

In immunocompromised patients, these DNA viruses may produce generalized illness that classically involves the nervous system, respiratory system, gastrointestinal tract, and liver. This class of viruses has recently emerged as a major problem in some bone marrow transplant units, and the infections may have a fulminant course, which may result in death. No drug has been shown to be definitively beneficial in these patients although intravenous ribavirin may be effective in some.

Measles Virus

Because individuals are protected against measles by cell-mediated immunity and since measles may cause severe illness in HIV-infected persons, protection via vaccine is an important consideration. A basic tenet in infectious diseases has been that live-virus vaccines should not be administered to immunocompromised patients. An exception has been use of measles vaccine, which is a live virus vaccine, in asymptomatic HIV-infected individuals and potentially in those with symptomatic HIV-infection. Fatal giant-cell pneumonitis has been described in a young male measles vaccine recipient with AIDS (*Ann Intern Med* 1998; 129:104-106). Even with the overwhelming success of measles immunization programs, this case has prompted reappraisal of recommendations and some have suggested that it may be prudent to withhold measles-containing vaccines from HIV-infected persons with evidence of severe immunosuppression.

Emerging Viral Pathogens in Persons with Defects in Cell-mediated Immunity

There have been increasing reports of infections caused by respiratory syncytial virus or parainfluenza virus, particularly in persons who have received bone marrow or solid organ transplantation. The spectrum of disease caused by these pathogens is evolving, with the lung being an important target organ. These viruses should be considered among the pathogens which may cause pneumonia in patients with defects in cell-mediated immunity.

Parasites and Protozoa

Pneumocystis carinii: The clinical setting in which *P. carinii* pneumonia (PCP) develops continues to evolve. In the pre-AIDS era, this pathogen was described as a cause of rapidly progressive infection in patients with malignant diseases especially during the time of steroid withdrawal. Following the onset of the AIDS epidemic in the early 1980s, PCP was most often diagnosed in HIV-infected persons. Following the widespread use of highly active antiretroviral therapy (HAART) in the mid-1990s, HIV-associated PCP has decreased, and it has been recently reported that PCP may in certain settings be diagnosed more often in non-HIV immunocompromised patients than in those with HIV infection (*JAMA* 2001; 286:2450-2460). Host defense against *Pneumocystis* includes humoral immunity; however, because of the overwhelming predominance of infection by this pathogen in HIV-infected persons, it has been included in this section of pathogens that infect patients with defective cell-mediated immunity. Although diffuse interstitial infiltrates are the most characteristic pulmonary finding with PCP, patients may present with focal infiltrates, cavitary lesions, or nodular lung lesions. Findings which support, but do not prove, the diagnosis of PCP in an HIV-infected patient with pulmonary infiltrates include a CD4 cell count <250 cells/mm^3, a white blood cell count <8,000 cells/mm^3, and an elevated serum lactate dehydrogenase (LDH). PCP may occur as part of the presentation of the acute retroviral syndrome. In a recent review of PCP from the Clinical Center at the National Institutes of Health (*JAMA* 2001; 286:2450-2460), diagnostic studies for PCP were reviewed. It was noted that traditional stains on sputum or from bronchoalveolar lavage specimens for the cyst form of *P. carinii* have been the mainstay for diagnosis in most settings. Direct immunofluorescent staining using monoclonal antibody 2G2 (which detects both cysts and trophozoites) has been used for many years in the algorithm of the NIH Clinic Center for diagnosing PCP. This stain is performed first on induced sputum, and if that smear is negative, then a BAL specimen is obtained for the same study. On-going investigation has been focused on the development of a quantitative PCR assay that can be performed on oral washes or gargles and that might allow a clinician not only to diagnose PCP at an earlier stage than has traditionally been possible but also to distinguish between colonization and disease with *P. carinii*. Trimethoprim-sulfamethoxazole is the current first-line therapeutic agent with pentamidine an alternative form of therapy. Clindamycin/primaquine has been compared to trimethoprim-sulfamethoxazole in a clinical trial and found to be a reasonable alternative therapy for mild to moderately severe PCP. Adjunctive corticosteroid therapy is recommended for patients with PCP whose room air p_aO_2 is <70 mg Hg or whose arterial-alveolar oxygen gradient is >35 mm Hg (*J Infect Dis* 1990; 162:1365-1369). It is important that steroids are started at the time antipneumocystis therapy is initiated in an attempt to prevent the lung injury that may occur when this pathogen is killed. The dramatic decrease in the number of cases of PCP relative to the number of patients with HIV infection has been attributable to prophylaxis, which is recommended for those patients with a $CD4^+$ cell count <200 cells/mm^3, $CD4^+$ cells less than 20% of total lymphocyte count, constitutional symptoms such as thrush or unexplained fever >100° F for >2 weeks (irrespective of the $CD4^+$ count), or a previous history of PCP. On the basis of several clinical investigations, it seems that discontinuing prophylaxis in patients with adequate immune recovery is a useful strategy that should be widely considered (*Clin Infect Dis* 2001; 33:1901-1909).

Toxoplasma   gondii:
Immunocompromised patients at higher risk for toxoplasmosis include those with hematologic malignancies (particularly patients with lymphoma), bone marrow transplant, solid organ transplant (including heart, lung, liver, or kidney), or AIDS (*J Infect Dis* 2002; 185[Suppl1]:S73-S82). In the vast majority of immunocompromised patients, toxoplasmosis results from reactivation of latent infection, but in heart transplant patients and in a small number of other immunocompromised patients, the highest risk of developing disease is in the setting of primary infection (i.e., a seronegative recipient who acquires the parasite from a seropositive donor via a graft). Although pulmonary disease due to this pathogen is associated with nonspecific radiographic findings of which bilateral pulmonary interstitial infiltrates are most common, neurologic disease is the classic pattern. In HIV-infected persons, it classically presents as fever, headache, altered mental status, and focal neurologic deficits, especially in individuals whose CD4 count falls below 100 cells/mm^3. Since the disease is due to reactivation of latent infection in about 95% of cases, IgG antibody to *Toxoplasma* is generally present. Imaging studies of the brain show multiple (usually ≥3) nodular contrast-enhancing lesions found most commonly in the basal ganglia and at the gray-white matter junction. In the classic setting, empiric therapy with sulfadiazine and pyrimethamine is recommended. Clindamycin-containing regimens may be considered in sulfa-allergic patients. Brain biopsy should be considered in immunocompromised patients with presumed CNS toxoplasmosis if there is a single lesion on MRI, a negative IgG antibody test result, or inadequate clinical response to an optimal treatment regimen or to what the physician considers to be an effective prophylactic regimen against *T. gondii* (*J Infect Dis* 2002; 185[Suppl1]:S73-S82). Trimethoprim-sulfamethoxazole given for PCP prophylaxis serves as primary prophylaxis for toxoplasmosis but should not be used for therapy. After acute therapy for toxoplasmic encephalitis, maintenance therapy is recommended.

Strongyloides stercoralis: Infection with this parasite has often been described in patients with COPD who have been on chronic steroid therapy and who present with Gram-negative bacteremia. The bacteremia occurs because of this organism's hyperinfection cycle, during which filariform larvae penetrate the intestinal mucosa, pass by way of the bloodstream to the lungs, break into alveolar spaces, and ascend to the glottis where they are swallowed into the intestinal tract to continue their process of autoinfection. Infection with this pathogen should be suspected in a patient with a defect in cell-mediated immunity who presents with clinical features, which include generalized abdominal pain, diffuse pulmonary infiltrates, ileus, shock, and meningitis. Eosinophilia is often absent in steroid-treated patients. In recent years, recommendations for therapy have changed based on the recognition that thiabendazole may not be consistently efficacious and that albendazole may be superior. Ivermectin may also be more effective than thiabendazole.

Cryptosporidium parvum: Although self-limited diarrhea associated with water-borne outbreaks has been noted in normal hosts, the clinical presentation of watery diarrhea, cramping, epigastric pain, anorexia, flatulence, and malaise in an HIV-infected patient suggests the diagnosis of cryptosporidiosis. Four clinical syndromes have been identified (*Clin Infect Dis* 1998; 27:536-542): chronic diarrhea (in 36% of patients); choleralike disease (33%); transient diarrhea (15%); and relapsing illness (15%). Biliary tract symptoms similar to cholecystitis have been noted to be present in 10% of cases. Diagnosis is confirmed by finding the characteristic acid-fast oocysts on examination of feces. No predictably effective antimicrobial therapy is available, and management is largely supportive.

Isospora belli: Like cryptosporidiosis, this pathogen is acid-fast and can cause a very similar diarrheal illness. In contrast to cryptosporidiosis, the pathogen is larger, oval, and cystic, and very importantly, responds to therapy with trimethoprim-sulfamethoxazole.

Microsporidia: These obligate intracellular protozoa are transmitted to humans probably through the ingestion of food contaminated with its spores, which are resistant to environmental extremes. *Enterocytozoon bieneusi* produces a protracted diarrheal illness

accompanied by fever and weight loss similar to that caused by *Cryptosporidium* and which is reported to occur in 20 to 30% of patients with chronic diarrhea not attributable to other causes. *Encephalitozoon cuniculi* has been described as an etiologic agent for hepatitis, peritonitis, and keratoconjunctivitis. Transmission electron microscopy with observation of the polar filament is considered the gold standard for diagnosis, but the Brown Brenn stain and the Warthin-Starry silver stain are commonly used for detecting microsporidia in tissue culture. The modified trichrome stain has been used in clinical diagnostic laboratories to detect microsporidia in fluids (*Clin Infect Dis* 1998; 27:1-8). Albendazole may be the most effective drug to treat infections due to most species of microsporidia.

Amebae: Naegleria and *Acanthamoeba* are free-living amebae that have the potential to infect humans. Of these, *Acanthamoeba* spp. may infect individuals with defects in cell-mediated immunity (including patients with AIDS or after organ transplantation) and result in granulomatous amebic encephalitis. Clinical manifestations include mental status abnormalities, seizures, fever, headache, focal neurologic deficits, meningismus, visual disturbances, and ataxia. An important clinical clue may be pre-existing skin lesions, which have been present for months before CNS disease is clinically manifested and which may take the form of ulcerative, nodular, or subcutaneous abscesses. Pneumonitis may also be a part of the clinical presentation. There are few data regarding therapy for granulomatous amebic encephalitis, but it appears that the diamidine derivatives pentamidine, propamidine, and dibromopropamidine have the greatest activity against *Acanthamoeba*.

Leishmania Species: In endemic areas of the world, these pathogens infect patients with defective cell-mediated immunity and cause a febrile illness with visceral involvement, most notably hepatomegaly and splenomegaly. Recently, leishmaniasis has been increasingly described in HIV-infected persons from endemic regions and may take a chronic relapsing course. Pentavalent antimonials (with stibogluconate sodium as the representative agent) may be useful for this infection. Notable is that the drug may cause dose-related QT prolongation on ECG, with arrhythmias (atrial and ventricular) and sudden death occasionally. It is contraindicated in patients with myocarditis, hepatitis, or nephritis. Antimony resistance has been noted in some HIV-infected patients, and in such situations liposomal amphotericin B has been shown to be potentially effective since it targets infected macrophages and reaches high levels in plasma and tissues.

Of the relevant disease models influencing the understanding of the clinical significance of type 1 and type 2 immunity, leishmaniasis is important. Biopsy specimens from patients with localized infection with *Leishmania braziliensis* were consistent with a protective type 1 immune response that included prominent mRNA coding for interleukin-2 and interferon-γ (*J Clin Invest* 1993; 91:1390-1395). As the lesions in patients became more destructive, there was a switch to a marked increase in the level of interleukin-4 mRNA, which is consistent with a failed type 2 immune response. Such data have been interpreted as an eloquent demonstration of the facts that type 1 immunity is the key to protection against *Leishmania* infections in humans and that a high infectious burden suppresses the human immune system from mounting type 1 responses. This has implications for therapy, which has included the use of interferon-γ as an adjunctive agent for visceral leishmaniasis.

Trypanosoma cruzi: With immunosuppression including HIV infection, reactivation of this pathogen can occur. In addition to the characteristic lesions seen with Chagas disease, immunosuppressed patients have an increased incidence of neurologic disease, with brain abscess being an increasingly reported finding in AIDS patients.

Miscellaneous Pathogens

Chlamydiae: This group of intracellular pathogens has been listed in some recent reviews of pathogens defended against by cell-mediated immunity. Although patients with a defect in this host defense system may be at increased risk

for chlamydial infections, such problems have not been classically described.

Rickettsiae: As with chlamydiae, rickettsiae are intracellular pathogens defended against by cell-mediated immunity. Recent reviews have not described immunocompromised patients as being at increased risk for infection by pathogens in this group.

Treponema pallidum: Defense against this pathogen may include a role for macrophages and other antigen-presenting cells such as dendritic cells which process and present treponemal antigens to helper T cells. HIV-infected patients can have abnormal serologic test results, including unusually high, unusually low, and fluctuating titers. However, aberrant serologic responses are uncommon, and most specialists believe that both treponemal and nontreponemal serologic tests for syphilis can be interpreted in the usual manner for patients who are infected with both HIV and *Treponema pallidum* (*MMWR* 2002; 51[RR-6]:1-80) With HIV infection, treponemal infection is more likely to have an atypical clinical presentation, to be aggressive, or to invade sites such as the central nervous system. When neurosyphilis is present, the CSF leukocyte count usually is elevated to >5 WBCs/mm^3. Although the VDRL-CSF is the standard serologic test for neurosyphilis, it may be nonreactive when neurosyphilis is present. The CSF FTA-ABS is less specific for neurosyphilis than the VDRL-CSF, but the high sensitivity of the study has lead some experts to believe that a negative CSF FTA-ABS test excludes neurosyphilis (*MMWR* 2002; 51[RR-6]:1-80). In addition to meningitis, a characteristic clinical presentation of syphilis in the central nervous system is stroke in a young person. The recommended regimen for the treatment of patients with neurosyphilis is aqueous penicillin G 18-24 million units per day, administered as 3-4 million units IV every 4 hours or as continuous infusion, for 10-14 days (*MMWR* 2002; 51[RR-6]:1-80). If compliance with therapy can be insured, an alternative regimen is procaine penicillin 2.4 million units IM once daily plus probenecid 500 mg orally four times a day, both for 10-14 days. Since the duration recommended for neurosyphilis is shorter than those for latent syphilis, some experts recommend administering benzathine penicillin 2.4 millions IM once weekly for up to 3 weeks upon completion of the neurosyphilis regimen to provide a comparable total duration of therapy. It is recommended that all HIV-infected persons be tested for syphilis and that all persons with syphilis be tested for HIV. Spinal fluid examination has been recommended for all HIV-infected persons with latent syphilis or with neurologic abnormalities. Some experts have recommended spinal fluid examination for any HIV-infected person with primary or secondary syphilis. Such recommendations, however, are not specifically noted in the CDC's 2002 guidelines (*MMWR* 2002; 51[RR-6]:1-80).

SUMMARY

The identification of a defect in neutrophil function, humoral immunity, or cell-mediated immunity allows the clinician to better focus on the most likely pathogens involved in an infectious process. An approach to the immunocompromised patient based on pathogenesis of disease should result in more directed, cost-effective therapy and in improved patient outcome.

SUGGESTED READINGS

Overview

1. Speller B, Edwards JE, Jr. Type1/Type 2 Immunity in infectious diseases. *Clin Infect Dis* 2001; 32:76-102
   An overview of type 1 and type 2 immunity, providing insight into forms of adaptive host defenses and their implications for therapy.

Neutropenia

2. Macron A, Carratala, Gonzales-Bacca E, et al: Serious complications of bacteremia caused by viridans streptococci in neutropenic patients with cancer. *Clin Infect Dis* 2000; 31:1126-1130
   A description of a life-threatening Gram-positive infection in neutropenic patients,

including the predispositions to such infection.

3. Hughes WT, Armstrong D, Bodey GP et al: 2002 guidelines for the use of antimicrobial agents in neutropenic patients with cancer. *Clin Infect Dis* 2002; 34:730-751
   A position paper from the Infectious Diseases Society of America, written by leaders in the field of infection in neutropenic patients, that in an exemplary fashion gives definite clinical opinions regarding various aspects of the management of febrile neutropenic patients.

4. Gold HS, Moldering RC Jr: Antimicrobial-drug resistance. *N Engl J Med* 1996; 335:1445-1452
   A recent and clinically useful review of the subject of antibiotic resistance, with clinical applicability in the management of febrile neutropenic patients.

5. Over H, Armitage JO, Bennett CL, et al: 2000 update of recommendations for the use of hematopoietic colony-stimulating factors: Evidence-based, clinical practice guidelines. *J Clin Onc* 2000; 18:3558-3585
   A set of recommendations which includes the role of granulocyte-colony stimulating factor in the management of febrile neutropenic patients.

6. Rex JH, Walsh TJ, Sobel JD, et al: Practice guidelines for the treatment of candidiasis. *Clin Infect Dis* 2000; 30:662-678
   Guidelines of the Infectious Diseases Society of America for the management of infections caused by Candida species.

7. Stevens DA, Kan VL, Judson MA, et al: Practice guidelines for diseases caused by Aspergillus. *Clin Infect Dis* 2000; 30:696-709
   Guidelines of the Infectious Diseases Society of America for the management of infections caused by Aspergillus species.

Humoral Immunity

8. Kingston ME, Mackey D: Skin clues in the diagnosis of life-threatening infections. *Rev Infect Dis* 1986; 8:1-11
   Includes a description of the types of skin lesions, which may occur in patients with

overwhelming pneumococcal bacteremia that occurs after splenectomy.

9. Centers for Disease Control and Prevention: Recommendations of the advisory committee on immunization practices (ACIP): Use of vaccines and immune globulins for persons with altered immunocompetence. *MMWR* 1993; 42(RR-4):1-12
A summary statement regarding patients with altered immunocompetence that addresses the principles for vaccination, how specific immunocompromising conditions may alter recommendations for vaccination, use of vaccine based on underlying conditions, and the role of immune globulins in persons with alterations in immunocompetence.

10. Centers for Disease Control and Prevention. Prevention of pneumococcal disease. Recommendations of the Advisory Committee on Immunization Practices (ACIP). *MMWR* 1997; 46(RR-8):1-24
A review of pneumococcal vaccination, including new recommendations for revaccination.

11. Centers for Disease Control and Prevention: Prevention and control of meningococcal disease: Recommendations of the Advisory Committee on Immunization Practices (ACIP). *MMWR* 2000; 49(RR-7):1-20
Data regarding meningococcal infection, including the role of vaccine in asplenic persons.

Cell-Mediated Immunity

12. Centers for Disease Control and Prevention: Prevention and treatment of tuberculosis among patients infected with human immunodeficiency virus: Principles of therapy and revised recommendations. *MMWR* 1998; 47(RR-20):1-58
A summary document that includes definitive therapy and prophylaxis for M. tuberculosis infection in HIV-infected patients.

13. Havlir DV, Barnes PF: Tuberculosis in patients with human immunodeficiency virus infection. *N Engl J Med* 1999; 340:367-373

A review of relevant issues related to the diagnosis and management of HIV-infected persons who are infected with M. tuberculosis.

14. American Thoracic Society: Targeted tuberculin testing and treatment of latent tuberculosis infection. *Am J Respir Crit Care Med* 2000; 161:S221-S247
Recent guidelines emphasizing the terminology "latent tuberculosis infection" (previously referred to as "preventive therapy") and outlining patient treatment groups based on tuberculin skin testing.

15. Masur H and the Public Health Service Task Force on Prophylaxis and Therapy for *Mycobacterium avium* Complex: Recommendations on prophylaxis and therapy for disseminated *Mycobacterium avium* Complex disease in patients infected with the human immunodeficiency virus. *N Engl J Med* 1993; 329:898-904
The opinions of an expert panel regarding the diagnosis, treatment, and prophylaxis of infection due to MAC in patients infected with HIV.

16. van der Hurst CM, Saag MS, Cloud GA, et al: Treatment of cryptococcal meningitis associated with the acquired immunodeficiency syndrome. *N Engl J Med* 1997; 337:15-21
Results of a multicenter trial that evaluated initial treatment of AIDS-associated cryptococcal meningitis.

17. Wheat J, Sarosi G, McKinsey D, et al: Practice guidelines for the management of patients with histoplasmosis. *Clin Infect Dis* 2000; 30:688-695
Guidelines of the Infectious Diseases Society of America for the management of histoplasmosis.

18. van der Bij, Speich R. Management of cytomegalovirus infection and disease after solid-organ transplantation. *Clin Infect Dis* 2001; 33(Suppl 1):S33-S37
An approach to the management of patients infected with CMV, with emphasis on the concept of preemptive therapy.

19. Cohen JI, Brunell PA, Staus SE, et al: Recent advances in varicella-zoster virus infection. *Ann Intern Med* 1999; 130:922-932

A *review of the infection with varicella-zoster virus, including a table summarizing the treatment of both chickenpox and shingles in immunocompromised patients.*

20. Kovacs JA, Gill VJ, Meshnick S, Masur H: New insights into transmission, diagnosis, and drug treatment of *Pneumocystis carinii* pneumonia. *JAMA* 2001; 286:2450-2460
    A *summary of established and evolving information about P. carinii, including potential options for more effective diagnostic studies.*

21. USPHS/IDSA Prevention of Opportunistic Infections Working Group. 2001 USPHS/IDSA guidelines for the prevention of opportunistic infections in persons infected with human immunodeficiency virus. (http://ww.hivatis.org) November 28, 2001
    A *clinically relevant summary for primary and secondary prophylaxis in HIV-infected persons.*

NERVOUS SYSTEM INFECTIONS, CATHETER INFECTIONS

George H. Karam, MD, FCCP

Objectives

- To review clinical presentations of nervous system infections which may present as a serious or life-threatening process
- To outline principles influencing diagnosis and management of nervous system infections
- To present an approach to infections related to catheters placed in the vasculature, urinary bladder, or peritoneum
- To summarize existing opinions and data about management of catheter-related infections

Key Words*:* meningitis; encephalitis; spinal epidural abscess; brain abscess; cavernous sinus thrombosis; rabies; botulism; catheter-related infections

TABLE OF ABBREVIATIONS

ADH	antidiuretic hormone
AIDS	acquired immunodeficiency syndrome
CSF	cerebrospinal fluid
EEE	Eastern equine encephalitis
HIV	human immunodeficiency virus
HSV	herpes simplex virus
LCD	lymphocytic choriomeningitis
MIC	minimal inhibitory concentration
PEP	postexposure prophylaxis
PML	progressive multifocal leukoencephalopathy
RMSF	Rocky Mountain Spotted Fever
SCMD	serogroup C meningococcal disease
SLE	St. Louis encephalitis
TEE	transesophageal echocardiography
WNV	West Nile virus

INTRODUCTION

Infection affecting various parts of the nervous system has the potential to be life-threatening or to result in severe sequelae if the infection is not appropriately diagnosed and treated. Although infections such as meningitis, encephalitis, and brain abscess are the most frequently encountered, processes such as spinal epidural abscess, septic intracranial thrombophlebitis, rabies, and botulism may present as emergent problems which require a high level of clinical suspicion for prompt diagnoses to be made. In addition to infections of the nervous system, infections associated with catheters placed in the vasculature, urinary bladder, or peritoneum can result in morbidity and create diagnostic or therapeutic dilemmas for the clinician. This review will attempt to summarize these infections as they relate to the critical care setting.

NERVOUS SYSTEM INFECTIONS

Meningitis

From 1986 until 1995, the median age of persons with bacterial meningitis increased from 15 months to 25 years, making meningitis in the United States a disease predominantly of adults rather than of infants and young children.

The basic diagnostic tool in the diagnosis of meningitis is examination of cerebrospinal fluid (CSF). When such fluid is obtained, important clinical studies include a) stains and cultures, b) glucose, c) protein, and d) cell count with differential. Gram stain and culture of CSF are highly specific but may have a median sensitivity of about 75%. Helpful in understanding the pathogenesis of meningitis due to varied processes is the CSF glucose level. Glucose enters the CSF by facilitated transport across the choroid plexus and capillaries lining the CSF. Normally, the CSF-to-blood glucose ratio is 0.6. Although consumption of glucose by white blood cells and organisms may contribute to low CSF glucose levels (which is referred to as hypoglycorrhachia), the major mechanism for low glucose is impaired transport into the CSF that classically occurs because of acute inflammation or with infiltration of the meninges by granulomas or malignant cells. Protein is usually excluded from the CSF but rises following disruption of the blood-brain barrier. Levels are lower in cisternal and ventricular CSF than in lumbar CSF. When protein levels exceed 150 mg/dL, the fluid may appear xanthochromic. In the absence of other CSF changes, the CSF protein level has little specific value.

The diagnosis of meningitis is made by the finding of a CSF pleocytosis and may occur on the basis of both infectious and noninfectious processes. In the absence of a positive stain on the CSF, the most helpful study in the initial approach to the patient with meningitis is a cell count with differential on the cerebrospinal fluid. As summarized in Table 1, an approach for diagnosing the etiology of meningitis based on the CSF analysis would include 3 common categories: a) polymorphonuclear meningitis; b) lymphocytic meningitis with a normal glucose;

and c) lymphocytic meningitis with a low glucose. In addition, on rare occasions patients may have a predominance of eosinophils in the CSF, but eosinophilic meningitis is uncommon.

Polymorphonuclear Meningitis

Because of the acute inflammation, this process is usually associated with a low CSF glucose due to impaired transport across the meninges. This is most notable with bacterial meningitis. In the differential diagnosis of polymorphonuclear meningitis are 4 major groups of disease: a) bacterial infection; b) the early meningeal response to any type of infection or inflammation; c) parameningeal foci; and d) persistent neutrophilic meningitis. Because of the sequella that may be associated with a delay in therapy, the single most important cause of a polymorphonuclear meningitis is bacterial infection. Discussion in this syllabus will be limited to this topic.

Table 1. An approach to cerebrospinal fluid pleocytosis[a]

Polymorphonuclear	Lymphocytic With Normal Glucose	Lymphocytic With Low Glucose
Bacterial (see Table 2)	Viral meningitis	Fungal
Early Meningitis	Enteroviruses, including poliovirus	Tuberculous
Tuberculosis	Herpes simplex virus (usually type 2)	Certain forms of
Fungal	Human immunodeficiency virus	meningoencephalitis
Viral	Adenovirus	(e.g., herpes simplex)
Drug-induced	Tick-borne viruses	or viral meningitis
Parameningeal Foci	Meningoencephalitis, including	Partially treated
Brain abscess	viral causes	bacterial meningitis
Subdural empyema	Parameningeal foci	Carcinomatous
Epidural abscess	Partially treated bacterial meningitis	meningitis
Sinusitis	Listeria meningitis	Subarachnoid
Mastoiditis	Spirochetal Infections	hemorrhage
Osteomyelitis	Syphilis	Chemical meningitis
Persistent neutrophilic meningitis	Leptospirosis	
	Lyme disease	
	Rickettsial Infections	
	Rocky Mountain Spotted Fever	
	Ehrlichiosis	
	Infective endocarditis	
	Immune-mediated diseases	
	Sarcoidosis	
	Drug-induced	

[a]Although not clinically common in the United States, eosinophilic meningitis can occur, and the characteristic pathogens causing such a process are *Angiostrongylus cantonesis, Trichinella spiralis, Taenia solium, Toxocara canis, Gnathostoma spinigerum,* and *Paragonimus westermani.*

Likely etiologic agents for bacterial meningitis are summarized in Table 2 from the perspectives of a) the age of the patient and b) underlying predispositions to meningitis.

Presented in a different manner, rates of meningitis per 100,000 population in 22 counties of 4 states revealed the following: *Streptococcus pneumoniae* 1.1; *Neisseria*

Table 2. Likely pathogens in bacterial meningitis based on patient's age or underlying conditions

Neonates	Enterobacteriaceae Group B streptococci *Listeria monocytogenes*
<6 years	*Neisseria meningitidis* *Streptococcus pneumoniae* *Haemophilus influenzae*
6 years to young adult	*N. meningitidis* *S. pneumoniae* *H. influenzae*
Adults <50 years	*S. pneumoniae* *N. meningitidis*
Alcoholic and elderly	*S. pneumoniae* *N. meningitidis* Enterobacteriaceae *L. monocytogenes*
Closed skull fracture	*S. pneumoniae* *H. influenzae* *Staphylococcus aureus* Coagulase-negative staphylococci Gram-negative bacilli

Open skull fracture	Gram-negative bacilli, including *Klebsiella pneumonia* ande
	    Acinetobacter calcoaceticus (when meningitis
	    develops from a contiguous postoperative traumatic
	    wound infection)
	S. aureus

Cerebrospinal fluid leak	*S. pneumoniae* *H. influenzae* Gram-negative bacilli Staphylococci
Cerebrospinal fluid shunt-associated	Coagulase-negative staphylococci
Diabetes	*S. pneumoniae* Gram-negative bacilli *S. aureus*
Defects in cell-mediated immunity	*L. monocytogenes*
Concern of bioterrorism	*Bacillus anthracis*

meningitidis 0.6; Group B streptococci 0.3; *Listeria monocytogenes* 0.2; and *Haemophilus influenzae* 0.2 (*N Engl J Med* 1997; 337:970-976). The most notable change in etiologic agents over the past decade has been the dramatic decrease in the incidence of *H. influenzae* meningitis, which has occurred as a result of vaccination against this pathogen.

Although pneumococci are the most common pathogens in bacterial meningitis, an emerging problem is infection caused by strains of *Streptococcus pneumoniae* that are penicillin resistant. Strains with relative, or intermediate, resistance will have a penicillin MIC of 0.12 to 1.0 µg/mL. High-level resistance to penicillin is defined as an MIC ≥2 µg/mL. Although rates of pneumococcal resistance to penicillin vary geographically, a recent survey of 34 medical centers in the United States noted that 29.5% of isolates of *S. pneumoniae* were penicillin-resistant, with 17.4% having intermediate resistance. Compounding this problem is the inability of antibiotics to cross the blood-brain barrier in an effective enough way to yield CSF levels significantly above the minimal inhibitory concentration (MIC) for the infecting organism. For pneumococcal meningitis caused by penicillin-susceptible strains, penicillin G and ampicillin are equally effective. Although high-dose penicillin (150,000 to 250,000 units/kg/day) has been useful in patients with pneumonia caused by strains of pneumococci with intermediate resistance, such high doses do not predictably lead to cerebrospinal fluid levels of penicillin that exceed the MIC of intermediately-resistant strains. For such isolates, cefotaxime or ceftriaxone has been recommended, but clinical failures when these agents have been used for strains with intermediate resistance have been reported. For isolates with high-level resistance, vancomycin is the drug of choice. Impacting this therapeutic option is the less-than-optimal penetration of vancomycin into cerebrospinal fluid. Steroids given concomitantly for meningitis may further decrease this penetration. A recent review, outlined in Table 3, summarizes recommendations for the management of meningitis that may be caused by pneumococci. It has been suggested that the regimen of a broad-spectrum cephalosporin plus vancomycin

should be continued if the *S. pneumoniae* isolate is resistant to penicillin (MIC ≥0.1 µg/mL) and to ceftriaxone and cefotaxime (MIC >0.5 µg/mL). In adults who receive adjunctive dexamethasone, ceftriaxone or cefotaxime plus rifampin has been suggested as the preferred combination pending susceptibility studies. The usual duration of therapy for pneumococcal meningitis is generally stated to be 10 to 14 days.

The role for steroids in adults with meningitis has not been definitively established. An opinion by experts in the field has suggested that those adult patients who might be candidates for steroid therapy in meningitis are those with a high CSF concentration of bacteria (i.e., demonstrable bacteria on Gram's stain of CSF), especially if there is increased intracranial pressure (*Clin Infect Dis* 1993; 17:603-610). In a recent discussion of pneumococcal meningitis, the issue of adjunctive steroid therapy in adults with meningitis was discussed (*Hosp Pract* [off ed] 2001; 36[2]:43-51). It was the opinion of the authors that adjunctive dexamethasone should be considered in adults who have a positive CSF Gram stain for bacteria and who have at clinical presentation at least 2 of the 3 prognostic features for an adverse clinical outcome (i.e., altered mental status, seizures, hypotension). When steroids have been recommended for meningitis, a suggested dose of dexamethasone has been 0.15 mg/kg given intravenously every 6 hours for 4 days.

The infectious syndromes caused by *N. meningitidis* are somewhat broad and include meningococcal meningitis, meningococcal bacteremia, meningococcemia (purpura fulminans and the Waterhouse-Friderichsen syndrome), respiratory tract infections (pneumonia, epiglottitis, otitis media), focal infection (conjunctivitis, septic arthritis, urethritis, purulent pericarditis), and chronic meningococcemia (*Clin Infect Dis* 2001; 355:1378-1388). Important in the pathogenesis of the clinical illnesses caused by the meningococcus is the organism's natural reservoir in the nasopharynx. It is this site from which disease may develop. The epidemiology of meningococcal meningitis is evolving. The traditional groups of patients at risk have included children and young adults, especially college students or military recruits who have relatively confined quarters. A recent report from Argentina (*J Infect Dis* 1998; 178:266-269) described epidemic meningococcal disease in the northeastern part of that country associated with disco patronage, supporting the pathogenetic point that close confinement allows aerosolization and spread of the organism from the nasopharynx. An additional observation from this study, which has been raised in previous studies, is the association with passive or active cigarette smoking. This report, which was subtitled "Disco Fever," expands the closed settings in which meningococcal meningitis originates to include dance clubs and discos. Pneumonia, sinusitis, and tracheobronchitis are important sources of bacteremic meningococcal disease. Although meningitis is the characteristic infection caused by *N. meningitidis*, a report from Atlanta (*Ann Intern Med* 1995; 123:937-940) noted that only 14 (32%) of the 44 adult patients with meningococcal infection had meningitis. When it occurs, meningococcal meningitis is usually acute and often associated with purpuric skin lesions (although the Atlanta report noted that only 10 of the 14 adults with meningitis [71%] had a generalized rash). During the very early stages of infection, the CSF analysis may be relatively normal even though the clinical course is hyperacute with fever, nuchal rigidity, and coma. Although variably reported through the years, the potential for *N. meningitidis* to cause purulent pericarditis should be noted. The illness may progress to acidosis, tissue hypoxia, shock, disseminated intravascular coagulopathy, and hemorrhagic adrenal infarction. The potential for β-lactamase-producing strains remains a concern, as does the existence of relatively resistant strains, presumably caused by alterations in the penicillin-binding proteins; however, active surveillance among a large, diverse population in the United States has failed to identify any such strains (*Clin Infect Dis* 2000; 30:212-213). Penicillin or ampicillin, therefore, remains a drug of choice for treating meningitis caused by this pathogen. The usual duration of therapy is generally 7 to 10 days, but duration is best based on clinical response. With meningococcemia, a fulminant complication is acute, massive adrenal hemorrhage with the resultant clinical entity of the Waterhouse-Friderichsen syndrome. However, not all patients who die of meningococcemia have evidence of adrenal hemorrhage at autopsy, and many steroid-treated patients succumb despite therapy, implying that adrenal insufficiency may not be the primary cause of circulatory collapse. Because of the implications of such a complication, it would be helpful to have definitive recommendations about the role, if any, of steroids in management of patients with meningococcal meningitis. There are anecdotal reports in the literature of improved outcome in such patients treated with corticosteroids. In some patients with meningococcal infection, cortisol levels may be elevated. In contrast, other reports have noted that not all patients with severe meningococcal infection who have been given ACTH have responded to ACTH stimulation of cortisol production, and this raises the issues of whether adrenal reserves may be decreased in certain patients and whether steroids may have a role. In 1992, the Infectious Diseases Society of America published a review of the role of steroids in patients with infectious diseases (*J Infect Dis* 1992; 165:1-13). Of the 10 infections for which steroids were strongly supported or suggested as having a role, meningococcemia was not one of those listed. At the present time, the role of steroids in meningococcemia is unresolved. Since fulminant meningococcal septicemia represents an extreme form of endotoxin-induced sepsis and coagulopathy, with clinical consequences that include amputations and organ failure, investigators have addressed other potential therapeutic modalities that may be beneficial in patients with overwhelming meningococcal infection. The dual function of protein C as an anticoagulant and as a modulator of the inflammatory response was recently reviewed in the context of experimental data showing that activated protein C replacement therapy reduces the mortality rate for fulminant meningococcemia (*Clin Infect Dis* 2001; 32:1338-1346). Such data become especially noteworthy given the efficacy and safety data about recombinant human activated protein C in patients with severe sepsis (*N Engl J Med* 2001; 344:699-709).

In patients treated with penicillin for meningococcal meningitis, posttreatment with rifampin, ciprofloxacin, or ceftriaxone has been recommended to eradicate the nasal carrier state, since penicillin will not eliminate organisms at this site *(MMWR* 2000; 49[RR-7]:1-20). Since 1991, there have been increased numbers of outbreaks of serogroup C meningococcal disease (SCMD) in the United States. A recent trial has shown that meningococcal polysaccharide vaccine was effective against SCMD in a community outbreak, with vaccine efficacy among 2- to 29-year-olds of 85% (*JAMA* 1998; 279:435-439). Based on this observation, it has been recommended for future outbreaks that emphasis be placed on achieving high vaccination coverage, with special efforts to vaccinate young adults. The Advisory Committee on Immunization Practices and the American Academy of Pediatrics have recommended that healthcare providers and colleges educate freshmen college students, especially those who live in dormatories, and their parents about the increased risk of meningococcal diseases and the potential benefits of immunization so that informed decisions about vaccination can be made (*MMWR* 2000; 49[RR-7]:11-20). In individuals with recurrent episodes of neisserial infections like meningococcal meningitis, deficiencies in the late complement components (i.e., C_5-C_8) may be the underlying predisposition. Such a deficiency is best screened for using the total hemolytic complement (CH_{50}) assay, with a normal study essentially excluding complement deficiency.

Like the meningococcus, *H. influenzae* may be isolated from the nasopharynx, and this may be the immediate source of invading pathogens. Rates of infection caused by this pathogen have decreased because of vaccine against *H. influenzae*. In patients with meningitis due to this organism, a contiguous focus of infection like sinusitis or otitis media should be investigated. In adults without these underlying processes, a search for a CSF leak, which may be the basis for the meningitis, is necessary. Since about one-third of *H. influenzae* isolates are β-lactamase producers, agents that are stable in the presence of these enzymes and that cross the blood-brain barrier should be used. The

third-generation cephalosporins cefotaxime and ceftriaxone have had the most successful record of use in this regard. Even though the second-generation cephalosporin cefuroxime is active against *H. influenzae*, it has been shown to result in delayed sterilization of the CSF when compared to ceftriaxone. A lower incidence of sensorineural hearing loss was demonstrated in children who adjunctively received dexamethasone (3.3%) versus those who did not receive steroids (15.5%). Similar findings have not been corroborated in adults. The usual duration of therapy for *H. influenzae* meningitis is generally 10 to 14 days.

Meningitis due to Gram-negative bacilli occurs most characteristically after neurosurgical procedures, with head trauma being a less likely predisposition. Medical conditions, including urosepsis, account for about 20% of episodes of this infection. In patients who develop Gram-negative meningitis in the setting of immunosuppressive therapy that impairs cell-mediated immunity, one should exclude *Strongyloides stercoralis* infection as the underlying predisposing cause. Parenterally administered aminoglycosides do not cross the blood-brain barrier after the 28th day of life. For these antibiotics to be useful beyond the neonatal period, they need to be administered intrathecally or intraventricularly. Chloramphenicol has activity against some Gram-negative bacilli, and it crosses the blood-brain barrier. Concern about toxicity issues such as aplastic anemia has over the years decreased the use of this agent, although it still occupies an important role in persons with meningitis and Type I (IgE-mediated) hypersensitivity to penicillins. Third-generation cephalosporins have become the mainstay of therapy for Gram-negative meningitis because of their spectrum and their penetration into the CSF. All of the presently available third-generation agents, except for cefoperazone, have an indication for meningitis due to susceptible pathogens. For meningitis due to *Pseudomonas aeruginosa*, ceftazidime is the most efficacious agent. It is usually administered with a parenteral aminoglycoside, recognizing that this latter agent will not cross the blood-brain barrier in adults but that it might help to eradicate the site of infection outside the central nervous system that served as the focus for the meningitis. For meningitis due to Gram-negative pathogens, therapy is generally given for 10 days after the CSF becomes sterile.

Pharmacologic and microbiologic issues are important for 2 important pathogens that cause meningitis. *L. monocytogenes* is an intracellular Gram-positive rod that characteristically infects persons with defects in cell-mediated immunity. It may also cause disease in diabetics and elderly persons, and about 30% of infected adults have no apparent risk. Acquisition has been associated with consumption of contaminated coleslaw, milk, and cheese. Although the CSF cellular response is usually polymorphonuclear, some patients present either with lymphocytes or with a normal glucose. Like fungal and tuberculous meningitis, *Listeria* meningitis has a predilection for involving the meninges at the base of the brain. This may lead to hydrocephalus. Ampicillin or penicillin is the drug of choice, and there is no significant activity by third-generation cephalosporins against this pathogen. Some experts suggest the addition of an aminoglycoside given parenterally because of *in vitro* synergy. For those patients who are penicillin allergic, trimethoprim-sulfamethoxazole is the agent of choice. Because of the intracellular location of this pathogen, therapy should be continued for 3 weeks or longer. A review of *S. aureus* meningitis divided this disease entity into 2 categories: a) hospital-acquired and b) community-acquired (*Scand J Infect Dis* 1995; 27:569-573). It was noted that hospital-acquired infection occurred as an occasional complication of neurosurgical procedures, with the presence of medical devices, or with certain skin infections; it generally had a favorable prognosis and a relatively low mortality rate. In contrast, community-acquired *S. aureus* meningitis was associated with valvular heart disease, diabetes mellitus, or drug or alcohol abuse, and it had mortality significantly higher than nosocomial infection. In this review of 28 patients with community-acquired *S. aureus* meningitis, 8 had negative or no CSF culture. Of these 8 patients, 4 had received antibiotics prior to lumbar puncture. This finding is consistent with the observation that an important presentation of *S.*

aureus is in patients with addict-associated infective endocarditis. For *S. aureus*, nafcillin or oxacillin has better activity against methicillin-sensitive strains than does vancomycin. In addition, the penetration of vancomycin into CSF may be variable even in the setting of meningeal inflammation.

Beginning with the September 11, 2001 episode of terrorism in the United States, an important new consideration entered the differential diagnosis of patients with a life-threatening illness that includes a meningeal component: anthrax. Inhalational anthrax is a biphasic clinical syndrome with initial nonspecific flu-like symptoms (fatique, malaise, myalgia, headache, nonproductive cough, and nausea/vomiting) followed by a second phase with hemodynamic collapse, septic shock/MODS, and rapid death with overwhelming bacterial spread. It is during the stage of bacteremia that there is a strong likelihood of meningitis, which some sources cite as occurring in 50% of cases. The index case of bioterrorism anthrax in Florida presented with hemorrhagic meningitis (*N Engl J Med* 2001; 345:1607-1610), which is characteristic of disseminated anthrax; however, meningitis without hemorrhage can occur with anthrax. In patients suspected of having infection with *Bacillus anthracis* as the cause of meningitis, some have suggested the addition of either penicillin or chloramphicol to the multidrug regimen that would be given for inhalational anthrax (*JAMA* 2001; 286:2549-2553).

Empiric therapy for meningitis has changed in recent years. In previously healthy individuals with acute pyogenic community-acquired meningitis in whom little information is available, ampicillin was suggested in a 1993 review (*N Engl J Med* 1993; 328:21-28) as a reasonable empiric agent in the absence of penicillin allergy. For those patients with Type I (IgE-mediated) allergy to penicillin but who were previously healthy with acute pyogenic community-acquired meningitis, chloramphenicol was offered in that review as appropriate therapy. As listed in Table 3, a broad-spectrum cephalosporin (e.g., cefotaxime or ceftriaxone) has been more recently suggested as empiric therapy for individuals that are age 18 to 50 years with a nondiagnostic Gram's stain.

The addition of ampicillin to a broad-spectrum cephalosporin is reasonable empiric therapy for polymorphonuclear meningitis undiagnosed by Gram's stain in patient populations with the following underlying conditions: a) advanced age; b) alcoholism; and c) immunocompromised states. The activity by ampicillin against *Listeria* is an important component of the coverage in this regimen.

Certain epidemiologic situations may exist which influence the acquisition of specific pathogens that may then cause meningitis. Those conditions (including skull fractures and shunt-associated infections), and the pathogens likely to occur in their setting, are summarized in Table 2.

Lymphocytic Meningitis with Normal Glucose

The meningeal response to infection or inflammation may be less marked in certain conditions, and the response may therefore be less associated with the inability to transport glucose across the meninges. Those conditions associated with the findings of lymphocytes and normal glucose in the CSF are listed in Table 1. The classic consideration in this differential has been viral meningitis. Enteroviruses, which are recognized causes of pleurodynia and pericarditis, are the most common cause of aseptic meningitis and characteristically cause a self-limited form of meningitis that presents with fever, headache, and lymphocytic pleocytosis, most often in the late summer or early fall. Recently, however, 2 other viruses have gained importance in the differential diagnosis of viral meningitis. With initial episodes or flares of genital herpes simplex virus infection, patients may develop meningitis as a systemic manifestation of their herpes infection. This process is distinctly different from the life-threatening entity of herpes encephalitis in that it is self-limited and does not require therapy. Because of the propensity for herpes genitalis to recur, this form of meningitis may similarly present as a recurrent form of lymphocytic meningitis. HIV has a predilection for neural tissue, and patients, including those with the acute retroviral syndrome, may present with viral meningitis that may resolve spontaneously. In those individuals with risk factors for HIV

and who present with an illness consistent with viral meningitis, HIV infection is an important consideration.

Encephalitis may occur on the basis of both infectious and noninfectious causes. When these conditions are associated with white blood cells in the CSF, the diagnosis of meningoencephalitis may be made. Traditional teaching has been that meningoencephalitis, like viral encephalitis, will give a normal glucose in association with lymphocytes. As outlined in Table 1, herpes encephalitis may result in a low glucose level.

Spirochetal infections are an important cause of lymphocytic meningitis with normal glucose. *Treponema pallidum*, the etiologic agent of syphilis, is a recognized cause of asymptomatic infection of the central nervous system in nonimmunocompromised hosts. Increasingly diagnosed in the era of HIV infection has been meningovascular syphilis, which may take the forms of syphilitic meningitis or of a stroke syndrome. In May 2002, the Centers for Disease Control and Prevention published its most recent guidelines for the management of sexually transmitted diseases (*MMWR* 2002; 51[RR-6]:1-80). Several important points were made regarding neurosyphilis. Since CNS disease can occur during any stage of syphilis, a patient who has clinical evidence of neurologic involvement with syphilis (e.g., cognitive dysfunction, motor or sensory deficits, ophthalmic or auditory symptoms, cranial nerve palsies, and symptoms or signs of meningitis) should have a CSF examination. Because it is highly specific although insensitive, the VDRL-CSF is the standard serologic test for CSF. When reactive in the absence of substantial contamination of CSF with blood, it is considered diagnostic of neurosyphilis. However, with syphilitic meningitis, patients may present without symptoms of nervous system disease and may have on CSF analysis only a few lymphocytes and a negative VDRL-CSF. The FTA-ABS test on CSF is less specific for neurosyphilis than the VDRL-CSF, but the high sensitivity of the study has led some experts to believe that a negative CSF FTA-ABS test excludes neurosyphilis (*MMWR* 2002; 51[RR-6]:1-80). Based on these facts, individuals whose peripheral blood

Table 3. Recommendations for empiric therapy for meningitis based on Gram stain of cerebrospinal fluid (CSF)

In Patients with a Nondiagnostic Gram Stain of CSF		In Patients with a Positive Gram Stain or Culture of CSF	
Age <3 months	Ampicillin plus a broad-spectrum cephalosporin	Gram-positive cocci	Vancomycin plus broad-spectrum cephalosporin
Age 3 months to <18 years	Broad-spectrum cephalosporin	Gram-negative cocci	Penicillin G
Age 18 to 50 years	Broad-spectrum cephalosporin	Gram-positive bacilli	Ampicillin (or penicillin) plus aminoglycoside
Age >50 years	Ampicillin plus broad-spectrum cephalosporin	Gram-negative bacilli	Broad-spectrum cephalosporin plus aminoglycoside
Impaired cell-mediated immunity	Ampicillin plus ceftazidime		
Head trauma, neurosurgery, or CSF shunt	Vancomycin plus ceftazidime		

For the recommendations used in Table 3, broad-spectrum cephalosporin was used to refer to either cefotaxime or ceftriaxone. Specific comments regarding these recommendations are included in the paper.

Adapted from Quagliarello VJ and Scheld WM: Treatment of bacterial meningitis. *N Engl J Med* 1997; 336:708–716

serology is positive for syphilis and who have >5 WBCs/mm^3 in their CSF without another identified etiology for this pleocytosis should be treated for neurosyphilis, regardless of the VDRL-CSF. Similar findings may also occur with cerebrovascular disease caused by syphilis. These patients, often young, may present with a stroke syndrome due to an endarteritis, which most characteristically involves the middle cerebral artery.

According to recent guidelines (*MMWR* 2002; 51[RR-6]:1-80), the recommended regimen for patients with neurosyphilis is aqueous crystalline penicillin G 18-24 million units per day, administered as 3-4 million units IV every 4 hours or continuous infusion, for 10-14 days. If compliance with therapy can be ensured, patients may be treated with procaine penicillin 2.4 million units IM once daily plus probenecid 500 mg orally 4 times a day, both for 10-14 days. Since these durations are shorter than the regimen used for late syphilis in the absence of neurosyphilis, some specialists administer benzathine penicillin, 2.4 million units IM once per week for up to 3 weeks after completion of these neurosyphilis treatment regimens to provide a comparable total duration of therapy. The CSF leukocyte count has been stated to be a sensitive measure of the effectiveness of therapy.

The classic presentation of neurologic Lyme disease, which is caused by *Borrelia burgdorferi*, is seventh nerve palsy (which may be bilateral), in association with a lymphocytic meningitis.

Leptospirosis, caused by *Leptospira interrogans*, is epidemiologically linked to such factors as infected rat urine or exposure to infected dogs. It presents as 2 distinct clinical syndromes. Anicteric leptospirosis is a self-limiting illness, which progresses through 2 well-defined stages: a septicemic stage and an immune stage. The septicemic stage occurs after a 7- to 12-day incubation period and is primarily manifested as fever, chills, nausea, vomiting, and headache. The most characteristic physical finding during this stage is conjunctival suffusion. The causative organism can be isolated from blood or CSF at this point. Following a 1- to 3-day asymptomatic period, the immune stage develops, and it is characterized by aseptic meningitis. Leptospira are present in the urine during this stage and may persist for up to 3 weeks. Icteric leptospirosis, or Weil's syndrome, is a less common but potentially fatal syndrome that occurs in 5% to 10% of cases. Jaundice, renal involvement, hypotension, and hemorrhage are the hallmarks of this form of leptospirosis; however, the severity of these manifestations can vary greatly, and renal involvement is not universal. In icteric leptospirosis, the biphasic nature of the disease is somewhat obscured by the persistence of jaundice and azotemia throughout the illness, but septicemic and immune stages do occur. Leptospires can be isolated from blood or cerebrospinal fluid during the first week and from the urine during the second week of illness. Additionally, the diagnosis can be made by demonstrating rising antibody titers. Treatment of leptospirosis involves intense supportive care as well as antibiotic coverage. The use of intravenous penicillin (1.5 million units every 6 hours) has been shown to shorten the duration of fever, renal dysfunction, and hospital stay.

Over the years, Rocky Mountain Spotted Fever, which is caused by *Rickettsia rickettsii*, has been considered the classic rickettsial infection in the United States. CSF analysis is usually normal unless patients have stupor or coma, in which case there may be a lymphocytic pleocytosis with normal glucose and elevated protein. An important emerging infection in the United States is ehrlichiosis. The clinical illness attributable to this infection is

discussed in this syllabus in the section on encephalitis. The characteristic CSF abnormalities in patients with ehrlichiosis have been a lymphocytic pleocytosis with elevated protein. In a recent review of the subject, CSF glucose was normal in the majority of patients, with 24% of the patients having borderline low CSF glucose concentrations. In this review, morulae were seen in CSF white cells in only a small minority of the patients. Clinical features supporting the diagnosis of ehrlichiosis are leukopenia (because of the intracellular location of the organism), thrombocytopenia, and elevated liver enzymes. From the limited clinical data available, it appears that chloramphenicol or tetracycline is the agent most frequently used for this infection.

Certain infectious diseases such as infective endocarditis may cause a lymphocytic pleocytosis with normal glucose that is the result of a vasculitis, which the infectious process causes in the central nervous system. A review of a 12-year experience at the Cleveland Clinic included the results of lumbar punctures done on 23 of 175 patients with endocarditis (*Neurology* 1989; 39:173-178). There was a CSF pleocytosis in 14 and no CSF white blood cells in 9. Of the 14 patients who had a pleocytosis, the etiology was attributed to a stroke in 8 and to encephalopathy in 5; the remaining patient only had isolated headaches described. No positive CSF cultures were reported in any of these 14 patients. Such information underscores a dilemma for the clinician managing a patient with endocarditis who has a CSF pleocytosis: Is the pleocytosis due to secondary bacterial seeding of the meninges, or is it due to other events associated with endocarditis that lead to a central nervous system response that is associated with a secondary cellular response?

A group of noninfectious causes of lymphocytic meningitis with normal glucose are described in Table 1.

Lymphocytic Meningitis with Low Glucose

With chronic processes, it is not surprising that the cellular CSF response would be lymphocytes. Low CSF glucose has been described in this syllabus as occurring due to impaired transport based on acute inflammation of the meninges. In certain conditions, glucose transport may be associated with infiltration of the meninges by either granulomatous processes or malignant cells. Such is the situation for several of the conditions summarized in Table 1 which cause lymphocytic meningitis with low glucose.

Viral meningitis due to mumps and lymphocytic choriomeningitis (LCM) has characteristically been associated with a low CSF glucose. As previously discussed, certain forms of meningoencephalitis, including that due to herpes simplex virus, may present in this manner. Partially-treated bacterial meningitis and certain chemical-induced meningitides may have similar findings. Four other groups of conditions are important in this setting: a) tuberculous meningitis; b) fungal meningitis; c) carcinomatous meningitis; and d) subarachnoid hemorrhage.

A review of 48 adult patients with tuberculous meningitis who were admitted to an intensive care unit demonstrates the potential for this infectious process to cause serious disease (*Clin Infect Dis* 1996; 22:982-988). It also emphasizes the difficulty often encountered in establishing the diagnosis. Repeated large-volumes (10-20 mL) of CSF have a higher yield for acid-fast bacilli (*Clin Infect Dis* 1993; 17:987-994). When 4 CSF smears for acid-fast bacilli are obtained, positive findings may occur in up to 90% of patients with tuberculous meningitis. Some studies have shown that elevated CSF titers of adenosine deaminase (*Clin Infect Dis* 1995; 20:525-530) or that CSF chloride levels <110 mEq/L in the absence of bacterial infection support the diagnosis of tuberculous meningitis. ELISA assays are felt by some to be helpful with this diagnosis. PCR for *Mycobacterium tuberculosis* may be helpful when performed on CSF, but false negatives have been reported. Because of a predilection for tuberculous meningitis to involve the base of the brain, imaging studies of the central nervous system may reveal an obstructing hydrocephalus. In addition to antituberculous therapy with agents such as isoniazid, rifampin, pyrazinamide, and ethambutol, corticosteroids may play a role, especially in situations of increased intracranial pressure or obstruction resulting from the infection. From the series of

patients with tuberculous meningitis admitted to an intensive care unit, several important clinical points can be extracted. a) Ischemic lesions with signs of localization may be present. b) Extrameningeal tuberculous infection may support the diagnosis. (Overall, the rate has been stated to be 40% to 45%, but in this review it was 66%.) c) Clinical features and CSF profiles did not appear to be modified in the HIV-infected patients. d) Delay to onset of treatment and the neurological status at admission were identified as the main clinical prognostic factors.

Although fungal meningitis may be due to several etiologic agents, the 2 most common ones are *Cryptococcus neoformans* and *Coccidioides immitis*. Although both of these pathogens have been increasingly diagnosed as a cause of meningitis because of HIV infection, both caused meningitis in normal hosts prior to the AIDS era. Both organisms gain access to the body via the lungs. In HIV-infected persons with cryptococcal meningitis, there may be a lack of inflammation in the CSF, and therefore findings may include <20 CSF white cells/mm^3 and a normal glucose. Important, therefore, in the diagnosis are the India ink, latex agglutination, and fungal culture of the CSF. Potentially helpful in establishing the diagnosis are other sites of involvement including lung, skin, and blood. Based on data from the Mycoses Study Group of the National Institutes of Health (*N Engl J Med* 1997; 337:15-21), it appears that therapy for cryptococcal meningitis in HIV-infected patients should begin with amphotericin B (0.7 mg/kg/day) in combination with flucytosine (100 mg/kg/day in persons with normal renal function) for the initial 2 weeks of therapy followed by fluconazole (400 mg/day orally) for a further 8 to 10 weeks. In the 381 patients with cryptococcal meningitis treated in this double-blind multicenter trial, 13 of 14 early deaths and 40% of deaths during weeks 3 through 10 were associated with elevated intracranial pressure. Based on the association of elevated intracranial pressure and mortality in patients with cryptococcal meningitis, it was suggested that measurement of intracranial pressure be included in the management of such patients. Included in the recommendations were daily lumbar punctures, use of acetazolamide, and ventriculoperitoneal shunts for asymptomatic patients with intracranial CSF pressure >320 mm and for symptomatic patients with pressures >180 mm. More recently (*Clin Infect Dis* 2000; 30:47-54), it was recommended in the absence of focal lesions that opening pressures ≥250 mm H_2O be treated with large-volume CSF drainage (defined in this report as allowing CSF to drain until a satisfactory closing pressure had been achieved, commonly <200 mm H_2O. Maintenance therapy is required following completion of primary therapy, and studies have defined fluconazole (200 mg/day orally) as the agent of choice.

Meningitis due to *Coccidioides immitis* commonly presents with headache, vomiting, and altered mental status. Although the CSF formula is usually one of lymphocytes with low glucose, eosinophils are occasionally present. In addition to direct examination and culture of CSF, complement-fixing antibodies in the CSF may be an especially important aid to the diagnosis of coccidioidal meningitis. As with cryptococcal meningitis, the epidemiologic history and the other body sites of involvement (including lung, skin, joints, and bone) are important in making the diagnosis. In contrast to cryptococcal meningitis, management strategies for coccidioidal meningitis may vary from patient to patient. Recent guidelines of the Infectious Diseases Society of America (*Clin Infect Dis* 2000; 30:658-661) noted that oral fluconazole is currently preferred therapy, with itraconazole being listed as having comparable efficacy. It was acknowledged that some physicians initiate therapy with intrathecal amphotericin B in addition to an azole on the basis of their belief that responses may be more prompt with this approach. Since *Coccidioides* has a predilection for the basilar meninges, hydrocephalus may occur. Regardless of the regimen being used, this potential complication nearly always requires a shunt for decompression

Other fungi have the capability of causing meningitis, but they are less likely to do so. As a general rule, fungal meningitis like tuberculous meningitis may involve the base of the brain and cause obstruction of CSF flow with resulting hydrocephalus.

Eosinophilic Meningitis

Angiostrongylus cantonesis is a nematode that can infect humans who ingest poorly cooked or raw intermediate mollusc hosts such as snails, slugs, and prawns. Infection can also occur when fresh vegetables contaminated with infective larvae are eaten. Once ingested, the infective larvae penetrate the gut wall and migrate to the small vessels of the meninges to cause a clinical picture of fever, meningismus and headache. CSF analysis reveals an eosinophilic pleocytosis, and larvae are usually not found. Such a process has been most characteristically described in Asia and the South Pacific. A recent report described an outbreak of meningitis due to *A. cantonesis* that developed in 12 travelers who traveled to the Caribbean and whose clinical illness was strongly associated with the consumption of a Caesar salad at a meal (*N Engl J Med* 2002; 346:668-675). From this outbreak, it was suggested that *A. cantonensis* infection should be suspected among travelers at risk who present with headache, elevated intracranial pressure, and pleocytosis, with or without eosinophilia, particularly in association with paresthesias or hyperesthesias. Less classic causes of eosinophilic meningitis include *Trichinella spiralis, Taenia solium, Toxocara canis, Gnathostoma spinigerum,* and *Paragonimus westermani.*

Meningitis Caused by Protozoa or Helminths

Of the causes of nervous system disease due to protozoa or helminths, 5 deserve special comment. The most common is due to *Toxoplasma gondii* and presents most often as multiple ring-enhancing lesions in HIV-infected patients. Because this usually represents reactivation disease, the IgG antibody to *Toxoplasma* is positive in about 95% of these individuals. Therapy is with sulfadiazine and pyrimethamine. *Naegleria fowleri* is a free-living amoeba that enters the CNS by invading the nasal mucosa at the level of the cribriform plate. The classic presentation is of an acute pyogenic meningitis in a person who recently swam in fresh water. The CSF analysis shows a polymorphonuclear pleocytosis, many red blood cells, and hypoglycorrhachia. The diagnosis is confirmed by identifying the organism on CSF wet mount as motile amoeba, or it can be made by biopsy of brain tissue. Amphotericin B administered systemically and intraventricularly is the drug of choice. Another amoebic pathogen infecting the nervous system is *Acanthamoeba*, which may infect individuals with defects in cell-mediated immunity (including patients with AIDS or after organ transplantation) and result in a granulomatous amoebic encephalitis. Clinical manifestations include mental status abnormalities, seizures, fever, headache, focal neurologic deficits, meningismus, visual disturbances, and ataxia. An important clinical clue may be pre-existing skin lesions which have been present for months before CNS disease and which may take the form of ulcerative, nodular, or subcutaneous abscesses. Pneumonitis may also be a part of the clinical presentation. Neurocysticercosis, which is caused by the pork tapeworm *Taenia solium*, is an important cause of new-onset seizures in patients from Mexico. Brain imaging studies may reveal intracranial lesions, which may be cystic or calcified; because of chronic inflammation at the base of the brain, hydrocephalus may be present. The epidemiologic history combined with brain imaging studies and serologies (ELISA or hemagglutination) help make the diagnosis. Steroids may be useful adjunctively in patients with severe symptoms or seizures during therapy. Traditional treatment has been with praziquantel for cystic lesions or with increased intracranial pressure, but albendazole may be preferred for medical treatment with concurrent corticosteroids and for resection of ventricular cysts. As previously noted, *Angiostrongylus cantonesis* may be a cause of eosinophilic meningitis.

Miscellaneous Issues in the Diagnosis and Management of Meningitis

The timing of diagnostic studies in patients with meningitis is of critical importance. An important issue is focality. Over the last several decades, many have limited the designation of focality to such processes as hemiparesis, isolated abnormalities on an imaging study of the brain, or an abnormal focus on an electroencephalogram. More recently, it has been stated that altered mental status indicates bilateral hemispheric or brainstem dysfunction and severely compromises the ability to determine whether the patient's neurologic assessment is nonfocal.

Because of the potential for severe neurologic sequella in individuals with bacterial meningitis who are treated in a suboptimal manner, attention has been focused in recent years on the appropriate sequencing of diagnostic studies. As was stated in the paper referenced in Table 3, patients with coma, papilledema, or focal neurologic findings require cranial imaging before lumbar puncture. Some would consider altered mental status as an additional reason for cranial imaging before lumbar puncture. More recently, a prospective study of 301 adults with suspected meningitis was conducted to determine whether clinical characteristics present before CT of the head was performed could be used to identify patients who were unlikely to have abnormalities on CT (*N Engl J Med* 2001; 345:1727-1733). Thirteen base-line clinical characteristics were used to predict abnormal findings on head CT: age ≥ 60 yr; immunocompromised state; history of CNS disease; seizure within 1 week before presentation; abnormal level of consciousness; inability to answer 2 questions correctly; inability to follow 2 commands correctly; gaze palsy; abnormal visual fields; facial palsy; arm drift; leg drift; and abnormal language (i.e., aphasia, dysarthria, and extinction). From the results of the study, the authors concluded that adults with suspected meningitis who have none of the noted baseline features are good candidates for immediate lumbar puncture since they have a low risk of brain herniation as a result of lumbar puncture. It was acknowledged that such an approach would have resulted in a 41% decrease in the frequency of CT scans performed in the study cohort. When imaging is indicated, the following sequence of evaluation and management has been suggested: a) obtain blood cultures; b) institute empiric antibiotic therapy; c) perform lumbar puncture immediately after the imaging study if no intracranial mass lesion is present (*N Engl J Med* 1997; 336:708-716).

Supporting the importance of the timing of antibiotics in patients with meningitis are the findings of a retrospective, observational cohort study of patients with community-acquired bacterial meningitis (*Ann Intern Med* 1998; 129:862-869). In this study, patients with microbiologically-proven, community-acquired bacterial meningitis were stratified into 3 groups based on the clinical findings of hypotension, altered mental status, and seizures. Patients with none of these 3 predictor variables were Stage I, with 1 predictor variable were Stage II, and with 2 or more predictor variables were Stage III. Delay in therapy after arrival in the emergency department was associated with adverse clinical outcome when the patient's condition advanced from Stage I or II to Stage III before the initial antibiotic dose was given, a finding which underscores the need for prompt administration of antibiotics in patients with bacterial meningitis. This study was further interpreted as suggesting that the risk for adverse outcome is influenced more by the severity of illness than the timing of initial antibiotic therapy for patients who arrive in the emergency department at Stage III.

A recent analysis of the causes of death in adults hospitalized with community-acquired bacterial meningitis provides some important insights (*Clin Infect Dis* 2001; 33:969-975). Although 50% of the 74 patients had meningitis as the underlying and immediate cause of death, 18% of patients had meningitis as the underlying but not immediate cause of death and 23% had meningitis as neither the underlying nor immediate cause of death. A 14-day survival end point discriminated between deaths attributable to meningitis and those with another cause. It was concluded that such an end point will facilitate greater accuracy of epidemiological statistics and will assist investigations of the impact of new therapeutic interventions. For many years, clinicians have relied on a cerebrospinal fluid pleocytosis for diagnosing meningitis. In the *Medical Knowledge Self-Assessment Program IX (MKSAP IX)* of the American College of Physicians, it was acknowledged that there are at least 4 clinical entities in which patients may have fever, coma, and nuchal ridigity but a normal cerebrospinal fluid analysis: a) early bacterial meningitis; b) cryptococcal meningitis with concomitant HIV infection; c) parameningeal foci; and d) herpes simplex encephalitis.

Encephalitis

Characteristic of processes involving cortical brain matter are alterations of consciousness and/or cognitive dysfunction. A representative clinical entity with such findings is acute viral encephalitis, which occurs on the basis of direct infection of neural cells with associated perivascular inflammation, neuronal destruction, and tissue necrosis. Pathologically, the involvement in acute viral encephalitis is in the gray matter. This may be associated with evidence of meningeal irritation and CSF mononuclear pleocytosis, in which the process is referred to as meningoencephalitis. In addition to infectious agents, which may cause direct brain injury, there are indirect mechanisms including induction of autoimmune diseases. This process is referred to as postinfectious encephalomyelitis and is characterized by widespread perivenular inflammation with demyelination localized to the white matter of the brain. The list of infectious and noninfectious processes causing encephalitis is lengthy and is partially summarized in Table 4. An additional process, which represents the sequella of an infection, is production of neurotoxins as occurs with shigellosis, melioidosis, and cat-scratch disease.

Of all the mechanisms by which an infectious process leads to involvement of the brain, direct viral invasion of neural cells is the most classic. Although the most common cause of acute viral meningitis is enteroviral infection (notably coxsackie A and B viruses and echoviruses), it has been stated that <3% of the central nervous system complications from such infections would be classified as encephalitis. Diagnostic studies should include viral pharyngeal, rectal, and urine cultures, but confirmation using acute and convalescent phase serology is important because viral shedding from the sites of culture may occur without clinical disease. No specific therapy is available for enteroviral encephalitis.

From the clinical perspective, the most emergent encephalitis to diagnose is that due to herpes simplex virus (HSV). This infection is characteristically caused by HSV Type 1 and

Table 4. Encephalitis

Infectious	Postinfectious Encephalomyelitis	Noninfectious Diseases Simulating Viral Encephalitis
Viral	Vaccinia virus	Systemic lupus erythematosus
Rabies	Measles virus	Granulomatous angiitis
Herpes viruses (herpes simplex 1	Varicella-zoster virus	Behcet's disease
and 2, varicella-zoster, herpes B	Rubella virus	Neoplastic diseases, including
[Simian herpes], Epstein-Barr,	Epstein-Barr virus	carcinomatous meningitis
CMV, human herpes 6)	Mumps virus	Sarcoid
Arthropod-borne (See Table 5)	Influenza virus	Reye syndrome
Mumps	Nonspecific respiratory	Adrenal leukodystrophy
Lymphocytic choriomeningitis	disease	Metabolic encephalopathies
Enteroviruses (coxsackie, echo		Cerebrovascular disease
hepatitis A)		Subdural hematoma
Human immunodeficiency virus		Subarachnoid hemorrhage
Bacterial (including *Brucella, Listeria*		Acute multiple sclerosis
Nocardia, Actinomyces,		Toxic encephalopathy,
relapsing fever, cat scratch		including cocaine-induced
disease, Whipple's disease,		Drug reactions
infective endocarditis,		
parameningeal foci)		
Mycobacterium tuberculosis		
Mycoplasma pneumoniae		
Spirochetes (syphilis, Lyme disease,		
leptospirosis)		
Fungal (including *Cryptococcus*		
Coccidioides, Histoplasma,		
Blastomyces, Candida)		
Rickettsial (RMSF, typhus, *Ehrlichia,*		
Q fever)		
Parasites		
Toxoplasma		
Naegleria		
Acanthamoeba		
Plasmodium falciparum		
Trichinella		
Echinococcus		
Cysticercus		
Trypanosoma cruzii		

CMV, cytomegalovirus; RMSF, Rocky Mountain spotted fever.

results in inflammation or necrosis localized to the medial-temporal and orbital-frontal lobes. Although it may have an insidious onset, in its most classic form HSV encephalitis presents as an acute, febrile, focal illness. Because of the temporal lobe localization, personality change may be prominent for a few days to as long as a week before other manifestations. Headache is also a prominent early symptom. Patients may progress rapidly from a nonspecific prodrome of fever and malaise, to findings such as behavioral abnormalities and seizures, to coma. A hallmark of the diagnosis is focality, which may be demonstrated with history (e.g., changes in personality or in olfaction), physical exam, imaging studies of the brain, or electroencephalography. These findings most characteristically involve the temporal lobes. Subtle clues to focality may include abnormalities such as changes in olfaction, which may be influenced by the fact that HSV might access the brain via the olfactory tract. CSF analysis may initially be unrevealing even in some acutely ill patients who have fever, nuchal rigidity, and coma. Characteristic features with lumbar puncture include increased intracranial pressure, CSF lymphocytosis, and the presence of red blood cells in the CSF. Although CSF glucose is characteristically normal, patients may have hypoglycorrhachia. For many years, brain biopsy with viral culture was considered the gold standard diagnostic study. In suspected cases, such pathologic examination of brain tissue often yielded another treatable diagnosis. Because of the invasiveness of the procedure and since neurosurgical services are not available at all hospitals, there has been attention to noninvasive diagnostic procedures. PCR analysis of CSF (when performed with optimal techniques in an experienced laboratory) has been reported to be 100% specific and 75% to 98% sensitive. In a decision model comparing a PCR-based approach with empiric therapy, the PCR-based approach yielded better outcomes with reduced acyclovir use (*Am J Med* 1998; 105:287-295). Prompt initiation of intravenous therapy with acyclovir is critical in management of patients suspected of having this infection, since prognosis is influenced by the level of consciousness at the time therapy is begun. It

has been stated that one cannot anticipate an accuracy of >50% in the diagnosis of HSV encephalitis in the early course of the infection, even when one uses physical examination, spinal fluid analysis, and neuroimaging studies. Relapse of HSV encephalitis has been stated to occur in some patients 1 week to 3 months after initial improvement and completion of a full course of acyclovir therapy. Retreatment may be indicated in these patients.

The arthropod-borne encephalitides are a group of central nervous system infections in which the viral pathogen is transmitted to humans via a mosquito or tick vector. Of those described in Table 5, all are mosquito-borne except for Powassan encephalitis, which is transmitted by the tick *Ixodes cookei*. The distinguishing features of these illnesses are summarized in this table. Of these, Eastern equine encephalitis (EEE) is associated with the highest mortality rate (30%-70%), and this fulminant process results in neurological sequella in >80% of survivors. St. Louis encephalitis (SLE) is caused by a flavivirus, which induces clinical disease in about 1% of those infected. Following a nonspecific prodrome, patients may experience the abrupt onset of headache, nausea, vomiting, disorientation, and stupor. Common laboratory findings include inappropriate secretion of antidiuretic hormone (ADH) and pyuria. In contrast to EEE, the overall mortality due to SLE is about 2% with the highest rate being in elderly persons. Emotional disturbances are the most common sequella. The outbreak of arboviral encephalitis described in metropolitan New York City in the late summer and fall of 1999 was caused by West Nile virus (WNV), a flavivirus that is serologically closely related to SLE virus and that was responsible for 61 human cases, including 7 deaths (*MMWR* 2000; 49:25-28). In addition to the encephalitis caused by this virus, notable features included profound muscle weakness. Like SLE virus, WNV is transmitted principally by *Culex* mosquitoes.

Healthcare providers should consider arboviruses in the differential diagnosis of aseptic meningitis and encephalitis cases during the summer months. According to recommendations by the Centers for Disease Control and Prevention, serum (acute and

Table 5. Arthropod-borne encephalitis

	Mortality	Neurologic Sequella
Eastern Equine Encephalitis	30-70%	80%
St. Louis Encephalitis	2-20%	20%
California Encephalitis	a	a
West Nile Encephalitis	11% [b]	NA
Western Equine Encephalitis	5-15%	30%
Venezuelan Equine Encephalitis	1%	Rare
Powassan Encephalitis	15%	

[a]Uneventful recovery in most patients; abnormal electroencephalograms in 75%, with seizures in 6% to 10%.
[b]Based on the 1999 outbreak in metropolitan New York (MMWR 2000; 49:25-28).

convalescent) and CSF samples should be obtained for serologic testing, and cases should be promptly reported to state health departments (*MMWR* 1995; 44:641-644). Diagnosis of arbovirus encephalitis may be rapidly facilitated by testing acute serum or spinal fluid for virus-specific IgM antibody. In its revised guidelines for surveillance, prevention, and control of West Nile virus infection, the CDC noted that the indirect immunofluorescence assay (IFA) using well-defined murine monoclonal antibodies is the most efficient, economical, and rapid method to identify flaviviruses (http://www.cdc.gov/ncidod/dvbid/westnile/reso urces/wnv-guidelines-apr-2001.pdf). Unfortunately no effective specific therapy is available for any of these infections. Supportive measures should focus on cerebral edema, seizures, or ventilation if problems related to any of these occur.

Human immunodeficiency virus (HIV) has tropism for neural tissue, and a significant number of patients will develop involvement of the central nervous system. As a part of the acute retroviral syndrome that follows initial infection with HIV, patients may develop an acute encephalitis that can include seizures and delirium and from which patients may spontaneously recover with little if any neurologic sequela. On a chronic basis and occurring later in the course of HIV infection, patients may develop an encephalopathy associated with cerebral atrophy and widened sulci on computerized tomographic studies of the brain. Clinical features may initially include forgetfulness and impaired cognitive function, and these may progress to include weakness, ataxia, spasticity, and myoclonus.

The DNA polyoma virus JC is the etiologic agent in progressive multifocal leukoencephalopathy (PML). In this primary demyelinating process involving white matter of cerebral hemispheres, patients present subacutely with confusion, disorientation, and visual disturbances, which may progress to cortical blindness or ataxia. Cerebrospinal fluid is characteristically acellular. A feature on neuroradiology imaging studies is lack of mass effect. No definitive therapy is presently available for this infection, and clinical efforts have recently focused on the role of immune reconstitution in modifying the clinical course of the illness. In a multicenter analysis of 57 consecutive HIV-positive patients with PML, neurologic improvement or stability at 2 months after therapy was demonstrated in 26% of patients who received highly active antiretroviral therapy (HAART) in contrast to improvement in only 4% of patients who did not receive HAART (*P*=0.03) (*J Infect Dis* 2000; 182:1077-1083). In this study, decreases in JC virus DNA to undetectable levels predicted a longer survival. In the context that untreated PML may be fatal within 3 to 6 months, such potential for preventing neurologic progression and improving survival by controlling JC virus replication becomes clinically relevant.

In recent months, there have been increasing reports of human rabies in the United States. Although this infection does not occur very often, it raises some important points about epidemiology, transmission, clinical presentation, and prevention. Rabies is probably best considered to be an encephalomyelopathy. After inoculation, the virus replicates in myocytes and then enters the nervous system via unmyelinated sensory and motor nerves. It spreads until the spinal cord is reached, and it is at this point in the clinical course that paresthesias may begin at the wound site. The virus then moves from the central nervous system along peripheral nerves to skin and intestine as well as into salivary glands, where it is released into the saliva (*Clin Infect Dis* 2000; 30:4-12). Knowledge of these factors allows one to understand both clinical presentation and prevention. In a recent review of the topic by the Centers for Disease Control and Prevention (*MMWR* 1997; 46:770-774), it was stated that ". . . . this infection should be considered in the differential diagnosis of persons presenting with unexplained rapidly progressive encephalitis." It is the CNS involvement that leads to the cognitive dysfunction characteristic in encephalitis. Because the rabies virus may in the early stages localize to limbic structures, changes in behavior may result. Although an ascending paralysis simulating the Guillain-Barre syndrome has been described, the most classic presentation is of encephalitis associated with hypertonicity and hypersalivation. Noteworthy in Table 6 is that all 5 of the patients had pain and/or weakness, explainable since rabies is a myelopathic infection.

There have been 21 cases of bat-related rabies reported in the United States since 1980. Of those, only 1 was definitively related to an animal bite. Four of the 5 cases reported in the recent *Morbidity and Mortality Weekly Reports* cited in Table 6 and 8 of the 17 previously reported cases were ascribed to nonbite contact with bats.

In individuals not previously vaccinated against rabies but who have an indication for rabies postexposure prophylaxis, the treatment regimen includes local wound cleansing, human rabies immune globulin, and vaccine. The doses of human rabies immune globulin and vaccine have been recently summarized (*MMWR* 1998; 47:1-5). The administration of rabies immune globulin has been modified, and recommendations now are that as much as possible of the 20 IU/kg body weight dose should be infiltrated into and around the wound(s), with the remainder administered intramuscularly at an anatomical site distant from the vaccine administration. An important consideration is the prevention of rabies infection after exposure of family members or health care providers to an index case. Possible percutaneous or mucous membrane exposure to a patient's saliva or cerebrospinal fluid is an indication for postexposure prophylaxis (PEP). In the reports of the 5 patients summarized in Table 6, 46 persons received PEP after possible exposure to case 1, 50 persons after exposure to case 2, 60 persons after exposure to case 3, 53 persons after exposure to case 4, and 48 persons after exposure to case 5.

A group of viruses, including dengue virus, enteroviruses, adenoviruses, and cytomegalovirus, may cause direct infection that results in encephalitis. In addition to viruses producing direct infection of the brain, certain viruses may cause a postinfectious encephalomyelitis. At one time this form of central nervous system pathology accounted for about one-third of fatal cases of encephalitis (with acute viral encephalitis being the major cause of infectious mortality in this category). With the elimination of vaccinia virus by vaccination for smallpox, the mortality attributable to postinfectious encephalomyelitis is now estimated to be 10% to 15% of cases of acute encephalitis in the United States. The pathogenesis of this process has not been definitively elucidated. The pathologic changes have been compared to those which occurred in persons who developed acute encephalomyelitis following rabies immunization, which used vaccine prepared in central nervous system tissue. It has been suggested that certain viral infections may cause a disruption of normal immune regulation with resultant release of autoimmune responses. The viruses, which have been associated with postinfectious encephalomyelitis, are summarized in Table 4. Treatment of patients with such problems is limited to supportive care.

Table 6. Clinical presentation of rabies

Clinical Feature	Case 1	Case 2	Case 3	Case 4	Case 5
Encephalitis symptoms	Visual hallucinations	Hypersalivation	Confusion	Hallucinations	Confusion
Pain and weakness	Left arm	Left arm	Left face, ear	Right shoulder	Right wrist
Findings of cerebro-vascular insufficiency	Yes	Yes	Yes	Yes	No
Myoclonus	Yes	Yes	Yes	No	Yes
Paralysis	Complete muscular	No	Vocal cord; oculomotor	No	No
Autonomic instability	No	Yes	No	Yes	Yes

Cases 1 and 2 reported in *MMWR* 1997; 46:770–774; Cases 3 and 4 reported in *MMWR* 1998; 47:1–5. Case 5 reported in *MMWR* 1999; 48:95-97.

Two common infections, which usually have benign courses in adolescents and young adults, may progress to serious disease which may include involvement of the central nervous system. Mononucleosis due to Epstein-Barr virus may, on rare occasions, cause direct infection of the brain and an encephalitic process, which is the most common cause of death resulting from this infection. Central nervous system infection is the most significant extrarespiratory manifestation of infection caused by *Mycoplasma pneumoniae*. Even though this organism has been isolated from the CSF, the mechanism by which it causes encephalitis is felt to be an autoimmune one.

Rickettsiae have the ability to produce infection of the central nervous system. Of these, the most characteristic is Rocky Mountain spotted fever (RMSF), caused by *R. rickettsii*. After being transmitted to humans via a tick bite, this intracellular pathogen can produce a constellation of symptoms and signs that includes fever, petechial skin lesions (involving the palms, soles, wrists, and ankles), and a meningoencephalitis. Because of the skin lesions and neurologic involvement, acute forms of this infection may mimic disease caused by *N. meningitidis*. Chloramphenicol is effective against both of these pathogens, but tetracycline

is considered the usual first line drug when only RMSF is suspected. In contrast to the distal skin lesions that progress centrally in RMSF, epidemic typhus caused by *Rickettsia prowazekii* is characterized by central lesions that move distally. This infection is more likely to occur during the winter months than is RMSF, which usually occurs during the late summer and early fall. The emerging rickettsial pathogen identified as a cause of nervous system involvement is *Ehrlichia*. Pathogens within the genus *Ehrlichia* have the propensity to parasitize either mononuclear or granulocytic leukocytes with the resultant infection respectively referred to as human monocytic ehrlichiosis or human granulocytic ehrlichiosis. The epidemiology of ehrlichiosis, including outdoor activity and exposure to ticks, is similar to that of RMSF, but in contrast to RMSF, ehrlichiosis is only associated with rash in about 20% of cases. In addition to causing the characteristic findings of fever, leukopenia, thrombocytopenia, and abnormal liver enzymes, nervous system involvement in ehrlichiosis may include severe headache, confusion, lethargy, broad-based gait, hyperreflexia, clonus, photophobia, cranial nerve palsy, seizures, blurred vision, nuchal rigidity, and ataxia. The characteristic CSF abnormalities have been a lymphocytic pleocytosis with elevated protein. In a recent review of the subject, CSF glucose was normal in the majority of patients, with 24% of the patients having borderline low CSF glucose concentrations. In this review, morulae were seen in CSF white cells in only a small minority of the patients. Radiographic and encephalographic studies did not reveal any lesions that supported a specific diagnosis. Although the definitive agent for treating this infection has not been established by clinical trials, it appears that chloramphenicol or tetracycline is the agent most frequently used. The clinical experience with this process has been limited, and the outcome in patients with nervous system involvement is not well established.

As summarized in Table 4, certain noninfectious diseases may mimic viral encephalitis.

Brain Abscess

Of bacterial infections of the central nervous system, brain abscess is the second most common. On a pathogenetic basis, this infection may develop after hematogenous dissemination of organisms during systemic infection (which often occurs in the context of such conditions as infective endocarditis, cyanotic congenital heart disease, and lung abscess), with extension from infected cranial structures (e.g., sinuses or middle ear) along emissary veins, or as a consequence of trauma or neurosurgery. The classic presentation may include recent onset of severe headache, new focal or generalized seizures, and clinical evidence of an intracranial mass. In the nonimmunocompromised host, brain abscess represents a deviation from the classic tenet that *Bacteroides fragilis* is not a significant pathogen above the diaphragm. In the patient without predisposing factors, streptococci (including the *Streptococcus intermedius [milleri]* group) along with anaerobes (including *B. fragilis)* are the predominant pathogens. Excision or stereotactic aspiration of the abscess is used to identify the etiologic agents and has been recommended for lesions >2.5 cm (Mandell, Douglas, Bennett [Eds.]: *Principles and Practice of Infectious Diseases.* 5th Edition. 2000, Philadelphia, Churchill Livingstone, pp 1016-1028). Some

experts have advocated using empiric antimicrobial therapy without aspiration of the abscess in patients who are neurologically stable and who have an abscess <3 cm in diameter that is not encroaching on the ventricular system; however, if such a decision is made, they have advised that the patient must be meticulously followed with a brain imaging study such as CT or MRI, and enlargement of the abscess during therapy mandates surgery. Because of the lack of consistent efficacy of metronidazole against streptococci and upper airway anaerobic cocci, penicillin or a third-generation cephalosporin (e.g., cefotaxime or ceftriaxone) is usually combined with this agent. An alternative to metronidazole in this regimen would be chloramphenicol. In the settings of penetrating head trauma, following neurosurgical procedures, or with acute bacterial endocarditis, therapy for *S. aureus* should be included. Those patients with a presumed otic or sinus origin for their abscess should have coverage against enterobacteriaceae and *H. influenzae* using a third-generation cephalosporin.

In HIV-infected persons, *Toxoplasma gondii* classically presents as fever, headache, altered mental status, and focal neurologic deficits, especially in individuals whose CD4 count falls below 100 cells/mm^3. Since the disease is due to reactivation of latent infection in about 95% of cases, IgG antibody to *Toxoplasma* is generally present. A review of neuroimaging studies in patients with AIDS is summarized in Table 7, with a key point being whether or not mass effect is present. Imaging studies of the brain in AIDS patients with *Toxoplasma* brain abscess show multiple (usually ≥3) nodular contrast-enhancing lesions with mass effect found most commonly in the basal ganglia and at the gray-white matter junction. In the classic setting described above, empiric therapy with sulfadiazine and pyrimethamine is recommended, with brain biopsy being reserved for atypical presentations and for patients who do not respond to initial therapy. Clindamycin-containing regimens may be considered in sulfa-allergic patients. Brain biopsy is reserved for atypical presentations and for patients who do not respond to initial therapy. After acute therapy for toxoplasmic encephalitis, prophylaxis to prevent recurrence

Table 7. Approach to mass lesions in human immunodeficiency virus (HIV)-infected persons

Focal Lesions with Mass Effect in HIV-Infected Persons	Focal Lesion without Mass Effect in HIV-Infected Persons
• Toxoplasmosis	• Progressive multifocal leukoencephalopathy
• Primary lymphoma of the CNS	
• Cerebral cryptococcosis[a]	
• Neurotuberculosis[a]	
• Syphilitic gumma[b]	

CNS, central nervous system.
[a]Rarely present as abscesses; [b]rare presentation of neurosyphilis.
Adapted from *Clin Infect Dis* 1996; 22:906–919.

has been recommended with a regimen like sulfadiazine plus pyrimethamine plus leukovorin (*MMWR* 1999; 48[RR-10]:1-66). The lesions of toxoplasmosis may be confused with primary central nervous system lymphoma, which also causes a mass effect due to surrounding edema and which may undergo central necrosis and present as ring-enhancing masses.

Spinal Epidural Abscess and Subdural Empyema

A review of spinal epidural abscess provides the basis for understanding 2 common threads included in literature published about this infection: reports of poor prognosis and appeals for rapid treatment (*Medicine* 1992; 71:369-385). Spinal epidural abscess represents a neurosurgical emergency since neurologic deficits may become irreversible when there is a delay in evacuating the purulent material. Although the basis for this irreversibility has not been definitively established, mechanisms for the associated spinal cord necrosis include a decrease in arterial blood flow, venous thrombosis, or direct compression of the spinal cord. The triad of findings that supports the diagnosis is fever, point tenderness over the spine, and focal neurologic deficits. The predisposing factors to this infection shed light on the likely pathogens. Skin and soft tissue are the most probable source of infection and provide an understanding of why *S. aureus* is the most common pathogen in this infection. Spinal

epidural abscess has been reported to follow surgery, trauma, urinary tract infections, and respiratory diseases. Of increasing importance are the reports of this infection occurring as a complication of lumbar puncture and epidural anesthesia. In 16% of cases, the source of infection may be unknown. Usual pathogens include *S. aureus*, streptococci (both aerobic and anaerobic), and Gram-negative bacilli.

Gadolinium-enhanced magnetic resonance imaging has replaced myelography as the diagnostic study of choice because it identifies not only mass lesions, but also signal abnormalities that are consistent with acute transverse myelopathy and spinal cord ischemia.

Subdural empyema is an infection that occurs between the dura and arachnoid, and which results as organisms are spread via emissary veins or by extension of osteomyelitis of the skull. The paranasal sinuses are the source in over half the cases, with otitis another likely predisposing condition. In young children, it is usually a complication of meningitis. The clinical features include fever, headache, vomiting, signs of meningeal irritation, alteration in mental status, and focal neurologic deficits that progress to focal seizures. The usual pathogens are aerobic streptococci (including *S. pneumoniae*), staphylococci, *H. influenzae*, Gram-negative bacilli, and anaerobes (including *B. fragilis*). The diagnosis is often made using magnetic resonance imaging, but CT scan with contrast enhancement may offer the advantage of imaging bone. Antibiotics directed against the likely pathogens and surgical interventions are mainstays of therapy.

Septic Intracranial Thrombophlebitis

Thrombosis of the cortical vein may occur as a complication of meningitis and is associated with progressive neurologic deficits, including hemiparesis, bilateral weakness, or aphasia. Thrombosis of the intracranial venous sinuses classically follows infections of the paranasal sinuses, middle ear, mastoid, face, or oropharynx, although the process may be metastatic from lungs or other sites. The most frequent pathogens are *S. aureus*, coagulase-negative staphylococci, streptococci, Gram-negative bacilli, and anaerobes. Five anatomic sites may be involved with varying clinical presentations. Superior sagittal sinus thrombosis results in bilateral leg weakness or in communicating hydrocephalus. Lateral sinus thrombosis produces pain over the ear and mastoid, with possible edema over the mastoid. Superior petrosal sinus thrombosis causes ipsilateral pain, sensory deficit, or temporal lobe seizures. Inferior petrosal sinus thrombosis may produce the syndrome of ipsilateral facial pain and lateral rectus weakness that is referred to as Gradenigo syndrome.

Of the forms of venous sinus thrombosis, cavernous sinus thrombosis is the most frequently discussed. Within this sinus lie the internal carotid artery with its sympathetic plexus and the sixth cranial nerve. In the lateral wall of the sinus are the third and fourth cranial nerves along with the ophthalmic and sometimes maxillary divisions of the trigeminal nerve. The clinical presentation is influenced by these anatomic considerations. The process, which is considered life-threatening, begins unilaterally but usually becomes bilateral within hours. High fever, headaches, malaise, nausea, and vomiting are the predominant findings. Patients progress to develop proptosis, chemosis, periorbital edema, and cyanosis of the ipsilateral forehead, eyelids, and root of the nose. Ophthalmoplegia may develop, with the sixth cranial nerve usually involved first. Trigeminal nerve involvement may manifest itself as decreased sensation about the eye. Ophthalmic nerve involvement may present as photophobia and persistent eye pain. Papilledema, diminished pupillary reactivity, and diminished corneal reflexes may also develop. The disease may be relentless in its progression to alteration in level of consciousness, meningitis, and seizures. The mainstays of therapy include broad-spectrum antibiotics and surgical drainage with removal of infected bone or abscess. The issue of anticoagulation in patients with suppurative intracranial thrombophlebitis is controversial. It is the opinion of some experts in the field that heparin followed by warfarin may be beneficial (Mandell, Douglas, Bennett [Eds.]: *Principles and Practice of Infectious Diseases*. 5ᵗʰ Edition. 2000, Philadelphia, Churchill Livingstone, pp 1034-1036), but heparin-induced thrombocytopenia has been noted as a potential complication. Steroids may be necessary if involvement of the pituitary gland leads to adrenal insufficiency and circulatory collapse.

Neuritis

Infection of nervous tissue outside of the central nervous system can take place on the basis of several pathogenetic mechanisms. Certain pathogens such as *Borrelia burgdorferi* (the etiologic agent of Lyme disease), HIV, cytomegalovirus, HSV Type 2, and varicella-zoster virus can produce peripheral neuropathy. Direct infection of nerves may occur with *Mycobacterium leprae* and *Trypanosoma* species. *Corynebacterium diphtheriae*, *Clostridium tetani*, and *Clostridium botulinum* can produce toxins, which can injure peripheral nerves.

C. diphtheriae produces a toxin that directly involves nerves to cause a noninflammatory demyelination. Clinical sequella of such a process initially include local paralysis of the soft palate and posterior pharyngeal wall, followed by cranial nerve involvement, and culminating in involvement of peripheral nerves. Myocarditis occurs in as many as two-thirds of patients but <25% develop clinical evidence of cardiac dysfunction. Antitoxin is indicated in infected patients along with antibacterial therapy. Both penicillin and erythromycin have been recommended as treatment of diphtheria by the World Health

Organization (WHO). In a study in Vietnamese children with diphtheria that compared intramuscular benzylpenicillin to erythromycin, both antibiotics were efficacious, but there were slower fever clearance and a higher incidence of gastrointestinal side effects associated with erythromycin (*Clin Infect Dis* 1998; 27:845-850). Erythromycin resistance was noted in some of the isolates tested, but all were susceptible to penicillin. Both *C. tetani* and *C. botulinum* cause indirect nerve involvement on the basis of toxin production. The epidemiology of tetanus has changed somewhat in recent years. Joining elderly patients as a patient population at risk for tetanus, are injection drug users (IDUs) who inject drug subcutaneously (i.e., "skin pop"). The toxin of *C. tetani* is transported up axons and binds to presynaptic endings on motor neurons in anterior horn cells of the spinal cord. This blocks inhibitory input and results in uncontrolled motor input to skeletal muscle and tetanic spasm. Antitoxin is not available for this disorder, but tetanus immune globulin and tetanus toxoid are given for clinical disease. Prevention plays a pivotal role in controlling the number of cases of tetanus. A population-based serologic survey of immunity to tetanus in the United States revealed protective levels of tetanus antibodies which ranged from 87.7% among those 6 to 11 years of age to 27.8% among those 70 years of age or older (*N Engl J Med* 1995; 332:761-766). Although there is an excellent correlation between vaccination rates (96%) and immunity (96%) among 6-year-olds, antibody levels decline over time such that one-fifth of older children (10-16 years of age) do not have protective antibody levels. Such data argue strongly for ongoing tetanus immunization throughout a person's life in an attempt to prevent this potentially fatal disease.

The toxin of *C. botulinum* binds to the presynaptic axon terminal of the neuromuscular junction with inhibition of acetylcholine release. This results in a symmetric, descending, flaccid paralysis of motor and autonomic nerves, usually beginning with the cranial nerves. Recent reports of botulism have noted not only foodborne outbreaks associated with consumption of contaminated fish, commercial cheese sauce, and baked potatoes held in

aluminum foil for several days at room temperature, but also wound botulism in injection drug users who injected Mexican black tar heroin subcutaneously. The classic presentation includes neurological and gastrointestinal findings. Nausea and vomiting may be followed by diminished salivation and extreme dryness of the mouth, and by difficulty focusing eyes that occur due to interruption of cholinergic autonomic transmission. Patients progress to cranial nerve palsies (with common presentations being diplopia, dysarthria, or dysphagia) and then to a descending flaccid paralysis. The largest outbreak in the United States since 1978 occurred in 1994 in El Paso, Texas and was traced to a dip prepared in a restaurant from potatoes which had been baked in aluminum foil and which had then been left at room temperature for several days (*J Infect Dis* 1998; 178:172-177). In that report, the following criteria were used for making the diagnosis of botulism: a) an electromyography study showing a ≥50% increase in the evoked train of compound muscle action potentials with rapid repetitive stimulation (20 -50 Hz); b) stool culture positive for *C. botulinum*; and c) blurred vision, dysphagia, or dysarthria in a person who did not have electromyography findings indicating botulism and who did not have *C. botulinum* detected in stool (findings consistent with the diagnosis of "suspected case"). In addition, the mouse inoculation test for toxin using serum, stool, or food may be positive.

Along with the traditional forms of botulism, there are 2 additional forms of importance. Since 1978, the CDC has recorded cases of botulism in which extensive investigation failed to implicate a specific food as the cause. These have been referred to as cases of "undetermined origin." Investigation has shown that some of these cases were caused by colonization of the gastrointestal tract by *C. botulinum* or *C. baratii* with in vivo production of toxin, analogous to the pathogenesis of infant botulism. In some cases of botulism strongly suspected of representing intestinal colonization, the patients had a history of gastrointestinal surgery or illnesses such as inflammatory bowel disease, which might have predisposed them to enteric colonization. This form of botulism has been referred to as intestinal colonization botulism (also termed by some as adult-type infant botulism). Of more recent interest is inhalational botulism, which could occur as a component of bioterrorism with intentional release of aerosolized botulinum toxin.

As summarized in Table 8, antitoxin is indicated for adult botulism, which occurs on the basis of ingestion of preformed toxin, and for wound botulism, in which toxin is produced locally at the infected wound. A recent review of botulism has noted that antitoxin is released from the CDC for cases of intestinal colonization botulism (*Ann Intern Med* 1998; 129:221-228). With inhalational botulism, it has been suggested that antitoxin be given as early as possible based on clinical suspicion and should not be delayed while awaiting microbiological testing (*JAMA* 2001; 285:1059-1070). It has been suggested with this form of botulism that antitoxin might only prevent progression of disease but not reverse paralysis once it occurs. It is important to note that skin testing should be performed to test for sensitivity to serum or antitoxin prior to administration of antitoxin. In contrast, infant botulism, which occurs when the ingested organism produces toxin within the gastrointestinal tract, does not respond to antitoxin. A human-derived human botulism immune globulin has been administered to infants with botulism. Although this product is not yet commercially available, it may be obtained for the treatment of infant botulism under a Treatment Investigational New Drug protocol by contacting the California Department of Health Services (phone 510/540-2646). The acute, simultaneous onset of neurologic symptoms in multiple individuals should suggest a common source for the problem and increase the suspicion of botulism.

Certain toxins produced by fish and shellfish have been associated with neurologic involvement. Ciguatera fish poisoning (CFP) follows consumption of marine fish (most characteristically grouper, red snapper, and barracuda) that have been contaminated with toxins produced by microalgae known as dinoflagellates. The classic constellation of findings involves gastrointestinal, cardiovascular, and neurological systems. The characteristic neurologic findings include paresthesias (which may be chronic) periorally

and in distal extremities, often associated with a debilitating hot-to-cold reversal dysesthesia. Taste sensation is often altered. Implicated toxins include ciguatoxin (which induces membrane depolarization by opening voltage-dependent sodium channels), maitotoxin (which opens calcium channels), and palytoxin (which causes muscle injury). Therapy is primarily symptomatic and supportive. Paralytic shellfish poisoning (PSP) is caused by consumption of shellfish (most characteristically butter clams, mussels, cockles, steamer clams, sea snails, razor clams) or broth from cooked shellfish that contain either concentrated saxitoxin (a heat-stable alkaloid neurotoxin) or related compounds, with resultant sensory, cerebellar, and motor dysfunction. Characteristic neurologic findings include paresthesias of the mouth and extremities, ataxia, dysphagia, muscle paralysis, coma, and total muscular paralysis. Treatment is supportive.

The ascending paralysis that comprises the Guillain-Barré syndrome characteristically follows respiratory infection, gastrointestinal infection (notably, *Campylobacter* infection), or immunization. The pathology is segmental inflammation with perivascular mononuclear cells and demyelination. An exact etiology for this process has not been elucidated.

Table 8. Toxin-mediated peripheral neuritis

Direct Toxin Injury
    Corynebacterium diphtheriae[a]

Indirect Toxin Injury
    Clostridium tetani
    Clostridium botulinum
        Traditional categories
            Adult botulism[a]
            Infant botulism
            Wound botulism[a]
            Intestinal colonization botulism*
        New category
            Inhalational botulism*

[a]Antitoxin indicated.
*See text

CATHETER-RELATED INFECTIONS

Urinary Bladder Catheters

A clinical situation frequently associated with injudicious use of antibiotics in the critical care setting is asymptomatic bacteriuria. Table 9 summarizes those situations where therapy for asymptomatic bacteriuria is indicated and reviews situations where the data are evolving but not conclusive. A clinically important area, but one in which there are not definitive data, relates to renal transplant recipients. It has been acknowledged that urine culture surveillance and periodic renal scan or ultrasound examinations are recommended by some authors, at least during the first months after transplantation. Based on cited references that treatment of asymptomatic UTIs in renal transplant recipients are largely unsuccessful and that such therapy

may not have observable effect on graft function, it was noted that asymptomatic UTIs in this immunocompromised patient population may be left untreated (*Clin Infect Dis* 2001; 33 (Suppl 1):S53-S57). Frequent or inappropriate use of antibiotics exerts selective pressures that are responsible for the increasing prevalence of bacterial resistance. Because of this, it is important to use antibiotics in situations where the clinical benefits exceed risks such as adverse effects and the selection of resistant organisms. A recent report of the NIH-sponsored Mycoses Study Group evaluated the issue of treatment for candiduria that was asymptomatic or minimally symptomatic (*Clin Infect Dis* 2000; 30:19-24). Patients were randomized to fluconazole (200 mg/day) or placebo for 14 days. In 50% of cases, the isolate was *C. albicans*. At the end of treatment, urine was cleared in 50% of patients given fluconazole versus 29% of those given

Table 9. Treatment of asymptomatic bacteriuria (note: 2 cultures should be positive before treating)

Persons in Whom Therapy Is Recommended

Pregnant women (N Engl J Med 1961; 265:667-672. Clin Infect Dis 1992; 14:927-932.
J Infect Dis 1994; 169:1390-1392)

Men about to undergo urologic surgery (Gorbach, Bartlett, Blacklow [Eds]: Infectious Dieseases. 2nd Edition.
1998:950)

Children with vesicoureteral reflux

Persons in Whom Definitive Recommendations Are Not Available but for Whom Some Provide Therapy

Persons with positive urine cultures both at the time of catheter removal and then again 1-2 weeks after catheter removal (Infect Dis Clin North Am 1987; 1:823-824)

Patients with diabetes mellitus (Rev Infect Dis 1991; 13:150-154)

Certain immunocompromised patients, especially those who are neutropenic or who have undergone renal transplantation (see comments in text about renal transplant patients)

Elderly persons with obstructive uropathy (N Engl J Med 1986; 314:1152-1156 and 309:1420-1425. Ann Intern Med 1984; 120:827-833 and 1987; 106:764-766)

Some patients with struvite stones

Those undergoing certain types of surgery, particularly when prostheses or foreign bodies (notably vascular grafts) may be left in place

---

placebo. However, cure rate was about 70% in both groups at 2 weeks posttreatment. Although these data represented short-term eradication of candiduria (especially following catheter removal), the long-term eradication rates were not associated with clinical benefit. Notable in this study were the observations in the placebo group that candiduria resolved in about 20% of chronically catheterized patients when their catheter was only changed and in 41% of untreated patients when the catheter was removed.

Peritoneal Dialysis Catheters

The presentation of abdominal pain and/or fever and/or cloudy peritoneal fluid are the clinical features usually found in patients who are undergoing either continuous ambulatory peritoneal dialysis (CAPD) or automated peritoneal dialysis (APD) and who develop peritonitis. The organisms most frequently isolated in such processes have been coagulase-negative staphylococci (e.g., *S. epidermidis*) or *S. aureus*, but the incidence of Gram-negative pathogens has increased in patients utilizing disconnect systems. When caused by *S. aureus*, a toxic shock-like syndrome has been occasionally noted. The finding of >100 WBCs/mm^3, of which at least 50% are polymorphonuclear neutrophils, is supportive of the diagnosis of peritonitis. Recent trends in management of this infection have been impacted by the emergence of vancomycin resistance, both in enterococci as well as in *S. aureus*. Influencing such resistance has been vancomycin use. In a review of vancomycin intermediate *S. aureus* (VISA), it was noted that of the first 6 patients reported in the United States with this pathogen, all but 1 had had exposure to dialysis for renal insufficiency, with the resultant potential for recurrent vancomycin use (*Clin Infect Dis* 2001; 32:108-115). In recognition of the contribution of injudicious use of vancomycin to the development of vancomycin-resistance in Gram-positive organisms, it was recommended by the Advisory Committee on Peritonitis Management of the International Society for Peritoneal Dialysis (ISPD) that traditional empiric therapy of catheter-associated peritonitis be changed from

the regimen of vancomycin and gentamicin to a first-generation cephalosporin (e.g., cefazolin or cephalothin in a loading dose of 500 mg/L and a maintenance dose of 125 mg/L) in combination with an aminoglycoside (*Perit Dial Int* 1996; 16:557-573). It was further stated that modifications to this regimen could be made based on the organism isolated or on sensitivity patterns. In its more recent iteration of recommendations for treatment of adult peritoneal dialysis-related peritonitis (*Perit Dial Int* 2000; 20:396-411), the ISPD suggested the substitution of ceftazidime for the aminoglycoside. Residual renal function is an independent predictor of patient survival. It is especially noteworthy that use of any aminoglycoside (*Am J Kidney Dis* 1999; 34:14-20), even when given for short periods, and the rate of peritonitis (*Perit Dial Int* 1999; 19:138-142) are independent risk factors for the decline of residual renal function in CAPD patients. A concern about ceftazidime is its risk of selecting resistant Gram-negative organisms, including those that produce either type I β-lactamases or extended-spectrum β-lactamases (ESBLs). The role of empiric therapy with cefazolin has also been reported in potentially infected hemodialysis patients (*Am J Kidney Dis* 1998; 32:410-414 and 521-523), with vancomycin being reserved for confirmed resistant organisms. Many episodes of catheter-associated peritonitis may be managed without removal of the catheter, but peritonitis that does not respond to antibiotic therapy or peritonitis associated with tunnel infections may be indications for catheter removal. Infection with *Pseudomonas,* a fungal pathogen, or mycobacteria often requires catheter removal for cure (*Clin Infect Dis* 1997; 24:1035-1047). Also influencing the decision for catheter removal is relapsing peritonitis, defined as an episode of peritonitis caused by the same genus/species that caused the immediately preceding episode, occurring within 4 weeks of completion of the antibiotic course. If no clinical response is noted after 96 hours of therapy for relapsing peritonitis, catheter removal is indicated; if the patient responds clinically, but subsequently relapses an additional time, catheter removal and replacement are recommended (*Perit Dial Int* 2000; 20:396-411).

Vascular Catheters

Of the 200,000 nosocomial bloodstream infections that occur each year in the United States, most are related to different types of intravascular devices. The Infectious Diseases Society of America, the Society of Critical Care Medicine, and the Society for Healthcare Epidemiology of America have recently published guidelines for management of intravascular catheter-related infections (*Clin Infect Dis* 2001; 32:1249-1272). In their review, the following recommendations were made regarding blood cultures in cases of suspected catheter-associated bacteremia: a) that 2 sets of blood samples for culture, with a least 1 drawn percutaneously, be obtained with a new episode of suspected central venous catheter-related bloodstream infection; and b) that paired quantitative blood cultures or paired qualitative blood cultures with a continuously monitored differential time to positivity be collected for the diagnosis of catheter-related infection, especially when the long-term catheter cannot be removed. Quantitative blood cultures simultaneously obtained through a central venous catheter and a peripheral vein and demonstrating a 5- to 10-fold increase in concentration of an organism in catheter blood compared to peripheral blood have been reported to correlate well with catheter-related infections; however, some studies have not supported such a correlation. For tunneled catheters, a quantitative culture of blood from the central venous catheter that yields at least 100 cfu/mL may be diagnostic without a companion culture of a peripheral blood sample (*Eur J Microbiol Infect Dis* 1992; 11:403-407). A new diagnostic method has been made possible by continuous blood culture monitoring systems and compares the time to positive cultures of blood drawn from the catheter and from a peripheral vein. One study has shown a sensitivity of 91% and a specificity of 94% in determining catheter-related infection when a blood culture drawn from a central venous catheter became positive at least 2 hours earlier than the culture drawn from a peripheral vein (*J Clin Microbiol* 1998; 36:105-109). These data have most applicability to tunneled catheters.

Over the past 2 decades, the medical literature has proposed several predictors of sepsis from a catheter. Although Gram stain of material from the tip of a catheter may be helpful with diagnosis of local infection, it is significantly less sensitive than are quantitative methods. The most traditionally quoted study regarding predictors of catheter-related infection suggests that the presence of ≥15 colonies on a semiquantitative roll culture of the tip of a catheter or needle is most useful (*N Engl J Med* 1977; 296:1305-1309). Although such techniques are relied on at present to assist in the determination of an infected catheter, some data have suggested that the semiquantitative culture may not be predictive of clinical outcome. When compared with qualitative cultures, quantitative methods which, include either a) flushing the segment with broth or b) vortexing or sonicating the segment in broth, followed by serial dilutions and surface plating on blood agar, have greater specificity in the identification of catheter-related infections. In the recently published guidelines for management of intravascular catheter-related infections (*Clin Infect Dis* 2001; 32:1249-1272), the sensitivities of these 3 methods were listed as follows: sonication, 80%; roll plate method, 60%; and flush culture, 40%-50%.

The guidelines (*Clin Infect Dis* 2001; 3 2:1249-1272) also discussed alternative routes of antibiotic administration. An important consideration is whether the infection is intraluminal or extraluminal. Catheters that have been in place for <2 weeks are most often infected extraluminally, whereas catheters in place for longer duration were more likely to have intraluminal infection. Antibiotic solutions that contain the desired antimicrobial agent in a concentration of 1-5 mg/mL are usually mixed with 50-100 units of heparin (or normal saline) and are installed or "locked" into the catheter lumen during periods when the catheter is not used (e.g., for a 12-hour period each night). The volume of installed antibiotic is removed before infusion of the next dose of an antibiotic or intravenous medication or solution, and the most often used duration of such therapy is 2 weeks. Summarized in this review are some reports of cure of patients with infected tunneled catheters who were treated with both parenteral and lock therapy.

Of the pathogens most characteristically isolated as a complication of indwelling vascular catheters, coagulase-negative staphylococci, *Staphylococcus aureus*, and *Candida* species have been most frequently reported. In immunocompromised patients with long-term indwelling catheters, *Corynebacterium jeikeium* and *Bacillus* species are important, and notably both have vancomycin as their drug of choice for therapy. Gram-negative bacilli and atypical mycobacteria are also included as possible pathogens in this setting.

An important and common clinical question is whether a catheter-related intravascular infection can be cured with a long-term indwelling catheter left in place. The medical literature suggests that catheter-related coagulase-negative staphylococcal bacteremia may be successfully treated without recurrence in up to 80% of patients whose catheters remained in place and in whom antibiotics were given (*Infect Control Hosp Epidemiol* 1992; 13:215-221). In the 20% of patients who remained bacteremic while on antibiotics with their catheters in place, metastatic infection was not a significant problem. For patients with vascular catheter-associated coagulase-negative staphylococcal bacteremia, the following recommendations have been made (*Clin Infect Dis* 2001; 32:1249-1272): a) that if a central venous catheter is removed, appropriate systemic antibiotic therapy is recommended for 5-7 days; b) that if a nontunneled central venous catheter is retained and intraluminal infection is suspected, systemic antibiotic therapy for 10-14 days and antibiotic lock therapy are recommended; and c) that if a tunneled central venous catheter or an intravascular device are retained in patients with uncomplicated, catheter-related, bloodstream infection, patients should be treated with systemic antibiotic therapy for 7 days and with antibiotic lock therapy for 14 days.

Although some authors have suggested that infections caused by *Staphylococcus aureus* in the setting of a vascular catheter may respond to treatment with the catheter left in place, there are increasing reports of metastatic sites of infection by this organism when the catheter is not removed. As a result, it seems most prudent to remove the catheter when *S. aureus* is isolated from the bloodstream. Because of the potentially devastating complications that may occur when *S. aureus* seeds heart valves or bone, the issue of duration of therapy for bacteremia due to this pathogen in catheter-associated bacteremia is exceedingly important. It is well accepted that individuals with endocarditis or osteomyelitis occurring as complications of metastatic *S. aureus* infection require a prolonged course of parenteral antimicrobial therapy, with 6 weeks as the frequently stated duration of therapy in these settings. The duration of therapy for patients with *S. aureus* bacteremia that is catheter-related may be similar to that for *S. aureus* bacteremia due to a drainable focus. Discussed frequently in the medical literature, therapy for this clinical problem has not been definitively established by clinical trials. Based on the available data, the most frequently noted minimum duration of parenteral therapy in such settings is 2 weeks. However, before one makes the decision to limit parenteral therapy to this short course, all 4 of the following criteria should probably be met: a) that there is removal of the intravascular catheter or drainage of the abscess that was presumed to be the source of the bacteremia; b) that the bacteremia is demonstrated to promptly resolve with the removal or drainage; c) that there is prompt clinical response, including resolution of fever; and d) that heart valves are demonstrated to be normal. Some have suggested that transesophageal echocardiography (TEE) may be a cost-effective means of stratifying patients with catheter-associated *S. aureus* bacteremia to a specific duration of therapy (*Ann Intern Med* 1999; 130:810-820). With infectious disease consultation as 1 of the 6 components of the evaluation, it has been suggested that a 7-day course of antibiotics may be appropriate for patients with what has been termed "simple bacteremia" with *S. aureus* if all of the other criteria are met: a) TEE on day 5-7 of therapy was negative for both vegetations and predisposing valvular abnormalities; b) negative surveillance culture of blood obtained 2-4 days after beginning appropriate antibiotic therapy and removal of focus; c) removable focus of infection; d) clinical resolution (afebrile and no localizing complaints attributable to metastatic staphylococcal infections within 72 hours of initiating therapy and removal of focus); and e) no indwelling prosthetic devices (*Clin Infect Dis* 1998; 27:478-486). Even in such settings, patients with diabetes mellitus may still be at an increased risk for developing *S. aureus* endocarditis, and some experts have suggested 4 weeks of therapy in this patient population even if heart valves are normal. Removal is suggested in the following settings of *S. aureus* bacteremia: a) nontunneled central vascular catheters; and b) tunneled central vascular catheters or intravascular devices when there is evidence of tunnel, pocket, or exit-site infection (*Clin Infect Dis* 2001; 32:1249-1272). In the recommendations just cited, it was noted that tunneled central vascular catheters or intravascular devices with uncomplicated intraluminal infection and *S. aureus* bacteremia should be removed or, in selected cases, retained and treated with appropriate systemic and antibiotic lock therapy for 14 days. For patients who remain febrile and/or have bacteremia for >3 days after catheter removal and/or initiation of antibiotic therapy, a longer course of therapy and an aggressive workup for septic thrombosis and infective endocarditis should be instituted. Since the sensitivity of transthoracic echocardiography is low, it is not recommended for excluding a diagnosis of catheter-related endocarditis if TEE can be done (*Clin Infect Dis* 2001; 32:1249-1272). It is important to reiterate that not all of the recommendations listed in this discussion of *S. aureus* bacteremia have been definitively validated by clinical trials.

Like *S. aureus* and enterococci, *Candida* species have a predilection to cause metastatic infection on heart valves and in bone when these organisms are bloodborne. In addition to the complications of endocarditis and osteomyelitis, *Candida* may seed the retina of the eye to cause retinal abscesses that proliferate into the vitreous and result in the clinical entity of *Candida* endophthalmitis. Because of the significant complications associated with candidemia, there are now 2 basic recommendations for all patients with a positive blood culture for *Candida*: a) that the patient receive a course of antifungal therapy (*Clin Infect Dis* 1992; 14[Suppl 1]:S106-S113); and b) that intravascular lines be removed (*Clin

Infect Dis* 1996; 22:467-470). The risk factors cited for candidemia vary by reports, but the following is a representative list from a group of international experts in the field: antibiotics; indwelling catheters; hyperalimentation; cancer therapy; immunosuppressive therapy after organ transplantation; hospitalization in intensive care units; candiduria; and colonization with *Candida* species (*Clin Infect Dis* 1997; 25:43-59). A clinical trial conducted by the Mycoses Study Group of the National Institutes of Health compared amphotericin B with fluconazole in the treatment of candidemia in non-neutropenic and non-immunocompromised patients (*N Engl J Med* 1994; 331:1325-1330). In the 194 patients who had a single species of *Candida* isolated, 69% of the organisms were *C. albicans*. The study concluded that fluconazole and amphotericin B were not significantly different in their effectiveness in treating candidemia. Since that study was performed, there has been an increasing prevalence of non-*albicans* strains of *Candida* in the bloodborne isolates from certain hospitals, and some of these strains may not respond to traditional doses of fluconazole. In their guidelines for the treatment of candidemia (*Clin Infect Dis* 2000; 30:662-678), the Infectious Diseases Society of America noted that most experts would initiate therapy with fluconazole in stable patients who had not recently received azole therapy. In the clinically unstable patient infected with an isolate of unknown species, it was acknowledged that fluconazole has been used successfully, but that amphotericin B is preferred by some authorities because of its broader spectrum. Definitive data regarding the role of fluconazole versus amphotericin B in treating neutropenic patients with candidemia are not available at this time.

Other clinical situations for which catheter removal is necessary for cure of a catheter-related infection include a) bacteremia due to *Corynebacterium jeikeium* and *Bacillus* species, b) bacteremia with gram-negative bacilli; c) fungemia; d) persistence of fever or bacteremia during therapy, e) evidence of tunnel infection, and f) rapid relapse after treatment. Currently available data do not support the need for scheduled replacement of short-term central venous catheters, either by guidewire exchange or through insertion at a new site (*N Engl J Med* 1992; 327:1062-1068).

SUGGESTED READINGS

1. Quagliarello V, Scheld WM: Treatment of bacterial meningitis. *N Engl J Med* 1997; 336:708-716
   A review of therapy for bacterial meningitis, which includes a discussion of changes in empiric therapy based on the increasing prevalence of penicillin-resistant Streptococcus pneumoniae.

2. Hasbun R, Abrahams J, Jekel J, Quagliarello VJ: Computed tomography of the head before lumbar puncture in adults with suspected meningitis. *N Engl J Med* 2001; 345:1727-1733
   A clinically relevant review that addresses the commonly encountered question of when to do computed imaging of the head prior to performing lumbar puncture

3. Rosenstein NE, Perkins BA, Stephens DS et al: Meningococcal disease. *N Engl J Med* 2001; 344:1378-1388
   A comprehensive review of Neisseria meningitidis, which includes epidemiology, risk factors, clinical manifestations, diagnosis, management, control, and prevention.

4. Alberio L, Lämmle B, Esmon CT: Protein C replacement in severe meningococcemia: Rationale and clinical experience. *Clin Infect Dis* 2001; 32:1338-1346
   A timely review of the experimental data, which describe the pathophysiology in severe meningococcemia and the potential role for protein C replacement in preventing some of the significant clinical consequences in this infection.

5. Verdon R, Chevret S, Laissy J-P, et al: Tuberculous meningitis in adults: Review of 48 cases. *Clin Infect Dis* 1996; 22:982-988
   A review of 48 adults patients with tuberculous meningitis who were admitted to an intensive care unit, with emphasis on diagnostic studies and on outcome.

6. Cintron R, Pachner AR: Spirochetal diseases of the nervous system. *Curr Opin Neurol* 1994; 7:217-222
   A review of the salient features of neurosyphilis and of Lyme disease involving the nervous system, with emphasis on epidemiology, clinical manifestations, laboratory diagnosis, and clinical management.

7. Ratnasamy N, Everett ED, Roland WE, et al: Central nervous system manifestations of human ehrlichiosis. *Clin Infect Dis* 1996; 23:314-319
   A report of the CSF analysis obtained from 15 of 57 patients with a confirmed diagnosis of human ehrlichiosis, and a review of 21 additional cases identified from a search of the English-language literature.

8. Johnson RT: Acute encephalitis. *Clin Infect Dis* 1996; 23:219-226
   A concise review that focuses on both acute viral encephalitis and postinfectious encephalomyelitis.

9. Mathisen GE, Johnson JP: Brain abscess. *Clin Infect Dis* 1997; 25:763-781
   A review of the clinical entity of brain abscess that focuses on epidemiology, pathogenesis, microbiology, clinical presentation, diagnosis, and therapy.

10. Walot I, Miller BL, Chang L, et al: Neuroimaging findings in patients with AIDS. *Clin Infect Dis* 1996; 22:906-919
    A clinical discussion of the neuroradiographic findings in patients with AIDS and central nervous system involvement, with a clinical differentiation between focal lesions with and without mass effect.

11. Darouiche RO, Hamill RJ, Greenberg SB, et al: Bacterial spinal epidural abscess: Review of 43 cases and literature survey. *Medicine* 1992; 71:369-385
    A summary of the epidemiology, clinical presentations, microbiology, diagnosis (including an opinion regarding the role of magnetic resonance imaging), and treatment of spinal epidural abscess based on a series of 43 patients combined with a literature review.

12. Southwick FS, Richardson EP, Swartz MN: Septic thrombosis of the dural venous sinuses. *Medicine* 1986; 65:82-106
    An excellent presentation of the anatomy of the various dural venous sinuses that allows

the reader to more fully appreciate the *pathogenetic, clinical, microbiologic and therapeutic aspects of septic thrombosis related to these structures.*

13. Keane WF, Bailie GR, Boeschoten E, et al: Adult peritoneal dialysis-related peritonitis treatment recommendations: 2000 update. *Perit Dial Int* 2000; 20:396-411
The recommendations of the Advisory Committee on Peritonitis Management of the International Society for Peritoneal Dialysis on the diagnosis and managements of infections associated with peritoneal catheters in patients on peritoneal dialysis.

14. Raad I: Intravascular-catheter-related infections. *Lancet* 1998; 351:893-898

A review of infections involving intravascular catheters, including an analysis based on specific pathogens that includes recommendations for duration of therapy and for whether catheter removal is indicated.

15. Mermel LA, Farr BM, Sherertz RJ, et al: Guidelines for the management of intravascular catheter-related infections. *Clin Infect Dis* 2001; 32:1249-1272
A comprehensive, practical review of infections related to intravascular catheters, with exceptionally helpful recommendations for dealing with commonly encountered dilemmas that occur in clinical practice.

ACUTE RESPIRATORY DISTRESS SYNDROME

Jesse B. Hall, MD

INTRODUCTION

Type I or acute hypoxemic respiratory failure (AHRF) arises from diseases causing collapse and/or filling of alveoli with the result that a substantial fraction of mixed venous blood traverses nonventilated airspaces, effecting a right-to-left intrapulmonary shunt. (see Figure 1, panel b). In addition to the adverse consequences upon gas exchange, interstitial and alveolar fluid accumulation result in an increase in lung stiffness, imposing a mechanical load with a resulting increase in the work of breathing (see Figure 1, panel a). Uncorrected, the gas exchange and lung mechanical abnormalities may eventuate in tissue hypoxia, respiratory arrest, and death (see Figure 2). When this form of respiratory failure arises from acute lung injury with diffuse alveolar damage and flooding, it is termed the acute respiratory distress syndrome (ARDS).

Classification and Definition

To a first approximation, the disorders causing AHRF may be divided into diffuse lesions such as pulmonary edema, and focal lung lesions such as lobar pneumonia (see Table 1).

Since the distribution of airspace involvement may have implications for the response to interventions such as positive end expiratory pressure (PEEP), this nosology is of both therapeutic and didactic value.

Low pressure pulmonary edema, also termed pulmonary capillary leak or ARDS when encountered clinically, results from injury to the lung microcirculation sustained from direct lung insults (e.g., aspiration, inhalation, or infectious agents) or indirectly by systemic processes (e.g., sepsis, traumatic shock with large volume blood product resuscitation). Regardless of initiating event, the result is a "leak" of fluid and protein into the interstitium (and eventually alveolar spaces) despite normal microvascular hydrostatic and oncotic pressures.

In cases of ARDS, it is useful to distinguish between the early phases of acute lung injury and events occurring subsequently (see Figure 3).

By light microscopy, the early appearance is of flooding of the lung with proteinaceous fluid and minimal evidence of cellular injury. By electron microscopy, changes of endothelial cell swelling, widening of intercellular junctions, increased numbers of pinocytotic vesicles, and disruption and

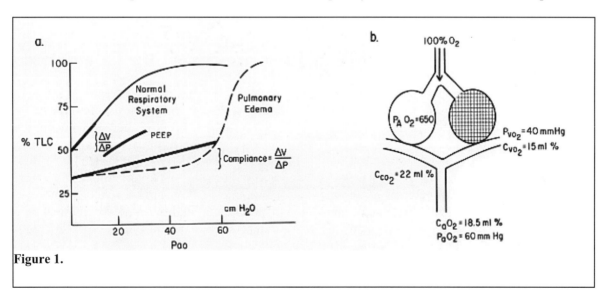

Figure 1.

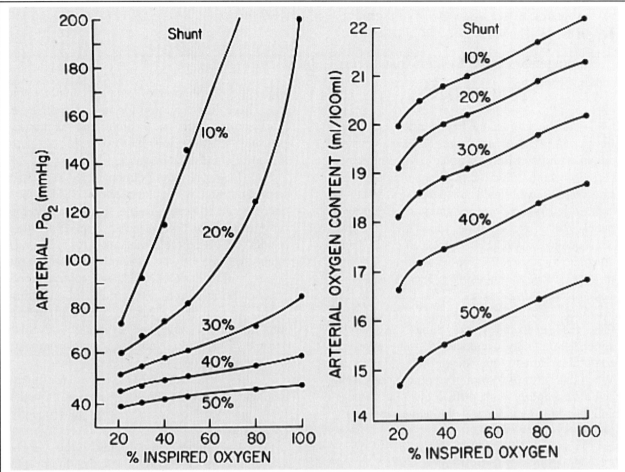

Figure 2. Left panel: The impact of shunt fraction on oxygenation—note that when shunt is 30% and above, the response to oxygen as judged by arterial PO₂ is minimal. Right panel: Even though the arterial PO₂ changes with oxygen are minimized by large shunt fraction, the increase in arterial oxygen content are large given the steep slope of the hemoglobin-oxygen dissociation curve in this range.

denudation of the basement membrane are prominent. This early phase of diffuse alveolar damage (DAD) has been termed *exudative*, and is a period of time during which pulmonary edema and its effects are most pronounced and intrapulmonary shunt is a primary problem dictating ventilatory strategies.

Over the ensuing days hyaline membrane formation in the alveolar spaces is prominent, attributed to precipitation of serum proteins. Inflammatory cells become more numerous and as DAD progresses, there is extensive necrosis of Type I alveolar cells. The latter phase of DAD is dominated by disordered healing. This can occur as early as 7 to 10 days

after initial injury and may result in extensive pulmonary fibrosis. This has been termed the *proliferative* phase of DAD. Type II alveolar cells proliferate along alveolar septae, and within the alveolar wall fibroblasts and myofibroblasts become more prominent. Lung flooding may be minimal at this point, and the clinical picture is often dominated by large dead space fraction and high minute ventilation requirements, progressive pulmonary hypertension, slightly improved intrapulmonary shunt, which is less responsive to PEEP, further reduction in

Table 1. Causes of Acute Hypoxemic Respiratory Failure

Homogenous Lung Lesions (producing pulmonary edema)

Cardiogenic or Hydrostatic Edema
Left ventricular (LV) failure
Acute LV ischemia
Accelerated or malignant hypertension
Mitral regurgitation
Mitral stenosis
Ball-valve thrombus
Volume overload, particularly with co-
existing renal and cardiac disease

Permeability or Low Pressure Edema (ARDS)
Most Common
Sepsis and sepsis syndrome
Acid aspiration
Multiple transfusions for hypovolemic shock
Less Common
Near drowning
Pancreatitis
Air or fat emboli
Cardiopulmonary bypass
Pneumonia
Drug reaction or overdose
Leukoagglutination
Inhalation injury
Infusion of biologics (e.g.,Interleukin 2)
Ischemia-reperfusion (e.g., postthrombectomy, posttransplant)

Edema of Unclear or `Mixed' Etiology
Re-expansion
Neurogenic
Postictal
Tocolysis-associated

Diffuse Alveolar Hemorrhage
Microscopic angiitis
Collagen vascular diseases
Goodpasture's syndrome
Severe coagulopathy and bone marrow transplant
Retinoic-acid syndrome

Focal Lung Lesions

Lobar Pneumonia

Lung Contusion

Lobar Atelectasis (acutely)

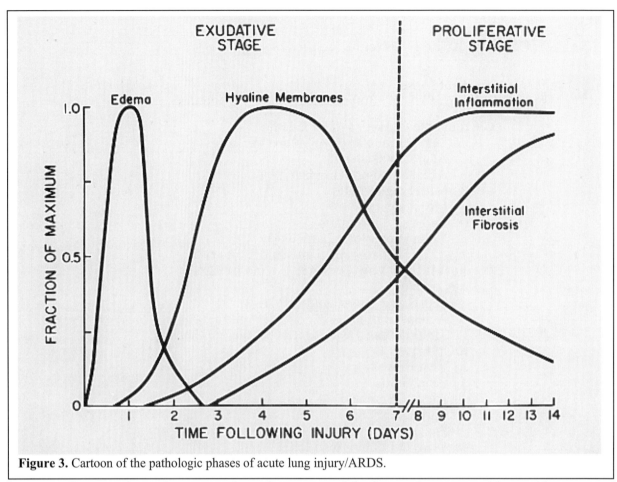

Figure 3. Cartoon of the pathologic phases of acute lung injury/ARDS.

lung compliance, and a tendency toward creation of Zone I conditions of the lung if the patient develops hypovolemia.

Although it is useful didactically to make a distinction between focal and diffuse causes of AHRF, this classification has arisen largely from chest radiograph assessment, a relatively insensitive measure of fluid distribution. When patients with ARDS have been imaged with computerized chest tomography, marked inhomogeneity of alveolar flooding has been noted. Consolidation is frequently most pronounced in dependent lung regions, and if patients are prone positioned, lung consolidation redistributes to the newly dependent lung regions. Such findings support the notion of ARDS as a disease with small or "baby" lungs of relatively preserved function. This provides a rationale for ventilator strategies that avoid over-distension and hence injury of normal lung regions yet still achieve recruitment of flooded and collapsed lung regions.

Since patients with ARDS have a large number of underlying medical and surgical etiologies, and present with a wide range of severity of lung injury, there has been a longstanding recognition of a need for definition and assessment of severity that can help standardize patient groups for comparison. One such attempt was made by a joint American-European Consensus Conference which published its deliberations in 1994 and recommended using the term "acute lung injury" (ALI) to describe the milder manifestations of evolving diffuse lung damage, and ARDS to describe the more severe end of the spectrum. Both ALI and ARDS were defined by relatively simple timing, oxygenation, chest radiographic, and hemodynamic criteria, which are given in Table 2.

In addition to these attempts to define ALI/ARDS, a number of scoring systems have been developed which attempt to gauge the severity of the lung injury in a given patient. Interestingly, initial physiologic derangements in general have not been very useful to predict mortality in these patients, although 1 recent report indicated that the dead space fraction

Table 2.

	Timing	Oxygenation	CXR	Ppw
ALI Criteria	Acute onset	PaO2/FiO2 < 300 mm hg (regardless of PEEP level)	Bilateral infiltrates	< 18 mm Hg or no clinical evidence right atrial hypertension
ARDS Criteria	Acute onset	PaO2/FiO2 < 200 mm hg (regardless of PEEP level)	Bilateral infiltrates	< 18 mm Hg or no clinical evidence right atrial hypertension

measured during the first day of mechanical ventilation was a powerful determinant of survival—the odds ratio for mortality associated with each increase of dead-space fraction of .05 was 1.45 (95% CI 1.15-1.83, p=.002).

Treatment of ARDS

While the attention of the critical care physician is often focused upon the details of supportive therapy for patients with ARDS, it cannot be overemphasized that simultaneously a search for and treatment of the underlying cause of the lung failure must be conducted. Absent an identification and treatment of the underlying process(es) causing lung injury, supportive therapy alone will likely ultimately result in mounting complications and irreversible organ failures. ARDS represents a syndrome defined by bedside, radiologic, and physiologic criteria—it is not a specific diagnosis. The management principles detailed below are intended to stabilize the patient and provide a window of opportunity to perform the diagnostic and therapeutic interventions to treat underlying diseases.

Ventilatory Management of ARDS

Lung Mechanics, Ventilator-Induced Lung Injury (VILI), and Ventilator-Associated Lung Injury (VALI)

Over the past decade or more, a body of knowledge has accrued from both bench and clinical investigations that has motivated intensivists to reconsider how they ventilate patients with ARDS. Much of this work was based upon early observations that mechanical ventilation using large tidal volumes and high inflation pressures could cause a fatal lung injury in animals with otherwise normal lungs. The term ventilator-induced lung injury (VILI) has been applied to acute lung injury directly induced by mechanical ventilation in animal models. VILI is indistinguishable morphologically, physiologically, and radiologically from diffuse alveolar damage caused by other etiologies of acute lung injury. VILI is unique because one can identify that mechanical ventilation is the cause of lung injury, and hence the term *ventilator-induced* lung injury. Ventilator-associated lung injury (VALI) is defined as lung injury which resembles ARDS and which occurs in patients on mechanical ventilation. VALI is invariably associated with pre-existing lung pathology such as ARDS. However, while the experimental data is overwhelming in demonstrating the existence of VILI, one cannot be sure in any particular case whether and to what extent VALI is caused by a particular ventilator strategy, rather VALI is only *associated* with mechanical ventilation.

Studies in animal models of VILI have demonstrated that lung injury during mechanical ventilatory support appears related to the

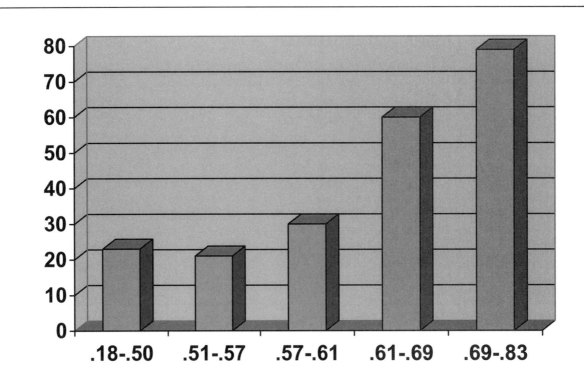

Figure 4. The observed mortality according to the quintile of dead-space fraction in 179 patients with ARDS (from Nuckton et al: *New Engl J Med* 2002; 346:1281)

distending volume to which the lung is subjected, rather than the distending pressure as measured at the mouth. For instance, in animal experiments in which the chest is banded and mechanical ventilation is conducted with high airway pressures but low tidal volumes resulting from the restricted chest wall, lung injury is not present. Such observations have caused the term "volutrauma" to be coined for this form of microstructural injury, a refinement of the standard term "barotrauma" applied to the grosser forms of extra-alveolar air collections that are sought on routine radiographs obtained on patients undergoing mechanical ventilation.

In addition to the detrimental effects of over-distension, numerous investigations have suggested a protective or ameliorating effect of positive end expiratory pressure (PEEP) on VILI. This protective effect has been postulated to result from the action of PEEP to avoid alveolar collapse and reopening. In the aggregate, these studies offer a view of VILI that is portrayed in Figure 5—that during the respiratory cycle, alveolar opening and collapse occur if end expiratory pressure is zero or only modestly positive, and depending on end

inspiratory lung volume, alveolar over-distension may occur.

In both animal models of lung injury and patients with ARDS, the respiratory system inflation PV curve exhibits a sigmoidal shape, with a lower inflection point (LIP) and an upper inflection point (UIP). Marked hysteresis is often noted when the inflation and deflation limbs are compared. The presence of the LIP is consistent with the edematous lung behaving as a2 compartment structure, with a population of alveoli exhibiting near normal compliance and another recruitable only at higher transpulmonary pressure. As transpulmonary pressure is raised to the LIP, effecting alveolar recruitment, lung compliance improves as reflected by the increase in the slope of the PV curve. Volume tends to increase in a nearly linear fashion as pressure is increased, until the UIP is reached, with a flattening of the curve taken to represent alveolar over-distension with the attendant risks of alveolar injury.

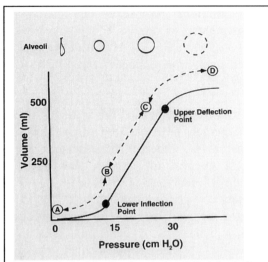

Figure 5. An idealized and simplified depiction of the pressure volume curve of the injured lung during inflation, with the state of alveolar collapse and inflation.

Clinical Studies of Ventilator Strategies for ARDS

These descriptions of VILI in animals and physiologic observations in patients resulted in strategies that have been tested at the bedside and demonstrated improved patient outcome. In the field of critical care medicine, this is one of the most substantive examples of bench-to-bedside transfer of knowledge that now provides an evidence-based approach to patient care.

Hickling and colleagues reported a favorable impact on survival of tidal volume reduction and permissive hypercapnea in the management of patients with ARDS, comparing outcome to historical controls. These studies were limited by the lack of a randomized prospective controlled design, particularly in light of findings that the survival of patients with ARDS in the same timeframe is likely improving apart from the details of mechanical ventilatory support.

The first prospective randomized trial testing a strategy of limiting tidal volume and utilizing PEEP to avoid alveolar recruitment-derecruitment (so called "open lung" ventilation) was conducted by Amato and colleagues, who randomized patients with ARDS to two treatments: a) assist-control ventilation with tidal volumes of 12 ml/kg, PEEP sufficient to maintain an adequate SaO_2 on $FiO_2 < 0.6$), and

respiratory rates sufficient to maintain arterial carbon dioxide levels of 25-38 mm Hg; no efforts were made to control peak inspiratory or plateau airway pressures ("conventional" approach); or b) pressure-controlled inverse ratio ventilation, pressure-support ventilation, or volume-assured pressure-support ventilation with tidal volumes less than 6 ml/kg, recruitment maneuver, peak pressures less than 40 cm H_2O, and PEEP titrated to maintain lung inflation above the lower inflection point ("open-lung" approach). Patients managed with the "open-lung" approach demonstrated a more rapid recovery of pulmonary compliance, decreased requirement for high FiO_2, a lower rate of barotrauma, a higher rate of liberation from the ventilator, decreased death associated with respiratory failure, and a decreased mortality at 28 days (although not at hospital discharge).

While these results were striking, a number of concerns regarding this study deserve consideration. The number of patients included in the study was small (only 53). Further, there were multiple treatment differences between the two groups, including PEEP strategy, tidal volume, PCO_2, minute ventilation, lung recruitment maneuvers, and mode of ventilation. Importantly, mortality was extremely high in the conventional ventilation group (71%), and the early differences in mortality seen between the groups did not seem consistent with the 2 ventilator strategies differing by the accrual of progressive lung injury. Finally, patients with severe metabolic acidosis, a common feature of patients with overwhelming sepsis and ARDS, were excluded from study. Even if one accepts the results of this study, perhaps the benefit was simply due to tidal volume reduction, not to the PEEP strategy. Even if this PEEP strategy prevented VILI, the PEEP value selected from the LIP on inflation of edematous lungs from zero end expiratory pressure is considerably larger than the PEEP value required to maintain alveolar recruitment during tidal ventilation on PEEP. In addition, several other investigations evaluating the effect of tidal volume manipulation on outcome did not show a similar salutary effect of low tidal volume ventilation.

The controversy over proper tidal volumes for ventilation of patients with ARDS has been largely resolved by the performance of a trial conducted by the NIH funded ARDSnet, a network of 10 centers in 24 hospitals comprising 75 intensive care units that enrolled 861 patients. Patients were randomized to a strategy of either 12 ml/kg tidal volume or 6 ml/kg tidal volume tidal volume, based on ideal body weight. If plateau airway pressure (Pplat), used as a surrogate of end inspiratory lung "stretch," exceeded 30 cm H_2O water pressure in the low tidal volume group, tidal volume was further reduced as necessary to reduce Pplat to this target value. The experimental protocol could be summarized as:

The trial was stopped sooner than the anticipated endpoint since the findings were striking. The strategy achieved a significant difference in tidal volumes as intended—the mean tidal volumes on days 1 to 3 were 6.2 and 11.8 ml/kg in the low and high groups respectively (p<.001), associated with Pplat of 25 and 33 cm H2O respectively (p<.001). PEEP levels were minimally higher in the low tidal volume group from days 1 to 3 (averaging less than 1 cm H_2O and lower on day 7). The low tidal volume group had a modest increase in $PaCO_2$ relative to the traditional group and a very modest decrease in pH; the potential for greater degrees of respiratory acidosis between the groups was minimized by the higher respiratory rates used in the low tidal volume group. The primary endpoint of the study, 28-day mortality—was significantly improved with low tidal volume ventilation, falling from 39.8% in the traditional group to 31.0% with low tidal volume ventilation (p = .007). In addition, the number of ventilator free-days in the first 28 days was greater in the low tidal volume group.

This trial is a benchmark and confirms earlier basic and clinical studies suggesting low tidal volume ventilation can be protective for patients with ARDS and will improve outcome. Perhaps the best evidenced-based recommendation for routine management of patients with ARDS undergoing mechanical ventilation is to implement the ARDSnet protocol. While questions surround other elements of ventilatory strategy—the "best PEEP" level, the trade-off between FiO_2 and PEEP, the use of recruitment maneuvers, patient positioning—the current evidence strongly supports the use of the ARDSnet strategy

pending additional information to guide these other components of ventilatory support.

Practical points for managing the patient with ALI/ARDS

Upon presentation the patient should receive oxygen provided by high flow or rebreather mask, although these devices rarely achieve a tracheal FiO_2 much above 0.6 in dyspneic, tachypneic patients. The administration of supplemental oxygen is a diagnostic as well as therapeutic maneuver. Patients whose oxygenation improves dramatically with supplemental oxygen generally have a small shunt and a larger component of ventilation-perfusion mismatch (or hypoventilation). Even when the PaO_2 improves only slightly, indicating a large shunt, oxygen delivery may rise importantly, due to the steep nature of the hemoglobin saturation relationship at low PaO_2 (see Figure 2). The role of noninvasive positive-pressure ventilation (NIPPV) has not been established in ARDS. Although we have used NIPPV successfully in this setting, we believe it is generally not a good choice and patients must be carefully selected. Since the course of ARDS is usually longer than patients will tolerate NIPPV, and since ARDS is so often associated with hemodynamic instability, coma, and multiorgan system failure (including ileus), we believe all but exceptional patients should be endotracheally intubated.

Intubation should be performed early and electively when it is clear that mechanical ventilation will be required, rather than waiting for frank respiratory failure. If hypoperfusion is present, as in the patient with hypotension, cardiovascular instability, or the hyperdynamic circulation of sepsis, oxygen delivery may be compromised not only by hypoxemia but by an inadequate cardiac output as well. In this circumstance, sedation and muscle relaxation should be considered as a means to diminish the oxygen requirement of the skeletal muscles. Patients with extreme hypoxemia despite ventilator management as described below may also benefit from sedation or paralysis.

The initial ventilator settings should pursue the protocol given in Table 3 above. While the use of low tidal volume is strongly

Table 3. ARDSnet Low Tidal Volume Protocol

Variable	Protocol
Ventilator mode	**Volume assist-control**
Tidal volume	**≤ 6 mL/kg predicted body weight**
Plateau airway pressure	**≤ 30 cm H2O**
Vent rate/pH goal	**6-35/min, adjusted to achieve arterial pH > 7.30 if possible**
Inspiratory flow	**Adjust for I:E of 1.1:1.3**
Oxygenation	**55 ≤ PaO2 ≤ 80 mm Hg or 88 ≤ SaO2 ≤ 95%**
FiO2/PEEP combinations	**.3/5, .4/5, .4/8, .5/8, .5/10, .6/10, .7/10, .7/12, .7/14, .8/14, .9/14, .9/16, .9/18, 1.0/18, 1.0/22, 1.0/24**
Weaning	**Attempt by PS when FiO2/PEEP < .4/8**

Predicted body weight for males = 50 + (2.3 x (height in inches – 60)) or 50 + (.91 x (height in cm – 152.4))
Predicted body weight for females = 45 + (2.3 x (height in inches –60)) or 45 + (.91 x (height in cm – 152.4))

supported by current evidence, the proper PEEP level is less clear. Some intensivists recommend a "least PEEP" approach, using PEEP only as necessary to achieve adequate oxygenation and avoid toxic levels of FiO_2 (although these thresholds are not well established). Others would recommend higher PEEP levels with a goal of achieving maximal lung recruitment and avoiding mechanical events such as collapse-reinflation that could lead to VALI. Some even advocate the use of the pressure-volume curve of the lung measured during the respiratory cycle as a guide to this PEEP titration. Data do not support one or another approach strongly, and the ARDSnet is currently completing a trial comparing low and high PEEP strategies. In the interim, use of the ARDSnet protocol seems prudent.

Regardless of specific strategy, reducing PEEP, even for short periods of time, is often associated with alveolar derecruitment and hence rapid arterial hemoglobin desaturation. Thus, once endotracheal tube suctioning has been accomplished for diagnostic purposes, nursing and respiratory therapy staff should be instructed to keep airway disconnections to a minimum, or to use an in-line suctioning system that maintains sterility and positive pressure, usually via the suctioning catheter residing in a sterile sheath and entering the endotracheal tube via a tight-sealing diaphragm. These suctioning systems are generally effective for lesser levels of PEEP (< 15 cm H_2O) but often leak if higher levels are attempted.

Innovative Therapies for ARDS

While the general strategy described above will provide adequate ventilatory support for the majority of patients with ALI/ARDS, a fraction of patients will have severe hypoxemia or other adverse consequences of these approaches, and innovative or salvage therapies have been reported in the literature. In general these approaches are not supported by large prospective trials (or trials have been conducted without benefit seen) but they may have some role in individual patient management.

Prone Position

Multiple studies have shown that a substantial fraction of patients with ARDS exhibit improved oxygenation with prone positioning. Some studies suggest this maneuver enhances lower lobe recruitment and thus would have the potential to not only improve gas exchange but perhaps reduced VALI and ultimate patient outcome. A recent large prospective trial evaluated proning in patients with ALI/ARDS and did not see a benefit. In subset analysis, there did appear to be a trend to improved outcome in patients with more severe physiologic derangement. In addition, this study has been criticized for the relatively short periods of proning that were employed. Further studies of this strategy are ongoing.

High Frequency Ventilation

If excessive lung excursion is associated with injury to the lung, then it seems reasonable that ventilation with very small tidal volumes at high frequencies would be associated with the least possible ventilator induced-lung injury, and would be associated with improved outcome. High frequency jet ventilation (HFV) typically employs tidal volumes of 1-5 ml (or higher) and respiratory rates of 60 to 300 breaths/min. Gas exchange is poorly understood under these conditions, but is thought to occur as much through augmented axial diffusion as through bulk flow. Unfortunately, multiple trials of high frequency ventilation in adults have failed to demonstrate any benefit compared to mechanical ventilation. It is interesting to note that high frequency jet ventilation has never been associated with either improved oxygenation, reduced barotrauma, or decreased days of mechanical ventilation. These are all outcomes that would be reasonably expected as a logical extension of the physiology and concerns driving open lung ventilation. That they have not been observed suggests that all previous investigations of high frequency jet ventilation were conducted using the wrong guidelines for ventilation (i.e., striving to maintain normocarbia), or that some other effect not yet understood precludes benefit from this technique. Future studies of HFV should compare this technique to ventilation using the low tidal volume ventilation as described in the

ARDSnet trial and will have to demonstrate benefit compared to these strategies to gain acceptance

ECMO

The use of extracorporeal gas exchange (ECMO) to adequately oxygenate and ventilate the blood while allowing the lung to rest remains an attractive strategy for the management of patients with acute lung injury, but has not been supported by clinical outcome studies. There is little apparent future for this technique in adult patients with ARDS. ECMO is best regarded at this time as heroic salvage therapy for patients with isolated respiratory failure in whom all other supportive measures have failed.

Inhaled Nitric Oxide

Nitric oxide is a potent endogenous vasodilator which, when given by inhalation, selectively vasodilates the pulmonary circulation. iNO has several potentially salutary effects in ARDS: it selectively vasodilates pulmonary vessels which subserve *ventilated* alveoli, diverting blood flow to these alveoli (and away from areas of shunt). The first effect, the lowering of the pulmonary vascular resistance, accompanied by a lowering of the pulmonary artery pressure, appears maximal at very low concentrations (approx 0.1ppm) in patients with ARDS. The beneficial effects on oxygenation take place at somewhat higher inspired concentrations of NO (1-10 ppm). The rapid inactivation of iNO via hemoglobin binding prevents unwanted systemic hemodynamic side effects, but also mandates the continuous delivery of gas to the ventilator circuit. In the numerous studies evaluating the acute response to iNO, there has been a consistent finding of approximately 50-70% of patients improving oxygenation. However, 2 recent prospective trials have failed to demonstrate improved long-term outcome from iNO administration in ARDS ventilation, and thus this remains a salvage therapy at best.

Circulatory Management of ARDS

Debate has surrounded the proper circulatory management of patients with ARDS for decades. On the one hand, animal and some clinical studies suggest that edemagenesis can be reduced by reducing pulmonary microvascular pressures in acute lung injury, in a fashion similar to the management of cardiogenic pulmonary edema. Of course, since these microvascular pressures are normal in these patients despite their lung flooding, the possibility of reducing cardiac preload exists, thus engendering inadequate organ perfusion in a patient population known to be a risk of multiple organ failure and indeed in whom outcome appears dictated in large part by the accrual of organ failures.

In addition, the proper monitoring tools for assessing the adequacy of the circulation in these patients and whether monitoring should include invasive hemodynamic measurement is equally controversial. It seems reasonable to state that mere monitoring with invasive measurements that is not coupled to a strategy to achieve predefined goals is not warranted.

It is difficult to make firm recommendations in the current state of knowledge. The ARDSnet is currently conducting a trial which enrolls and randomizes patients to management with either a central venous catheter or right heart catheter, and then each group is additionally randomized to receive a fluid liberal or fluid conservative strategy. Hopefully information from this study will help guide the circulatory management of these patients and will determine how that strategy can be best conducted.

Management of Proliferative Phase ARDS

A subset patients with ARDS will progress over the first week of mechanical ventilation to disordered healing and severe lung fibrosis. This is usually characterized by increasing airway pressures or a falling tidal volume on pressure control ventilation, a further fall in lung compliance, less response to PEEP, a "honey-comb" appearance on the chest radiograph, progressive pulmonary hypertension, and rising minute ventilation requirements (> 20 L/min). Barotrauma is a prominent feature and multiple organ failures often accrue. A number of observations regarding their supportive therapy should be made. Increased vascular permeability at this

point in the course may be minimal, and strategies to reduce preload and edema are fraught with complications. Patients are prone to increases in Zone I lung conditions, and attempts to reduce the pulmonary capillary wedge pressure (Ppw) may result in increased dead space and hypoperfusion. Thus, seeking the lowest Ppw providing adequate cardiac output is no longer appropriate; instead, liberalization of fluid intake to provide a circulating volume in excess of that just adequate is a better strategy in this later phase of ARDS.

Interventions to directly influence the course of lung fibrosis are not well established but high-dose corticosteroid therapy has its advocates. One recent prospective trial has shown an improved survival with the use of corticosteroids in late ARDS, but routine use in late ARDS remains controversial. The utility of corticosteroids in this setting will hopefully be determined by a trial currently underway under the auspices of the ARDSnet.

If corticosteroids are used in this setting, aggressive measures to monitor for ventilator-associated pneumonia are warranted. This complication of mechanical ventilation has a high incidence and high mortality in patients with ARDS. In view of the abnormal chest radiograph and gas exchange, multiple causes of fever and leukocytosis, and high incidence of colonization of the airway, diagnosis is difficult and maybe aided by various techniques to obtain protected specimens.

Pulmonary Sequelae of ARDS

Although there are a limited number of long-term follow-up studies of patients with ARDS, it appears that the range of outcomes is rather wide: patients may recover with minimal or no abnormality by routine lung function testing shortly after acute lung insult, or they may remain substantially impaired for a year or longer, if not permanently. In most studies, approximately a fourth of patients show no impairment at 1 year, a fourth moderate impairment, roughly half only mild impairment, and a very small fraction severe impairment. Exertional dyspnea is the most commonly reported symptom, although cough and wheezing are common as well. A reduced single-breath carbon monoxide diffusing capacity is the most common pulmonary function abnormality. Spirometry and lung volumes tend to reveal mixed restrictive-obstructive abnormalities. Determining the prognosis after ARDS may be aided by obtaining complete lung functions at the time of discharge. Those patients with substantial abnormalities should be referred for appropriate follow-up.

REFERENCES

1. O'Connor M, Hall, JB, Schmidt GA, Wood, LDH: Acute hypoxemic respiratory failure. *In:* Principles of Critical Care. Hall JB, Schmidt GA, Wood LDH (Eds): New York, McGraw-Hill Publishers, 1998, pp 537-559
   Useful overview of ALI/ARDS in the context of all forms of acute hypoxemic respiratory failure, including lung hemorrhage syndromes, cardiogenic pulmonary edema, and focal lesions such as lobar pneumonia.

2. Bernard GR, Artigas A, Brigham KL, et al: The American-European Consensus Conference on ARDS: Definitions, mechanisms, relevant outcomes, and clinical trial coordination. *Am J Respir Crit Care Med* 1994; 149:818-24
   Deliberations of a consensus group achieving definitions for ARDS/ALI that shaped future study design and enrollment.

3. Ware LB, Matthay MA: The Acute Respiratory Distress Syndrome. *New Engl J Med* 2000; 342:1334-1347
   Excellent and current review of the topic.

4. The Acute Respiratory Distress Syndrome Network. Ventilation with lower tidal volumes as compared with traditional tidal volumes for acute lung injury and ARDS. *New Engl J Med* 2000; 342:1301-1308
   Seminal investigation demonstrating improved outcome for patients ventilated with low tidal volumes during support for ALI/ARDS.

5. Brower RG, Ware LB, Berthiaume Y, Matthay MA: Treatment of ARDS. *Chest* 2001; 120:13470-1367
   Up-to-date review emphasizing therapeutic approach to patients with ARDS.

6. Nuckton TJ, Alonso JA, Kallet RH, et al: Pulmonary dead space fraction as a risk factor for death in the acute respiratory distress syndrome. *New Engl J Med* 2002; 346:1281-1286
   Unlike earlier studies indicating little correlation between early physiologic derangement and outcome in patients with ARDS, this study indicates dead space fraction to be a reasonable predictor of mortality.

7. Anzueto A, Baughman RP, Guntupalli KK, et al: Aerosolized surfactant in adults with sepsis induced acute respiratory distress syndrome. *N Engl J Med* 1996; 334:1417-21
   Largest trial of surfactant in adults, showing no benefit. Many have questioned the delivery technique used as well as the specific surfactant replacement agent.

8. Dreyfuss D, Saumon G: Ventilator-induced lung injury: Lessons from experimental studies. *Am J Resp Crit Care Med* 1998; 157:294-323
   Comprehensive review of a large number of basic investigations identifying the nature of ventilator induced lung injury and its specific determinants.

9. Hickling KG: The pressure-volume curve is greatly modified by recruitment: A mathematical model of ARDS lungs. *Am J Resp Crit Care Med* 1998; 158:194-199
   Mathematical modeling of the pressure volume curve from basic assumptions about lung mechanics in ARDS predicts a number of recruitment and distension events.

10. Slutsky AR, Tremblay LN: Multiple system organ failure: Is mechanical ventilation a contributing factor? *Am J Resp Crit Care Med* 1998; 157:1721-1725
    The concept that mechanical injury of the lung may result in inflammatory events with systemic effects is presented along with a review of the literature supporting this notion.

11. Amato MRP, Barbas CSV, Medeiros DM, et al: Effect of a protective ventilation strategy on mortality in the acute respiratory distress syndrome. *N Eng J Med* 1998; 338:347-354
    The earliest prospective study demonstrating improved outcome from the use of a lung

protective ventilatory strategy in patients with ARDS.

12. Gattinoni L, Pelosi P, Suter PM, Pedoto A, et al: Acute respiratory distress syndrome due to pulmonary and extra-pulmonary disease: different syndromes? *Am J Resp Crit Care Med* 1998; 158:3-11
Provocative study suggesting causes of ARDS that are pulmonary (e.g., lung infection) result in a lung injury that is different with regard to lung mechanics and PEEP response than ARDS arising from extrapulmonary processes (e.g., intra-abdominal sepsis or pancreatitis).

13. Dellinger RP, Zimmerman JL, Taylor RW, Straube RC, et al: Effects of inhaled nitric oxide in patients with acute respiratory distress syndrome: results of a randomized phase II trial. *Crit Care Med* 1998; 26:15-23
Prospective trial with no benefit seen from the use of inhaled nitric oxide during ventilatory management of patients with ARDS.

14. Meduri GU, Headley AS, Golden E, Carson SJ, et al: Effect of prolonged methylprednisolone therapy in unresolving acute respiratory distress syndrome: a randomized controlled trial. *JAMA* 1998; 280:159-165
Small trial demonstrating improved outcome from high dose corticosteroids used in late phase ARDS.

15. Chastre J, Trouillet JL, Vuagnat A, Joly-Guillou ML, et al: Nosocomial pneumonia in patients with acute respiratory distress syndrome. *Am J Resp Crit Care Med* 1998; 157:1165-1172
Study demonstrating high incidence of ventilator-associated pneumonia in patients with ARDS.

ANTIBIOTIC THERAPY IN CRITICAL ILLNESS

Michael S. Niederman, MD

INTRODUCTION

The therapy of severe pneumonia can be used as a paradigm to demonstrate the principles of antibiotic therapy of critically ill patients. The focus of this discussion will be on empiric antibiotic therapy, but the principles of antibiotic penetration and concentration in the lung are summarized in Table 1.

MECHANISMS OF ACTION

Antibiotics interfere with the growth of bacteria by undermining the integrity of their cell wall or by interfering with bacterial protein synthesis or common metabolic pathways. The terms "bactericidal" and "bacteriostatic" are broad categorizations, and may not apply for a given agent against all organisms, with certain antimicrobials being bactericidal for one bacterial pathogen, but bacteriostatic for another. Bactericidal antibiotics kill bacteria, generally by inhibiting cell wall synthesis or by interrupting a key metabolic function of the organism and include: the penicillins, cephalosporins, aminoglycosides, flourquinolones, vancomycin, rifampin and metronidazole. Bacteriostatic agents inhibit bacterial growth, do not interfere with cell wall synthesis, and rely on host defenses to eliminate bacteria. They include: the macrolides, tetracycline, sulfa drugs, chloramphenicol, and clindamycin. The distinction between these 2 types of agents may not be important in the therapy of lung infections since either can be effective. When neutropenia is present, or if there is accompanying endocarditis, meningitis, or osteomyelitis, then the use of a bactericidal agent may be advantageous.

Antimicrobial activity is often described by the terms MIC and MBC. The term MIC defines the minimum concentration of an antibiotic that inhibits the growth of 90% of a standard sized innoculum, leading to no visible growth in a broth culture. The term MBC refers to the minimum concentration needed to cause a 3-log drop (99.9% killing) in the size of the standard innoculum. These terms must be interpreted cautiously, and, if pneumonia is the infection being treated, the clinician must consider MIC and MBC data with a knowledge of how well an agent can reach the lung. The MIC is used to define the "sensitivity" of a pathogen to a specific antibiotic, under the assumption that the concentration required for killing can be reached *in vivo*, but lung concentrations may be substantially lower than serum concentrations—the latter being the site that is generally used to define antimicrobial susceptibility patterns.

Penetration Issues (Table 1)

The concentration of an antibiotic in the lung depends on the permeability of the capillary bed at the site of infection (the bronchial circulation), the degree of protein binding of the drug, and the presence or absence of an active transport site for the antibiotic in the lung. In the lung, the relevant site to consider for antibiotic penetration is controversial and not clearly defined. Sputum and bronchial concentrations are considered most relevant for bronchial infections, while concentrations in lung parenchyma, epithleial lining fluid, and in cells such as macrophages, neutrophils are probably more important for pneumonic infections. The localization of the pathogen may also be important, and intracellular organisms such as *Legionella pneumophila* and *Chlamydia pneumonia* are probably best eradicated by agents that achieve high concentrations in macrophages. Although local concentration of an antibiotic is important, it is also necessary to consider the activity of an agent at the site that it reaches. For example, antibiotics can be inactivated by certain local conditions. Aminoglycosides have reduced activity at acidic

Table 1. Penetration of antibiotics into respiratory secretions

---

Lipid: Soluble, concentrate independent of inflammation, good penetration

Quinolones:
    New macrolides: azithromycin, clarithromycin, tetracyclines, clindamycin, trimethoprim/sulfamethoxizole

Relatively lipid: Insoluble, inflammation dependent for concentration in the lung, poor penetration

Aminoglycosides:
    Beta-lactams: penicillins, cephalosporins, monobactams, carbapenems

---

pH's, and some pneumonic areas of lung are acidic. Bacteria can produce beta-lactamase enzymes, which can render a number of common penicillins and cephalosporins inactive. In addition, bacteria can become resistant to an agent (requiring that higher concentrations than are possible to achieve be present in order to be killed) because they become impermeable to antibiotic entry, or because they modify the site to which the antibiotic must bind in order to be active.

SPECIFIC ANTIBIOTICS

Beta-lactam Antibiotics

These bactericidal antibiotics have in common the presence of a beta lactam ring, which is bound to a 5-membered thiazolidine ring in the case of the penicillins and to a 6-membered dihydrothiazine ring in the case of the cephalosporins. Modifications in the thiazolidine ring can lead to agents such as the penems (imipenem and meropenem), while absence of the second ring structure characterizes the monobactams (aztreonam). These agents can also be combined with beta lactamase inhibitors such as sulbactam, tazobactam, or clavulanic acid, to create the beta-lactam/beta-lactamase inhibitor drugs. These agents extend the antimicrobial spectrum of the beta-lactams by providing a substrate for the bacterial beta lactamases (sulbactam, clavulanic acid, tazobactam), thereby preserving the antibacterial activity of the parent compound. Beta lactam antibiotics work by interfering with the synthesis of bacterial cell wall acquired and nosocomial,

and may be effective as monotherapy, taking into account the caveats discussed above. Aztreonam is a monobactam that is so antigenically different from the rest of the beta-lactams, that it can be used in penicillin allergic patients. It is only active against gram-negative organisms, having a spectrum very similar to the aminoglycosides.

Fluoroquinolones

These bactericidal agents act by interfering with bacterial DNA gyrase, leading to impaired DNA synthesis repair, transcription and other cellular processes, resulting in bacterial cell lysis. DNA gyrase is 1 form of bacterial topoisomerase enzyme that is inhibited by the quinolones, but activity against other similar enzymes is part of the effect of a variety of quinolones. As mentioned above, quinolones kill in a concentration-dependent fashion, related to the Cmax/MIC ratio and to the AUC/MIC ratio of drug concentration relative to organism susceptibility.

There are 2 features of quinolones which make them well-suited to respiratory infections. First, they penetrate well into secretions and inflammatory cells within the lung, achieving concentrations that exceed serum levels in many instances. Thus, these agents may be clinically more effective than predicted by MIC values. Secondly, these agents are highly bioavailable with oral administration, thus similar levels can be reached if administered orally or intravenously. This allows for some "borderline" patients (such as nursing home patients) with pneumonia to be

Table 2. Severe Community Acquired Pneumonia

Hospitalized Patients with Severe Community-Acquired Pneumonia

No Pseudomonal Risk Factors
    Streptococcus pneumoniae (ncluding DRSP)
      Legionella species
      H. influenzae
      Enteric gram-negatives
      S. aureus
      M. pneumoniae or *C. pneumoniae*
        Respiratory viruses
        Miscellaneous: *M. tuberculosis*, Endemic fungi
Therapy
      Macrolide OR Anti-pneumococcal quinolone
                 PLUS
     Selected beta-lactam with anti-pneumococcal activity (ceftriaxone, cefotaxime,
ampicillin/sulbactam)

Hospitalized Patients with Severe Community-Acquired Pneumonia

Pseudomonal risks
    Streptococcus pneumoniae (including DRSP)
      Legionella species
      H. influenzae
      Enteric gram-negatives (including *P. aeruginosa*)
      S. aureus
      M. pneumoniae or *C. pneumoniae*
        Respiratory viruses
        Miscellaneous: *M. tuberculosis*, Endemic fungi
Therapy
      Ciprofloxacin PLUS anti-Pseudomonal, anti-pneumococcal beta lactam (imipenem,
meropenem, cefepime, piperacillin/tazobactam)
                OR
      Non-pseudomonal quinolone (levofloxacin , gatifloxacin, moxifloxacin) or macrolide
      PLUS anti-Pseudomonal, anti-pneumococcal beta lactam (imipenem, meropenem, cefepime,
piperacillin/tazobactam) PLUS aminoglycoside

Table 3. Severe hospital-acquired pneumonia, no specific risks, early onset infection

Likely Pathogens
"Core Pathogens"
       S. pneumoniae
       H. influenzae
       Methicillin-sensitive *S. aureus*
       Enteric gram-negatives
              Enterobacter spp.
              E. coli
              Klebsiella spp.
              Proteus spp.
              S. marcescens

Suggested Therapy
Any of the following:
       Second-generation cephalosporin (cefuroxime)
       Non-pseudomonal third-generation cephalosporin (cefotaxime, ceftriaxone)
       Beta-lactam/beta lactamase inhibitor combination (ampicillin/sulbactam, piperacillin/tazobactam,
           Ticarcillin/clavulanate)
       Fluoroquinolone (ciprofloxacin or ofloxacin)**
       Clindamycin and aztreonam**

**If penicillin and cephalosporin allergic

managed with outpatient oral therapy and not to be admitted solely for the purpose of intravenous therapy to achieve high serum levels of antibiotics. In addition, the high bioavailability of these agents permits an easy transition from intravenous to oral therapy of inpatients with pneumonia, facilitating early discharge when the patient is doing well, and permitting ongoing oral therapy with maintenance of high serum levels of antibiotics.

Currently, the quinolones fall into several "generations." The first generation agents had gram-negative activity only and were used for urinary tract infections, epitomized by the agent nalidixic acid. The second-generation agents had added gram-positive activity and could be used for systemic infections and included ciprofloxacin, ofloxacin, pefloxacin, fleroxacin, and lomefloxacin. These agents had limited value for respiratory infections because of relatively high MIC values among pneumococci, making it necessary to use high doses to achieve efficacy against this pathogen. The third-generation agents are characterized by better gram-positive activity, particularly against pneumococcus. These agents include levofloxacin, gatifloxacin and moxifloxacin, which are currently available. Among the third-generation agents, the most active against pneumococcus is moxifloxacin, followed by gatifloxacin, and then levofloxacin. These new agents also have long half-lives, allowing once-daily dosing with most of the third-generation agents. In addition, quinolones that are active against pneumococcus are likely to be effective regardless of penicillin susceptibility patterns since penicillin and quinolone resistance do not generally occur together in the same organisms, and pneumococcal resistance rates to new quinolones are low. However, some coexistence of quinolone resistance with penicillin resistance has been reported, and the most active pneumococcal agents (on an MIC basis) are the least likely to develop resistance. With this in mind, it is not surprising that there have been reports of failures of therapy for pneumococcal CAP using levofloxacin. When quinolones are used for severe CAP, the current recommendation is not to use them as monotherapy.

AMINOGLYCOSIDES

These bactericidal agents act by binding to the 30S ribosomal subunit of bacteria, thus interfering with protein synthesis.

Table 4. Severe HAP, anytime with risk factors, or late onset in the absence of risk factors

Likely Pathogens:
"Core organisms" PLUS
  P. aeruginosa
  Acinetobacter spp.
  Methicillin-resistant *S. aureus*

Suggested Therapy
Dual anti-pseudomonal therapy:
  Aminoglycoside or ciprofloxacin PLUS ONE OF THE FOLLOWING:
    Third-generation cephalosporin with anti-Pseudomonal activity or cefepime
    Anti-pseudomonal penicillin
    Imipenem, Meropenem
    Aztreonam
    Ticarcillin/clavulanate or piperacillin/tazobactam
    PLUS CONSIDER: Vacomycin or alternatives

Aminoglycosides have primarily a gram-negative spectrum of activity, and are usually used in combination with other agents targeting difficult organisms such as *P. aeruginosa* or other resistant gram-negatives. When combined with certain beta-lactam agents they can achieve antibacterial synergy against *P. aeruginosa*. Amikacin is the least susceptible to enzymatic inactivation by bacteria, while tobramycin is more active than gentamicin against *P. aeruginosa*. Aminoglycosides penetrate poorly into lung tissue, and can be inactivated by acid pH's, which are common in pneumonic lung tissue. Thus, in 1 clinical trial of nosocomial pneumonia therapy, the use of an aminoglycoside with a beta-lactam was no more effective than a beta-lactam alone, and the combination regimen was not more effective in preventing the emergence of Pseudomonal resistance during therapy than was the monotherapy regimen with a beta-lactam (63). In the treatment of bacteremic Pseudomonal pneumonia, aminoglycoside combination therapy may be more effective than monotherapy.

As discussed above, aminoglycosides kill in a concentration-dependent fashion, and can be dosed once daily to optimize killing while minimizing toxicity. In clinical practice, this has not been proven to occur, and once-daily dosing is comparable in efficacy and nephrotoxicity to multiple dose regimens. When aminoglycosides are used, it is necessary to monitor serum levels to minimize the occurrence of acute renal failure. Peak concentrations correlate with efficacy, but only have meaning with multiple daily doses, and their utility in once-daily regimens has not been established. Trough concentrations are monitored to minimize toxicity and probably should be followed regardless of dosing regimen.

Because of poor penetration into tissues, some investigators have used nebulized aminoglycosides for the therapy and/or prevention of gram-negative pneumonia. This approach has been effective in the treatment of infectious exacerbations of cystic fibrosis, but has not been effective as adjunctive therapy to systemic antibiotics in patients with serious respiratory tract infections.

Oxazolidinones (Linezolid)

*Acts to inhibit bacterial protein synthesis
–Binds to the 50S subunit and prevents binding of tRNA and prevents formation of the 70S initiation complex
–Unique mechanism and no cross-resistance to other agents
•Active versus MRSA, DRSP, and VRE (BOTH faecium and faecalis). Bacteriostatic, but bactericidal against some pneumoccci
•Susceptibility with MIC of 4 mg/L or less. MRSA, PRSP, VRE all fall in this range.

•600 mg twice daily. Oral and IV bioequivalent. Half-life 4.5 - 5.5 hours. Peak concentration = 18 mg/L. Renal and non-renal clearance
•Efficacy for nosocomial pneumonia, CAP, complicated skin/soft tissue infections, VRE.
•Side effects: well-tolerated. nausea, diarrhea, anemia, and thrombocytopenia (with prolonged use, < 1%). Weak MAO inhibitor.
•*Drugs* 2000; 59: 815-827

EMPIRIC THERAPY OF PNEUMONIA: AN EXAMPLE OF ANTIBIOTIC USAGE

Severe pneumonia patients can be divided into 3 different categories (Tables 2 - 4), each with their own list of likely pathogens, and from this list follows suggested antibiotic regimens. In order to decide which category a patient falls into, it is first necessary to determine if the pneumonia is community-acquired or hospital-acquired. Patients with severe CAP are likely to be infected with the organisms listed in Table 2 and should receive the therapy suggested. In the setting of severe HAP, stratification is identical whether the patient is intubated or not, but patients are separated on the basis of whether or not they have risk factors for resistant pathogens. If no risk factors are present and if the pneumonia is early onset (within the first 4 days of admission), then the patient is at risk for the organisms in Table 3 and should receive the therapy listed. If the patient has a late onset HAP (day 5 or later) in the absence of risk factors, or pneumonia of any time of onset in the presence of risk factors, then the patient is treated according to Table 4.

Although all patients undergo some diagnostic testing, empiric antibiotic therapy must be initiated before the results of diagnostic testing become available. Empiric therapy is needed for CAP patients because: even with extensive diagnostic testing, no diagnosis is found in up to half of all patients; the bacteriology of severe CAP is predictable, making empiric therapy possible; and in the setting of severe CAP, accurate empiric therapy has been shown to improve outcome. Similarly, empiric therapy, based on a clinical diagnosis of infection, is necessary for patients with severe HAP because: clinical criteria are sensitive to early and potentially treatable forms of pneumonia; algorithms can be used to predict the likely pathogens and to guide therapy; and empiric therapy can be modified once the results of tracheal aspirates or sputum cultures become available.

Severe CAP. Because the spectrum of likely pathogens is so broad and includes not only pneumococcus but also *Legionella spp.* and enteric gram-negatives, it is necessary to use multiple intravenous agents, as outlined in Table 2. This includes an intravenous macrolide or quinolone with the addition of other agents, the type and number being determined by whether risk factors for *P. aerugionosa* are present.

The initial empiric regimen for severe CAP should be adequate for a penicillin-resistant pneumococcal infection. Recent studies have shown that most resistance is of the intermediate, and not high-level type. As many as 85 - 90% of penicillin resistant organisms are still macrolide sensitive, and high-dose beta-lactam therapy, with a penicillin or third-generation cephalosporin, is also adequate for most resistant pneumococci. If penicillin resistance is especially likely, then cefotaxime or ceftriaxone should be used instead of an anti-Pseudomonal third-generation cephalosporin. If a resistant pneumococcal infection is suspected and cultures of blood or sputum show high-level resistance to both cephalosporins and penicillin, then therapy should include either vancomycin or a new anti-pneumococcal quinolone.

One organism that is not well covered by the suggested empiric regimen in Table 2 is *S. aureus*. This organism is not a common cause of severe CAP, but is a concern in patients with diabetes mellitus, renal failure, or after influenza infection. In these settings, the use of an anti-staphylococcal penicillin or vancomycin should be considered, possibly in place of one of the anti-Pseudomonal agents.

Severe HAP. Patients with no risk factors for resistant pathogens and early onset of HAP are only at risk for the core pathogens listed in Table 3, and they can often be treated with only a single antimicrobial agent. However, when patients are at risk for *P. aeruginosa* or other resistant pathogens, because of the presence of risk factors such as prior antibiotics, corticosteroid use, or malnutrition, or because of prolonged mechanical ventilation ($\geq$ 5 days) leading to late onset pneumonia, then combination therapy is necessary. Combination anti-Pseudomonal therapy should be started in these patients, and continued if *P. aeruginosa* or other resistant gram-negatives (such as *Enterobacter spp.*) are present. In immune compromised patients, combination therapy can provide synergism against *P. aeruginosa*, but this is not the usual reason for using combination regimens in other types of patients. The rationale for combination therapy is to prevent the emergence of resistance during treatment, a common event when only a single antimicrobial agent is used for these pathogens. In addition, there is evidence that dual agent therapy can improve the outcome of patients with bacteremic *P. aeruginosa* pneumonia.

The antimicrobials that are anti-Pseudomonal are either beta lactams (penicillins, cephalosporins, monobactams, and carbapenems), or agents from other drug classes. These include: penicillins such as piperacillin and mezlocillin; the beta-lactam/beta-lactamase inhibitor combination ticarcillin/clavulanate; the third-generation cephalosporins ceftazidime and cefoperazone; the monobactam, aztreonam; the carbapenem, imipenem; a fluoroquinolone, ciprofloxacin; and the aminoglycosides. When these agents are combined, 3 general approaches can be used. The traditional combination includes a beta lactam and an aminoglycoside, which can achieve antibacterial synergy. This is rarely an important benefit for the non-neutropenic patient, and it requires the use of an aminoglycoside, which has several limitations in the critically ill pneumonia patient. Aminoglycosides should be administered once daily, to take advantage of their enhanced killing when high peak levels are achieved, but even with this type of regimen, nephrotoxicity can occur. In addition, aminoglycosides penetrate poorly into the lung and may not be active at the acid pH's that are common in pneumonic lung tissue.

Recently, Hatala and associates conducted a meta-analysis of once-daily aminoglycoside dosing studies and concluded that, compared with standard dosing regimens, bacteriologic cure rates are identical, but once-daily dosing regimens may have reduced toxicity (*Ann Intern Med* 1996; 124: 717-725).

Given the ease of using these agents in a single daily dose and the associated reduced costs of this approach, the findings in this analysis may be sufficient to justify the widespread use of such dosing regimens.

An alternative type of combination regimen is to use 2 beta-lactam agents, but this approach can lead to antagonism in the mechanism of action of the 2 drugs, and if one drug induces a bacterial beta-lactamase, both drugs may be simultaneously inactivated. A third type of combination is to use ciprofloxacin with a beta-lactam, thus avoiding a dual beta-lactam regimen and avoiding the use of an aminoglycoside. This regimen also has the advantage of excellent respiratory tract penetration by the quinolone agent, ciprofloxacin.

In some patients with severe HAP, additional empiric therapy with vancomycin may be needed for possible methicillin-resistant *S. aureus* infection, another organism seen in patients with late onset pneumonia following prolonged intubation or prior antibiotic therapy. In the intubated patient, tracheal aspirates can be used to identify the pathogen(s) present, and therapy can be reduced to a single agent if *P. aeruginosa*, other resistant gram-negatives, or methicillin-resistant *S. aureus* are not present. One recent multi-center trial showed that when such organisms were absent, patients with severe HAP could be successfully treated with a single agent such as ciprofloxacin or imipenem.

ANTIBIOTIC RESISTANCE

Mechanisms of Resistance

- Decreased permeability of microbial cell wall permeability through alteration of cell wall porin channels
  –primary mechanism of gram-negatives to b-lactamases
- Antibiotic inactivation
  –beta-lactamases, AG inactivating enzymes, other inactivating enzymes
- Alteration of antibiotic target site
  –PBP, DNA gyrase, RNA polymerase
- Active efflux of the antibiotic

REFERENCES

1. Craig W: Pharmacodynamics of antimicrobial agents as a basis for determining dosage regimens. *Eur J Clin Microbiol Infect Dis* 1993; 12:6-8

2. Fink MP, Snydman DR, Niederman MS, Leeper KV, Johnson RH, Heard SO, Wunderink RG, Caldwell JW, Schentag JJ, Siami GA, Zameck RL, Haverstock DC, Reinhart HH, Echols RM, and the Severe Pneumonia Study Group: Treatment of severe pneumonia in hospitalized patients: Results of a multicenter, randomized, double-blind trial comparing intravenous ciprofloxacin with imipenem-cilastatin. *Antimicrobial Agents and Chemotherapy* 1994; 38:547-557
   Multi-center randomized trial comparing ciprofloxacin 400 mg q 8H to imipenem 1 gm q 8 H and showing both to be effective monotherapy for severe VAP, provided no highly resistant organisms were present.

3. Honeybourne D: Antibiotic penetration into lung tissues. *Thorax* 1994; 49:104-106

4. Mandell LA: Antibiotics for pneumonia therapy. *Med Clin North Am* 1994; 78:997-1014

5. Niederman MS: An approach to empiric therapy of nosocomial pneumonia. *Med Clin North Am* 1994; 78:1123-1141

6. Prins JM, Van Deventer S, Kuijper EJ, Speelman P: Clinical relevance of antibiotic-induced endotoxin release. *Antimicrobial Agents and Chemotherapy* 1994; 38:1211-1218

7. Campbell GD, Niederman MS, Broughton WA, Craven DE, Fein AM, Fink MP, et al: Hospital-acquired pneumonia in adults: Diagnosis, assessment of severity, initial antimicrobial therapy, and preventative strategies: A consensus statement. *Am J Respir Crit Care Med* 1996; 153: 1711-1725

8. Hilf M, Yu VL, Sharp J, Zuravleff JJ, Korvick JA, Muder RR: Antibiotic therapy for *Pseudomonas aeruginosa* bacteremia: Outcome correlations in a prospective study of 200 patients. *Am J Med* 1989; 87:540-546
   Study showing a mortality benefit for combination therapy versus monotherapy in patients with bacteremic P. aeruginosa pneumonia.

9. Sieger B, Berman SJ, Geckler RW, Farakas SA for the Meropenem Lower Respiratory Tract Infection Group: Empiric treatment of hospital-acquired lower respiratory tract infections with merepenem or ceftazidime with trobramycin: A randomized study. *Crit Care Med* 1997; 25:1663-1670

10. Chow JW, Fine MJ, Shlaes DM, Quinn JP, Hooper DC, Johnson MP, Ramphal R, Wagener MM, Miyashira DK, Yu VL: Enterobacter bacteremia: Clinical features and emergence of antibiotic resistance during therapy. *Ann Intern Med* 1991; 115:585-590
    Classic article showing that third-generation cephalosporins can promote the emergence of resistance during therapy of Enterobacter bacteremia, and are also a risk factor for resistance that is present prior to therapy.

11. Niederman MS: The principles of antibiotic use and the selection of empiric therapy for pneumonia. *In*: Pulmonary Diseases and Disorders, 3rd ed. Fishman A (Ed). New York, McGraw-Hill, 1997; p 1939-1949

12. Craig WA: Pharmacokinetic/pharmacodynamic parameters: Rationale for antimicrobial dosing of mice and men. *Clin Infect Dis* 26:1-12, 1998

13. Preston SL, Drusano GL, Berman AL, Fowler CL, Chow AT, Dornseif B, Reichl V, Natarajan J, Corrado M: Pharmacodynamcis of levofloxacin: A new paradigm for early clinical trials. *JAMA* 279:125-129, 1998
    Study that documents the need to achieve a peak to MIC ratio of 10 - 12 to optimize outcomes in the therapy of CAP due to pneumococcus.

14. Forest A, Nix DE, Ballow CH, Goss TF, Birmingham MC, Schentag JJ: Pharmacodynamics of intravenous ciprofloxacin in seriously ill patients. *Antimicrob Agents Chemother* 1993; 37:1073-1081
    Landmark study showing that outcome in nosocomial pneumonia is improved if the

AUIC of the drug used is 125 or greater, especially for gram–negative infections.

15. Hatala R, Dinh T, Cook DJ: Once-daily aminoglycoside dosing in immunocompetent adults: A meta-analysis. *Ann Intern Med* 1996; 124:717-725

16. Gold HS, Moellering RC: Antimicrobial - drug resistance. *N Engl J Med* 1996; 335: 1445-1453

17. Cometta A, Baumgartner JD, Lew D, et al: Prosptective randomized comparison of imipenem monotherapy with imipenem plus netilmicin for treatment of severe infections in nonneutropenic patients. *Antimicrobial Agents and Chemotherapy* 1994; 38:1309-1313

Addition of an aminoglycoside to imipenem for the therapy of nosocomial pneumonia was not associated with improved outcomes, but only with a higher rate of nephrotoxicity.

SEIZURES, STROKE, AND OTHER NEUROLOGIC EMERGENCIES

Thomas P. Bleck, MD, FACP, FCCM, FCCP

Objectives

- Improve the recognition, differential diagnosis, and management of seizures occurring in critically ill patients
- Understand the pharmacology and application of newer anticonvulsant drugs in the ICU
- Recognize and manage status epilepticus
- Understand the special diagnostic and management issues of refractory status epilepticus
- Improve recognition of patients with acute subarachnoid hemorrhage (SAH)
- Recognize and manage the major CNS complications of SAH
- Recognize the common systemic complications of SAH
- Review the role of the critical care service in the management of stroke
- Briefly review other neurologic emergencies in the ICU setting

Key Words: Seizure, status epilepticus, nonconvulsive status epilepticus, lorazepam, diazepam, propofol, ketamine, subarachnoid hemorrhage, stroke, rt-PA, meningitis, encephalitis, herpes simplex, polymerase chain reaction, brain abscess, neurogenic respiratory failure, myasthenia gravis, Guillain-Barré syndrome

INTRODUCTION

Seizures complicate about 3% of adult intensive care unit (ICU) admissions for non-neurologic conditions. The medical and economic impact of these seizures confers importance on them out of proportion to their incidence. A seizure is often the first indication of a central nervous system (CNS) complication; thus, their rapid etiologic diagnosis is mandatory. In addition, since epilepsy affects 2% of the population, patients with pre-existing seizures occasionally enter the ICU for other problems. Since the initial treatment of these patients is the province of the intensivist, he or she must be familiar with seizure management as it affects the critically ill patient. Patients developing status epilepticus (SE) will often require the care of a critical care specialist in addition to a neurologist.

Seizures have been recognized at least since Hippocratic times. Their relatively high rate of occurrence in critically ill patients has only recently been recognized. Seizures complicating critical care treatments (e.g., lidocaine) are also a recent phenomenon. Early attempts at treatment included bromide (1), morphine (2), and ice applications. Barbiturates were first employed in 1912, and phenytoin in 1937 (3). Paraldehyde was popular in the next decades (4). More recently, emphasis has shifted to the benzodiazepines, which were pioneered in the 1960s (5).

Epidemiology

Limited data are available on the epidemiology of seizures in the ICU. A 10-year retrospective study of all ICU patients with seizures at the Mayo Clinic found 7 patients per 1000 ICU admissions (6). Our 2-year prospective study of medical ICU patients acquired 35 with seizures per 1000 admissions (7). These studies are not exactly comparable, as the patient populations and methods of detection differed. Seizures are probably even more frequent in pediatric ICUs.

Certain ICU patients are at higher risk for seizures, but the degree of that increase has not been quantitated. Renal failure or an altered blood-brain barrier increases the seizure likelihood for patients receiving imipenem-cilastatin, but other patients receiving this antibiotic (or GABA antagonists like penicillin) are also at risk. Transplant recipients, especially receiving cyclosporine, are also at increased risk, as are those who rapidly become hypo-osmolar from any etiology. Nonketotic hyperglycemia patients have an unusual

Table 1. Etiologies of status epilepticus at San Francisco Hospital (11). *Indicates conditions most likely to result in ICU admission.

Etiology	1970-1980 (n=78)		1980-1989 (n=152)	
	Prior Seizures	No Prior Seizures	Prior Seizures	NoPrior Seizures
Ethanol-related	11%	4%	25%	12%
Anticonvulsant noncompliance	27%	0	41%	0
Drug toxicity	0	10%	5%	10%
Refractory epilepsy	(not used)	(not used)	8%	0
CNS infection*	0	4%	2%	10%
Trauma	1%	2%	2%	6%
Tumor	0	4%	2%	7%
Metabolic*	3%	5%	2%	4%
Stroke*	4%	11%	2%	5%
Anoxia*	0	4%	0	6%
Other	11%	5%	3%	5%

predisposition toward partial seizures and partial SE.

Incidence estimates for generalized convulsive SE (GCSE) in the United States vary from 50,000 cases/year (8) to 250,000 cases/year (9). Some portion of this difference is due to different definitions; however, the latter estimate represents the only population-based data available, however, and may be more accurate. Mortality estimates similarly vary from 1-2% in the former study to 22% in the latter. This disagreement follows from a conceptual discordance: the smaller number describes mortality which the authors directly attribute to SE, while the larger figure estimates the overall mortality rate, even though death was frequently due to the cause of the underlying disease rather than SE itself. For example, the DeLorenzo study included SE due to anoxia in its SE mortality estimate. In many of the reports surveyed in the earlier review, such patients would not have been counted.

Many risk factors emerged from the Richmond study. SE lasting longer than 1 hour carried a mortality of 32%, compared with 2.7% for a duration less than 1 hour. SE caused by anoxia resulted in 70% mortality in adults, but less than 10% in children. The most common cause of SE in adults was stroke, followed by withdrawal from antiepileptic drug therapy, cryptogenic SE; and that related to alcohol withdrawal, anoxia, and metabolic disorders. Systemic infection was the most common cause of childhood SE, followed by congenital anomalies, anoxia, metabolic problems, anticonvulsant withdrawal, CNS infections, and trauma.

The data in Table 1, based upon 20 years of experience at the San Francisco General Hospital (10-12), are of interest since almost all patients with SE in the city of San Francisco who begin to seize outside of a hospital are transported there. About 10% of epilepsy patients present with SE (13), and nearly 20% of

Table 2. International classification of epilectic seizures (16)

I.   Parial seizures (seizures beginning locally)
      A. Simple partial seizures (consciousness not impaired; SPS)
            1. with motor symptoms
            2. with somatosensory or special sensory symptoms
            3. with autonomic symptoms
            4. with psychic symptoms
      B. Complex partial seizures (with impairment of consciousness; CPS)
            1. beginning as SPS and progressing to impairment of consciousness
                a. without automatisms
                b. with automatisms
            2. with impairment of consciousness at onset
                a. with no other features
                b. with features of SPS
                c. with automatisms
      C. Partial seizures (simple or complex), secondarily generalized
II.   Primary generalized seizures (bilaterally symmetric, without localized onset)
      A. Absence seizures
            1. true absence ("petit mal")
            2. atypical absence
      B. Myoclonic seizures
      C. Clonic seizures
      D. Tonic seizures
      E. Tonic-clonic seizures ("grand mal;" GTC)
      F. Atonic seizures
III.   Unclassified seizures

seizure patients experience an episode of SE within 5 years of their first seizure (9).

Classification

The most frequently used classification schema is that of the International League Against Epilepsy (14) (Table 2). This allows classification on clinical criteria without inferring etiology. *Simple partial* seizures start focally in the cerebral cortex without invading other structures. The patient is aware throughout the episode and appears otherwise unchanged. Bilateral limbic dysfunction produces a *complex partial* seizure; awareness and ability to interact are diminished (but may not be completely abolished). *Automatisms* (movements which the patient makes without awareness) may occur. *Secondary generalization* results from invasion of the other hemisphere or subcortical structures.

Primary generalized seizures arise from the cerebral cortex and diencephalon at the same time; no focal phenomena are visible, and consciousness is lost at the onset. *Absence* seizures are frequently confined to childhood, consisting of the abrupt onset of a blank stare, usually lasting 5 - 15 seconds, from which the patient abruptly returns to normal. Atypical absence occurs in children with the Lennox-Gastaut syndrome. *Myoclonic* seizures start with brief synchronous jerking without initially altered consciousness, followed by a generalized convulsion. They frequently occur in the genetic epilepsies; in the ICU, they commonly follow anoxia or metabolic disturbances (15). *Tonic-clonic* seizures start with tonic extension and evolve to bilaterally synchronous clonus, and conclude with a postictal phase. Clinical judgment is required to apply this system in the ICU. Patients in whom consciousness has already been altered by drugs, hypotension,

Table 3. Clinical classification of status epilepticus (SE) (17)

I.   Generalized seizures
    A. Generalized convulsive SE (GCSE)
            1. Primary generalized SE
                a. tonic-clonic SE
                b. myoclonic SE
                c. clonic-tonic-clonic SE
            2. Secondarily generalized SE
                a. partial seizure with secondary generalization
                b. tonic SE
    B. Nonconvulsive SE (NCSE)
            1. absence SE (petit mal status)
            2. atypical absence SE (e.g., in the Lennox-Gastaut syndrome)
            3. atonic SE
            4. NCSE as a sequel of partially treated GCSE
II.   Partial SE
    A. Simple partial SE
            1. typical
            2. epilepsia partialis continua (EPC)
    B. Complex partial SE (CPSE)
III.   Neonatal SE

sepsis, or intracranial pathology may be difficult to classify concerning the nature of their partial seizures.

SE is classified by a similar system, altered to match observable clinical phenomena (Table 3) (16). *Generalized convulsive SE* (GCSE) is the most common type encountered in the ICU, and poses the greatest risk to the patient. It may either be primarily generalized, as in the drug-intoxicated patient, or secondarily generalized, as in the brain abscess patient who develops GCSE. *Nonconvulsive* SE (NCSE) in the ICU frequently follows partially treated GCSE. Some use the term for all SE involving altered consciousness without convulsive movements; this blurs the distinctions among absence SE, partially treated GCSE, and *complex partial SE* (CPSE), which have different etiologies and treatments. *Epilepsia partialis continua* (EPC, a special form of partial SE in which repetitive movements affect a small area of the body) sometimes last for months or years.

Pathogenesis and Pathophysiology

The reported "causes" of SE can be divided into predispositions and precipitants. *Predispositions* are static conditions increasing the likelihood of SE in the presence of a precipitant. *Precipitants* are events which can produce SE in most, if not all, people, but tend to affect those with predispositions at lesser degrees of severity (e.g., barbiturate withdrawal). The causes and effects of SE at the cellular, brain, and systemic levels are interrelated, but their individual analysis is useful for understanding them and their therapeutic implications. Longer SE durations produce more profound alterations, with an increasing likelihood of permanence, and of becoming refractory to treatment. The processes involved in a single seizure and the transition to SE have recently been reviewed (17).

The ionic events of a seizure follow the opening of ion channels coupled to excitatory amino acid (EAA) receptors. From the standpoint of the intensivist, 3 channels are particularly important because their activation may raise intracellular free calcium to toxic

Table 4. Electrographic-clinical correlations in generalized convulsive status epilepticus (20)

Stage	Typical Clinical Manifestations*	Electroencephalographic Features
1	Tonic-clonic convulsions; hypertension and hyperglycemia common	Discrete seizures with interictal slowing
2	Low or medium amplitude clonic activity, with rare convulsions	Waxing and waning of ictal discharges
3	Slight but frequent clonic activity, often confined to the eyes, face, or hands	Continuous ictal discharges
4	Rare episodes of slight clonic activity; hypotension and hypoglycemia become manifest	Continuous ictal discharges punctuated by periods
5	Coma without other manifestations of seizure activity	Periodic epileptiform discharges on a flat background

*The clinical manifestations may vary considerably, depending on the underlying neuropathophysiologic process (and its anatomy), systemic diseases, and medications. In particular, stages of the electrographic progression may be sufficiently overlooked. Partially treating SE may dissociate the clinical and electrographic features.

concentrations: AMPA channels, NMDA channels, and metabotropic channels. These EAA systems are crucial for learning and memory. Many drugs affect these systems but are too toxic for chronic use. The deleterious consequences of SE, and the brief period for which they would be needed, suggest that such agents may have a role in SE. Counterregulatory ionic events are triggered by the epileptiform discharge as well, such as the activation of inhibitory interneurons, which suppress excited neurons via $GABA_A$ synapses.

The cellular effects of excessive EAA channel activity include: (1) generating toxic conentrations of intracellular free calcium; (2) activating autolytic enzyme systems; (3) producing oxygen free radicals; (4) generating nitric oxide, which both enhances subsequent excitation and serves as a toxin; (5) phosphorylating enzyme and receptor systems, making seizures likely; and (6) increasing intracellular osmolality, producing neuronal swelling. If ATP production fails, membrane ion exchange ceases, and the neuron swells further. These events produce the neuronal damage associated with SE.

Many other biophysical and biochemical alterations occur during and after SE. The intense neuronal activity activates immediate-early genes and produces heat shock proteins, providing indications of the deleterious effects of SE and insight into the mechanisms of neuronal protection (18). Wasterlain's group has summarized mechanisms by which SE damages the nervous system (19). Absence SE is an exception among these conditions; it consists of rhythmically increased inhibition and does not produce clinical or pathologic abnormalities.

The mechanisms which terminate seizure activity are poorly understood. The leading candidates are inhibitory mechanisms, primarily GABAergic neuronal systems. Clinical observation supports the contention that human SE frequently follows withdrawal from GABA agonists (e.g., benzodiazepines).

The electrical phenomena of SE at the whole brain level, as seen in the scalp EEG, reflect the seizure type which initiates SE, e.g., absence SE begins with a 3-Hz wave-and-spike pattern. During SE, there is slowing of this rhythm, but the wave-and-spike characteristic remains. GCSE goes through a sequence of electrographic changes (Table 4) (20). The initial discharge becomes less well formed, implying that neuronal firing is losing synchrony. The sustained depolarizations which characterize SE alter the extracellular milieu, most importantly by raising extracellular potassium. The excess potassium ejected during SE exceeds the buffering ability of astrocytes. Raising extracellular potassium potentiates more seizures.

The increased cellular activity of SE elevates demand for oxygen and glucose, and blood flow initially increases. After about 20 minutes, however, energy supplies become exhausted. This causes local catabolism to support ion pumps (attempting to restore the internal milieu). This is a major cause of epileptic brain damage.

The brain contains systems to terminate seizure activity; GABAergic interneurons and inhibitory thalamic neurons are both important.

SE produces neuropathology even in patients who are paralyzed, ventilated, and maintained at normal temperature and blood pressure. The hippocampus, a crucial area for memory, contains the most susceptible neurons, but other regions are also vulnerable. In addition to damaging the CNS, GCSE produces life-threatening systemic effects (21). Systemic and pulmonary arterial pressures rise dramatically at seizure onset. Epinephrine and cortisol prompt further elevations and also produce hyperglycemia. Muscular work raises blood lactate. Breathing suffers from both airway obstruction and abnormal diaphragmatic contractions. CO_2 excretion falls while its production increases markedly. Muscular work accelerates heat production; skin blood flow falls concomitantly, sometimes raising core temperature dangerously.

After about 20 minutes, motor activity begins to diminish, and ventilation usually improves Body temperature may rise further, however. Hyperglycemia diminishes; after 1 hour, gluconeogenesis can fail, producing hypoglycemia. GCSE patients often aspirate oral or gastric contents, producing pneumonia. Rhabdomyolysis is common and may lead to renal failure. Compression fractures, joint dislocations, and tendon avulsions are other sequelae.

Clinical Manifestations

Three problems occur in seizure recognition: (1) complex partial seizures in the

setting of impaired awareness, (2) seizures in patients receiving pharmacologic paralysis, and (3) misinterpretation of other abnormal movements as seizures. ICU patients often have depressed consciousness in the absence of seizures due to their disease, its complications (such as septic encephalopathy[22]), or drugs. A further decline in alertness may reflect a seizure; an EEG is required to diagnose one.

Patients receiving NMJ blocking agents do not manifest the usual signs of seizures. Since most such patients receive sedation with GABA agonists, the likelihood of seizures is small. Autonomic signs of seizures (hypertension, tachycardia, pupillary dilation) may also be the effects of pain or the response to inadequate sedation. Hence, patients manifesting these findings who have a potential for seizures (e.g., intracranial pathology) should have an EEG. The actual incidence of this problem is unknown.

Abnormal movements can occur in patients with metabolic disturbances or anoxia. Some can be distinguished from seizures by observation, but if doubt about their nature persists, an EEG should be performed. Psychiatric disturbances in the ICU occasionally resemble complex partial seizures. Prolonged EEG monitoring may be required if the problem is intermittent.

Manifestations of Status Epilepticus

The manifestations of SE depend on the type and, for partial SE, the cortical area of abnormality. Table 3 depicts the types of SE encountered. This focuses on those seen most in the ICU.

Primary GCSE begins as tonic extension of the trunk and extremities without preceding focal activity. No aura is reported and consciousness is immediately lost. After several seconds of tonic extension, the extremities start to vibrate, quickly giving way to clonic (rhythmic) extension of the extremities. This phase wanes in intensity over a few minutes. The patient may then repeat the cycle of tonus followed by clonic movements, or continue to have intermittent bursts of clonic activity without recovery. Less common forms of GCSE are *myoclonic SE*, (bursts of myoclonic jerks increasing in intensity, leading to a convulsion) and *clonic-tonic-clonic SE* (clonic activity precedes the first tonic contraction). Myoclonic SE is usually seen in patients with anoxic encephalopathy or metabolic disturbances.

Secondarily generalized SE begins with a partial seizure and progresses to a convulsion. The initial focal clinical activity may be overlooked. This seizure type implies a structural lesion, so care must be taken to elicit evidence of lateralized movements.

Of the several forms of generalized *nonconvulsive SE*, the one of greatest importance to intensivists is NCSE as a sequel of inadequately treated GCSE. When a patient with GCSE is treated with anticonvulsants (often in inadequate doses), visible convulsive activity may stop while the electrochemical seizure continues. Patients begin to awaken within 15 - 20 minutes after the successful termination of SE; many regain consciousness much faster. Patients who do not start to awaken after 20 minutes should be assumed to have entered NCSE. Careful observation may disclose slight clonic activity. NCSE is an extremely dangerous problem because the destructive effects of SE continue even without obvious motor activity. NCSE demands emergent treatment *under EEG monitoring* to prevent further cerebral damage, since there are no clinical criteria to indicate when therapy is effective.

Partial SE in ICU patients often follows a stroke or occurs with rapidly expanding brain masses. Clonic motor activity is most easily recognized, but the seizure takes on the characteristics of adjacent functional tissue. Therefore, somatosensory or special sensory manifestations occur, and the ICU patient may be unable to report such symptoms. Aphasic SE occurs when a seizure begins in a language area and may resemble a stroke. *Epilepsia partialis continua* involves repetitive movements confined to a small region of the body. It may be seen with nonketotic hyperglycemia or with focal brain disease; anticonvulsant treatment is seldom useful. *Complex partial SE* presents with diminished awareness. The diagnosis often comes as a surprise when an EEG is obtained.

Diagnostic Approach

When an ICU patient seizes, one has a natural tendency to try to stop the event. This leads to both diagnostic obscuration and iatrogenic complication. Beyond protecting the patient from harm, very little can be done sufficiently rapidly to influence the course of the seizure. Padded tongue blades or similar items should not be placed in the mouth; they are more likely to obstruct the airway than to preserve it. Most patients stop seizing before any medication can reach the brain in an effective concentration.

Observation is the most important activity during a single seizure. This is the time to collect evidence of a partial onset, in order to implicate structural brain disease. The postictal examination is similarly valuable; language, motor, sensory, or reflex abnormalities after an apparently generalized seizure are evidence of focal pathology.

The ICU patient has several potential seizure etiologies which must be investigated. Drugs are a major cause of ICU seizures, especially in the setting of diminished renal or hepatic function, or when the blood-brain barrier is breached. Drug withdrawal is also a frequent offender. While ethanol withdrawal is common, discontinuing any hypnosedative agent may prompt convulsions 1 to 3 days later. A recent report suggests that narcotic withdrawal may produce seizures in the critically ill (9).

The physical examination should emphasize the areas listed for the postictal exam. Evidence of cardiovascular disease or systemic infection should be sought, and the skin and fundi closely examined.

Illicit drug screening should be performed on patients with unexplained seizures. Cocaine is becoming a major cause of seizures (23). Electrolytes and serum osmolality should also be measured. However, hypocalcemia rarely causes seizures beyond the neonatal period; its discovery must not end the diagnostic workup. Hypomagnesemia has an equally unwarranted reputation as the cause of seizures in malnourished alcoholic patients.

The need for imaging studies for these patients has been an area of uncertainty. A prospective study of neurologic complications in MICU patients determined that 38 of 61 patients (62%) had a vascular, infectious, or neoplastic explanation for their fits. Hence, CT or MRI should be performed on most ICU patients with new seizures. Hypoglycemia and nonketotic hyperglycemia can produce seizures, and such patients might be treated for metabolic disturbances and observed if they lack other evidence of focal disease. With current technology, there are almost no patients who cannot undergo CT scanning. While MRI is preferable in most situations, the magnetic field precludes infusion pumps and other metallic devices. Whether to administer contrast for a CT depends on the clinical setting and on the appearance of the plain scan.

The EEG is a vital diagnostic tool for the seizure patient. Partial seizures usually have EEG abnormalities which begin in the area of cortex producing the seizures. Primary generalized seizures appear to start over the entire cortex simultaneously. Postictal slowing or depressed amplitude provide clues to the focal etiology of the seizures, and epileptiform activity helps to classify the type of seizure and guide treatment. In patients who do not begin to awaken soon after seizures have apparently been controlled, an emergent EEG is necessary to exclude NCSE.

Considering the etiologies of seizures in the ICU setting, patients who need CSF analysis usually require a CT scan first. When CNS infection is suspected, empiric antibiotic treatment should be started while these studies are being performed.

In contrast to the patient with a single or a few seizures, the SE patient requires concomitant diagnostic and therapeutic efforts. Although 20 minutes of continuous or recurrent seizure activity usually define SE, one does not stand by waiting for this period to start treatment. Since most seizures stop within 2 to 3 minutes, it is reasonable to treat after 5 minutes of continuous seizure activity, or after the second or third seizure occurring without recovery between the spells.

GCSE can rarely be confused with decerebrate posturing, but observation usually makes the distinction straightforward. Tetanus patients are awake during their spasms and flex their arms rather than extending them as seizure patients do (18).

Treatment for SE should not be delayed to obtain an EEG. A variety of findings may be present on the EEG depending on the type of SE and its duration (see Table 4). CPSE patients often lack such organized discharges of GCSE, but instead have waxing and waning rhythmic activity in 1 or several head regions. A

diagnostic trial of an intravenous benzodiazepine is often necessary to diagnose CPSE. Patients developing refractory SE or having seizures during NMJ blockade require continuous EEG monitoring.

Management Approach

Deciding to administer anticonvulsants to an ICU patient who experiences one or a few seizures requires a provisional etiology, estimation of the recurrence likelihood, and recognition of the utility and limitations of anticonvulsants. For example, seizures during ethanol withdrawal do not indicate chronic treatment, and giving phenytoin will not prevent more withdrawal convulsions. The patient may need prophylaxis against delirium tremens, but the few seizures themselves seldom require treatment. Convulsions during barbiturate or benzodiazepine withdrawal, in contrast, should usually receive short-term treatment with lorazepam (LRZ) to prevent SE. Seizures due to drugs or metabolic disorders should also be treated briefly but not chronically.

The ICU patient with CNS disease who has even 1 seizure should usually start chronic anticonvulsant therapy, with review of this decision before discharge. Initiating this treatment after the first *unprovoked* seizure helps prevent subsequent epilepsy (24). Starting after the first seizure in a critically ill patient at risk for seizure recurrence may be even more important, especially in conditions which would be seriously complicated by a convulsion. In the ICU setting, phenytoin (PHT) is frequently selected for ease of administration and lack of sedation. The hypotension and arrhythmias which may complicate rapid administration can usually be prevented by slowing the infusion to less than 25 mg/min. Because of the rare occurrence of third-degree AV block, an external pacemaker should be available when patients with conduction abnormalities receive intravenous PHT. Fosphenytoin is safer to administer from an extravasation standpoint, but still carries risks of hypotension and arrhythmias. The PHT concentration should be kept in the "therapeutic" range of 10-20 µg/mL unless further seizures occur; the level may then be increased until signs of toxicity occur. Failure to prevent seizures at a concentration of 25 μg/mL is usually an indication to add phenobarbital (PB).

PHT is usually 90% protein bound. Patients with renal dysfunction have lower total PHT levels at a given dose because the drug is displaced from binding sites, but the unbound level is not affected. Thus, renal failure patients, and perhaps others who are receiving highly protein bound drugs (which compete for binding), may benefit from free PHT level determination. Only the free fraction is metabolized, so the dose is not altered with changing renal function. The clearance half-time with normal liver function varies from about 12 - 20 hours (intravenous form) to over 24 hours (extended-release capsules), so a new steady-state serum concenration occurs in 3 to 6 days. PHT need not be given more frequently than every 12 hours. Hepatic dysfunction mandates decreasing the maintenance dose.

Hypersensitivity is the major adverse effect of concern to the intensivist. This may manifest itself solely as fever, but commonly includes rash and eosinophilia. Adverse reactions to PHT and other anticonvulsants have been reviewed (25).

Phenobarbital (PB) remains a useful anticonvulsant for those intolerant to PHT or who have persistent seizures after *adequate* PHT. The target for PB in the ICU should be 20 - 40 μg/mL. Hepatic and renal dysfunction alter PB metabolism. Since its usual clearance half-time is about 96 hours, give maintenance doses of this agent once a day. A steady-state level takes about 3 weeks to be established. Sedation is the major adverse effect; allergy occurs rarely.

Carbamazepine is seldom started in the ICU because its insolubility precludes parenteral formulation. Oral loading in conscious patients may produce coma lasting several days. This drug causes hyponatremia in patients receiving it chronically.

Management Issues in Acute Repetitive (Serial) Seizures

Despite the near-certainty that acute repetitive seizures not meeting a definition of SE must occur more frequently than SE itself, and that many cases of SE emerge from such a state, there has been little study of the issue of treatment. Although the use of intravenous benzodiazepines has become common in many inpatient settings, the choice of drug and the appropriate dose are uncertain. Many clinicians use intravenous diazepam, perhaps more out of tradition than pharmacokinetics. The anticonvulsant effect of a single dose of diazepam is very brief (about 20 minutes), while that of lorazepam is much longer (4 hours or longer). Since the risk of serious adverse effects (e.g., respiratory depression) is potentially greater for diazepam, lorazepam may represent a better choice (26). If a shorter-acting agent is desired for diagnostic purposes when the diagnosis of a seizure is uncertain, midazolam may represent a better choice. The role of other agents, such as intranasal or buccal midazolam or intravenous valproate, remain to be determined ((27).

Outside of the hospital setting, there is reasonably good evidence that rectal diazepam is effective and safe in the management of serial seizures, especially in children, at a dose of 0.2 – 0.5 mg/kg, with the dose repeated as necessary according to an age-based protocol (28).

Management Issues in SE

Once the decision is made to treat the patient for SE, considerations for therapy should proceed on 4 fronts simultaneously: (1) termination of SE; (2) prevention of seizure recurrence once SE is terminated; (3) management of potential precipitating causes for SE; and (4) management of the complications of SE and of underlying conditions ((29).

There is an implicit assumption here that the forms of SE that can produce neuronal damage should be terminated as rapidly as is safely possible. While there is no direct proof of this contention in humans, it appears to be the most reasonable approach.

The intensity of treatment for SE should reflect the risk that the patient experiences from the SE and its etiology. For example, generalized convulsive SE (GCSE) puts the patient at risk for a panoply of neurologic, cardiac, respiratory, renal, hepatic, and orthopedic disorders, and should be terminated as rapidly one can safely accomplish the task, even if such termination requires the full support of a critical care unit. Typical absence SE, in contrast, probably only poses a risk to the patient

Table 5. Treatment results for first agents in the Veteran's Affairs Cooperative Study (30)

Agent	Overt SE Success Rate (%)	Subtle SE Success Rate (%)
Lorazepam	64.9	17.9
Phenobarbital	58.2	24.2
Diazepam/phenytoin	55.8	8.3
Phenytoin alone	43.6	7.7

if it occurs during a potentially dangerous activity (e.g., driving an automobile), and initial attempts at its termination should probably not include agents likely to profoundly depress respiration and blood pressure. Treatment of complex partial SE, in which the risk of neurologic sequelae is considerable, should probably be similar to that recommended for GCSE. Simple partial SE appears to pose less risk to the patient than complex partial SE, and furthermore, attempts at therapy along the lines recommended for GCSE seldom result in prolonged seizure control. Therefore, therapy for simple partial SE is often pursued with somewhat less vigor that GCSE or complex partial SE.

The following recommendations were developed for patients in GCSE. There is very limited evidence regarding the optimal therapy for other types of SE. Because of the life-threatening nature of GCSE and of the risks associated with its treatment, physicians caring for these patients must be constantly vigilant for respiratory and cardiovascular compromise, which may develop abruptly. Thus, neurologists and others caring for these patients should be adept at basic aspects of airway and blood pressure management. During the termination of SE, the patient should be constantly attended by personnel who can effectively perform bag-valve-mask ventilation, and plans for the rapid endotracheal intubation of such patients when necessary should be devised before they are necessary.

Termination of SE

The lynchpin of treatment for SE is the rapid, safe termination of ictal activity. Numerous treatment modalities are available for this goal, and until recently there were little data to guide a decision among the various possible choices. The publication of the Veterans' Affairs (VA) cooperative trial allows a much greater degree of rational choice, and raises many new questions for study ((30).

Within the VA trial, patients were divided into the categories of "overt" and "subtle" SE. All patients were felt to have GCSE, which could be either primarily or secondarily generalized; the distinction of overt from subtle depended on the intensity of the clinically viewed convulsive activity. The subtle SE patients were much more likely to have a serious underlying medical condition, and in general responded poorly to therapy. This discussion will concentrate on the overt SE patients, since their results underlie the treatment paradigm developed herein.

The study randomized 384 patients with overt SE into 4 treatment arms, which were chosen based upon a survey of North American neurologists prior to the study's inception. These arms were a) lorazepam, 0.1 mg/kg; b) diazepam, 0.15 mg/kg, followed by phenytoin, 18 mg/kg; c) phenytoin alone, 18 mg/kg; and d) phenobarbital, 15 mg/kg. Successful treatment required both clinical and electroencephalographic (EEG) termination of seizures within 20 minutes of the start of therapy, without seizure recurrence within 60 minutes from the start of therapy. Patients who failed the first treatment received a second, and if necessary, a third choice of study drug. These latter choices were not randomized, as this would have resulted in some patients receiving 2 loading doses of phenytoin, but the treating physician remained blinded to the treatments being given.

The overall success rates for patients whose diagnosis of overt SE was confirmed by subsequent review of clinical and EEG data are presented in Table 1. The results for patients with subtle SE are included for reference. Treatment with lorazepam demonstrated a statistically significant advantage over phenytoin (p = 0.002); there were no significant differences among the other agents. This differs from the intention-to-treat analysis, which showed similar trends but did not find a statistically significant difference among the treatment arms.

The results of this study may be compared to those of Leppik and colleagues, who found lorazepam to be successful in about 85% of cases ((31). However, this study used only clinical cessation of seizures as the criterion of success; preliminary data from the VA trial indicates that 20% of patients in whom SE appears to have been terminated actually remain in electrographic SE.

Preliminary analysis of the results of subsequent treatments in patients who failed the first line agents indicates that the aggregate response rate to the second line was 7.0%, and to the third line 2.3% (Treiman DM, personal communication, 1998). These results call into question the common practice of using 3 conventional agents (e.g., lorazepam, phenytoin, and phenobarbital) in the management of SE prior to using a more definitive approach.

Based upon these results and the experience of many workers in the field, we recommend that treatment for GCSE begin with a single dose of lorazepam, 0.1 mg/kg. The limited data available do not suggest that administration of further conventional doses of lorazepam will be useful (31). The drug should be administered after dilution with an equal volume of the intravenous solution through which it will be administered. If this fails to control SE within 5 to 7 minutes, a second agent should be chosen. The results of the VA trial suggest that a second conventional agent is unlikely to be successful. At this time, however, we still recommend the use of phenytoin (or

fosphenytoin), 20 mg/kg, as the second drug. This approach carries the advantage that if it is effective, the patient may not require endotracheal intubation and extended critical care. However, it may delay the eventual termination of SE by more definitive treatment.

The introduction of the phenytoin prodrug fosphenytoin as a safer way of rapidly achieving an effective serum phenytoin concentration may prompt some reconsideration of the way in which this drug is used (32). At its maximal rate of administration (150 mg phenytoin equivalent/min), and its 7-minute half-time of conversion to phenytoin, a free phenytoin level of about 2 μg/mL can be achieved with fosphenytoin in about 15 minutes, as opposed to about 25 minutes for phenytoin itself. Whether this greater speed of administration will produce a higher rate of SE control remains to be demonstrated. It is clear that fosphenytoin administration is safer, in that the risk of hypotension may be somewhat less, and the adverse effects of extravasation are nil with the newer drug. The much greater cost of fosphenytoin has discouraged many from using it, although pharmacoeconomic simulations suggest that its use may be cost effective (33).

Valproate is available in an intravenous form; its role in the termination of SE remains to be defined. Experimental data suggest that a serum valproate concentration of 250 μg/mL or greater may be necessary to control secondarily generalized SE (34). We have limited experience using doses of 60 – 70 mg/kg to obtain such a concentration in patients, and have found the drug effective on occasion in situations where in was necessary to avoid the risks of hypotension and respiratory depression associated with other treatment modalities. However, more information is required before the role of this agent in SE becomes clear.

Patients who continue in SE after lorazepam and phenytoin have traditionally been treated with conventional doses of phenobarbital, but the results of the VA study suggest that this is very unlikely to result in the rapid termination of SE. At this point, we consider SE to be refractory, and go on to 1 of the more definitive forms of treatment (35). These treatment modalities are very likely to result in termination of SE, but are also likely to carry higher risks of respiratory depression, hypotension, and secondary complications such as infection. Patients who are to undergo 1 of these definitive therapies should be in a critical care unit and be endotracheally intubated if this has not yet been accomplished.

Discussion of the entire range of proposed definitive treatments for SE is beyond the scope of this paper. Three categories will be considered: high-dose barbiturates, high-dose benzodiazepines, and propofol.

It is our contention that patients reaching this stage in the treatment of SE should undergo continuous EEG monitoring. The technologic aspects of continuous EEG monitoring have been reviewed elsewhere (36). What the goal regarding the activity on the EEG should be remains a matter of debate. There is no prospectively collected evidence that a burst-suppression EEG pattern is required for, or is efficacious for, the termination of SE. Many patients can achieve complete seizure control with a background of continuous slow activity, and do not thereby incur the greater risks associated with the higher doses of medication required to achieve a burst-suppression pattern. Conversely, a few patients will continue to have frequent seizures which emerge out of a burst-suppression background, and presumably need even higher doses of medication, which may result in very long periods of suppression or even a "flat" EEG. Without continuous EEG monitoring, one must rely on occasional samples of the EEG, which are thus associated with risks of under- and over-treatment.

Most of the published experience with high-dose barbiturates involves pentobarbital, although some of the earlier investigators used thiopental, and a few reports discuss phenobarbital. There are few data regarding efficacy rates and adverse effects of these drugs. Thiopental is the most rapidly acting of these drugs, but may produce more hypotension. Pentobarbital has emerged as 1 of the standard choices for refractory SE. A loading dose of 5–12 mg/kg is usually given intravenously, followed by an infusion of the drug at a dose chosen to achieve the desired effect on the EEG; this is usually in the range of 1–10 mg/kg/hr. We usually increase the infusion rate, along with an additional 3–5 mg/kg loading dose, when a seizure occurs (almost all seizures at this stage of treatment are electrographic, probably as a

consequence of the medications suppressing clinical seizure activity [twitchless electrical activity]), and perhaps also as a consequence of the prolonged duration of SE by the time definitive treatment has commenced). After 12 hours free of seizures, the pentobarbital infusion rate is decreased by 50%. If seizures recur, the patient again receives the smaller loading dose, and the infusion rate is raised to obtain another 12-hour seizure-free period. Other medications (e.g., phenytoin) are continued. Many patients reaching this point will require substantial maintenance anticonvulsant treatment in order to be weaned from the pentobarbital; we commonly maintain the serum phenytoin concentration in excess of 20 µg/mL, and load with phenobarbital to achieve a concentration in excess of 40 µg/mL (often, 100 µg/mL or even higher concentrations are required to successfully wean severely refractory patients, such as those with encephalitis, from their pentobarbital infusions). High doses of barbiturates are potently immunosuppressive, indicating extra care to avoid nosocomial infection and aggressive treatment if it is suspected.

High-dose benzodiazepine strategies for SE usually employ either midazolam or lorazepam. Midazolam has the advantages of rapid onset of activity and greater water solubility, avoiding the problem of metabolic acidosis from the propylene glycol vehicle of the other benzodiazepines and the barbiturates. Its major disadvantage is tachyphylaxis; over 24–48 hours, the dose of the drug must often be increased several-fold in order to maintain seizure control. A loading dose of 0.2 mg/kg is followed by an infusion of 0.1–2.0 mg/kg/hr, titrated to produce seizure suppression by continuous EEG monitoring (37). High dose-lorazepam was the subject of a report by Labar and colleagues, used in doses up to 9 mg/hr (38).

Propofol is a pharmacologically unique GABA$_A$ agonist, which may also have other mechanisms of anticonvulsant action. Soon after its introduction as a general anesthetic agent, concerns about a potential proconvulsant effect arose; this apparently represented myoclonus rather than seizure activity. At the doses used to control SE, it has a very potent anticonvulsant action. A loading dose of 3-5 mg/kg is frequently administered, followed by an infusion of 1–15 mg/kg/hr (39), titrated to EEG seizure suppression. After 12 hours of seizure suppression, we taper the dose as outlined above for pentobarbital. There is evidence that rapid discontinuation of propofol can induce withdrawal seizures.

In our experience, propofol is more likely than midazolam to provide rapid control of refractory SE, exhibits less tachyphylaxis than midazolam, and produces less hypotension than pentobarbital for an equivalent degree of seizure control (40). However, a recent retrospective analysis of our patients suggests that those with APACHE II scores > 20 may have better survival when treatment is started with midazolam (41). There are few data addressing the immunosuppressive effects of the benzodiazepines or propofol (42); clinically, these drugs appear associated with fewer nosocomial infections than high-dose pentobarbital. Although it is difficult to determine functionally equivalent doses of these agents because of differing rates of tachyphylaxis, in our institution the patient charge for midazolam appears to be about 10 times that for pentobarbital, and propofol about 2.5 times that for pentobarbital.

Many other agents have been employed for the control of refractory SE (43). The information above represents a distillation of our experience; the available published data are inadequate to support more definite treatment recommendations.

Prevention of Seizure Recurrence Once SE is Terminated

Once SE is controlled, attention turns to preventing its recurrence. The best regimen for an individual patient will depend upon the cause of the patient's seizures and any previous history of anticonvulsant therapy. For example, a patient developing SE in the course of ethanol withdrawal may not need anticonvulsant therapy once the withdrawal phenomena have run their course. SE following changes in a previously effective anticonvulsant regimen will often mandate a return to the former successful mode of treatment. In contrast, patients with a new,

ongoing epileptogenic stimulus (e.g., encephalitis) may require extraordinarily high serum concentrations of anticonvulsant drugs to control their seizures as therapy for refractory SE is decreased.

Management of the Complications of SE and of Underlying Conditions

The major systemic complications of GCSE include rhabdomyolysis and hyperthermia. Patients presenting with GCSE should be screened at presentation for myoglobinuria (most effectively by a dipstick evaluation of the urine for occult blood; the reagent will react with myoglobin as well as hemoglobin, and if the reaction is present, a microscopic examination will determine whether red blood cells are present) and elevation of serum creatine kinase (CK). If myoglobinuria is present, or if the CK concentration is more than 10 times the upper limit of normal, one should consider instituting a saline diuresis as well as urinary alkalinization.

If the patient's core temperature exceeds 40°C, the patient should be cooled. The techniques available for managing hyperthermic patients have been reviewed elsewhere (44).

Cerebral edema may complicate SE. Vasogenic edema may develop as a consequence of the seizures themselves, and the underlying cause of SE may also produce either vasogenic or cytotoxic edema. The management of secondary cerebral edema with increased intracranial pressure depends upon the etiology; edema due solely to seizures rarely causes problems with intracranial pressure.

Prognosis

Wijdicks and Sharbrough report that 34% of patients experiencing a seizure died during that hospitalization (9). Our prospective study of neurologic complications in MICU patients found that having even 1 seizure if in the unit for a non-neurologic reason doubled in-hospital mortality (10). This effect on prognosis primarily reflected the etiology of the seizure.

Three major factors determine outcome in SE: the type of SE, its etiology, and its duration. GCSE has the worst prognosis for neurologic recovery; in contrast, myoclonic SE

Table 6. Suggested management protocol for status epilepticus

I. *Establish an airway.* Whether to perform endotracheal intubation emergently depends primarily on the safety with which the airway can be maintained during the control of SE. Should NMJ blockade be needed, one must assume that the patient is still in SE despite the appearance of relaxation, unless EEG monitoring is available to demonstrate the actual state of brain function. Use a nondepolarizing agent (e.g., vecuronium).

II. *Determine the blood pressure.* If the patient is hypotensive, begin volume replacement and/or vasoactive agents as clinically indicated. GCSE patients who present with hypotension will usually require admission to a critical care unit. (Hypertension should not be treated until SE is controlled, since terminating SE will usually substantially correct it, and many of the agents used to terminate SE can produce hypotension).

III. *Rapidly determine the blood glucose.* Unless the patient is known to be normo- or hyper-glycemic, administer dextrose (1 mg/kg) and thiamine (1 mg/kg).

IV. *Terminate SE.* We recommend the following sequence:

    A. Lorazepam, 0.1 mg/kg at 0.04 mg/kg/min. This drug should be diluted in an equal volume of the solution being used for intravenous infusion, as it is quite viscous. Most adult patients who will respond have done so by a total dose of 8 mg. The latency of effect is debated, but lack of response after 5 minutes should be considered a failure.

    B. If SE persists after lorazepam, begin phenytoin 20 mg/kg at 0.3 mg/kg/min. If the patient tolerates this infusion rate, it may be increased to a maximum of 50 mg/min. Alternatively, administer fosphenytoin at the same dose, but at a rate up to 150 mg/min. Hypotension and arrhythmias are the major concern. Many investigators believe that an additional 5 mg/kg dose of phenytoin or fosphenytoin should be administered before advancing to the next line of therapy.

    C. If SE persists, administer either midazolam or propofol. Midazolam can be given with a loading dose of 0.2 mg/kg, followed by an infusion of 0.1-2.0 mg/kg/hr to achieve seizure control (as determined by EEG monitoring). Propofol can be given with a loading dose of 1–3 mg/kg, followed by an infusion of 1–15 mg/kg/hr. We routinely intubate patients at this stage if this has not already been accomplished. Patients reaching this stage should be treated in a critical care unit.

    D. Should the patient not be controlled with propofol or midazolam, administer pentobarbital 12 mg/kg at 0.2–0.4 mg/kg/min as tolerated, followed by an infusion of 0.25-2.0 mg/kg/hr as determined by EEG monitoring (with a goal of seizure suppression). Most patients will require systemic and pulmonary arterial catheterization, with fluid and vasoactive therapy as indicated to maintain blood pressure.

    E. Ketamine (1 mg/kg, followed by 10–50 μg/kg/min) is a potent NMDA antagonist (1) with intrinsic sympathomimetic properties which may be useful in patients who have become refractory to $GABA_A$ agonists.

V. *Prevent recurrence of SE.* The choice of drugs depends greatly on the etiology of SE and the patient's medical and social situation. In general, patients not previously receiving anticonvulsants whose SE is easily controlled often respond well to chronic treatment with phenytoin or carbamazepine. In contrast, others (e.g., patients with acute encephalitis) will require 2 or 3 anticonvulsants at "toxic" levels (e.g., phenobarbital at greater than 100 μg/mL) to be weaned from midazolam or pentobarbital, and may still have occasional seizures.

VI. *Treat complications.*

    A. Rhabdomyolysis should be treated with a vigorous saline diuresis to prevent acute renal failure; urinary alkalinization may be a useful adjunct.

    B. Hyperthermia usually remits rapidly after termination of SE. External cooling usually suffices if the core temperature remains elevated. In rare instances, cool peritoneal lavage or extracorporeal blood cooling may be required. High dose pentobarbital generally produces poikilothermia.

    C. The treatment of cerebral edema secondary to SE has not been well studied. When substantial edema is present, one should suspect that SE and cerebral edema are both manifestations of the same underlying condition. Hyperventilation and mannitol may be valuable if edema is life threatening. Edema due to SE is vasogenic, so steroids may be useful as well.

following an anoxic episode carries a very poor prognosis for survival. CPSE can produce limbic system damage, usually manifested as a memory disturbance. Most studies of outcome concentrate on GCSE mortality. Hauser, summarizing data available in 1990, suggested that mortality rates vary from 1% to 53%. Those studies attempting to distinguish mortality due to SE from that of the underlying disease attribute rates of 1% to 7% to SE and 2% to 25% to its cause. Population-based studies in Richmond, VA showed the mortality of SE lasting longer than 1 hour increased 10-fold over SE lasting less than 1 hour. Etiologies associated with increased morality included anoxia, intracranial hemorrhages, tumors, infections, and trauma.

Limited data are available concerning the functional abilities of GCSE survivors, and none reliably permit a distinction between the effects of SE and of its etiologies. One review concluded that intellectual ability declined as a consequence of SE (45). Survivors of SE frequently seem to have memory and behavioral disorders out of proportion to structural damage produced by the etiology of their seizures. A wealth of experimental data support this observation, arguing strongly for rapid and effective control of SE. Case reports of severe memory deficits following prolonged CPSE have also been published (46). Whether treatment of SE reduces the risk of subsequent epilepsy remains uncertain. Recent experimental studies indicate that SE lowers the threshold for subsequent seizures (47).

SUBARACHNOID HEMORRHAGE
Introduction

The management of patients following acute aneurysmal subarachnoid hemorrhage (SAH) has changed substantially in the past 2 decades. Previously, patients were typically put to bed rest for 2 weeks, until the periods of maximal risk for rebleeding and vasospasm had passed, and if they survived were then given the option of surgical treatment. Current management strategies recognize a) improvements in surgical technique which make early definitive obliteration of the aneurysm more feasible and safer; b) the consequent ability to use induced hypertension and hypervolemia to treat cerebral vasospasm; c) the

introduction of nitrendipine-class calcium channel blockers to relieve or ameliorate the effects of vasospasm; d) the development of interventional neuroradiologic techniques (e.g., angioplasty and intra-arterial papaverine infusion) to treat symptomatic vasospasm; e) the use of ventricular drainage to treat communicating hydrocephalus; and f) the introduction in several countries, although not in North America, of a free radical scavenger which appears to improve outcome in patients who present with high-grade SAH.

Future directions in the medical management of patients following SAH will probably depend primarily on the ability to recognize and manage cerebral vasospasm before it becomes symptomatic and before it produces cerebral infarction.

Epidemiology

The principal medical complications of aneurysmal SAH include rebleeding, cerebral vasospasm, and volume and osmolar disturbances. The risk of rebleeding from unsecured aneurysms varies with time after the initial hemorrhage, being about 4% on the first post-bleed day and about 1.5% per day up to day 28 (48). The mortality of rebleeding following the diagnosis of SAH exceeds 75% (49). This complication is more frequent in patients with higher grades of SAH, in women, and in those with systolic blood pressures exceeding 170 mmHg.[1] Cerebral vasospasm exceeding 170 mm Hg (50. Cerebral vasospasm produces symptoms in up to 45% of patients (51), but is noted angiographically in another 25%, who appear asymptomatic (52). Vasospasm usually starts to occur between post-bleed days 4 and 6; the risk of its development is minimal after day 14. Volume and osmolar disturbances are reported in about 30% of patients (53).

A number of other complications occur in this group of patients, which are less directly related to the SAH itself (51). Life-threatening cardiac arrhythmias are found in 5%, with less ominous rhythm disturbances in 30%. Pulmonary edema is diagnosed in 23%, with 6% experiencing a severe form. Some degree of hepatic dysfunction is noted in 24% of patients, predominantly mild elevation of transaminases without symptoms; 4% experience severe hepatic dysfunction. Many of these patients are probably manifesting hepatic toxicity from anticonvulsants or other medications. Thrombocytopenia is reported in 4% of patients, usually related to sepsis or medications. Renal dysfunction is seen in 7%, but rarely requires dialysis.

Although this paper deals primarily with aneurysmal SAH, there are other causes of SAH, and their epidemiology is different. SAH following rupture of an arteriovenous malformation (AVM) tends to occur at a younger age, with a peak incidence in the mid-20s. Traumatic SAH is a common accompaniment of severe head trauma, occurring in 15% to 40% of patients with severe head trauma. The incidence of the major complications of SAH in these patients appears to be less than in patients suffering aneurysmal SAH, but data are scarce. Following AVM rupture, the time course of angiographically-diagnosable vasospasm is similar to that seen in aneurysmal SAH patients; it is usually asymptomatic (54), except in rare cases (55). The significance of vasospasm related to traumatic SAH continues to be debated, but in 1 series, 7 of 29 patients with large amounts of subarachnoid blood (detected by CT scanning) developed symptomatic vasospasm (detected angiographically) with subsequent infarction (56). In patients with penetrating head trauma, the incidence (detected by transcranial Doppler (TCD) flow velocity measurements) may be as high as 40% (57).

Pathophysiology

Rebleeding

Rebleeding of an aneurysm prior to its obliteration presumably reflects further leakage of blood at the site of the initial rupture. The tendency for this to occur appears to increase with arterial hypertension, which increases the stress on the aneurysm wall and the clot that occludes the original rupture site. Lowering the pressure in the subarachnoid space (e.g., by lumbar puncture, or by allowing a ventriculostomy system to have a low pop-off pressure) similarly increases the pressure gradient across the aneurysm wall. Whether these procedures actually increase the risk of

rebleeding is uncertain, and this theoretical concern does not militate against performing diagnostic lumbar punctures if needed either to prove the diagnosis of SAH or to exclude meningitis. Systemic factors which alter the balance between thrombosis and fibrinolysis (e.g., disseminated intravascular coagulation) would presumably affect the risk of rebleeding as well.

Cerebral Vasospasm

Vasospasm appears to be a 2-stage process, with an initial vasoconstrictive phase followed by a proliferative arteriopathy, associated with smooth muscle cell necrosis and fibrosis of the arterial wall (58, 59). Vasospasm appears to depend primarily upon the presence of erythrocytes in the subarachnoid space (60), but why it occurs more frequently and more symptomatically after aneurysmal SAH than after SAH due to other causes remains unexplained. The list of potential mediators contributing to the development of vasospasm is substantial, but the vasoconstrictor peptide endothelin-1 appears to be one of the most important (61). Endothelin antagonists are promising experimental agents for the prevention and treatment of this condition (62).

The maximal risk for vasospasm occurs from day 4 through day 14 after SAH, although about 10% of patients may have some angiographic signs of vasospasm at the time of the initial angiogram (63).

The risk of developing vasospasm is related to the amount of blood in the subarachnoid space. Fisher and colleagues reported that patients with thick subarachnoid clots were much more likely to develop vasospasm than those without such clots (64). Antifibrinolytic agents (e.g., ε-aminocaproic acid, tranexamic acid) used to prevent rebleeding raise the risk of symptomatic vasospasm and delayed ischemic deficits (65), but whether there is an actual increase in the rate of vasospasm, or an increase in the rate of occlusion of already spastic vessels, is uncertain.

Hyperglycemia probably worsens outcome in stroke patients (66), and, therefore, presumably in SAH patients developing delayed ischemia. Plasma glucose concentrations exceeding 120 mg/dL in the first post-bleed week are associated with poor outcome (67). All of these studies suffer from the confounding effect of severity of illness on intrinsic plasma glucose regulation, but they do suggest that maintenance of normoglycemia is a reasonable goal.

Volume and Osmolar Disturbances

Although earlier studies attributed the hyponatremia and hypo-osmolality occurring after SAH to the syndrome of inappropriate antidiuretic hormone secretion (SIADH) (68), most investigators now believe that these disturbances are the result of cerebral salt wasting (69). The pathophysiology of this condition remains to be completely elucidated, but probably begins with the release of atrial, brain, and c-type natriuretic factors from the brain (70). These peptides produce isotonic volume loss by their renal effects, resulting in hypovolemia. This hypovolemic state then prompts an appropriate ADH response, causing a fall in free water clearance and thereby producing hyponatremia and hypo-osmolality. Hypovolemia appears to increase the risk of cerebral infarction (delayed ischemic deficits) in patients with vasospasm, and should therefore be prevented with prophylactic volume replacement (71).

Physical signs of hypovolemia are rare in SAH patients, who are usually kept flat in bed, and in whom a putative increase in adrenal catecholamine secretion and increased sympathetic nervous system activity often produce hypertension. Overly vigorous treatment of this hypertension after the aneurysm is secured appears to worsen outcome (72).

Seizures

Following SAH, patients may experience any of 4 patterns of seizures. About 6% of patients appear to suffer a seizure at the time of the hemorrhage (73), although the distinction between a generalized convulsion and an episode of decerebrate posturing may be difficult to establish from the reports of non-medical observers. Postoperative seizures occur in about 1.5% of SAH patients despite anticonvulsant prophylaxis (usually phenytoin)

(74). Patients developing delayed ischemia from vasospasm may seize following reperfusion by angioplasty (75). Late seizures occur in about 3% of patients over several years of follow-up (74).

SAH patients are somewhat more likely to have a seizure at the time of presentation than are patients with other types of stroke (76).

Cardiovascular Complications

Cardiac arrhythmias and electrocardiographic signs of ischemia are frequent in SAH patients (77). In 1 series, all 61 patients had a least 1 such abnormal finding (78). The most serious of such problems is the development of ventricular tachycardia, typically of the torsade de pointes form (79).

Electrocardiographic changes resembling acute myocardial infarction, and elevation of the MB isoenzyme of creatine kinase (CK; and, by inference, elevation of troponins) occur without evidence of coronary arterial occlusion. About 10% of patients will have an ECG suggesting acute myocardial infarction during the first 3 post-SAH days (80). In 1 study, elevation of CK was associated with left ventricular wall motion abnormalities (81). Histopathologically, these findings correspond to myocardial contraction band necrosis, which resembles the cardiomyopathic changes associated with pheochromocytomas.

Pulmonary edema occurring in SAH patients may be either cardiogenic or noncardiogenic in origin. Some patients have echocardiographic evidence of left ventricular dysfunction at the time their pulmonary edema is severe (82). However, the majority of SAH patients have a defect in pulmonary gas exchange in the absence of evidence of cardiac dysfunction or aspiration, suggesting that neurogenic pulmonary edema is responsible (83). This probably occurs as the consequence of a neurally-mediated increase in extravascular lung water (84).

Central Nervous System Infection

Excepting cases of ruptured mycotic aneurysms, central nervous system infections in SAH patients are almost always iatrogenic, either from organisms introduced during aneurysm clipping or, much more commonly, from ventriculostomy systems which become colonized with bacteria.

Other Infectious Complications

The non-CNS infectious complications of SAH patients vary with the severity of their illness. Patients remaining in Hunt and Hess grades 1 and 2 do not seem to be at particular risk for aspiration, and may not need urinary catheters, feeding tubes, or central venous lines, which are the proximate causes of many ICU infections. Higher-grade patients are susceptible to the typical infectious complications of critical care. The contribution of corticosteroids in decreasing resistance to infection in these patients is unquantified. SAH patients in the trials of tirilazad mesylate (85), a steroid free radical scavenger without glucocorticoid effects, were not given glucocorticoids either before or after procedures to secure their aneurysms; they did not appear to suffer intracranial pressure problems. Although this question has not been formally tested, it raises the possibility that routine dexamethasone administration may not be necessary in this population. Withholding this agent would be expected to decrease both infectious and metabolic complications in these patients.

Higher-grade patients may need feeding tubes for nutritional support, or larger bore gastric tubes should an ileus develop. Placing these tubes via the nasal route appears to increase the risk of nosocomial sinusitis, and probably of pneumonia as well (86).

Seizures

The mechanisms producing seizures in SAH patients are uncertain. Patients in whom aneurysmal rupture produces a concomitant intracerebral hematoma probably have a direct epileptogenic stimulus. Irritation from the aneurysm clipping appears to account for some postoperative seizures. Reperfusion injury accounts for a small percentage (75). Late seizures may reflect the epileptogenic effects of iron on the cerebral cortex (87).

Deep Venous Thrombosis and Pulmonary Embolism

SAH patients are at risk for the development of deep venous thromboses and subsequent pulmonary embolism by virtue of immobilization. Whether the use of antifibrinolytic agents increases the risk of deep venous thrombosis has long been debated; the use of these agents for 2 weeks in patients undergoing late aneurysm surgery probably does increase these risks (88). Brief use of these agents to decrease the risk of rebleeding prior to early surgery probably carries a lower risk (89). Although the concentration of circulating fibrinogen complexes is increased in SAH patients (and other stroke patients) compared with controls (90), the role of this finding in the genesis of venous thrombosis remains speculative.

Nutrition

Although standard critical care practice emphasizes the early institution of nutritional support to maintain muscle mass and gut integrity, the importance of nutritional support for SAH patients remains unproven. Starvation prior to experimental ischemia may result in a shift to the metabolism of fuels other than glucose, even in the brain, and potentially result in an improved outcome after delayed ischemia (91). However, the balance between risks and benefits of this approach remains to be established. SAH patients are markedly catabolic, and may have a defect in the utilization of amino acids (92); the mechanism of this defect is unknown.

Management

The higher-grade SAH patient may require all of the skills a critical care team can muster. The sickest of these patients can still attain a good functional outcome despite what appear to be overwhelming difficulties. Thus, attention to all of the details of care in these patients is essential. Guidelines for the care of SAH patients have recently been published by the American Heart Association(93) and the Canadian Neurosurgical Society (94).

Table 7. Selected drugs useful in the management of SAH patients

Agent	Dose	Comments
Enalaprilat	0.625-1.25 mg 6 hrs	May decrease renal plasma flow and raise creatinine
Esmolol	250-500 μg/kg, then 50-200 mg/kg/min	May produce congestive heart failure
Hydralazine	10-20 mg q 3-4 hrs	Theoretical risk of increasing shear forces
Labetalol	10 mg q 10 min, up to 300 mg	Oral form lacks significant α-adrenergic blocking effect
Nicardipine	0.075-0.15 mg/kg/hr	May produce congestive heart failure
Nimodipine	60 mg q 4 hrs for 14-21 days	Duration of therapy uncertain
Nitroprusside	0.25-10 μg/kg/min	Rarely necessary
Phenytoin	15-20 mg/kg loading doses, then 5-8 mg/kg/day maintenance (q 12 hrs for suspension, q 24 hrs for Dilantin® capsules	Duration of therapy uncertain; maintain serum concentration between 10-20 μg/mL. feeding 1 hr before and after dose.

Rebleeding

Although aneurysm obliteration is the most important method of preventing rebleeding, antihypertensive drugs and antifibrinolytic agents may be valuable prior to surgery or interventional radiologic approaches. Preoperative blood pressures are typically elevated; we strive to maintain systolic pressures below 150 mmHg and mean arterial pressures below 100 mmHg in these patients. Nimodipine, which is used to try to prevent delayed ischemic deficits (*vide infra*), often lowers the blood pressure to a modest degree. Labetalol (see the table), which has both α- and β-adrenergic blocking effects when given intravenously, is commonly the first drug employed for blood pressure control. Hydralazine is also commonly used, although there is a theoretical concern about the use of pure vasodilators in preoperative SAH patients (increasing pulse pressure may increase stress on the aneurysm wall). Enalaprilat may be useful for patients not responding to these agents. We tend to avoid

nitrates because of the potential for increased intracranial pressure, but rarely nitroprusside may be the only effective drug. Pain relief with acetaminophen, codeine, or fentanyl is often necessary, and is frequently helpful in lowering blood pressure as well.

Postoperatively, the blood pressure may be allowed to rise to higher levels. Patients at risk for vasospasm may require higher blood pressures for adequate cerebral perfusion. In patients with more than 1 aneurysm, the risk of producing a new SAH from a previously unruptured aneurysm appears to be small (but not absent [95]) during the first few post-bleed weeks.

Cerebral Vasospasm

Delayed ischemic deficits from vasospasm have emerged as the major cause of morbidity and mortality in patients undergoing early aneurysm obliteration. Management approaches attempt to prevent both spasm and its consequences, although it is not clear that any of the currently employed techniques actually prevent vasospasm. Rather, most attempt to preserve either perfusion or neuronal survival in areas affected by vasospasm.

Vasospasm is definitively diagnosed angiographically, although spasm in vessels below the resolution of angiography probably occurs in patients whose symptoms suggest vasospasm. The initial symptom of vasospasm is typically decreased interaction with the unit staff and the patient's family and visitors. The patient may then progress to an abulic state, or appear to have bilateral frontal lobe dysfunction. The etiology of these symptoms is uncertain, since they do not appear to depend on the location of the aneurysm, the localization of subarachnoid blood, or the development of complications such as hydrocephalus. At this point, the TCD velocity measurements are usually elevated (e.g., mean velocities above 120 cm/sec). Xenon-CT blood flow studies suggest that TCD may underestimate the incidence and severity of vasospasm (96). Lateralized motor findings suggest the development of delayed ischemic lesions.

Nimodipine, a voltage-sensitive calcium channel blocker, was introduced with the expectation that it would prevent vasospasm. Angiographic studies did not confirm this effect, at least on vessels visible by radiologic techniques, but clinical trials did confirm its utility in improving outcome (97). Nicardipine, a related agent, does appear to decrease angiographically diagnosed vasospasm (98). The outcome of patients treated with nicardipine did not differ statistically from those receiving placebo, but the placebo patients received "rescue" hypertensive-hypervolemic therapy (HHT; *vide infra*) more frequently.

Volume replacement and expansion, usually practiced by attempts to maintain either a fixed, relatively high saline intake (e.g., 3–6 L/d of normal or mildly hypertonic saline), or a positive fluid balance, is relatively standard in centers caring for SAH patients. While this usually prevents volume contraction due to cerebral salt wasting, it is unlikely that it prevents vasospasm *per se*. However, it appears to be very useful in preventing or decreasing the extent of symptomatic vasospasm and delayed ischemic deficits.

The free radical scavenger tirilazad may be effective in improving outcome in SAH patients, primarily those in higher grades. A European-Australian trial showed efficacy in men only at a dose of 6 mg/kg/d (99), presumably because the drug is more rapidly metabolized in women. A parallel North American trial did not achieve a statistically significant result (100). This appears at least in part to reflect a higher percentage of North American patients receiving phenytoin, which accelerates the metabolism of tirilazad. Higher dose trials have been concluded, but the results have not yet been published. This agent has been licensed for SAH in men in 13 countries. The drug has poor blood-brain barrier penetration; more lipophilic derivatives have been synthesized (101), and await clinical trials.

Treatment

Two approaches are currently employed for the management of vasospasm. The first is volume expansion, usually accompanied by induced hypertension (HHT) (102). Although some consider hemodilution (to hemoglobin concentrations between 10 and 11 gm/dL) to be part of this treatment as well, in the hope that decreasing blood viscosity will improve perfusion, this is the least consistently practiced part of this approach. HHT has not been subjected to a randomized clinical trial, and substantial debate persists regarding its utility (103, 104). If it is to be employed, careful patient monitoring is necessary, involving an arterial line and either a central venous line or, preferably, a pulmonary artery catheter to guide vasopressor and volume management. Angiographic confirmation of the diagnosis of vasospasm is usually obtained prior to instituting vasopressor therapy.

Because SAH patients appear to have low thresholds for the development of hydrostatic pulmonary edema, we try to maintain the pulmonary capillary wedge pressure (PCWP) between 15-18 mmHg. In some patients, this volume expansion alone is adequate to produce an increase in cardiac index and mean arterial pressure. What mixture of colloid and crystalloid to use for volume expansion in this setting is the subject of endless debate and absent data. If the patient's examination does not improve, we next raise the mean arterial pressure using phenylephrine, dopamine, norepinephrine, epinephrine, or a combination of phenylephrine and dobutamine, as suggested by the patient's heart rate, the cardiac index produced, and evidence of ectopy or cardiac ischemia or renal dysfunction. None of these medications has a proven advantage over the others in this setting, and each case provides individual challenges. Hypertensive encephalopathy can apparently complicate overly vigorous therapy (105).

The second approach to vasospasm patient management involves interventional radiologic techniques, either angioplasty or papaverine infusion (106). We employ both hemodynamic and radiologic techniques. Intraventricular infusion of nitroprusside may be useful in the future (107).

Volume and Osmolar Disturbances

Volume deficits are prevented or corrected as discussed above. If SAH patients receive adequate saline replacement, hypo-osmolality is an infrequent occurrence.

Evaluation of the SAH patient whose laboratory results indicate a low serum sodium concentration requires both clinical and laboratory evaluation. Prior to intervention, serum and urine osmolality measurements should be obtained. This will prevent the inadvertent treatment of the patient for hypo-osmolality when the real problem is, for example, a factitious hyponatremia due to hyperglycemia or pseudohyponatremia from hyperlipidemia. Truly hypo-osmolar SAH patients require careful thought, rather than just salt administration. Unless the patient has developed pulmonary edema or other signs suggesting congestive heart failure, one should not assume that hyponatremia is due to combined salt and water excess. The likely occurrence of cerebral salt wasting favors a diagnosis of salt loss with water retention. Osmolality measurements will usually indicate that the patient's urine is inappropriately concentrated for a patient with hypotonic serum. While this combination may suggest SIADH in many circumstances, this condition should rarely be diagnosed during the first 2 post-bleed weeks. Attempts to treat the patient with volume

restriction will likely lead to greater problems with delayed ischemic deficits. One potentially useful biochemical assay is the serum uric acid level, which tends to be low in SIADH but normal in cerebral salt wasting.

Management of hypo-osmolar states depends critically upon their rate of development (108). Rapidly developing (e.g., over hours) hypo-osmolality produces neuronal swelling and is associated with elevated intracranial pressure (ICP) and seizures. More slowly developing (over days) hypo-osmolality is accompanied by solute shifts out of neurons, which prevents ICP increases and is unlikely to produce seizures; the patient may become confused, lethargic, and weak, but seldom experiences any life-threatening complications from the osmolality itself. However, these are the patients at risk for central and extra-pontine myelinolysis if their osmolalities are raised too rapidly.

Patients who became rapidly hypo-osmolar may be treated with small doses of hypertonic (e.g., 100 mL of 3N) saline to begin correcting this problem. They usually respond quickly with lower ICP and resolution of seizures. Those who became hypo-osmolar more slowly must be corrected more slowly; a goal of 6 mOsm/L/day increases appears safe. Since these patients should not be allowed to become volume depleted, this is best performed by replacement of their urine output and insensible loss by mildly hypertonic solutions, or, in patients receiving enteral feeding, addition of salt to their food. Attempts to decrease the urine osmolality with loop diuretics are seldom sufficiently successful to be useful.

Cardiovascular Complications

Prevention of electrolyte disturbances and magnesium replacement are probably useful for the prevention of arrhythmias. Alpha- and β-adrenergic blockade may decrease or prevent myocardial contraction band necrosis, but this has not been tested.

Cardiac arrhythmias in SAH are seldom life threatening. Sinus tachycardia and other supraventricular tachycardias should lead to a reassessment of electrolytes, volume status, pain control, infection, and endocrine (especially thyroid) function. Depending on the arrhythmia and its hemodynamic consequences, treatment with adenosine, calcium antagonists, β-blocking agents, or digoxin may be indicated. Ventricular arrhythmias frequently reflect adrenergic drug administration (e.g., dopamine) or electrolyte disorders; alternatively, they may represent signs of myocardial ischemia. If possible, dopamine-induced rhythm disorders indicate switching to another agent. Lidocaine or procainamide may be required if runs of ventricular tachycardia appear. Torsade de pointes may respond to supplemental magnesium, or may require overdrive pacing.

SAH patients with heart failure who develop signs suggesting vasospasm will usually require pulmonary artery catheterization for volume and hemodynamic management.

Central Nervous System Infection

Infection is a major problem for SAH patients, because fever may increase the degree of damage produced by delayed ischemia. Another problem is the diagnosis of the etiology of fever in these patients. A preliminary analysis in our unit suggests that about 20% of SAH patients experience fever without evidence of infection on retrospective review, suggesting that they have developed "central fever (109)." These patients frequently receive antibiotics, putting them at risk for drug reactions and increasing expense, because it is difficult to prove that they do not have an infection. Drug-induced fevers are a major problem in all ICU patients, and SAH patients are not exceptions. Commonly implicated drugs include phenytoin, antibiotics, and, less frequently, agents such as H2-antagonists and stool softeners.

Whether patients with ventriculostomies or lumbar drains should receive antibiotic prophylaxis is an open question. If prophylaxis is to be given, a cephalosporin with activity against *Staphylococcus aureus* (e.g., cefazolin) is probably the most reasonable choice. Activity against coagulase-negative staphylococci does not seem important, nor does the brain or CSF penetration characteristics of the drug. A risk-benefit analysis suggests that ventriculostomy catheters should probably be changed every 5 days (110).

Treatment of ventriculostomy infections should be based initially on a gram stain of CSF.

If staphylococcal infection is suspected, initial treatment with vancomycin is appropriate pending culture and sensitivity results. Patients with gram-negative rods in the CSF should receive either a cephalosporin with antipseudomonal activity (e.g., cefepime) or meropenem until microbiologic results are available. If the CSF contains increasing numbers of white cells but the gram stain is negative, a combination of vancomycin and either meropenem or cefepime seems reasonable, although some of these patients will have an aseptic postoperative meningitis.

Other Infectious Complications

The question of routine changes of central venous catheters and pulmonary artery catheters is beyond the scope of this discussion. Whatever local practices control these policies for other critically ill patients should apply to SAH patients.

We attempt to place all tracheal and gastric tubes through the mouth, rather than the nose, to decrease the incidence of sinusitis (111) (*vide supra*).

Seizures

Since seizures in patients with unsecured aneurysms may promote rebleeding, it is a common, although by no means universal, practice to place SAH patients on anticonvulsants.

The standard agent for prophylaxis in North America is phenytoin. Fosphenytoin, a water-soluble prodrug, is safer to administer intravenously, and may be given intramuscularly if necessary. An adequate loading dose should be given.

Should seizures occur in an SAH patient, one should obtain a CT scan to look for new intracranial pathology. At the same time, one should give an additional dose of phenytoin to raise the serum concentration. If seizures recur, and the phenytoin has been pushed to the point of symptomatic toxicity (in the responsive patient) or a level of about 24 μg/mL (in patients with impaired ability to respond), adding either phenobarbital or carbamazepine have been standard approaches. The recent introduction of gabapentin, and of an intravenous form of valproate, increases the number of therapeutic options. This choice must be individualized.

Phenytoin is frequently implicated as a cause of drug-induced fever. When a rash and fever appear in a patient on this drug, it is typically discontinued. Because of its long half-life, several days will elapse before it is cleared from the patient. Substitution of another anticonvulsant (e.g., gabapentin) without sedative effects and without cross-sensitivity is a reasonable approach. Suspected allergy is the only circumstance in which most anticonvulsants should be stopped abruptly.

Deep Venous Thrombosis and Pulmonary Embolism

Prior to securing the aneurysm, many physicians are reticent to give prophylactic doses of heparin, and instead rely upon sequential compression devices to prevent deep venous thrombosis. These devices are effective in many circumstances, but have not been formally tested in SAH patients. Interestingly, sequential compression devices accelerate *in vitro* measurements of fibrinolysis (112), and part of their effectiveness probably stems from this mechanism. We continue to use these devices for prophylaxis in bedbound patients after the aneurysm is secured.

Deep venous thrombosis or pulmonary embolism in patients with either unsecured aneurysms or fresh craniotomies pose difficult management problems. Our approach is usually to place an inferior vena cava filter, and not to anticoagulate the patient until at least 1 week after surgery. The filter is generally held to be safer than immediate anticoagulation (113).

Nutrition and Gastrointestinal Bleeding Prophylaxis

Despite strongly held opinions, there are few data upon which to base recommendations for nutrition in SAH patients. In view of the likely deleterious effect of hyperglycemia on outcome after delayed ischemia, whatever nutritional approach is taken should include frequent measurements of blood glucose, and probably its tight control. So-called "trophic" feeding, in which a small volume (e.g., 5 ml/hr) of an enteral nutrition formula is constantly infused via a gastric or jejunal feeding tube, may maintain the structure of the intestinal villi and help to prevent both bacterial translocation and the subsequent incidence of diarrhea when full feedings are instituted.

If patients are NPO, some form of prophylaxis against gastrointestinal (GI) bleeding seems reasonable. Clinically important GI bleeding occurs in up to 6% of SAH patients (114). H_2-blocking agents such as ranitidine or nizatidine are commonly used. These agents are occasionally associated with neutropenia or thrombocytopenia; in this circumstance, sucralfate or omeprazole may be substituted. The use of nonsteroidal anti-inflammatory agents appears to increase the risk of GI bleeding; we routinely administer misoprostol with these agents. Once patients are fully fed, these prophylactic agents may no longer be necessary.

When feedings begin, patients frequently develop diarrhea. Because a large percentage of patients are receiving antibiotics, the possibility of antibiotic-induced *Clostridium difficile* infection must be considered. After sending specimens for fecal leukocyte, cytotoxin, and *C. difficile* cultures, we use kaolin and pectin to attempt to decrease the diarrhea. Some patients appear to have diarrhea induced by sorbitol, used in many solutions of drugs for tube administration.

STROKE

Stroke is the most common neurologic cause for hospital admission in the USA. About 80% of strokes are ischemic, with the remainder divided between intracerebral hemorrhage and subarachnoid hemorrhage. The incidence of stroke is declining, coincident with and probably in part reflecting improvement in the treatment of hypertension. The association of stroke with hypertension, particularly intracerebral hemorrhage, has been slightly overstated in the past (blood pressures were often measured when the patient presented with the stroke, rather than seeking a documented history of hypertension; the same is true of many studies of hyperglycemia in stroke). Other risk factors include diabetes, cardiac disease, previous cerebrovascular disease (TIA or stroke), age, gender, lipid disorders, excessive ethanol ingestion, elevated hematocrit, elevated fibrinogen, and cigarette smoking. Smoking is the most powerful risk factor for aneurysmal subarachnoid hemorrhage. In younger patients (usually defined as those less than 55 years old), one should consider abnormalities of antithrombin III, protein S, protein C, or antiphospholipid antibodies. Young stroke patients with Marfanoid habitus should be worked up for homocysteinuria; the heterozygous state is associated with stroke, and many patients respond to pyridoxine treatment.

The intensivist most commonly encounters potential stroke patients in the settings of a) suspected carotid artery disease, and b) cardiac disturbances, which are potentially emboligenic. Patients with *asymptomatic* carotid bruits have an approximately 2% annual risk of stroke, but the side of the bruit does not predict the side of the stroke. There are no data upon which to base the selection of patients for further workup. I tend to start these people on aspirin (80–325 mg/day), but not to investigate them further. If studies (noninvasive or angiographic) have already been obtained, I would *consider* endarterectomy for *otherwise healthy* patients who have > 70% stenosis or a large area of ulceration. The common practice of "prophylactic" endarterectomy before other vascular surgical procedures lacks validation; from the poor data available, the risk of stroke related to such procedures does not seem to exceed the risks related to endarterectomy itself. The results of the ACAS trial suggest that men with asymptomatic carotid stenosis of > 70% derive greater benefit from carotid endarteractomy than from medical therapy alone. Endarterectomy of the vertebral arteries, and angioplasty of any cerebral vessel, remain experimental techniques.

About 30% of untreated patients with new onset TIAs will suffer a stroke in the next 2 years. If the patient has 70-99% stenosis in the relevant carotid artery, endarterectomy reduces the risk of stroke or death to about 10%. Patients not appropriate for surgery should probably receive ticlopidine 250 mg bid (with appropriate monitoring of the WBC count); this drug appears effective in both men and women (aspirin has not been universally efficacious in women).

If a cardiac source of embolism is suspected, anticoagulation with warfarin is usually indicated. For patients with nonvalvular atrial fibrillation, a protime of 1.3-1.7 times control (or an INR about 3.0; should be > 2.0 and < 5.0) is probably adequate and has few side effects (in 3 recent studies of prophylaxis, minor bleeding was more common in the warfarin groups than in controls, but intracerebral hemorrhage or other major bleeding was not). One study suggested that aspirin also reduced stroke rates; it could be used for patients who are poor risks for warfarin. In patients with suspected embolism from other cardiac disorders (e.g., cardiomyopathies, LV aneurysms), low-dose warfarin has not been well studied. The aortic arch is a hitherto under-recognized source of emboli; management of this condition remains to be established.

Transesophageal echocardiography can detect clots and other lesions, which escape detection by transthoracic echo. In some series, the rate of detection of cardiac lesions is so high that their significance is uncertain.

In patients 6 hours or more into acute ischemic stroke, no treatment has been proven useful. Heparin may be indicated to prevent subsequent embolic strokes, but does not affect either a completed stroke or so-called stoke-in-evolution. If the patient is to be anticoagulated because of a suspected source of embolism, some investigators feel that patients with large infarcts should not be anticoagulated for several days because of a presumed risk of hemorrhage into the infarct. Other data suggest that the greatest risk of re-embolization occurs in the first few days after the initial stroke, which argues for early anticoagulation of this group. I favor the latter approach.

Patients who follow a stuttering course may benefit from induced hypertension to improve flow through stenotic vessels until collaterals can open. Spontaneous hypertension in these patients should be considered a compensatory response, and should not be treated in the first few post-stroke days unless evidence of end-organ damage develops. We avoid treating blood pressure unless the MEAN pressure exceeds 160 mm Hg. After the patient has stabilized neurologically, a course of chronic antihypertensive treatment can be instituted.

The role of hyperglycemia in worsening stroke outcome seems established, but no studies have been done to determine whether tight control of blood sugar will improve prognosis.

The NINDS study showed that thrombolysis was safe and effective if performed within 3 hours of stroke onset (this does not mean 3 hours after waking up with a new stroke; the time of stroke onset must be known) (115). The rt-PA dose in this study was 0.9 mg/kg, with 10% of the dose as a bolus and the remainder over 1 hour. The treated patients had a very significant improvement in functional outcome. There were more intracerebral hemorrhages in the treated group, but their mortality was actually lower (this did not reach statistical significance).

Patients who develop serious increases in intracranial pressure during the first 3-4 post-stroke days are at risk for herniation and death. The earliest sign is usually diminished consciousness, often followed by an ipsilateral third nerve palsy. Corticosteroids do not decrease the cytotoxic edema associated with strokes, and should not be used (unless the cause of the stroke is vasculitic). Although the routine use of hyperventilation in stroke patients is not indicated, this technique is appropriate to prevent herniation. Mannitol can also be used. If more drastic therapy is contemplated (e.g., high-dose barbiturates), an intracranial pressure monitor should be inserted. We now use hemicraniectomy to reduce ICP in these patients, with surprisingly good functional outcomes; this has not become the standard of care. Experimental results suggest that the skull should be removed before swelling occurs, in order to protect the cortex from loss of pial collaterals.

Intracerebral hemorrhage produces much more rapid rises in intracranial pressure because of the volume of the hematoma. The major concerns for the internist are a) exclusion or treatment of a bleeding diathesis, which should always be considered, and b) management of intracranial pressure. Although the edema around an intracerebral hemorrhage is vasogenic, it does not respond to steroids. Three controlled studies have documented poorer outcome in steroid-treated patients, due to the side effects of the steroids. In older patients, especially those with more than 1 episode of

hemorrhage and without a history of hypertension, amyloid angiopathy becomes a diagnostic consideration (about 15% of all ICH). In younger patients, ICH related to sympathomimetic agents (including cocaine) is becoming an increasingly frequent problem.

Although neurogenic pulmonary edema (NPE) may occur in any acute intracranial condition, SAH patients seem particularly prone to it; about 40% of our SAH patients have some degree of oxygenation difficulty not explained by other conditions. In NPE, the PCWP is normal, and the edema fluid has a high protein content; this reflects the presumed pathogenic mechanism of pulmonary venoconstriction. One must then attempt to balance the need to volume expand patients with the need to keep their lungs dry. We tend to keep the PCWP around 10 mmHg, and use vasopressors to improve cerebral perfusion if necessary.

NERVOUS SYSTEM INFECTIONS

Meningitis

The consensus of opinion seems to favor presumptive treatment for suspected meningitis in any situation in which lumbar puncture is delayed. This includes even delays to obtain CT scans, since the most common causes of meningitis in adults (pneumococcal and meningococcal) can kill the patient while waiting for the scan. I believe that patients who are alert and have normal fundi and neurologic exams can undergo LP without scanning, since the possibility of a patient in that setting herniating soon after LP is infinitesimally small, but presumptive treatment is clearly more important than intellectual purity. With the increasing prevalence of penicillin-resistant pneumococci, cefotaxime (2 gms q4h) or ceftriaxone (2 gms q12h) should be used for empiric therapy. A few pneumococci with significant resistance to third-generation cephalosporins have emerged, prompting some to add vancomycin until sensitivities are available. Cefuroxime is inferior to these third-generation cephalosporins and should no longer be used. Since ampicillin-resistant *H. influenzae* are common, children should also receive the third-generation agents. Chloramphenicol is often recommended for truly penicillin-allergic (e.g., anaphylactic) patients, although clinical failures have been reported in patients with penicillin-resistant pneumococci. In most cases, the initial dose of antibiotics will not sterilize the CSF within 30-60 minutes; even if this occurs, testing for bacterial antigens will reveal the etiology in the majority of cases. Blood cultures should be obtained before antibiotics are given. Further treatment decisions can be made based on the gram stain and antigen results. If listeriosis is suspected (immune compromised host, or negative gram stain and bacterial antigen tests), ampicillin or sulfa-trimethoprim should be added until an organism is isolated or blood and CSF cultures have been negative for at least 3 days. Because of its epileptogenic effects, imipenem should usually be avoided in CNS infections.

In infants and children, pretreatment with steroids (dexamethasone, 0.15 mg/kg q6h for 4 days) appears to decrease neurologic dysfunction after recovery from meningitis (predominantly that due to *H. influenzae)*. This is presumed to reflect a decrease in inflammation from lysis of organisms, with the subsequent host elaboration of TNF and other inflammatory mediators. The use of steroids in adult meningitides remains controversial, but does not appear to be deleterious in the few patients so far studied. I think that the evidence favors its use in adults as well, but this is still debated. A recent study in children suggests that 2 days of dexamethasone is as useful as 4 days. The issue is clouded when vancomycin is used for potential penicillin-resistant pneumococci, since steroids **may** decrease vancomycin penetration into the CSF (this is debated in humans).

Increased intracranial pressure in meningitis patients is treated as described above. Cerebral edema in children appears to respond to steroids; it is probably appropriate to treat adults in the same fashion if elevated ICP is a problem. Hyponatremia is common and may exacerbate vasogenic cerebral edema; it usually responds to fluid restriction. Whether this increases the rate of cerebral venous thrombosis is not clear. However, it is important not to let the cerebral perfusion pressure fall below about 60 mmHg; this is more important than fluid restriction. Seizures are initially managed with benzodiazepines and phenytoin; the treatment of SE is covered above.

Encephalitis

As in meningitis, the weight of expert opinion is shifting (albeit more slowly) to the "shoot first and ask questions later" approach. When encephalitis is suspected, acyclovir (10–15 mg/kg q 8 hrs) is begun while the workup is in progress; adequate hydration is necessary to prevent renal toxicity. The most sensitive test is CSF-PCR; MRI with gadolinium is second, with EEG third. Even though brain biopsy has a low complication rate (3%, most of which are minor), the relative safety of acyclovir has encouraged many physicians to treat presumptively, and only biopsy patients who do not respond or in whom the workup raises the question of another diagnosis. The commonly quoted list of "treatable disorders which mimic herpes simplex encephalitis" from the NIAID cooperative studies is not relevant in the MRI era. Seizures and elevated ICP are common.

Brain Abscess

Unless there is a strong suspicion of the etiology of a brain abscess (e.g., the patient had a proven bacteremia prior to developing the abscess), empiric treatment for suspected brain abscess should include a third-generation cephalosporin, vancomycin, and metronidazole. Vancomycin is probably adequate treatment for *Listeria*, but if there is a reason to suspect this organism one usually adds ampicillin or sulfa-trimethoprim. Although some surgeons have tried to avoid aspiration, biopsy, or resection of these patients on the grounds that empiric medical treatment seems effective, this contention is based on small numbers of patients. Furthermore, it is often difficult to be certain that a particular lesion is an abscess and not a high-grade astrocytoma. Surgery also offers some direct relief of intracranial pressure problems. For these reasons, I recommend early aspiration of suspected abscesses, with possible later debulking or resection.

NEUROGENIC RESPIRATORY FAILURE

Myasthenia Gravis

Although the standard teaching about myasthenia gravis stresses fatiguability with exercise, this is rarely what brings the patient to medical attention. The usual complaints are diplopia, ptosis, difficulty with speech and secretions, proximal limb weakness, and ventilatory dysfunction. The condition preferentially affects young women and older men. There is over-representation of HLA-A1, HLA-B8, and HLA-DRw3 (another place where HLA testing is not clinically useful). This is a true autoimmune disease in which antibodies directed at myoid cells in the thymus (which express acetylcholine receptors) attack the neuromuscular junction. There is a greater-than-expected incidence of other autoimmune diseases, including SLE, Sjögren's syndrome, polymyositis, and autoimmune thyroid disease. About 70% of patients have thymic hyperplasia, and 15% have thymomas. Anti-AChR antibodies are present in most patients with generalized myasthenia, and about 60% of those with ocular myasthenia. Anti-striated muscle antibodies are a marker for thymoma.

Diagnostic studies include the edrophonium test (for which change in ptosis is the only truly objective bedside parameter to follow), measurement of anti-AChR antibodies, EMG with repetitive stimulation, chest CT to evaluate the thymus. Patients with generalized myasthenia who are developing ventilatory failure should be followed with vital capacity (VC) and negative inspiratory force (NIF, or PI_{max}) measurements; hypercapnea is a late finding. We usually intubate and ventilate patients when the VC falls below about 12 mL/kg; some will require intubation because of upper airway problems but not need mechanical ventilation. Sometimes we will permit hypercapnea if the upper airway is intact and the patient is in the ICU. Edrophonium testing to distinguish myasthenic crisis from cholinergic crisis (too much anticholinesterase) is dangerous and should rarely be performed.

Treatment includes anticholinesterases (pyridostigmine), immunosuppressives (steroids, azathioprine, cyclophosphamide, sometimes cyclosporine), and thymectomy. Plasma exchange or IVIg can be dramatically effective but is only a short-term measure, primarily used for patients in crisis or to prepare them for thymectomy. Patients with purely ocular symptoms and normal thymic size on CT can be treated with anticholinesterases alone, but most other patients should be treated for the progressive autoimmune disease they have.

A large number of drugs have been reported to exacerbate myasthenia. The most important ones to remember are aminoglycosides, macrolides, lidocaine, propranolol, and quinidine. The effects of neuromuscular blocking agents are usually quite prolonged. Steroids often worsen the weakness before the patient improves.

Respiratory failure due to diseases of the nervous system is predominantly hypercapneic, except in the case of neurogenic pulmonary edema. The diagnosis of neuromuscular respiratory failure is usually straightforward if one considers this as a possibility. Many of these conditions will be apparent at presentation, but on occasion a diagnosis of ALS is made only when the patient has difficulty weaning from the ventilator. Critical illness polyneuropathy is a relatively recently described entity in which critically ill patients (most of whom have been septic) cannot be weaned from mechanical ventilation. EMG studies show an axonal neuropathy; the prognosis for eventual recovery is very good, but these patients commonly require 4-6 months of mechanical ventilation.

Roelofs and coworkers (116), Zochodne et al (117), and others described a unique peripheral neuropathy in patients who fail to wean from mechanical ventilation after an episode of critical illness, usually involving bacteremia. In a prospective study, Witt et al identified 43 patients with sepsis and multiple organ failure; electrophysiologic studies revealed sensorimotor axonal neuropathy in 70% of these patients, and 15 (30%) experienced difficulty in weaning from ventilatory support after improvement in their underlying conditions (118). Such patients display limb weakness on examination, with diminished or absent deep tendon reflexes. Twenty-three of Witt's patients (53%) survived; although all of the neuropathic patients improved, 3 with very severe neuropathy made incomplete recoveries. The authors suggested that the decrements in

Table 8. Findings regarding neuroleptic malignant syndrome by Kurlan et al (58)

Feature	% Affected
Systemic Findings:	
Fever	100
Tachycardia	79
Diaphoresis	60
Labile blood pressure	54
Tachypnea	25
Movement-Related Findings	98
Tremor	56
Dystonia	33*
Chorea	15
Other Neurologic Findings	
Dysphagia	40
Akinetic mutism	38
Stupor	27
Coma	27

*Includes 6% with oculogyric crises

peripheral nerve function were related to hyperglycemia and hypoalbuminemia. They speculated that the likely etiologies of this neuropathy include the metabolic stresses which accompany sepsis, as well as the microcirculatory abnormalities. A study of other neurologic causes of failure to wean from ventilatory support has been reported, and emphasizes the high frequency of neuromuscular diseases in ICU patients with respiratory failure (119). Interestingly, in general ICU patients, failure to wean from a neurologic cause carries a better prognosis than does similar failure due to a pulmonary cause (120).

Patients who have flaccid paralysis after the use of neuromuscular junction blockers have received considerable attention in recent years. One group, with a relatively brief duration of paralysis, represents patients who have accumulated large amounts of these agents and take days to clear them. A second group, most commonly including asthmatics and other patients treated with steroids in addition to NMJ blockade, appears to represent a myopathy, and the patients may take a very long time to recover. While earlier reports emphasized a

relationship with the steroid-based NMJ blocking drugs, this condition has been seen with atracurium as well.

Plasmapheresis is well established as a treatment for AIPN (Guillain-Barré syndrome) if it is started in the first 2 weeks after onset. Usually, 5 treatments are given over 10 days. Ventilatory support is initiated as described above for MG. Autonomic instability may appear in the second week of the illness, and has become a leading cause of death. Thus, patients need careful observation until they are clearly improving. IVIg is also commonly used for both AIPN and MG.

Neuroleptic Malignant Syndrome

The neuroleptic malignant syndrome (NMS) was recognized in the late 1950s (121). It occurs in less than 1% of patients exposed to these agents, but may be more frequent in patients requiring higher-than-normal doses or multiple agents (122). Although some agents have been more frequently associated with NMS than others (most prominently haloperidol, fluphenazine, and the thioxanthines), it has been reported with almost every neuroleptic agent and mixed dopamine-serotonin agents. Long-acting forms of haloperidol may result in more cases in the next several years. It may also occur in Parkinsonian patients from whom either dopaminergic agonists or anticholinergic agents are abruptly withdrawn (123), although the epidemiology of this problem is uncertain. Early studies cite a mortality rate of up to 20% (122), although more recent work suggests approximately 4% to be correct (124).

The condition appears to stem from central dopaminergic blockade in the majority of cases (125); the few reports of Parkinsonian patients who develop the condition when dopaminergic therapy is terminated suggest that lack of dopamine effect alone, rather than some other effect on the receptor, is necessary and sufficient to produce NMS. Drugs with stronger D2 receptor antagonist effects are more likely to produce NMS. A patient with a mutation in the D2 receptor has been reported (126). Dopaminergic blockade may also affect thermoregulation by altering the hypothalamic set-point for temperature.

Most cases occur within a few weeks of a dosage increase, or less commonly, of the start of neuroleptic treatment (127). Reported predispositions include strenuous exercise, dehydration, other central nervous system disorders, and the use of fluphenazine decanoate (128). States of diminished osmolality may contribute to the pathogenesis of NMS (129).

The major diagnostic findings of NMS include fever, severe rigidity (usually, but not always, accompanied by tremor), obtundation, and autonomic dysfunction (diaphoresis, pallor, unstable blood pressure, tachycardia, tachypnea, and pulmonary congestion) (130). Kurlan and colleagues reviewed 52 published cases (127); their observations are shown in Table 8.

NMS patients typically have a mild to marked leukocytosis. The combination of sustained muscular contraction and immobility predisposes these patients to rhabdomyolysis; in combination with volume depletion, this often produces acute renal failure. The differential diagnosis of rhabdomyolysis in association with acute CNS dysfunction is extensive; Table 9 is adapted from the review by Bertorini (131).

Other common systemic complications include disseminated intravascular coagulation and pulmonary embolism. Thrombocytopenia has recently been reported (132).

The major differential diagnostic concerns are malignant hyperthermia, the serotonin syndrome, and lethal catatonia (see below).

Once NMS is suspected, neuroleptic drugs should be withdrawn and the patient adequately hydrated. Whether to administer dopaminergic agonists (e.g., bromocriptine) or a direct muscle relaxant (133) (dantrolene) remains the subject of debate. Dantrolene relaxes muscle contraction by decreasing Ca^{2+} release from the sarcoplasmic reticulum. Electroconvulsive therapy has also been proposed as a treatment (134), blurring the distinction of NMS and lethal catatonia. Neuroleptic medications should not be restarted for at least 2 weeks because of the risk of recurrence (135).

Malignant Hyperthermia

Malignant hyperthermia (MH) was recognized as an anesthetic complication in the

Table 9. Differential diagnosis of rhabdomyolysis in association with acute central nervous system dysfunction

---

Myofiber Metabolic Exhaustion
Seizures
Delirium
Tetanus
Strychnine intoxication
Extremes of environmental temperature
Malignant hyperthermia
Neuroleptic malignant syndrome
Diabetic ketoacidosis
Electric shock

Infectious Myositides
Influenza
HIV
Toxic shock
Clostridial monectorsis (*Clostridium perfringens* bacteremia)

Toxins and Abused Drugs
Alcohol
Cocaine and other central stimulants
LSD
Narcotics
Phencyclidine
Envenomations (wasps, bees, spiders, snakes, etc.)

Medications
Salicylate overdose
Theophylline
Lithium

Fluid and Electrolyte Disturbances
Hyperosmolar states
Hypo-osmolar states
Severe hypophosphatemia

Trauma

1960s (136). It is an autosomal dominant disorder, which most typically follows exposure to anesthetic agents. A porcine model, and several clinical studies, implicate abnormally high levels of Ca^{2+} release from a sarcoplasmic calcium channel (also known as the ryanodine receptor). This results in Ca^{2+}- induced Ca^{2+} release, which lowers the threshold for sustained muscle contracture (137). (Most human cases are associated with a defect on chromosome 19, although a few cases are not associated with the defined ryanodine receptor abnormality [138].) The drugs that induce MH do so by triggering this Ca^{2+} release; the sustained contraction produced thereby causes excessive oxygen consumption and heat production. High-energy phosphate stores are quickly depleted, resulting in failure of Ca^{2+} reuptake. As in other cells, sustained excessive elevation of free intracellular Ca^{2+} produces membrane lysis, and, consequently, myoglobin leaks from muscle cells. MH begins with muscle contraction (classically, although not always, in the masseters) in response to a triggering agent (Table 10)

In a typical anesthetic-induced case, a rise in end-tidal CO_2 often signifies MH onset (139). Quickly thereafter, rapidly rising temperature, metabolic acidosis, hypoxemia, and cardiac arrhythmias may follow. The combination of muscle breakdown and acidosis results in hyperkalemia. On rare occasions, the condition may not arise until after the operation is over, or may occur in other situations of metabolic stress, such as exercise.A personal or appropriate family history of anesthetic complications is usually sufficient reason to suspect MH and to consider *in vitro* muscle testing where it is available. A muscle biopsy specimen (obtained under local anesthesia) is electrically stimulated during exposure to varying concentrations of caffeine or halothane. Patients with other muscle diseases, such as central core disease, dystrophinopathies, and several others, may be at risk for MH-like reactions. Muscle biopsies from MH patients are frequently abnormal, but not specifically so (131).

The major management issues in MH involve termination of exposure to the triggering agent and the use of dantrolene.

Serotonin Syndrome

In 1955, a patient died from the combination of iproniazid and meperidine (140). By 1960, the serotonin syndrome (SS) was well described (141). Most patients with SS are receiving more than 1 serotonergic agent (or a monoamine oxidase inhibitor [MAOI], raising extracellular serotonin concentrations), although overdoses of single agents may trigger the

syndrome (142). The newer reversible MAOIs, such as moclobemide, may be less likely to precipitate SS (143) but are not devoid of this potential. SS resembles NMS, but is frequently associated with myoclonus, and less frequently involves muscle rigidity (145). Autonomic instability is common in both conditions (146). The duration of SS is usually less than that of NMS. A case of SS also involving stroke in a young patient suggests that the spectrum of this disorder may involve precipitation of complicated migraine (147). Treatment is supportive.

Lethal Catatonia

Lethal catatonia was described by Stauder in 1934, almost half a decade before the introduction of neuroleptic agents. The presentation of lethal catatonia is essentially indistinguishable from NMS, although published case reports of the 2 syndromes indicate differences in mode of onset, signs and symptoms, and outcome (79). Lethal catatonia often begins with extreme psychotic excitement, which leads to fever, exhaustion, and death. In contrast, NMS begins with severe muscle rigidity. Lethal catatonia may require neuroleptic treatment, although electroconvulsive therapy is more commonly employed. Occasional reports of cases "requiring" treatment with both ECT and dantrolene serve to blur the distinction of lethal catatonia and NMS (80). The underlying pathophysiology of lethal catatonia remains unknown.

REFERENCES

1. Wilks S: Bromide and iodide of potassium in epilepsy. *Med Times and Gaz* (Lond) 1861; 2:635-636

2. Gowers WR: Epilepsy and other chronic convulsive diseases: Their causes, symptoms, and treatment. London: J. and A. Churchill, 1881

3. Bleck TP, Klawans HL: Mechanisms of epilepsy and anticonvulsant action. *In*: Textbook of clinical neuropharmacology. Klawans HL, Goetz CG, Tanner CM (Eds). New York: Raven Press, 1992, pp. 23-30

4. Weschler IS: Intravenous injection of paraldehyde for control of convulsions. *JAMA* 1940; 114:2198

5. Gastaut H, Naquet R, Poiré R, Tassinari CA: Treatment of status epilepticus with diazepam (Valium). *Epilepsia* 1965; 6:167-182

6. Wijdicks EFM, Sharbrough FW: New-onset seizures in critically ill patients. *Neurology* 1993; 43:1042-1044

7. Bleck TP, Smith MC, Pierre-Louis JC, Jares JJ, Murray J, Hansen CA: Neurologic complications of critical medical illnesses. *Crit Care Med* 1993; 21:98-103

8. Hauser WA: Status epilepticus: Epidemiologic considerations. *Neurology* 1990; 40(Suppl 2):9-13

9. DeLorenzo RJ, Towne AR, Pellock JM, et al: Status epilepticus in children, adults, and the elderly. *Epilepsia* 1992; 33(Suppl 4):S15-S25

10. Aminoff MJ, Simon RP: Status epilepticus: Causes, clinical features, and consequences in 98 patients. *Am J Med* 1980; 69:657-666

11. Lowenstein DH, Alldredge BK: Status epilepticus in an urban public hospital in the 1980s. *Neurology* 1993; 42:483-488

12. Bleck TP: Status epilepticus. University Reports on Epilepsy 1992; 1:1-7

13. Ettinger AB, Shinnar S: New-onset seizures in an elderly hospitalized population. *Neurology* 1993; 43:489-492

14. Commission on classification and terminology of the International League Against Epilepsy: Proposal for revised clinical and electroencephalographic classification of epileptic seizures. *Epilepsia* 1981; 22:489-501

15. Bleck TP: Metabolic encephalopathy. *In:* Emergent and urgent neurology. Weiner WJ (Ed). Philadelphia, Lippincott, 1991, pp 27-57

16. Bleck TP: Status epilepticus. *In:* Textbook of clinical neuropharmacology (second edition). Klawans HL, Goetz CG, Tanner CM (Eds). New York, Raven Press, 1992, pp 65-73

17. Lothman EW: The biochemical basis and pathophysiology of status epilepticus. *Neurology* 1990; 40 (Suppl 2):13-23

18. Lowenstein DH, Simon RP, Sharp FR: The pattern of 72-kDa heat shock protein-like immunoreactivity in the rat brain following fluothyl-induced status epilepticus. *Brain Res* 1990; 531:173-182

19. Wasterlain CG, Fujikawa DG, Penix L, Sankar R: Pathophysiological mechanisms of brain damage from status epilepticus. *Epilepsia* 1993; 34 (Suppl 1):S37-S53

20. Treiman DM: Generalized convulsive status epilepticus in the adult. *Epilepsia* 1993; 34 (Suppl 1):S2-S11

21. Walton NY: Systemic effects of generalized convulsive status epilepticus. *Epilepsia* 1993; 34(Suppl 1):S54-S58

22. Bolton CF, Young GB, Zochodne DW: The neurologic complications of sepsis. *Ann Neurol* 1993; 33:94-100

23. Rowbotham MC; Lowenstein DH: Neurologic complications of cocaine use. *Annu Rev Med* 1990; 41:417-422

24. First seizure trial group: Randomized clinical trial of the efficacy of antiepileptic drugs in reducing the risk of relapse after a first unprovoked tonic-clonic seizure. *Neurology* 1993; 43:478-483

25. Smith MC, Bleck TP: Toxicity of anticonvulsants. *In:* Textbook of clinical neuropharmacology (second edition). Klawans HL, Goetz CG, Tanner CM (Eds). New York, Raven Press, 1992, pp 45-64

26. Mitchell WG: Status epilepticus and acute repetitive seizures in children, adolescents, and young adults: Etiology, outcome, and treatment. *Epilepsia* 1996; 37 Suppl 1:S74-80

27. Bebin EM: Additional modalities for treating acute seizures in children: Overview. *J Child Neurol* 1998; 13 Suppl 1:S23-6

28. Dreifuss FE, Rosman NP, Cloyd JC, et al: A comparison of rectal diazepam gel and placebo for acute repetitive seizures. *N Engl J Med* 1998; 338:1869-75

29. Chang CWJ, Bleck TP: Status epilepticus. *Neurol Clin* 1995; 13:529-548

30. Treiman DM, Meyers PD, Walton NY, et al: A comparison of 4 treatments for generalized convulsive status epilepticus. Veterans Affairs Status Epilepticus Cooperative Study Group. *N Engl J Med* 1998 Sep 17; 339(12):792-8

31. Leppik IE, Derivan AT, Homan RW, Walker J, Ramsay RE, Patrick B: Double-blind study of lorazepam and diazepam in status epilepticus. *JAMA* 1983; 249:1452-4

32. Bebin M, Bleck TP: New anticonvulsant drugs. *Drugs* 1994; 48:153-171

33. Graves N: Pharmacoeconomic considerations in treatment options for acute seizures. *J Child Neurol* 1998; 13 Suppl 1:S27-9

34. Walton NY, Treiman DM: Valproic acid treatment of experimental status epilepticus. *Epilepsy Res* 1992 Sep; 12(3):199-205

35. Bleck TP: Refractory status epilepticus in 2001. *Arch Neurol* 2002; 59:18-189

36. Bleck TP: Electroencephalographic monitoring. *In*: Principles and Practice of Intensive Care Monitoring. Tobin MR (Ed). New York, McGraw Hill, 1998, pp 1035-1046

37. Kumar A, Bleck TP: Intravenous midazolam for the treatment of refractory status epilepticus. *Crit Care Med* 1992; 20:483-488

38. Labar DR, Ali A, Root J: High-dose intravenous lorazepam for the treatment of refractory status epilepticus. *Neurology* 1994; 44(8):1400-3

39. Stecker MM, Kramer TH, Raps EC, O'Meeghan R, Dulaney E, Skaar DJ: Treatment of refractory status epilepticus with propofol: Clinical and pharmacokinetic findings. *Epilepsia* 1998; 39:18-26

40. Huff JS, Bleck TP: Propofol in the treatment of refractory status epilepticus. *Acad Emerg Med* 1996; 3:179

41. Prasad A, Worrall BB, Bertram EB, Bleck TP: Propofol and midazolam in the treatment of refractory status epilepticus. *Epilepsia* 2001; 42: 380-386

42. Galley HF, Dubbels AM, Webster NR: The effect of midazolam and propofol on interleukin-8 from human polymorphonuclear leukocytes. *Anesth Analg* 1998; 86:1289-93

43. Weise KL, Bleck TP: Status epilepticus in children and adults. *Crit Care Clin* 1997; 14:629-646

44. Bertorini TE: Myoglobinuria, malignant hyperthermia, neuroleptic malignant syndrome, and serotonin syndrome. *Neurol Clin* 1997; 15:649-71

45. Dodrill CB, Wilensky AJ: Intellectual impairment as an outcome of status epilepticus. *Neurology* 1990; 40 (suppl 2):23-27

46. Treiman DM, Delgado-Escueta AV: Complex partial status epilepticus. *Adv Neurol* 1983; 34:69-81

47. Lothman EW, Bertram EH: Epileptogenic effects of status epilepticus. *Epilepsia* 1993; 34 (Suppl 1):S59-S70

48. Kassell NF, Torner JC: Aneurysmal rebleeding: A preliminary report from the Cooperative Aneurysm Study. *Neurosurgery* 1983; 13:479-481

49. Nishioka H, Torner JC, Graf CJ, Kassell NF, Sahs AL, Goettler LC: Cooperative study of intracranial aneurysms and subarachnoid hemorrhage: A long-term prognostic study. II. Ruptured intracranial aneurysms managed conservatively. *Arch Neurol* 1984; 41:1142-6

50. Torner JC, Kassell NF, Wallace RB, Adams HP Jr: Preoperative prognostic factors for rebleeding and survival in aneurysm patients receiving antifibrinolytic therapy: A report of the cooperative aneurysm study. *Neurosurgery* 1981; 9:506-13

51. Solenski NJ, Haley EC Jr, Kassell NF, et al: Medical complications of aneurysmal subarachnoid hemorrhage: A report of the multicenter, cooperative aneurysm study. *Crit Care Med* 1995; 23:1007-17

52. Biller J, Godersky JC, Adams HP Jr: Management of aneurysmal

subarachnoid hemorrhage. *Stroke* 1988; 19:1300-5

53. Hasan D, Wijdicks EF, Vermeulen M: Hyponatremia is associated with cerebral ischemia in patients with aneurysmal subarachnoid hemorrhage. *Ann Neurol* 1990; 27:106-8

54. von Holst H, Ericson K, Haberbeck-Modesto M, Steiner L: Angiographic investigation of cerebral vasospasm in subarachnoid haemorrhage due to arteriovenous malformation. *Acta Neurochir* (Wien) 1988; 94:129-32

55. Kothbauer K, Schroth G, Seiler RW, Do DD: Severe symptomatic vasospasm after rupture of an arteriovenous malformation. *AJNR* 1995; 16:1073-5

56. Taneda M, Kataoka K, Akai F, Asai T, Sakata I: Traumatic subarachnoid hemorrhage as a predictable indicator of delayed ischemic symptoms. *J Neurosurg* 1996; 84:762-8

57. Kordestani RK, Counelis GJ, McBride DQ, Martin NA: Cerebral arterial spasm after penetrating craniocerebral gunshot wounds: Transcranial Doppler and cerebral blood flow findings. *Neurosurgery* 1997; 41:351-9

58. Macdonald RL, Weir B: Cerebral vasospasm: Prevention and treatment. *In*: Cerebrovascular disease. Batjer HH (Ed). Philadelphia, Lippincott-Raven, 1997, pp 1111-1121

59. Vorkapic P, Bevan JA, Bevan RD: Longitudinal *in vivo* and *in vitro* time-course study of chronic cerebrovasospasm in the rabbit basilar artery. *Neurosurg Rev* 1991; 14:215-9

60. Macdonald RL, Weir BKA: A review of hemoglobin and the pathogenesis of cerebral vasospasm. *Stroke* 1991; 22:971-982

61. Pluta RM, Boock RJ, Afshar JK, Clouse K, Bacic M, Ehrenreich H, Oldfield EH: Source and cause of endothelin-1 release into cerebrospinal fluid after subarachnoid hemorrhage. *J Neurosurg* 1997; 87:287-93

62. Kwan AL, Bavbek M,; Jeng AY, et al: Prevention and reversal of cerebral vasospasm by an endothelin-converting enzyme inhibitor, CGS 26303, in an experimental model of subarachnoid hemorrhage. *J Neurosurg* 1997; 87:281-6

63. Qureshi AI, Sung GY, Suri MA, Straw RN, Guterman LR, Hopkins LN: Prognostic value and determinants of ultraearly angiographic vasospasm after aneurysmal subarachnoid hemorrhage. *Neurosurgery* 1999; 44:967-73

64. Fisher CM, Kistler JP, Davis JM: Relation of cerebral vasospasm to subarachnoid hemorrhage visualized by computerized tomographic canning. *Neurosurgery* 1980; 6:1-9

65. Haley EC Jr, Torner JC, Kassell NF: Antifibrinolytic therapy and cerebral vasospasm. *Neurosurg Clin N Am* 1990; 1:349-56

66. Wass CT, Lanier WL: Glucose modulation of ischemic brain injury: Review and clinical recommendations. *Mayo Clin Proc* 1996; 71:801-12

67. Lanzino G, Kassell NF, Germanson T, Truskowski L, Alves W: Plasma glucose levels and outcome after aneurysmal subarachnoid hemorrhage. *J Neurosurg* 1993; 79:885-91

68. Doczi T, Bende J, Huszka E, Kiss J: Syndrome of inappropriate secretion of antidiuretic hormone after subarachnoid hemorrhage. *Neurosurgery* 1981; 9:394-7

69. Harringan MR: Cerebral salt wasting syndrome: A review. *Neurosurgery* 1996; 38:152-160

70. Wijdicks EF, Schievink WI, Burnett JC Jr: Natriuretic peptide system and endothelin in aneurysmal subarachnoid hemorrhage. *J Neurosurg* 1997; 87:275-80

71. Wijdicks EF, Vermeulen M, ten Haaf JA, Hijdra A, Bakker WH, van Gijn J: Volume depletion and natriuresis in patients with a ruptured intracranial aneurysm. *Ann Neurol* 1985; 18:211-6

72. Hasan D, Vermeulen M, Wijdicks EF, Hijdra A, van Gijn J: Effect of fluid intake and antihypertensive treatment on cerebral ischemia after subarachnoid hemorrhage. *Stroke* 1989; 20:1511-5

73. Pinto AN, Canhao P Ferro JM: Seizures at the onset of subarachnoid haemorrhage. *J Neurol* 1996; 243:161-4

74. Baker CJ, Prestigiacomo CJ, Solomon RA: Short-term perioperative anticonvulsant prophylaxis for the surgical treatment of low-risk patients with intracranial aneurysms. *Neurosurgery* 1995;37:863-70

75. Schoser BG, Heesen C, Eckert B, Thie A: Cerebral hyperperfusion injury after percutaneous transluminal angioplasty of extracranial arteries. *J Neurol* 1997; 244:101-4

76. Talavera JO, Wacher NH, Laredo F, Halabe J, Rosales V, Madrazo I, Lifshitz A: Predictive value of signs and symptoms in the diagnosis of subarachnoid hemorrhage among stroke patients. *Arch Med Res* 1996; 27:353-7

77. Lanzino G, Kongable G, Kassell N: Electrographic abnormalities after nontraumatic subarachnoid hemorrhage. *J Neurosurg Anesth* 1994; 6:156-62

78. Brouwers PJ, Wijdicks EF, Hasan D, Vermeulen M, Wever EF, Frericks H, van Gijn J: Serial electrocardiographic recording in aneurysmal subarachnoid hemorrhage. *Stroke* 1989; 20:1162-7

79. Provencio JJ, Bleck TP: Cardiovascular disorders related to neurologic and neurosurgical emergencies. *In*: Neurologic and neurosurgical emergencies. Cruz J (Ed). Philadelphia, W.B. Saunders, 1997, pp 39-50

80. Zaroff JG, Rordorf GA, Newell JB, Ogilvy CS, Levinson JR: Cardiac outcome in patients with subarachnoid hemorrhage and electrocardiographic abnormalities. *Neurosurgery* 1999; 44:34-9

81. Mayer SA, Lin J, Homma S, et al: Myocardial injury and left ventricular performance after subarachnoid hemorrhage. *Stroke* 1999; 30:780-6

82. Mayer SA, LiMandri G, Sherman D, et al: Electrocardiographic markers of abnormal left ventricular wall motion in acute subarachnoid hemorrhage. *J Neurosurg* 1995; 83:889-96

83. Vespa P, Bleck TP, Brock DG, Chang C: Impaired oxygenation after acute aneurysmal subarachnoid hemorrhage. *Neurology* 1994; 44(Suppl 1):A344

84. Touho H, Karasawa J, Shishido H, Yamada K, Yamazaki Y: Neurogenic pulmonary edema in the acute stage of hemorrhagic cerebrovascular disease. *Neurosurgery* 1989; 25:762-8

85. Haley EC Jr, Kassell NF, Apperson-Hansen C, Maile MH, Alves WM: A randomized, double-blind, vehicle-controlled trial of tirilazad mesylate in patients with aneurysmal subarachnoid hemorrhage: A cooperative study in North America. *J Neurosurg* 1997; 86:467-74

86. Rouby JJ, Laurent P, Gosnach M, et al: Risk factors and clinical relevance of nosocomial maxillary sinusitis in the critically ill. *Am J Respir Crit Care Med* 1994; 150:776-83

87. Kabuto H, Yokoi I, Habu H, Willmore LJ, Mori A, Ogawa N: Reduction in nitric oxide synthase activity with development of an epileptogenic focus induced by ferric chloride in the rat brain. *Epilepsy Res* 1996; 25:65-8

88. Sundt TM Jr, Kobayashi S, Fode NC, Whisnant JP: Results and complications of surgical management of 809 intracranial aneurysms in 722 cases. Related and unrelated to grade of patient, type of aneurysm, and timing of surgery. *J Neurosurg* 1982; 56:753-65

89. Leipzig TJ, Redelman K, Horner TG: Reducing the risk of rebleeding before early aneurysm surgery: A possible role for antifibrinolytic therapy. *J Neurosurg* 1997; 86:220-5

90. Fletcher AP, Alkjaersig N, Davies A, et al: Blood coagulation and plasma fibrinolytic enzyme system pathophysiology in stroke. *Stroke* 1976; 7:337-48

91. Kirsch JR, D'Alecy LG: Effect of altered availability of energy-yielding substrates upon survival from hypoxia in mice. *Stroke* 1979; 10:288-91

92. Hersio K, Vapalahti M, Kari A, et al: Impaired utilization of exogenous amino acids after surgery for subarachnoid haemorrhage. *Acta Neurochir (Wien)* 1990; 106:13-7

93. Mayberg MR, Batjer HH, Dacey R, et al: Guidelines for the management of aneurysmal subarachnoid hemorrhage. A statement for healthcare professionals from a special writing group of the Stroke Council, American Heart Association. *Stroke* 1994; 25:2315-28

94. Findlay JM: Current management of aneurysmal subarachnoid hemorrhage guidelines from the Canadian Neurosurgical Society. *Can J Neurol Sci* 1997; 24:161-70

95. Levy M, Giannotta S: Cardiac performance indices during hypervolemic therapy for cerebral vasospasm. *J Neurosurg* 1991; 75:27-31

96. Clyde BL, Resnick DK, Yonas, H Smith HA, Kaufmann AM: The relationship of blood velocity as measured by transcranial doppler ultrasonography to cerebral blood flow as determined by stable xenon computed tomographic studies after aneurysmal subarachnoid hemorrhage. *Neurosurgery* 1996; 38:896-904

97. Adams HP Jr: Calcium antagonists in the management of patients with aneurysmal subarachnoid hemorrhage: A review. *Angiology* 1990; 41(11 Pt 2):1010-6

98. Haley EC Jr, Kassell NF, Torner JC: A randomized trial of nicardipine in subarachnoid hemorrhage: Angiographic and transcranial Doppler ultrasound results. A report of the Cooperative Aneurysm Study. *J Neurosurg* 1993; 78:548-53

99. Kassell NF, Haley EC Jr, Apperson-Hansen C, Alves WM: Randomized, double-blind, vehicle-controlled trial of tirilazad mesylate in patients with aneurysmal subarachnoid hemorrhage: A cooperative study in Europe, Australia, and New Zealand. *J Neurosurg* 1996; 84:221-8

100. Haley EC Jr, Kassell NF, Apperson-Hansen C, Maile MH, Alves WM: A randomized, double-blind, vehicle-controlled trial of tirilazad mesylate in patients with aneurysmal subarachnoid hemorrhage: A cooperative study in North America. *J Neurosurg* 1997; 86:467-74

101. Hall ED, Andrus PK, Smith SL, et al: Pyrrolopyrimidines: Novel brain-penetrating antioxidants with neuroprotective activity in brain injury and ischemia models. *J Pharmacol Exp Ther* 1997; 281:895-904

102. Kassell NF, Peerless SJ, Durward QJ, et al: Treatment of ischemic deficits from vasospasm with intravascular volume expansion and induced arterial hypertension. *Neurosurgery* 1982; 11:337-43

103. Oropello JM, Weiner L, Benjamin E: Hypertensive, hypervolemic, hemodilutional therapy for aneurysmal subarachnoid hemorrhage. Is it efficacious? No. *Crit Care Clin* 1996; 12:709-30

104. Ullman JS, Bederson JB: Hypertensive, hypervolemic, hemodilutional therapy for aneurysmal subarachnoid hemorrhage. Is it efficacious? Yes. *Crit Care Clin* 1996; 12:697-707

105. Amin-Hanjani S, Schwartz RB, Sathi S, Stieg PE: Hypertensive encephalopathy as a complication of hyperdynamic therapy for vasospasm: Report of 2 cases. *Neurosurgery* 1999; 44: 1113-6

106. Firlik KS, Kaufmann AM, Firlik AD, Jungreis CA, Yonas H: Intra-arterial papaverine for the treatment of cerebral vasospasm following aneurysmal subarachnoid hemorrhage. *Surg Neurol* 1999; 51:66-74

107. Thomas JE, Rosenwasser RH: Reversal of severe cerebral vasospasm in 3 patients after aneurysmal subarachnoid hemorrhage: Initial observations regarding the use of intraventricular sodium nitroprusside in humans. *Neurosurgery* 1999; 44:48-57

108. Bleck TP: Metabolic encephalopathy. *In*: Emergent and urgent neurology (2e). Weiner WJ, Shulman LM (Eds). Philadelphia, Lippincott, 1999, pp. 223-253

109. Bleck TP, Henson S: Sources of fever in patients after surgery for aneurysmal subarachnoid hemorrhage. *Crit Care Med* 1992; 20 (Suppl):S31

110. Paramore CG, Turner DA: Relative risks of ventriculostomy infection and morbidity. *Acta Neurochir (Wien)* 1994; 127:79-84

111. Deutschman CS, Wilton PB, Sinow J, Thienprasit P, Konstantinides FN, Cerra FB: Paranasal sinusitis: A common complication of nasotracheal intubation in neurosurgical patients. *Neurosurgery* 1985; 17:296-9

112. Jacobs DG, Piotrowski JJ, Hoppensteadt DA, Salvator AE, Fareed J: Hemodynamic and fibrinolytic consequences of intermittent pneumatic compression: Preliminary results. *J Trauma* 1996; 40:710-16

113. Swann KW, Black PM, Baker MF: Management of symptomatic deep venous thrombosis and pulmonary embolism on a neurosurgical service. *J Neurosurg* 1986; 64:563-7

114. Takaku A, Tanaka S, Mori T, Suzuki J: Postoperative complications in 1,000 cases of intracranial aneurysms. *Surg Neurol* 1979; 12:137-44

115. The National Institute of Neurological Diseases and Stroke rt-PA stroke study group: Tissue plasminogen activator for acute ischemic stroke. *N Engl J Med* 1995; 333:1581-1587

116. Roelofs RI, Cerra F, Bielka N, et al: Prolonged respiratory insufficiency due to acute motor neuropathy: A new syndrome. *Neurology* 1983; 33 (suppl 2):240

117. Zochodne W, Bolton CF, Wells GA, et al: Critical illness polyneuropathy: a complication of sepsis and multiple organ failure. *Brain* 1987; 110:819-842

118. Witt NJ, Zochodne DW, Bolton CF, et al: Peripheral nerve function in sepsis and multiple organ failure. *Chest* 1991; 99:176-184

119. Spitzer AR, Giancarlo T, Maher L, Awerbuch G, Bowles A: Neuromuscular causes of prolonged ventilator dependency. *Muscle Nerve* 1992; 15:682-686

120. Kelly BJ, Luce JM: The diagnosis and management of neuromuscular diseases causing respiratory failure. *Chest* 1991; 99:1485-1494.

121. Preston J: Central nervous system reaction to small doses of tranquilizers: report of one death. *AP-DT* 1959; 10:627

122. Caroff SN, Mann SC: The neuroleptic malignant syndrome. *J Clin Psychiatr* 1908;41:79-83

123. Keyser KL, Rodnitzky RL: Neuroleptic malignant syndrome in Parkinson's disease after withdrawal or alteration of dopaminergic therapy. *Arch Intern Med* 1977; 86:794

124. Addonizio G, Susman VL, Roth SD: Neuroleptic malignant syndrome – Review and analysis of 115 cases. *Biol Psychiatr* 1987; 22:1004-20

125. Henderson VM, Wooten GF: Neuroleptic malignant syndrome: a pathogenetic role for dopamine receptor blockade? *Neurology* 1981; 31:132-137

126. Ram A, Cao Q, Keck PE Jr, et al: Structural change in dopamine D2 receptor gene in a patient with neuroleptic malignant syndrome. *Am J Med Genet* 1995; 60:228-30

127. Kurlan R, Hamill R, Shoulson I: Neuroleptic malignant syndrome. Clin Neuropharmacol 1984; 7:109-120

128. Guzé BH, Baxter LR: Neuroleptic malignant syndrome. *New Engl J Med* 1985; 313:163-166

129. Wedzicha JA, Hoffbrand BI: Neuroleptic malignant syndrome and hyponatremia. *Lancet* 1984; 1:963

130. Weiner WJ, Lang AE: Movement disorders: A comprehensive survey. Mount Kisco, Futura Publishing Company, 1989, p. 617

131. Bertorini TE: Myoglobinuria, malignant hyperthermia, neuroleptic malignant syndrome and serotonin syndrome. *Neurol Clin* 1997; 15:649-71

132. Ray JG: Neuroleptic malignant syndrome associated with severe thrombocytopenia. *J Intern Med* 1997; 241:245-7

133. Buckley PF, Hutchinson M: Neuroleptic malignant syndrome. *J Neurol Neurosurg Psychiatr* 1995; 58:271-278

134. Addonizio G, Susman VL. ECT as a treatment alternative for patients with symptoms of neuroleptic malignant

syndrome. *J Clin Psychiatry* 1987; 48:102-5

135. Susman VL, Addonizio G: Recurrence of neuroleptic malignant syndrome. *J Nerv Ment Dis* 1988; 176:234-41

136. Denborough MA, Lovell RRH: Anaesthetic deaths in a family. *Lancet* 1960;2:45-6

137. El-Hayek R, Yano M, Antonui B, et al: Altered E-C coupling in trials isolated from malignant hyperthermia-susceptible porcine muscle. *Am J Physiol* 1995; 268(6Pt1):C1831

138. Gronert GA, Mott J, Lee J: Aetiology of malignant hyperthermia. *Br J Anaesth* 1988; 60:253-260

139. Struebing VL: Differential diagnosis of malignant hyperthermia: a case report. *AANA J* 1995; 63:455-460

140. Mitchell RS: Fatal toxic encephalitis occurring during iproniazid therapy in pulmonary tuberculosis. *Ann Intern Med* 1955; 42:417-9

141. Oates JA, Sjoerdsma A: Neurotoxic effects of tryptophan in patients receiving a monoamine oxidase inhibitor. *Neurology* 1960; 10:1076-80

142. Kolecki P: Isolated venlafaxine-induced serotonin syndrome. *J Emerg Med* 1997; 15:491-3

143. Hilton SE, Maradit H, Moller HJ: Serotonin syndrome and drug combinations: focus on MAOI and RIMA. *Eur Arch Psychiatry Clin Neurosci* 1997; 247:113-9

144. Singer PP, Jones GR: An uncommon fatality due to moclobemide and paroxetine. *J Anal Toxicol* 1997; 21:518-20

145. Kam PC, Chang GW: Selective serotonin reuptake inhibitors. Pharmacology and clinical implications in anaesthesia and critical care medicine. *Anaesthesia* 1997; 52:982-8

146. Halman M, Goldbloom DS: Fluoxitine and neuroleptic malignant syndrome. *Biol Psychiatr* 1990; 28:518-522

147. Molaie M: Serotonin syndrome presenting with migrainelike stroke. *Headache* 1997; 37:519-21

148. Castillo E, Rubin RT, Holsboer-Trachsler E: Clinical differentiation between lethal catatonia and neuroleptic malignant syndrome. *Am J Psychiatry* 1989; 146:324-8

149. WA, Zwaan WA: Treatment of lethal catatonia with electroconvulsive therapy and dantrolene sodium: a case report. *Acta Psychiatr Scand* 1990; 82:90-2

ACUTE RENAL FAILURE

Richard S. Muther, MD

Objectives

- To develop a systematic approach to the differential diagnosis of acute renal failure
- To learn prevention techniques for critically ill patients at high risk for acute renal failure
- To learn specific and supportive treatment options for acute renal failure
- To review various dialysis options and their indications

Key Words: prerenal azotemia; obstructive uropathy; interstitial nephritis; glomerulonephritis; glomerular hemodynamics; renal replacement therapies

TABLE OF ABBREVIATIONS

ANCA	antineutrophilic cytoplasmic antibodies
ARF	acute renal failure
ATN	acute tubular necrosis
AV	arteriovenous
BUN	blood urea nitrogen
ECV	extracellular fluid volume
FENa	fractional excretion of sodium
FEurea	fractional excretion of urea
GFR	glomerular filtration rate
NSAIDs	nonsteroidal anti-inflammatory drugs
PAN	polyarteritis nodosa
PEEP	positive end-expiratory pressure
PMMA	polymethyl methacrylate
RBF	renal blood flow
TTP	thrombotic thrombocytopenic purpura

Acute renal failure (ARF) is an abrupt decrease in glomerular filtration rate (GFR), caused by intrinsic renal parenchymal disease or an alteration in intrarenal hemodynamics. It is characterized by the accumulation of waste products (e.g., urea, creatinine, and potassium) in the serum and may be oliguric or nonoliguric.

Other factors may cause acute azotemia. Excluding these factors is essential before a diagnosis of ARF is made.

DIFFERENTIAL DIAGNOSIS OF ACUTE AZOTEMIA

In addition to ARF, acute azotemia may be due to various nonrenal factors (pseudorenal failure), decreased renal perfusion (prerenal azotemia), or urinary tract obstruction (postrenal azotemia) (Table 1).

Pseudorenal Failure. Pseudorenal failure may be caused by gastrointestinal bleeding, corticosteroid usage, severe catabolic states, or hyperalimentation. All may increase the blood urea nitrogen (BUN) without a change in GFR. The serum creatinine can increase with muscle breakdown (rhabdomyolysis), blocked renal tubular creatinine secretion (trimethoprim and cimetidine), or interference with the creatinine assay (cefoxitin, acetone, and α-methyldopa) (1). One should always consider these nonrenal factors as a potential explanation for acute azotemia.

Prerenal Azotemia. Prerenal azotemia occurs when renal perfusion is compromised by an absolute decrease in extracellular fluid volume (ECV) (e.g., hemorrhage, gastrointestinal fluid losses, and burns), a decrease in the "effective" circulating volume (heart failure and ascites), or the accumulation of fluid in a "third space" (e.g., pancreatitis, acute abdomen, bowel surgery, or muscle trauma). Correction of the intravascular volume deficit should result in improved renal perfusion and resolution of azotemia. In most series, prerenal azotemia has a 90% survival rate, but if unrecognized or untreated, this condition can evolve into ARF with a significantly worse prognosis.

The diagnosis of prerenal azotemia is based on the physical examination demonstrating ECV depletion and on several urinary indices (Table 2). Of these, the fractional

Table 1. Differential diagnosis of acute azotemia

1,   Nonrenal Factors
          Increased Blood Urea Nitrogen
              Catabolic states
              Corticosteroids
              Gastrointestinal bleeding
              Hyperalimentation
              Urinary leak
          Increased Creatinine Level
              Rhabdomyolysis
              Blocked Secretion
                  Trimethoprim
                  Cimetidine
              Assay Interference
                  Acetone
                  A-Methyldopa
                  Cefotoxin
2.   Prerenal Azotemia
          Decreased Extracellular Fluid Volume
              Burns
              Hemorrhage
              Gastrointestinal losses
              Renal losses
          Decreased "Effective" Volume
              Cardiac failure
              Cirrhosis/ascites
              Positive end-expiratoy pressure
          "Third Space" Fluids
              Abdominal catastrophes
              Soft-tissue trauma
              Severe hypoalbuminemia
3.   Postrenal Azotemia (Urinary Obstruction)
          Urethral stricture
          Prostatic hypertrophy or cancer
          Neurogenic bladder or tumor
          Ureteral stone, tumor, stricture
          Retroperitoneal tumor, fibrosis
4.   Renal Azotemia (Acute Renal Failure)
          Glomerular disease
          Interstitial nephritis
          Vascular disease
          Acute tubular necrosis

sepsis are all causes of ARF in which the FENa may be spuriously low, particularly early in the clinical course (3). In addition, patients with severe heart failure or cirrhosis often have an FENa of < 1%, despite ARF (4). Diuretics, glucosuria, or preexisting renal insufficiency will falsely increase the FENa in a patient with prerenal azotemia. When diuretics falsely elevate the FENa, a fractional excretion of urea (FEurea) of < 35% accurately indicates prerenal azotemia (5). The clinician must be alert to these potential pitfalls of the FENa when approaching the acutely azotemic patient.

In addition to a low FENa and FEurea, prerenal azotemia usually causes a low urinary Na level (< 20 mEq/L), high urine osmolarity (> 350 mOsm/L), and an elevated BUN/creatinine ratio (> 20). The urine sediment usually shows granular casts but is devoid of cellular elements. Oliguria is virtually universal unless a diuretic or glucosuria is present. ARF, on the other hand, causes a high urine Na level (> 30 mEq/L), isosthenuria (urine osmolarity ~ 300 mOsm/L), and a BUN/creatinine ratio near 10. Prerenal azotemia is confirmed if the urine output improves and the azotemia resolves with the administration of isotonic fluids or improvement in the underlying condition, e.g., heart failure.

Postrenal Azotemia. Postrenal azotemia is caused by an obstruction to urine flow. As long as the obstruction is relatively recent (days to weeks), and the serum creatinine level is

Table 2. Prerenal azotemia versus acute tubular necrosis (ATN)

	Prerenal	ATN
Urine specific gravity	> 1.020	± 1.012
Urine osmolarity (mOsm/L)	> 350	± 300
Urine/plasma osmolarity	> 1.5	1
Urine sodium (mEq/L)	< 20	> 30
FENa (%)	< 1	> 1
FEurea (%)	< 35	> 50
BUN/creatinine	20	10
Urine/plasma Cr	< 40	< 20
Urine volume (mL/day)	< 500	150 – 3000

FENa, fractional excretion of sodium; FEurea, fractional excretion of urea; BUN, blood urea nitrogen; Cr, creatinine.

excretion of sodium (FENa) is the most reliable (2). The FENa measures the ratio of the sodium excreted (urinary sodium × volume) to the sodium filtered (serum sodium × GFR) by the following formula: FENa = (UNa / SNa) ÷ (Ucr /Scr) × 100, in which U indicates urine; S, serum; cr, creatinine. The test can be done with spot samples of urine and blood. The FENa is < 1% when acute azotemia is due to prerenal azotemia but > 1% with ARF. A few exceptions must be kept in mind. Rhabdomyolysis, contrast nephropathy, acute glomerulonephritis, and

Table 3. Causes of acute renal failure in the ICU

Glomerulenephritis
    Bacterial endocarditis
    Staphylococcal sepsis (shunt nephritis)
    Visceral abscesses
    Hepatitis B antigenemia
    Lupus nephritis
    Goodpasture's syndrome
    Rapidlly progressing glomerulonephritis
Glomerular Hemodynamics
    Hepatorenal
    Nonsteroidal anti-inflammatory drugs
    Angiotensin-converting enzyme inhibitors
    Nifedipine
    Nitroprusside
    Sepsis
Interstitial Nephritis
    Allergic interstitial nephritis
    Pyelonephritis
    Myeloma
    Uric acid nephropathy
    Oxalate nephropathy
    Lymphoma/leukemia
    Sarcoidosis
Vascular Disease
    Malignant hypertension
    Thrombosis/thromboembolism
    Trauma atheroemboli (cholesterol emboli)
    Vasculitis (Wegener's disease, PAN, HSP)
    Microangiopathy (HUS, TTP)
Acute Tubular Necrosis
    Toxic
        Aminoglycosides
        Cisplatin
        Radiographic contrast
        Solvents (CCl_4, ethylene glycol)
        Rhabdomyolysis (trauma, alcohol,
          Seizures, cocaine, lovastatin)
    Ischemic
        Hemorrhage
        Hypotension/shock
        Sepsis

PAN, polyarteritis nodosa; HSP, Henoch Schönlein purpura; HUS, hemolytic uremic syndrome; TTP, thrombotic thrombocytopenic purpura.

relatively low (< 5 mg/dL), correcting the obstruction will improve the azotemia. With urethral or prostatic obstruction, a Foley catheter will suffice. This catheter and a renal ultrasound are required diagnostic steps in any patient with acute azotemia. For patients with 1 kidney, retrograde pyelogram may be necessary. Upper tract obstruction may require ureteral stent or percutaneous nephrostomy.

After excluding prerenal and postrenal azotemia, one must consider the various intrinsic renal parenchymal or hemodynamic derangements responsible for ARF. These include diseases that primarily affect the glomerulus (glomerulonephritis), interstitium (interstitial nephritis), blood vessels (vascular occlusion or vasculitis), or tubules (acute tubular necrosis [ATN]).

DIFFERENTIAL DIAGNOSIS OF ACUTE RENAL FAILURE IN THE ICU

Although ATN is the most common cause of hospital-acquired ARF, important glomerular, interstitial, and vascular diseases must be considered (Table 3). Fulminant *glomerulonephritis* due to bacterial endocarditis, lupus erythematosus, staphylococcal septicemia, visceral abscesses, hepatitis B antigenemia, Goodpasture's syndrome, or idiopathic rapidly progressive (crescentic) glomerulonephritis is common in a major ICU. Once considered, these diagnoses are not difficult to make. The urinalysis will show dysmorphic red blood cells (those with multiple surface irregularities), red blood cell casts, and moderate-to-heavy proteinuria. Hypertension is variably present. Blood cultures, serologic testing (antinuclear antibody, antineutrophilic cytoplasmic antibodies [ANCA], hepatitis B surface antigen, and antiglomerular basement membrane antibody), and a search for visceral abscess may be rewarding. An early renal biopsy is usually necessary when acute glomerulonephritis causes ARF.

Alterations in *glomerular hemodynamics* are increasingly recognized as a cause of ARF. These alterations include afferent arteriolar vasoconstriction (hepatorenal syndrome) or efferent arteriolar vasodilation (angiotensin-converting enzyme inhibitors). The latter is usually seen when renal blood flow is already compromised by diuretics, severe cardiac failure, or renal artery stenosis. In addition, less well-defined derangements in intrarenal hemodynamics are likely responsible for the ARF of sepsis, potent vasodilators (6) (nitroprusside and nifedipine), and the nonsteroidal anti-inflammatory drugs (NSAIDs). In these cases, the urine sediment is usually bland, and the renal biopsy (if performed) is normal. Recovery of renal function is expected, provided the offending drug is removed or the underlying condition is corrected.

Acute *interstitial nephritis* is usually due to drug allergy. Penicillins, cephalosporins, sulfonamides, diuretics, and NSAIDs are the most common agents. Patients typically have fever, rash, arthralgias, eosinophilia, and eosinophiluria (excepting NSAIDs) (7). Other causes of ARF due to interstitial nephritis are rare but include pyelonephritis, myeloma kidney, uric acid nephropathy, and occasionally infiltrative disorders, such as lymphoma, leukemia, and sarcoidosis. Oxalate nephropathy may complicate acute ethylene glycol ingestion. The urine sediment in these cases is usually bland, but crystalluria, pyuria, and white blood cell casts can be seen, even in the absence of infection.

Vascular disease is a frequently overlooked cause of ARF. Malignant hypertension usually accompanied by retinopathy, thrombocytopenia, and microangiopathy can cause ARF. Microangiopathy and thrombocytopenia also accompany hemolytic uremic syndrome or thrombotic thrombocytopenic purpura (TTP). Renal infarction due to trauma, arterial embolus, or thrombosis can cause ARF with fever, hematuria, acute flank pain, ileus, leukocytosis, and an increased LDH level. This syndrome often mimics an acute abdomen. Renal atherosclerotic or cholesterol microemboli commonly occur following aortic manipulation (surgery or catheterization) or systemic anticoagulation. Besides ARF, gastrointestinal bleeding (due to microinfarctions), livido reticularis of the lower extremities, patchy areas of ischemic necrosis in the toes, hypocomplementemia, and eosinophilia are common. Finally, renal vasculitis (Wegener's, polyarteritis nodosa [PAN], hypersensitivity vasculitis, and Henoch-Schönlein purpura) often causes ARF. These syndromes are identified by their multisystem manifestations, very active urine sediment (hematuria, pyuria, red and white blood cell casts, and proteinuria), and in the case of Wegener's and PAN, the presence of ANCA in the serum.

The most common cause of hospital- and ICU-acquired ARF remains ATN (8), which is broadly divided into toxic and ischemic causes. Among the more common toxins causing ATN are the aminoglycoside antibiotics. Risk factors for aminoglycoside nephrotoxicity include volume contraction, age, hypokalemia, concomitant use of other nephrotoxins, and a short-dosing interval. After an initial loading dose (2 to 3 mg/kg), the maintenance dose (1 mg/kg) should be adjusted based on the patient's creatinine clearance (Ccr) (estimated by the formula: Ccr = body weight [kg]/serum creatinine). The routine use of peak and trough serum levels does not decrease the likelihood of ATN.

Radiographic contrast agents may cause ARF in patients with preexisting renal insufficiency, diabetes mellitus, and poor left ventricular function, or when multiple studies are done in a 24-hour period. The volume of contrast used (> 1.5 mL/kg) appears directly related to nephrotoxicity. In patients at very high risk for contrast nephropathy, nonionic contrast may be slightly less nephrotoxic (9). However, volume expanding these high-risk patients with intravenous crystalloid (500 to 1000 mL) is the best prophylaxis (10). Intravenous mannitol, furosemide (either before or after contrast), and calcium-channel blockers do not appear to lessen nephrotoxicity, but theophylline may be of adjunctive value. Acetylcysteine appears to offer protection against contrast toxicity (11) though its use in very high-risk patients requires further study. Most cases of contrast nephrotoxicity are nonoliguric and resolve within a few days. Rarely, a patient will require acute dialysis. Permanent loss of renal function likely does not occur.

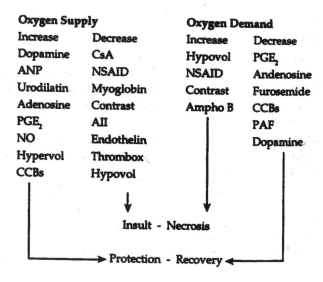

Figure 1. Factors affecting oxygen supply and demand in renal tubular cells. *ANP*, atrial natriuretic peptide; *PGE*, prostaglandin E; *NO*, nitric oxide; *Hypervol*, hypervolemia; *CCBs*, calcium-channel blockers; *CsA*, cyclosporine A; *NSAID*, nonsteroidal anti-inflammatory drug; *AII*, angiotensis II; *Thrombox*, thromboxane; *Ampho*, amphotericin; *PAF*, platelet-activating factor.

Rhabdomyolysis is producing ARF at an increasing rate. Drugs (e.g., heroin, cocaine, and lovastatin) and major crush injuries have joined alcohol, seizures, and muscle compression as common causes. All have the potential of producing myoglobinuria and ARF, particularly if ECV depletion or shock exists simultaneously. Hyperkalemia, hyperuricemia, hyperphosphatemia, and hypercreatinemia (low BUN/Cr ratio) also result. Hypocalcemia occurs early; hypercalcemia (often as high as 12 to14 mg/dL) appears during recovery (12). Dark heme-positive urine without red blood cells is a major diagnostic clue. Prophylaxis against ATN depends on aggressive intravenous crystalloid administration. The addition of mannitol and bicarbonate (½ NS with 12.5 g/L of mannitol and 50 mEq/L of NaHCO₃/L at 250 to 500 mL/hr) may be a useful adjunct.

Ischemic insults to the kidney occur with prolonged hypotension, suprarenal aortic or renal artery occlusion (either with clot or clamp), and sepsis. The renal tubular cells are particularly susceptible to ischemic insult because their baseline balance between oxygen supply and demand is tenuous (13). Thus, whenever systemic or intrarenal blood flow decreases slightly, ischemic insult to the tubular cells may occur. This imbalance of oxygen supply and demand may help to explain the beneficial effects attributed to loop diuretics shown in some studies. By inhibiting active chloride and sodium transport in the ascending limb of the loop, these agents decrease metabolic work and, therefore, oxygen requirements (13). Figure 1 diagrams the factors affecting oxygen supply and demand in the tubular cells of the renal medulla.

More than 50% of all cases of oliguric ARF in the hospital are due to sepsis. This condition appears related to a simultaneous decrease in systemic vascular resistance and increase in renal vascular resistance, reducing renal plasma flow and GFR. ARF occurs independently of systemic hypotension. Fever, leukocytosis, and other overt signs of sepsis may be absent. A mild alteration in mental status or respiratory akalosis may be the only clinical clue. Oliguria and/or azotemia in this setting should be considered occult septicemia unless disproved.

Table 4. Prevention of acute renal failure in high-risk patients

Risk Factors	Strategy for Prevention
Renal Hypoperfusion	Avoid nephrotoxins
ECV depletion	Isotonic crystalloids
Hypotension	Crystalloid, colloid, vasopressors
Congestive heart failure	Inotropic agents; cautious use of ACEI
Cirrhosis/ascites	Dopamine? Peritoneovenous shunt? Avoid NSAIDs
Third space	Colloid, isotonic crystalloids
PEEP	Isotonic crystalloids
Renal artery stenosis	Avoid ACEI with diuretics
Preexisting azotemia	Avoid ECV depletion; cautious use of nephrotoxins
Sepsis	Avoid ECV depletion; cautious use of nephrotoxins
Nephrotoxins	Avoid ECV depletion and other nephrotoxins
Aminoglycosides	Use alternative agent if possible; lengthen dosing interval; correct hypokalemia
Chemotherapy	Expand ECV; mannitol
Radiocontrast agents	Expand ECV; theophylline; limit dose; nonionic contrast with preexisting azotemia
Cyclosporine	Calcium-channel blockers
NSAIDs	Cautious use in congestive heart failure; cirrhosis; ECV depletion; avoid triamterene
Rhabdomyolysis	Expand ECV; mannitol; HCO_3
Hyperuricemia	Expand ECV; alkalinize urine; allopurinol
Electrolyte Disorders	
Hypokalemia	Correct
Hypophosphatemia	Correct
Hyperphosphatemia	Avoid calcium therapy; expand ECV
Hypercalcemia	Avoid phosphorus therapy; expand ECV; furosemide

ACEI, angiotensin-converting enzyme inhibitor; NSAIDs, nonsteroidal anti-inflammatory drugs; ECV, extracellular fluid volume; HCO_3, bicarbonate.

PREVENTION OF ACUTE RENAL FAILURE

Because the risk and the mortality of ARF are high in critically ill patients [14], prevention is the best therapy. Table 4 lists several common risk factors for ARF and suggestions for prophylaxis. The most common risk factor is ECV depletion. Volume expansion can minimize the risk of ARF from radiographic contrast agents, cisplatin, and NSAIDs. Mannitol appears to at least partially abrogate the ARF caused by rhabdomyolysis and cisplatin but not that caused by contrast agents. Limiting the dose and simultaneous exposure appears important in avoiding contrast, aminoglycoside, and cisplatin toxicity. Alkali may limit the nephrotoxicity of myoglobinuria and uric acid.

Allopurinol should be used before chemotherapy, whenever tumor lysis is anticipated. Adjusting dosing interval for changes in Ccr is important to prevent aminoglycoside toxicity. Polyuria or an increasing creatinine level should prompt additional widening of the dosing interval. Correcting hypokalemia and expanding ECV also are helpful. Although peak aminoglycoside level correlates with antibacterial effect, there is little evidence that monitoring trough levels minimizes or avoids nephrotoxicity.

Although some data support abdominal decompression with large volume paracentesis as a means of improving renal perfusion in patients with tense ascites, the clinician should be cautious about paracenteses > 0.5 L. Ascitic fluid may rapidly reaccumulate at the expense of intravascular volume, putting the patient at risk

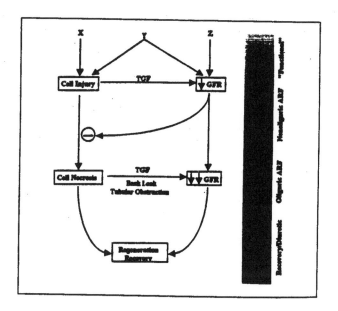

Figure 2. Pathophysiology of acute renal failure (*ARF*) with clinical correlation. Glomerular filtration rate (*GFR*) may fall after a cellular insult (*x*) stimulates tubuloglomerular feedback (*TGF*) or because of a direct hemodynamic alteration (*z*). Some etiologies (*y*) may directly affect tubular injury and GFR. In its mildest form, a functional renal failure results and resolves without oliguria or histologic evidence of cell necrosis. More severe and/or prolonged insults may cause call necrosis with tubular obstruction and backleak of ultrafiltrate contributing to oliguria. Tubular cell regeneration and recovery of GFR usually correspond to a diuretic phase clinically.

due to inadequate preload. Positive end-expiratory pressure (PEEP), as well as high intrathoracic pressure associated with mechanical ventilator support, may compromise cardiac output and renal perfusion. If possible, PEEP should be minimized and ECV should be expanded in high-risk patients.

There are animal data to suggest that hyperalimentation may increase the risk of ARF. However, the benefits of nutritional support seem to far outweigh this risk. Minimizing protein intake to between 0.6 and 0.8 g/kg/day during periods of very high risk may be prudent.

PATHOPHYSIOLOGY AND NATURAL HISTORY

Either a toxic or ischemic insult can initiate an intrarenal cascade that manifests as clinical ARF (Figure 2). The primary cellular event appears to be a decreased production and increased degradation of adenosine triphosphate, thus increasing local production of phospholipases, hypoxanthine, and adenosine. The phospholipases destabilize tubular cell membranes; xanthine oxidase catalyzes hypoxanthine to generate oxygen free radicals (15). Both processes may further injure renal tubular and endothelial cells. Local production of platelet-activating factor, vasoconstrictive prostaglandins, and endothelin are other factors that may affect intraglomerular hemodynamics (afferent arteriolar vasoconstriction or efferent arteriolar vasodilation) or glomerular capillary permeability in such a way as to decrease GFR (16). This phenomenon is known as tubuloglomerular feedback. Furthermore, injured cells or cell debris may cause intratubular obstruction and backleak of tubular fluid. The net result is a prolonged decrement in GFR with varying degrees of urine output. All of these events may occur without an alteration in systemic hemodynamics or even renal blood flow (RBF).

Simultaneous with these events causing renal functional decline, other factors appear to mediate a regenerative or repair process (17). Release of various cytokines from injured cells appears to recruit and activate macrophages, which synthesize growth factors (such as, epidermal and transforming growth factors), stimulating renal tubular cell regeneration and recovery. Production of vasodilatory prostaglandins and nitric oxide may aid this renal recovery.

Clinically, these pathophysiologic mechanisms appear to produce a brief initial decrease in RBF and GFR, followed by a prolonged (days to weeks) maintenance phase in which GFR remains low but RBF is normal. Oliguria may occur during this maintenance period, and dialysis is often necessary. The recovery phase is marked first by increasing urine volume, and finally, by return of GFR. This functional recovery may be delayed by intercurrent infection, repeated episodes of ischemia, or additional exposure to nephrotoxins

TREATMENT OF
ACUTE RENAL FAILURE

The above pathophysiology offers therapeutic potential. Restoration of ATP (ATP-MgCl$_2$; inhibition of 5' nucleotidase), free-radical scavengers, and adenosine inhibitors (theophylline) have all shown promise in experimental trials (15), as have antagonists to platelet-activating factor and endothelin (antiendothelin antibodies and endothelin receptor antagonists) (18). However, for most patients with ARF, treatment is largely supportive and expectant management is the rule.

Unfortunately, there are no specific therapies for most causes of ARF. Steroids and cyclophosphamides are indicated for polyarteritis, Wegener's disease, or diffuse proliferative lupus nephritis. Steroids also may be indicated for allergic interstitial nephritis. Plasmapheresis is indicated for Goodpasture's syndrome, TTP, and myeloma of the kidney. Antibiotics are useful for sepsis and infectious forms of glomerulonephritis.

Converting oliguria to nonoliguria appears helpful. Nonoliguric patients have fewer complications, a decreased dialysis requirement, and improved survival (19). Conversion to nonoliguria can often be accomplished by repleting intravascular volume (if deficient) and using high-dose loop diuretics (e.g., 200 mg iv of furosemide or continuous infusions at a rate of 10 to 40 mg/hr). The diuretic may have the additional advantage of decreasing tubular cell metabolic activity, thus lessening the oxygen requirement. A renal vasodilatory dose of dopamine (1.5 to 2.5 mg/kg/min) is sometimes helpful in stimulating urine volume. However, in a recent placebo-controlled trial in critically ill patients, low-dose dopamine failed to improve serum creatinine, dialysis requirement, ICU or hospital days (20). Neither furosemide nor dopamine has any utility as prophylaxis prior to major surgery.

Hyperalimentation preserves lean muscle mass, decreases protein breakdown, improves wound healing, and may improve immune competence. It appears to improve renal tubular cell regeneration in animals with ATN and improve survival in patients, particularly those with multiple complications. Whenever possible, enteral hyperalimentation is preferred. Regardless of the route, the hyperalimentation formula must be individualized and reevaluated daily in patients with ARF. Essential amino acid preparations offer no special advantage.

Potential drug toxicity must be avoided by adjusting antibiotic and other drug dosing in patients with renal failure. This includes potential dietary sources of potassium (salt substitutes) and phosphorus (dairy products), as well as the magnesium and aluminum contained in antacids.

Dialysis is often indicated when hyperkalemia, volume overload, or metabolic acidosis cannot be controlled medically or with signs and symptoms of severe uremia. Intermittent hemodialysis has been the standard therapy for many years because it is efficient, widely available, and generally well tolerated. However, hemodialysis is not without potential complications, bleeding (due to heparinization) and hypotension being the most severe. The bleeding can usually be avoided by using citrate as an alternative anticoagulant. Hypotension often can be modified by fluid removal (ultrafiltration) without simultaneous dialysis (dry ultrafiltration). However, the hypotension of hemodialysis is, at least in part, due to the use of bioincompatible (cellulose) dialysis membranes. Complement activation and alterations in immune function are observed when hemodialysis is performed with these dialyzers. Recent studies have established that hypotension and complement activation can be reduced by the use of the more compatible polysulfone, polyacrylonitrile, or polymethyl methacrylate (PMMA) dialysis membranes. Most importantly, survival is improved when ARF patients are dialyzed with these biocompatible membranes compared with cellulose membranes (21). Therefore, the use of polysulfone, polacrylonitrile, or PMMA membranes should be the standard of care for ARF patients requiring hemodialysis.

When hypotension limits the applicability of hemodialysis, peritoneal dialysis or continuous hemofiltration techniques can be used. Peritoneal dialysis requires no anticoagulation, and its slow continuous ultrafiltration rates are well suited to patients with baseline hypotension and/or poor cardiac output. However, its utility is limited after abdominal surgery and in severely catabolic patients because of relatively slow solute removal.

Continuous extracorporeal techniques for solute and fluid removal are valuable in hemodynamically unstable patients, particularly those with multiple organ failure (22). These include continuous arteriovenous (AV) hemofiltration in which the AV pressure gradient drives blood through an extracorporeal filter, the hydrostatic pressure producing ultrafiltration. If the AV pressure gradient is too low, a blood flow pump can be added. The pump also allows the use of continuous vein-to-vein hemofiltration, avoiding arterial puncture. Solute is removed by convection or "solute drag"; i.e., massive ultrafiltration (up to 2 L/hr) will remove solute with high-sieving coefficients (those with high-membrane permeability). The greater the membrane permeability, the greater will be the ultrafiltration rate and solute removal. Thus, replacement fluid (without urea, creatinine, etc.) must be simultaneously infused to avoid ECV

depletion. This technique has the theoretical advantage of being able to remove larger molecules (including tumor necrosis factor, interleukin-2, and myocardial depressant factor). In that regard, at least 2 studies have correlated survival with daily ultrafiltration volumes when this technique is used as the only renal replacement therapy for ARF. If additional solute removal is necessary to control uremia, peritoneal dialysate fluid can run through the filter simultaneously (1 to 2 L/hr), which enhances solute removal by diffusion. Membranes used for these dialysis techniques are biocompatible. All of these extracorporeal circuits may run continuously for several days. They usually require systemic heparinization or citrate for anticoagulation. There are as yet no convincing data that any specific dialysis technique improves survival, although the "dose" of dialysis does appear to directly affect patient survival and renal recovery.

PROGNOSIS AND RECOVERY

In most clinical series, the mortality rate from ARF continues to average 50%. The mortality rate in nonoliguric patients may be as low as 25%; with oliguric ARF, it approaches 70%. The major determinants of outcome are the precipitating event and preexisting disease. ARF associated with ventilatory failure, sepsis, trauma, abdominal catastrophe, and burns carries a mortality rate of 70% to 80%, but the mortality rate is 25% to 30% for patients with ARF due to aminoglycosides, radiographic contrast, or other drug reactions.

Mortality is highest in the very young and very old. The number of complications also influences prognosis. The mortality rate from ARF approaches 100% if 3 or more major organ systems have failed simultaneously. The dose of dialysis (solute removal) appears to directly improve survival, while the severity of azotemia and the choice of dialysis modality do not. Again, the use of biocompatible dialysis membranes improves survival in those patients who require dialysis.

Infection is the most common cause of death and is usually due to overwhelming sepsis from resistant gram-negative bacteria or yeast. Other common causes of death are cardiovascular compromise (e.g., strokes and myocardial infarction), respiratory failure (often with nosocomial pneumonia), and gastrointestinal bleeding.

If the patient with ARF survives, recovery is usually prompt and clinically complete. The period of oliguria averages 10 to 14 days. Urine volume recovers gradually during the next 3 to 7 days. Fluid therapy is needed to support this obligatory diuretic phase. Although the BUN and creatinine levels continue to increase during this phase, dialysis can usually be discontinued. Most survivors regain essentially complete renal function within 30 days; rarely, a patient requires 60 to 90 days (23). In 1 large series, 97% of survivors regained renal function, almost all within 30 days. Those patients who have delayed or no recovery are usually older, have preexisting renal insufficiency, or suffer severe ischemic insults to the kidney. Although renal recovery is usually clinically complete, as many as 50% of patients have minor decrements in GFR, decreasing concentrating ability, or defects in maximal urine acidification.

In patients

ANNOTATED REFERENCES

1. Muther RS: Drug interference with renal function tests. *Am J Kidney Dis* 1983; 3:118–120

2. Espinel CH, Gregory AW: Differential diagnosis of acute renal failure. *Clin Nephrol* 1980; 13:73–77
   A comparison of various serum and urinary indices used to differentiate prerenal azotemia from acute renal failure in oliguric patients.

3. Brosins FL, Lau K: Low fractional excretion of sodium in acute renal failure: Role timing of the test and ischemia. *Am J Nephrol* 1986; 6:450–457
   Various factors which may "spuriously" lower fractional excretion of sodium.

4. Diamond JR, Yoburn DC: Nonoliguric acute renal failure associated with a low fractional excretion of sodium. *Ann Intern Med* 1982; 96:597–600
   Congestive heart failure, nephrotic syndrome, and burns may spuriously lower fractional excretion of sodium.

5. Kaplan AA, Kohn OF: Fractional excretion of urea as a guide to renal dysfunction. *Am J Nephrol* 1992; 12:49–54

6. Reid GM, Muther RS: Nitroprusside-induced acute azotemia. *Am J Nephrol* 1987; 7:313–315
   Potent vasodilators can cause functional acute renal failure without systemic hypotension.

7. Nolan CR, Anger MS, Kelleher SP: Eosinophiluria: A new method of detection and definition of the clinical spectrum. *N Engl J Med* 1986; 315:1516–1519

8. Hou SH, Burshinsky DA, Wish JB, et al: Hospital-acquired acute renal insufficiency: A prospective study. *Am J Med* 1983; 74:243–248
   A prospective review of the risk factors and etiologies of hospital acquiredacute renal failure.

9. Rudnick MR, Goldfarb S, Wexler L, et al: Nephrotoxicity of ionic and nonionic contrast media in 1196 patients: A randomized trial. *Kidney Int* 1995; 47:254–261
   In patients with preexisting azotemia, nonionic contrast appears less nephrotoxic.

10. Solomon R, Werner C, Mann D, et al: Effects of saline, mannitol and furosemide on acute decreases in renal function induced by radiocontrast agents. *N Engl J Med* 1994; 331:1416–1420
    Volume expansion prior to contrast dye provides the best protection.

11. Tepel M, van der Giet M, Schwarzfeld C, et al: Prevention of radiographic-contrast-agent-induced reductions in renal function by acetylcysteine. *N Engl J Med* 2000; 343:180-184

12. Tadjis T, Grieff M, Locknat D, et al: Calcium metabolism in acute renal failure due to rhabdomyolysis. *Clin Nephrol* 1993; 39:22–27

13. Brezis M, Rosen SN: Hypoxemia of the renal medulla-its implications for disease. *N Engl J Med* 1995; 332:647–655
    A review of the unique physiologic aspects predisposing the kidney to injury and offering hope for therapeutic intervention.

14. Spiegel DM, Ullian ME, Zerbe GO, et al: Determinants of survival and recovery in

acute renal failure patients dialyzed in intensive-care units. *Am J Nephrol* 1991; 11:44–47

Predictors of mortality (#1 being ventilatory failure) in acute renal failure.

15. Bonventre JV: Mechanisms of ischemic acute renal failure. *Kidney Int* 1993; 43:1160–1178

    Comprehensive review of pathophysiology of acute renal failure.

16. Guignard JP, Semana D, John E, et al: Acute renal failure. *Crit Care Med* 1993; 21:S349–S351

    Brief summary of factors altering intraglomerular hemodynamics in acute renal failure.

17. Toback FG: Regeneration after acute tubular necrosis. *Kidney Int* 1992; 41:226–246

    Comprehensive review of mechanisms involved in renal recovery after acute insult.

18. Fischereder M, Trick W, Nath KA: Therapeutic strategies in the prevention of acute renal failure. *Semin Nephrol* 1994; 14:41–52

    Review of several potential future therapies for acute renal failure.

19. Anderson RJ, Linas SL, Berns AS, et al: Nonoliguric acute renal failure. *N Engl J Med* 1977; 296:1134–1138

    The classic and definitive article on nonoliguric acute renal failure.

20. Australian and New Zealand Intensive Care Society Clinical Trials Group: Low-dose dopamine in patients with early renal dysfunction: A placebo controlled trial. *Lancet* 2000; 356:2139-2143

21. Hakim RM, Wingard RL, Parker RA: Effect of the dialysis membrane in the treatment of patients with acute renal failure. *N Engl J Med* 1994; 331:1338–342

    Establishes a new standard of care for acute hemodialysis.

22. Hebbar S, Muther RS: Renal replacement therapy in the critically ill. *In:* Critical Care. Third Edition. Civetta JM, Taylor RW, Kirby RR (Eds). Philadelphia, JP Lippincott, 1997

    Review of various dialysis techniques for acute renal failure.

23. Spurney RF, Fulkerson WJ, Schwab SJ: Acute renal failure in critically ill patients:

Prognosis for recovery of kidney function after prolonged dialysis support. *Crit Care Med* 1991; 19:8–11

Don't give up! If your patient survives, renal function will usually return.

ACID-BASE DISORDERS

Gregory A. Schmidt, MD, FCCP

Objectives

- To describe the effects of acidemia and alkalemia in critically ill patients
- To present a structured approach to analyzing acid-base disorders
- To discuss the differential diagnosis of the fundamental acid-base derangements
- To discuss treatment of acid-base disorders

Key Words: Mechanical ventilation; ARDS; COPD; status asthmaticus; tidal volume; non-invasive ventilation; assist-control; pressure support; pressure control; SIMV; inverse ratio ventilation

TABLE OF ABBREVIATIONS

ACRF	acute-on-chronic respiratory failure
ACV	assist-control ventilation
ARDS	acute respiratory distress syndrome
COPD	chronic obstructive pulmonary disease
Crs	compliance of the respiratory system
f	respiratory rate
I:E	inspiratory to expiratory rate
IRV	inverse ratio ventilation
NIV	noninvasive ventilation
PCV	pressure-control ventilation
PEEP	positive end-expiratory pressure
Pinsp	inspiratory pressure
Ppeak	peak airway opening pressure
Pplat	plateau airway pressure
PSV	pressure-support ventilation
SIMV	synchronized intermittent mandatory ventilation
Ti	inspiratory time
Te	expiratory time
Vt	tidal volume

INTRODUCTION

Disturbances of acid-base equilibrium occur in a wide variety of critical illnesses and are among the most commonly encountered disorders in the ICU. In addition to reflecting the seriousness of the underlying disease, disturbances in H^+ concentration have important physiologic effects.

A blood pH less than normal is called *acidemia;* the underlying process causing acidemia is called *acidosis.* Similarly, *alkalemia* and *alkalosis* refer to the pH and the underlying process, respectively. While an acidosis and an alkalosis may coexist, there can be only one resulting pH. Therefore, acidemia and alkalemia are mutually exclusive conditions.

The approach to acid-base derangements should emphasize a search for the cause, rather than an immediate attempt to normalize the pH. Many disorders are mild and do not require treatment. Further, treatment may be more detrimental than the acid-base disorder itself. More important is a full consideration of the possible underlying pathologic states. This may facilitate a directed intervention that will benefit the patient more than normalization of the pH would.

APPROACH TO ACID-BASE DISTURBANCES

This discussion will generally follow the more widely accepted "bicarbonate-based" approach to understanding acid-base disturbances, although a superior method, developed by Peter Stewart, is available (1, 2). The Stewart method identifies the true determinants of the pH: the strong ion difference (the [SID]); the total concentration of weak acids (Atot); and the PCO_2. Using any method, diagnosing disorders of acid-base homeostasis in the ICU can be challenging. Many critically ill patients have combinations of disorders. In addition, patients admitted to the ICU often have preexisting disturbances—such as respiratory acidosis in patients with COPD, and metabolic alkalosis in patients on diuretics—that must be taken into account when one is evaluating subsequent changes.

A stepwise, conventional, approach follows:

Step 1: Do the numbers make sense? (Use the Henderson equation: $[H^+] = 24 \times PCO_2/HCO_3$);

Step 2: Determine whether an acidemia (pH < 7.36) or an alkalemia (pH > 7.44) is present. (In mixed disorders the pH may be in the normal range, but the bicarbonate level, the PCO_2, or the anion gap will signal the presence of an acid-base disturbance);

Step 3: Is the primary disturbance metabolic or respiratory? (That is, does any change in the PCO_2 account for the direction of the change in pH?);

Step 4: Is there appropriate compensation for the primary disturbance (See Table 1)?

Step 5: Is the anion gap elevated? If so, is the Δgap $\approx \Delta HCO_3^-$? If not, there is an additional non-gap acidosis or a metabolic alkalosis.

Step 6: Put it all together—what is the most likely diagnosis?

PHYSIOLOGIC EFFECTS OF ACIDEMIA AND ALKALEMIA

In patients the effects of acidemia and alkalemia are difficult to discern because any physiologic consequences may be obscured or modified by the severe illness causing the acid-base disorder.

Acidemia causes stimulation of the sympathetic-adrenal axis. In severe acidemia this effect is countered by a depressed responsiveness of adrenergic receptors to circulating catecholamines. The net effect on ventricular performance, heart rhythm, and

Table 1. Appropriate Compensation in Simple Acid-Base Disorders

Metabolic acidosis
$$PCO_2 = (1.5 \times HCO_3^-) + 8 \pm 2$$
Metabolic alkalosis
$$PCO_2 = (0.7 \times HCO_3^-) + 21 \pm 1.5*$$
Respiratory acidosis
Acute: $HCO_3^- = [(PCO_2 - 40)/10] + 24$
Chronic: $HCO_3^- = [(PCO_2 - 40)/3] + 24$
Respiratory alkalosis
Acute: $HCO_3^- = [(40 - PCO_2)/5] + 24$
Chronic: $HCO_3^- = [(40 - PCO_2)/2] + 24$

* For a bicarbonate (HCO_3^-) level greater than 40 the formula to be used is: $PCO_2 = (.75 \times HCO_3^-) + 19 \pm 7.5$

vascular tone depends on the relative effects of these competing influences. For example, mild acidemia causes increased cardiac output, a response that can be prevented by ß-adrenergic blockade. Severe acidemia typically causes a decrease in cardiac output and vasodilation despite sympathetic stimulation. Clinically no increase in arrhythmias is seen in patients with respiratory acidemia during permissive hypercapnia, except that attributable to hypoxia. Once ventricular fibrillation is established, acidemia has little or no effect on the success of conversion to sinus rhythm.

Acute respiratory acidemia causes marked increases in cerebral blood flow. When PCO_2 exceeds 70 mmHg, loss of consciousness and seizures can occur. This is likely due to an abrupt lowering of intracellular pH rather than to any effect of CO_2 per se. The encephalopathy of acute-on-chronic respiratory failure is poorly understood, but may include elements of intracellular acidosis, hypoxia, and endogenous neuropeptide secretion. Thus the term "CO_2 narcosis," which implies a direct effect of CO_2, is a misnomer.

Acute hypercapnia causes depression of diaphragmatic contractility and a decrease in endurance time. This effect may contribute to the downward spiral of respiratory failure in patients with acute CO_2 retention.

During intentional hypoventilation, as practiced in patients with status asthmaticus or

ARDS, hypercapnia has been quite well tolerated. No significant impact on systemic vascular resistance, pulmonary vascular resistance, cardiac output, or systemic oxygen delivery has been seen (3). There are several cautions, however. Patients are generally carefully chosen so as to have no increased intracranial pressure or cardiac ischemia, the inspired gas must be oxygen-enriched to prevent hypoxemia, and patients should be well-sedated (4). There is no agreement about the role of bicarbonate during permissive hypercapnia.

Alkalemia appears to increase myocardial contractility, at least to a pH of 7.7. Some animals exhibit spontaneous ventricular fibrillation at pH levels above 7.8. There are reports of alkalemic patients with atrial and ventricular arrhythmias that were refractory to treatment until the alkalemia was corrected. Respiratory alkalosis lowers blood pressure and calculated systemic vascular resistance. Most vascular beds demonstrate vasodilation but vasoconstriction predominates in the cerebral circulation. Cerebral blood flow falls maximally, to 50 percent of basal flow, at a PCO_2 of 20 mmHg, an effect which has been utilized to acutely lower intracranial pressure, but this effect lasts only 6 hours. Both respiratory and metabolic alkalemia can lead to seizures. Alkalemia can also cause coronary artery spasm with ECG evidence of ischemia. The clinical effect of alkalemia-induced changes in oxygen delivery is small but in patients with ongoing tissue hypoxia the increased hemoglobin oxygen affinity may be detrimental and clinically significant.

Metabolic Acidosis

Metabolic acidosis is characterized by a primary decrease in bicarbonate concentration and a compensatory reduction in the PCO_2. The etiologies of metabolic acidosis are divided into those that cause an increase in the anion gap and those associated with a normal anion gap (hyperchloremic acidosis). The *anion gap* is the difference between measured cations and measured anions, defined as $[Na^+] - [Cl^+] - [HCO_3^-]$, with a normal value traditionally defined as 8 to 14 meq/L. The majority of

unmeasured anion normally is accounted for by plasma proteins, primarily albumin. The remainder consists of phosphate, sulfates, lactate, and other organic anions. Seventy percent of patients with an anion gap greater than 20 meq/L will have an identifiable organic anion, as will virtually all of those with an anion gap greater than 30 meq/L.

Normal-anion-gap acidosis occurs from

Table 2. Etiologies of Renal Tubular Acidosis (RTA) in the ICU

Proximal RTA
    Primary renal disease
    Nephrotic syndrome
    Systemic diseases
        Amyloidosis
        Multiple myeloma
        Systemic lupus erythematosus (SLE)
    Drugs and toxins
        Heavy metal toxicity
        Carbonic anhydrase inhibitors
Type I Distal RTA
    Primary renal disease
        Obstructive uropathy
        Renal transplant rejection
        Nephrocalcinosis
        Pyelonephritis
        Allergic Interstitial Nephritis
    Systemic diseases
        Cirrhosis
        Multiple myeloma
        Sickle cell disease
        Amyloidosis
        SLE
    Drugs and toxins
        Amphotericin
        Lithium
        Analgesic abuse
Type IV Distal RTA
    Primary renal disease
        Obstructive uropathy
        Hyporeninemia
    Systemic diseases
        Diabetes mellitus
        Addison's disease
        Sickle cell disease
    Drugs and toxins
        Spironolactone
        Triamterene
        Amiloride
        Pentamidine

Table 3. Etiologies of Normal-Anion-Gap Metabolic Acidosis

Gastrointestinal Loss of Bicarbonate
     Diarrhea
     Urinary diversion
   Small bowel, pancreatic, or bile drainage
   (fistulas, surgical drains)
     Cholestyramine
Renal Loss of Bicarbonate (or Bicarbonate Equivalent)
     Renal tubular acidosis
     Recovery phase of DKA
     Renal insufficiency
     Post-Hypocapneic
Acidifying Substances
     HCl
     NH_4Cl
     Arginine HCl
     Lysine HCl
     $CaCl_2$ or $MgCl_2$ (oral)
     Sulfur

Table 4. Etiologies of Increased-Anion-Gap Metabolic Acidosis

Etiology	Anion
Ketoacidosis	Acetoacetate, β-hydroxybutyrate
Diabetic	
Alcoholic	
Starvation	
Lactic acidosis	Lactate
Uremia	Phosphates, sulfates, organic anions
Toxins	
Ethylene glycol	Glycolate, lactate
Methanol	Formate, lactate
Salicylate	Salicylate, lactate, organic anions
Paraldehyde	Unknown

the loss of bicarbonate, through the kidneys or through the gut, or from the addition of an acid with chloride as the accompanying anion. The most common cause of normal-gap metabolic acidosis in the ICU is diarrhea; in the absence of diarrhea a renal tubular acidosis is likely. The causes of renal tubular acidosis encountered in the ICU are listed in Table 2. The other causes of normal-anion-gap acidosis are usually obvious from the history and medication list. The etiologies of normal-anion-gap metabolic acidosis are listed in Table 3. The etiologies of increased-anion-gap metabolic acidosis are given in Table 4.

KETOACIDOSIS

Ketoacidosis occurs when free fatty acids are overproduced and preferentially shunted to form ketones, typically in states of low insulin and increased glucagon. Diabetic ketoacidosis is a common reason for ICU admission and is easily diagnosed from glucose and ketone measurement. Treatment involved rehydration, insulin administration, and attention to electrolyte disturbances. Alcoholic ketoacidosis (AKA) generally occurs after binge drinking in alcoholics who have no food intake and repeated vomiting. It is characterized by a normal or slightly elevated serum glucose level with increased ketones. Because of the altered redox state of the liver, much of the ketones in AKA occur in the form of ß-hydroxybutyrate, which is not measured by the Ketostix or Acetest. Specific enzymatic testing is necessary to detect ß-hydroxybutyrate. Rehydration and provision of glucose is generally sufficient therapy for AKA although insulin may be useful in some patients. Alkali therapy is not useful in ketoacidosis.

TOXINS

Toxin ingestion is an uncommon but important cause of increased-anion-gap acidosis. Any patient who presents with an anion-gap acidosis that is not explained by tests for ketones and lactate should be suspected of having ingested a toxin. However, it should also be remembered that lactic acidosis can occur with toxin ingestion so that an increased lactate level does not rule out an acidosis from toxins. Often the laboratory diagnosis of toxin ingestion is slow; thus the diagnosis must be suspected, and clinical clues sought, prior to laboratory confirmation. Specific tests must be ordered, since methanol and ethylene glycol are not included in a routine toxicology screen. Salicylate intoxication is the most common of these ingestions and often presents with a mixed respiratory alkalosis and metabolic acidosis, which can be an important diagnostic clue.

The toxic effects of ethylene glycol and methanol are mediated by metabolites—glycolate in the case of ethylene glycol, and formaldehyde and formate in the case of methanol. The osmolal gap, which is the difference between measured osmolality and that calculated from the formula $Osm = 2[Na^+] + [glucose]/ 18 + [BUN]/ 2.8 + [ethanol]/ 4.6$, is increased above its normal value of less than 10 mosmol/L. The osmolal gap may lack sensitivity, however, and its value as a screening test has been questioned. The loss of retinal sheen or even frank papilledema seen with methanol poisoning and the characteristic urinary oxalate crystals seen with methylene glycol poisoning can be important diagnostic clues.

The identification of the anion associated with an increased-anion-gap acidosis in the ICU is not as precise as it might seem from the relatively short list of possibilities. In some cases of acidosis, no anion is found or the rise in anions accounts for only a fraction of the rise in the anion gap; the identity of the offending anion, or anions, in these circumstances has not been determined.

LACTIC ACIDOSIS

Lactic acidosis, commonly defined as a lactate level greater than 5 mmol/L with an arterial pH less than 7.35, is the most common and most important metabolic acidosis encountered in the ICU. The acidemia serves as a marker for a diverse group of serious underlying conditions and has important prognostic implications. The etiologies of lactic acidosis are numerous and are listed in Table 5. Most cases of lactic acidosis encountered in the ICU occur secondarily to a handful of processes; shock is the most common cause, with hypoxia, seizures, regional ischemia (i.e., mesenteric or in an extremity), and toxin exposure account for a majority of the remaining cases.

Sepsis is a common cause of lactic acidosis in the ICU, but the mechanism is still debated. The belief that the lactic acidosis of sepsis is due to anaerobic metabolism has come under question based on several lines of evidence. If cellular oxygen lack were the basis of lactic acid production, the lactate to pyruvate ratio should be elevated, a finding that is lacking in resuscitated septic patients. Further, when the adequacy of cellular oxygenation has been assayed by various methods, it has been found to be adequate. Pathologic supply dependence, a finding which was often interpreted to support tissue hypoxia, now appears to be an artifact of mathematical coupling, at least regarding this phenomenon at the whole body level. No dependence of oxygen consumption on oxygen delivery can be found when each is measured by independent means. Additionally, various methods of boosting oxygen delivery fail to lower lactate levels. Finally, in an animal model of sepsis and lactic acidosis, hypoxic challenge failed to worsen lactic acidosis. Possible alternate mechanisms include hypermetabolism-induced protein catabolism, leading to increased circulating levels of alanine, pyruvate, and lactate (consistent with the normal lactate to pyruvate ratio), or regional (i.e., gut) production of lactate, possibly due to local hypoxia.

Bicarbonate had long been the standard therapy for lactic acidosis although its safety and efficacy only came under scrutiny in the early 1980's. The accumulated data has challenged the traditional arguments for bicarbonate use, and questioned the safety and efficacy in patients with lactic acidosis. Increased PCO_2 after bicarbonate administration may translate into an acute decrease in intracellular pH (pHi), since CO_2 equilibrates across cell membranes more rapidly than bicarbonate. Indeed, several animal studies have demonstrated a fall in pHi in the liver and in muscle following bicarbonate administration although this effect has not been seen in all studies. The rationale for bicarbonate use is to mitigate the adverse hemodynamic consequences of acidemia. Animal studies in numerous models have shown bicarbonate to be no more effective than saline in improving cardiac output, mean arterial pressure, or left ventricular contractility. In patients with lactic acidosis, bicarbonate effectively increases bicarbonate levels and arterial pH, but does not improve cardiac output, mean arterial pressure, or any other relevant hemodynamic parameter (5,6). In mechanically ventilated patients with acute lung injury being ventilated with a lung protection strategy, bicarbonate lowers the pH,

Table 5. Etiologies of Lactic Acidosis

Increased Oxygen Consumption
    Strenuous exercise
    Grand mal seizure
    Neuroleptic malignant syndrome
    Severe asthma
    Pheochromocytoma
Decreased Oxygen Delivery
    Decreased cardiac output
        Hypovolemia
        Cardiogenic shock (including pericardial and pulmonary vascular disease)
    Decreased arterial oxygen content
        Profound anemia
        Severe hypoxemia
    Regional ischemia (mesentery or extremity)
Alterations in Cellular Metabolism
    Sepsis
    Diabetes mellitus, hypoglycemia
    Thiamine deficiency
    Severe alkalemia
    Malignancy
    Mitochondrial myopathies
    AIDS?
Toxins and Drugs
    Carbon monoxide
    Ethanol, methanol
    Biguanides, e.g. metformin
    Ethylene glycol, propylene glycol
    Salicylates
    Isoniazid
    Streptozocin, nalidixic acid
    Cyanide, nitroprusside
    Papaverine
    Acetaminophen
    Ritodrine
    Terbutaline
    Fructose, sorbitol, xylitol
    Epinephrine, norepinephrine, cocaine
  Zidovudine and other highly active anti-retroviral drugs
    Kombucha tea?
    Propofol?
Congenital
    Glucose-6-phosphatase deficiency
    Fructose-1,6-diphosphatase deficiency
    Pyruvate carboxylase deficiency
    Pyruvate-dehydrogenase (PDH) deficiency
    Oxidative phosphorylation defects
Decreased Lactate Clearance
    Fulminant hepatic failure
d-Lactate
    Short gut syndrome
    Antibiotic-induced

largely because carbon dioxide excretion cannot be augmented in the face of limited ventilation and PCO_2 rises significantly (7). Alternative alkalinizing treatments (dialysis, THAM) are largely untested. THAM is effective in raising blood pH when bicarbonate is not (7), but whether this is beneficial is unknown.

The decision whether to use bicarbonate is a difficult one. It is the choice between a long-standing but unproven therapy with potential deleterious effects, and reliance on limited studies; neither is an entirely satisfactory choice. The debate will most likely continue until additional trials of bicarbonate therapy are conducted. With respect to the primary rationale for bicarbonate use, improvement in cardiovascular function, bicarbonate has shown no benefit. Because of the lack of data supporting bicarbonate use in human beings and the arguments reviewed above, I do not recommend the use of bicarbonate in lactic acidosis, *regardless of the pH* (8).

Metabolic Alkalosis

Metabolic alkalosis is characterized by a primary increase in the bicarbonate concentration and a compensatory increase in the PCO_2. The fact that patients will hypoventilate to compensate for metabolic alkalosis, even unto hypoxemia, is often not fully appreciated (9). For a metabolic alkalosis to persist there must be both a process that elevates serum bicarbonate concentration (generally gastric or renal loss) and a stimulus for renal bicarbonate reabsorption (typically hypovolemia, hypokalemia, or mineralocorticoid excess. The major causes of metabolic alkalosis in the ICU—vomiting, nasogastric suction, diuretics, corticosteroids, and overventilation of patients with chronically increased bicarbonate levels—are obvious (when present) from a patient's history and medication list. A careful search of all substances given to the patient is needed to disclose administration of compounds, such as citrate with blood products, and acetate in parenteral nutrition, that can raise the bicarbonate level. If the etiology is not clear, a trial of volume and chloride replacement, as well as correction of hypokalemia, can be attempted.

Table 6. Etiologies of Metabolic Alkalosis

Chloride-Responsive
    Renal H+ loss
        Diuretic therapy
        Posthypercapnia
        Penicillin, ampicillin, carbenicillin
        therapy
    Gastrointestinal H^+ losses
        Vomiting, nasogastric suction
        Villous adenoma, congenital
        chloridorrhea
        Watery diarrhea hypokalemia
        achlorhydria syndrome (VIPoma,
        pancreatic cholera)
    Alkali administration
        Bicarbonate
        Citrate in blood products
        Acetate in TPN
        Nonabsorbable alkali [$Mg(OH)_2$,
        $Al(OH)_3$] and exchange resins
Chloride-Resistant
    Increased mineralocorticoid activity
        Primary aldosteronism
        Cushing's syndrome
        Drugs with mineralocorticoid activity
    Profound hypokalemia
    Refeeding
    Bartter's syndrome
    Parathyroid disease
    Hypercalcemia

If this does not effect an improvement in the alkalosis, a search for increased mineralocorticoids may be warranted. The etiologies of metabolic alkalosis are listed in Table 6.

In patients who require continued diuresis but exhibit rising bicarbonate levels, acetazolamide can be used to reduce the bicarbonate level. When rapid correction of severe alkalosis is desired hemodialysis or hydrochloric acid infusion (0.1 to 0.2 *N* infused into a central vein at 20-50mEq/h with arterial pH monitored every hour) can be instituted.

Respiratory Acidosis

Respiratory acidosis is characterized by a primary increase in the arterial PCO_2 and a compensatory increase in the bicarbonate concentration. Respiratory acidosis represents ventilatory failure or disordered central control of ventilation, the pathophysiology, etiology, and treatment of which are described elsewhere. In mechanically ventilated patients with hypercapnia, it is important to consider the consequences of attempting to raise the minute ventilation. In many, normalizing the PCO_2 comes at the cost of alveolar overdistention (volutrauma) or exacerbation of autoPEEP. The point here is that normalizing the PCO_2 comes at a cost, that cost being volutrauma or frank barotrauma. The experience with permissive hypercapnia for patients with ARDS or status asthmaticus (10), in which hypercapnia and acidemia are tolerated in order to avoid alveolar overdistention, has changed many clinicians perspective about the adverse impact of acidemia. In sedated and ventilated patients with ARDS, rapid intentional hypoventilation (pH falling from 7.40 to 7.26 in 30-60 min) lowered systemic vascular resistance while cardiac output rose. Mean systemic arterial pressure and pulmonary vascular resistance were unchanged. Further, in many studies of patients undergoing permissive hypercapnia, a pH of well below 7.2 was tolerated well. The feared consequences of acidemia, projected from the experience with patients having lactic acidosis (and, usually, concomitant sepsis), failed to materialize. With data now available for many patients permissively hypoventilated, the systemic hemodynamic effects are quite small even as the pH falls to 7.15, with the typical patient experiencing no change or small increases in cardiac output and blood pressure. Patients whose pH falls far below 7.0 are fewer in number, so firm conclusions cannot be drawn, but they similarly tolerate their acidemia. The current practice of permissive hypercapnia does not generally include an attempt to alkalinize the blood to compensate for respiratory acidosis.

When the ventilator is used to correct respiratory acidosis, the end-inspiratory plateau and autoPEEP pressures should be monitored routinely to detect any adverse effects of ventilation.

Respiratory Alkalosis

Respiratory alkalosis is characterized by a primary reduction in the arterial PCO_2. Respiratory alkalosis is very common in the ICU and its causes range from benign (simple anxiety) to life-threatening (sepsis or pulmonary embolism). Distinguishing those respiratory alkaloses that are manifestations of serious disease requires a thorough clinical review. The etiologies of respiratory alkalosis are listed in Table 7.

The primary treatment of respiratory alkalosis is treatment of the underlying cause of hyperventilation. The alkalemia itself generally does not require treatment. In cases where a severe alkalemia is present—generally, when a respiratory alkalosis is superimposed on a metabolic alkalosis—sedation may be necessary. In sepsis, where a significant portion of cardiac output can go to the respiratory muscles, intubation and muscle relaxation are occasionally used to control hyperventilation and redirect blood flow.

Table 7. Etiologies of Respiratory Alkalosis

Hypoxia
    High altitude
    Pulmonary disease
    Decreased $F\underline{i}O_2$
    Profound anemia
Increased CNS Respiratory Drive
    Anxiety, pain, and voluntary hyperventilation
    CNS disease (CVA, tumor, infection, trauma)
    Fever, sepsis, and endotoxin
    Drugs (salicylates, catecholamines, progesterone) analeptics, doxapram
    Hyperthyroidism
    Liver disease
    Pregnancy, progesterone
    Epinephrine
    Exercise
Pulmonary Disorders
    Pneumonia
    Pulmonary embolism
    Restrictive lung disease
    Pulmonary edema
    Bronchospasm
    Pleural effusion
    Pneumothorax
Mechanical Ventilation

REFERENCES

1. Stewart PA: How to understand acid-base: a quantitative acid-base primer for biology and medicine. Elsevier, New York, 1981
   This outstanding text, now out of print, develops acid-base medicine from the ground up, replacing the unwieldy "bicarbonate-based" approach with a more accurate and computationally amenable method. Describes the determinants of the pH: the difference in the concentrations of strong ions (the [SID]); the total concentration of weak acids (Atot); and the PCO₂.

2. Fencl V, Jabor A, Kazda A, et al: Diagnosis of metabolic acid-base disturbances in critically ill patients. *Am J Respir Crit Care Med* 2000; 162:2246-51
   Compared two commonly used diagnostic approaches, one relying on plasma bicarbonate concentration and "anion gap," the other on "base excess," with Peter Stewart's approach, for their value in detecting complex metabolic acid-base disturbances. Of 152 patients, one-sixth had normal base excess and plasma bicarbonate. In a great majority of these apparently normal samples, the Stewart method detected simultaneous presence of acidifying and alkalinizing disturbances, many of them grave. The almost ubiquitous hypoalbuminemia confounded the interpretation of acid-base data when the customary approaches were applied.

3. Thorens J-B, Jolliet P, Ritz M, et al: Effects of rapid permissive hypercapnia on hemodynamics, gas exchange, and oxygen transport and consumption during mechanical ventilation for the acute respiratory distress syndrome. *Intensive Care Med* 1996; 22:182-191
   Describes the hemodynamic effects of acute respiratory acidosis in patients with ARDS, showing that permissive hypercapnia is well-tolerated.

4. Feihl F, Perret C: Permissive hypercapnia: how permissive should we be? *Am J Respir Crit Care Med* 1994; 150:1722-37
Commentary regarding the potential risks of permissive hypercapnia.

5. Cooper DJ, Walley KR, Wiggs BR, Russell JA: Bicarbonate does not improve hemodynamics in critically ill patients who have lactic acidosis: A prospective controlled clinical study. *Ann Intern Med* 1990; 112:492
Well-controlled study in patients with septic lactic acidosis, almost all of whom were on catecholamines, directly addressing the role of bicarbonate in these patients. These investigators showed that bicarbonate was no different thant control with respect to any relevant hemodynamic parameter, despite the known catecholamine unresponsiveness during acidemia.

6. Mathieu D, Neviere R, Billard V, et al: Effects of bicarbonate therapy on hemodynamics and tissue oxygenation in patients with lactic acidosis: A prospective, controlled clinical study. *Crit Care Med* 1991; 19:1352
Another study demonstrating the lack of efficacy of bicarbonate with regards to any hemodynamic benefit.

7. Kallet RH, Jasmer RM, Luce JM, et al: The treatment of acidosis in acute lung injury with tris-hydroxymethyl aminomethane (THAM). *Am J Respir Crit Care Med* 2000; 161:1149
Patients mechanically ventilated for acute lung injury who also had significant metabolic acidosis were given THAM. Arterial pH rose and PCO_2 fell, in contrast to the effects of sodium bicarbonate (which lowered the pH and raised the PCO_2).

8. Forsythe SM, Schmidt GA: Sodium bicarbonate for the treatment of lactic acidosis. *Chest* 2000; 117:260-67 *Critically reviews the clinical and laboratory data regarding bicarbonate therapy for metabolic acidosis, concluding that bicarbonate should not be given routinely for lactic acidosis, no matter what the pH.*

9. Javaheri S, Kazemi H: Metabolic alkalosis and hypoventilation in humans. *Am Rev Respir Dis* 1987; 136:1011-6
Study of patients with metabolic alkalosis showing that compensatory respiratory acidosis is a predictable response, even when the PO2 falls significantly.

10. Tuxen DV, Williams TJ, Scheinkestel CD, et al: Use of a measurement of pulmonary hyperinflation to control the level of mechanical ventilation in patients with acute severe asthma. *Am Rev Respir Dis* 1992; 146:1136-42
Key study validating the approach of intentionally hypoventilating patients with status asthmaticus to avoid the consequences of barotraumas.

ELECTROLYTE DISORDERS: DISORDERS OF SERUM SODIUM, CALCIUM, MAGNESIUM, AND POTASSIUM

Richard S. Muther, MD

Objectives

- To review the basic physiology affecting sodium, water, calcium, magnesium, and potassium balance
- To recognize the common critical care syndromes and causes of deranged serum cations
- To become facile with the acute treatment of disordered cation balance

Key Words: hypo/hyperosmolality; hypo/hypernatremia; hypo/hypercalcemia; hypo/hypermagnesemia; hypo/hyperkalemia

TABLE OF ABBREVIATIONS

ACE	angiotensin-converting enzyme
ANP	atrial natriuretic peptide
AV	atrioventricular
CHF	congestive heart failure
DI	diabetes insipidus
ECF	extracellular fluid
ECV	extracellular fluid volume
FEMg	fractional excretion of magnesium
FE Na	fractional excretion of sodium
GFR	glomerular filtration rate
GI	gastrointestinal
H^+	hydrogen ion
H_{GC}	transglomerular capillary hydrostatic pressure
JVD	jugular venous distention
K_f	permeability of glomerular capillary wall
MI	myocardial infarction
π_{GC}	transglomerular capillary oncotic pressure
PTH	parathyroid hormone
PTHrP	parathyroid hormone-related peptides
RTA	renal tubular acidosis
SIADH	syndrome of inappropriate antidiuretic hormone

DISORDERS OF SERUM SODIUM

Osmolality is the number of osmotically active particles (osmoles) per liter of solution. Osmolarity is expressed per kilogram. Osmolality is most useful as a measure of water balance, such that hypoosmolality indicates an excess of water; hyperosmolality indicates water deficiency (1, 2). The serum osmolality can be calculated by the following formula: Serum osmolality (mOsm/L) = 2 (Na + K) + (glucose / 18) + (urea / 2.8), where Na is sodium and K is potassium; 18 and 2.8 are derived from the conversion of mg/dL to mOsm/L.

One can see that serum osmolality is primarily due to the serum concentration of sodium and potassium (and their accompanying anions), glucose and urea. Of these, the serum sodium is most powerful, accounting for nearly 95% of serum osmolality. Therefore, in most clinical circumstances, the serum sodium can be used as a surrogate for osmolality and, therefore, an indicator of water balance. The serum sodium has no direct relationship to the total body sodium.

Tonicity refers to the force (ability to move water across a semipermeable membrane) exerted by osmotically active particles. Hypotonic solutions will lose water to, and hypertonic solutions will gain water from an isotonic solution. Not all osmoles are equivalent in tonicity. Urea, for example, readily crosses cell membranes and exerts no tonic force. Glucose will induce water movement from most cells. However, the major extracellular osmole sodium is responsible for the variation in serum tonicity in most cases, and, as such, is largely responsible for the volume of extracellular fluid (ECV). Therefore, an excess of body sodium causes water movement into the extracellular space and obligates an increase in ECV, although not an increase in sodium concentration.

Hyponatremia is not always equivalent to hypoosmolality (Figure 1). By stimulating water movement into the ECV, hyperglycemia physiologically lowers serum sodium (by 1.6 mEq/100 mg/dL glucose), causing hyponatremia with hyperosmolality. The same is true for hypertonic mannitol. Other molecules increasing serum osmolality (e.g., ethanol, isopropyl alcohol, ethylene glycol, and methanol) do not cause hyponatremia because of their small size and high membrane permeability. They will, however, cause an osmolar gap (a differemce of > 20 mOsm between the calculated and measured serum osmolality). Hyperproteinemia (usually > 10 g/dL) and hyperlipidemia produce an increase in the solid phase of the blood volume, causing "hyponatremia," as the sodium present is indexed to an artificially increased volume. The serum osmolality does not change. These "pseudohyponatremias" usually account

for small changes in serum sodium (e.g., 1 mEq of sodium/460 mg/dL of lipid). In most clinical situations, however, the serum sodium is directly related to the serum osmolality, such that hyponatremia indicates an excess and hypernatremia indicates a deficiency of water relative to total body sodium..

Regulation of Sodium Balance

As the major extracellular cation and osmole, sodium determines ECV. Changes in total body sodium are reflected as changes in the ECV and are best assessed by physical findings (Figure 2). Therefore, rales, jugular venous distention (JVD), edema, and an S3 gallop, indicate excess ECV and body sodium. Tachycardia, hypotension, dry mucous membranes, and skin tenting indicate ECV and body sodium depletion. In neither case will the serum sodium concentration necessarily change. Thus, the total body sodium or ECV has no direct relationship with the serum sodium concentration.

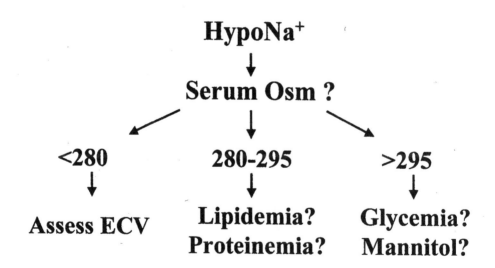

Figure 1. The serum osmolality helps distinguish the "pseudohyponatremias" in the hyponatremic patient. If the serum osmolality and serum sodium are both low, assessing the extracellular fluid volume (ECV) provides diagnostic help (see Table 1).

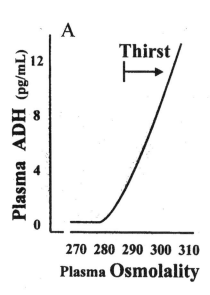 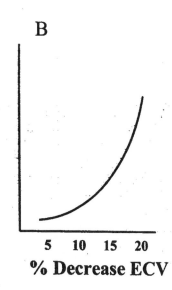

Figure 2. Increasing plasma osmolality (*A*) and decreasing extracellular fluid volume (ECV) (*B*) stimulate ADH secreation and thirst.

Dietary sodium intake is balanced by gastrointestinal (GI) and renal sodium loss. The renal excretion of sodium is dependent on the glomerular filtration rate (GFR), aldosterone, and a variety of "third factors," which affect renal tubular resorption of filtered sodium. These include natriuretic peptides (ANP), the renin angiotensin system, norepinephrine, prostaglandins, and intraglomerular and peritubular Starling forces. The GFR, in turn, is dependent on renal blood flow, the transglomerular capillary hydrostatic (H_{GC}), oncotic (π_{GC}) pressures, and the permeability (K_f) of the glomerular capillary wall. Intraglomerular Starling forces (H_{GC} and π_{GC}) are largely determined by the afferent and efferent glomerular arteriolar sphincters. Aldosterone enhances distal tubular sodium resorption coupled to hydrogen ion (H^+) and potassium secretion. Normally, $\sim$ 99% of filtered sodium is resorbed. The 1% excreted sodium is best measured by the fractional excretion of sodium (FENa).

Regulation of Water Balance

Thirst, antidiuretic hormone (ADH), and the kidneys control water balance. Hypothalamic receptors for hyperosmolality and hypovolemia stimulate thirst and ADH secretion (Figure 2). While hypoosmolality is the more common stimulus, hypovolemia is more potent. For example, the hypovolemic patient will continue to secrete ADH despite hypoosmolality and hyponatremia. ADH exerts its primary effect by enhancing and allowing renal water resorption across the collecting tubule, thus concentrating the urine (Figure 3). This passive resorption of water is dependent on the presence of a more highly concentrated renal medullary interstitium caused by active sodium and chloride resorption from the ascending limb of Henle. Sodium (but not water) resorption from the late ascending limb and early distal tubule dilutes the filtrate and generates free water. Free water excretion occurs in the absence of ADH. Both the GFR and proximal tubular resorption rate affect free water excretion (urine dilution) and resorption (urine concentration), as these factors control the quantity of glomerular filtrate delivered to the downstream nephron segments.

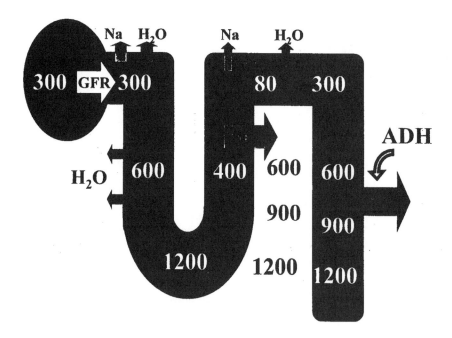

Figure 3. Renal handling of water. Water reabsorption (urine concentration) depends on the presence of ADH and a concentrated medullary interstitium due to active Na and Cl reabsorption in the ascending limb. Water excretion occurs in the absence of ADH as sodium, but no water is absorbed from the ascending limb and distal tubule (urine dilution). GFR and proximal tubular reabsorbtion affect both concentration and dilution by controlling the delivery of filtrate in the downstream nephron segments.

Clinical Disorders of Sodium Balance
(Disorders of the ECV)

Hemorrhage, GI (vomiting and/or diarrhea), or renal sodium loss depletes the ECV. Hypoaldosteronism, diuretics, or renal tubular defects decreasing sodium resorption (e.g., Bartter's syndrome, "salt-losing" nephropathy, and rarely, renal tubular acidosis [RTA]), are the usual causes of renal sodium loss. The volume lost in these cases is approximately isosmolar so that serum sodium concentration does not change. Patients manifest signs of ECV depletion on physical examination. Basic fluid therapy is isotonic saline. Accompanying potassium and acid-base disorders are outlined in Table 1.

Renal failure (decreased GFR), hyperaldosteronism or enhanced renal tubular sodium resorption due to congestive heart failure (CHF), cirrhosis with ascites, or nephrotic syndrome are the common causes of ECV excess and are termed the "edematous disorders." Physical findings of ECV excess (rales, JVD, edema) are usually present. When mild, the serum sodium is usually normal in these syndromes. Basic fluid therapy is salt and water restriction.

Clincal Disorders of
Water Balance: Hyponatremia

As a surrogate for serum osmolality, the serum sodium reflects changes in water balance relative to total body sodium. Therefore, after excluding pseudohyponatremias, one can best approach hyponatremia based on the patient's ECV (Figure 4; Table 1).

Hyponatremia can occur with ECV depletion when free water intake accompanies GI or renal sodium loss. The most common example is diuretic-associated hyponatremia. Although usually mild, severe hyponatremia can occur, particularly with polydipsic patients and those with significant hypokalemia. ECV depletion appropriately stimulates ADH

Table 1. Differential diagnosis of hyponatremia and hypoosmolality.

ECV	Hypovolemia (↓ ECV)		Euvolemia (Normal ECV)		Hypervolemia (↑ECV)
Diagnoses	Vomiting Diarrhea Fistula	Diuretics Hypoaldo RTA "Salt losing"	Polydipsia Malnutrition	SIADH Hypothyroid Hypocortisol	CHF Cirrhosis/Ascites Nephrotic syndrome Renal failure
U_{osm} mOsm/L	>300	300	<100	>100	>300*
U_{na} mEq/L	<20	>20	>30	>30	<10*
Other findings	Hypokalemia: Vomiting, diarrhea, diuretics, RTA Hyperkalemia: Hypoaldo Met Alk: Vomiting, diuretics Met Acid: Diarrhea, Hypoaldo		Hypokalemia: SIADH, polydipsia Hyperkalemia: Hypocortisol Hypouricemia		
Fluid Rx	Isotonic Saline		Restrict H_2O		Restrict H_2O and saline

Abbreviations: ECV,extracellular volume; SIADH, syndrome of inappropriate antidiuretic hormone; CHF, congestive heart failure; U_{osm}, urine Osmolality; U_{na},urine sodium; RTA, renal tubular acidosis; Met Alk, metabolic alkalosis; Met Acid, metabolic acidosis; Rx, therapy.

* Excludes renal failure.

secretion and water resorption, contributing to the hyponatremia. The syndrome is much more commonly seen with thiazides than with loop diuretics. Thiazides limit free water excretion by inhibiting distal tubular sodium resorption. Loop diuretics gradually diminish medullary interstitial solute and osmolarity, thereby limiting the osmolar gradient for water resorption. Elderly females and patients on nonsteroidal anti-inflammatory drugs are particularly prone to thiazide-induced hyponatremia. Treatment is to discontinue thiazides, restrict water, and replace potassium. Isotonic saline is indicated for those patients with moderate-to-severe volume depletion. Care must be taken to avoid a too-rapid correction of hyponatremia, since ADH secretion is abrogated as saline is replaced.

Other examples of hyponatremia with ECV depletion include GI disorders, osmotic diuretics, "salt-losing" nephropathies, proximal RTA, hypoaldosteronism, and ketonuria.

Hyponatremia with a normal ECV occurs with extreme polydipsia (psychogenic polydipsia) or the syndrome of inappropriate ADH (SIADH). In normal patients, 10 to 15 L of water intake is required to cause significant hyponatremia. However, hyponatremia occurs with significantly less water intake if ADH secretion is stimulated or if its renal tubular effect is enhanced by certain drugs (Table 2).

SIDAH refers to euvolemic (no edema) patients with hypoosmolality and high urine osmolality (less than maximally dilute urine osmolality or > 100 mOsm/L), hyponatremia, and increased urine sodium (> 30 mEq/L). Because ADH secretion or action is enhanced by hypothyroidism and cortisol deficiency, excluding these diagnoses is prerequisite to the diagnosis of SIDAH. The differential diagnosis of SIDAH is outlined in Table 3.

Hyponatremia often accompanies the edematous disorders, particularly CHF. The decrease in "effective" intravascular volume stimulates thirst, increases ADH secretion, limits GFR, and enhances proximal renal tubular resorption of sodium and water. The result is increased intake and limited excretion of free water. Hyponatremia is a marker of the severity of CHF. Hyponatremia is also commonly seen in

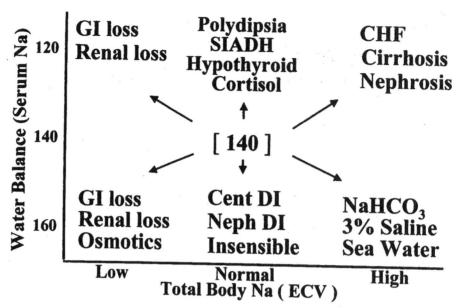

Figure 4. Differential diagnosis of hypo- and hypernatriemia based on water balance relative to total body sodium (ECV). See Tables 1 and 4 for additional details.

patients with cirrhosis (particularly those with ascites) and nephrotic syndrome. The urine sodium is low (< 30 mEq/L), and the urine osmolarity is high (> 300 mOsm/L), mimicking ECV depletion, although with very different physical findings. Basic fluid therapy for these disorders is salt and water restriction with diuretics.

Clinical Disorders of Water Balance: Hypernatremia

Because thirst provides excellent protection against hyperosmolality, hypernatremia is unusual unless access to water is impaired. Therefore, hypernatremic patients are usually elderly, have a decreased mental status, or are in some way incapacitated. The fact that hypernatremia mandates hypertonicity ensures cellular dehydration, particularly of the brain. Therefore, hypernatremic patients are usually quite ill. Since hypernatremia is synonymous with hyperosmolality, a water deficit relative to salt is always present. Therefore, an approach to the hypernatremic patient, based on his/her salt balance (ECV) is appropriate (Table 4; Figure 4).

Hypernatremia in patients with decreased ECV occurs with osmotic cathartics and diuretics. The osmotic effect ensures that water will be lost in excess of sodium and potassium (because of the presence of some other osmole). This water diuresis occurs with lactulose or sorbitol in the intestinal tract or in the urine with hyperglycemia, mannitol, low-molecular weight proteins (from hyperalimentation) and urea (postobstructive diuresis). The osmotic effect also causes variable salt depletion. Fluid therapy for these patients, therefore, requires water (to correct the free water deficit) and isotonic saline (to correct the decreased ECV).

Euvolemia with hypernatremia indicates isolated loss of free water. Free water loss can occur with massive insensible losses such as severe sweating or hyperventilation, or rarely, with primary hypodipsia. The most common cause of euvolemic hypernatremia, however, is diabetes insipidus (DI). These patients have an inappropriately low ADH level (central DI) or a blunted ADH effect (nephrogenic DI). The urine osmolality is inappropriately low (< 300

Table 2. Factors affecting the secretion or action of antidiuretic hormone (ADH)

Stimulate ADH Secretion	*Inhibit ADH Secretion*
Hyperosmolarity	Hypoosmolality
Hypovolemia	Hypervolemia
Pain/stress	Drugs
Nausea	Ethanol
Pregnancy	Phenytoin
Drugs	
Nicotine	*Enhance ADH Effect*
Morphine sulfate	Psychosis
Cyclophosphamide	Drugs
Vincristine/vinblastine	Chlorpropamide
Chlorpropamide	Carbamazepine
Thiothixene	Nonsteroidals
Thioridizine	Tolbutamide
Haldoperidol	
Amitriptylline	
MAO inhibitors	
Bromcriptine	

MAO, monoamine oxidase.

Table 3. Etiologies of syndrome of inappropriate antidiuretic hormone

CNS:	CVA, meningitis, encephalitis, trauma, psychosis, primary or metabolic tumors
Tumor:	Small cell lung, other lung, duodenal, pancreas neuroblastoma
Pulmonary:	Pneumonia, atelectasis, pheumonthorax, tuberculosis
Major Surgery:	Abdominal, thoracic, transphenoidal
Drugs:	See Table 2

CNS, central nervous system; CVA, cerebrovascular accident.

mOsm/L), despite hypernatremia. Patients with central DI will respond to parenteral administration of ADH by increasing urine osmolality and decreasing urine volume. Both central and nephrogenic DI can occur in either partial or complete forms and, therefore, a broad range of urine osmolalities following water deprivation or ADH. The differential diagnosis of both central and nephrogenic DI is shown in Table 5.

The rarest clinical salt and water problem is hypernatremia with increased ECV. Hypervolemic hypernatremia occurs with massive administration of hypertonic bicarbonate, hypertonic saline, or rarely, in those with salt-water ingestion. The urine osmolality is high and the patients are appropriately excreting increased urine sodium. Treatment is required to restrict the salt and administer free water and diuretics as needed.

Treatment Issues

The serum osmolality is the major determinant of brain water and, therefore, brain volume (Figure 5). Abrupt hypoosmolality causes brain edema; abrupt hyperosmolality causes brain shrinkage. The more rapidly the osmolality changes, the more likely symptoms will occur and the more urgent is the need for therapy. Over time (48-72 hours), adaptation to changes in osmolality occurs. With hypoosmolality, the brain loses electrolytes (osmolytes), thus lowering intracellular osmolality to that of plasma. With hyperosmolality, the brain will generate osmoles (idiogenic osmoles), thus increasing intracellular osmolality. Both adaptations tend to return brain volume toward normal, and a new steady state is reached. Any subsequent changes in plasma osmolality (e.g., those induced by therapy) will cause brain swelling or shrinkage once again. Potential complications of this include altered

Table 4. Differential diagnosis of hypernatremia.

ECV	Hypovolemia (↓ ECV)		Euvolemia (Normal ECV)		Hypervolemia (↑ECV)
Diagnoses	**GI loss:** Vomiting Diarrhea Fistula	**Renal Loss:** Hyperglycemia Mannitol High protein feedings Postobstructive diuesis	Sweating Hypodipsia	Cent DI Neph DI	Hypertonic NaHCO$_3$ Hypertonic saline Sea water ingestion
U$_{osm}$ mOsm/L	>800	300-800	>800	<300*	>800
U$_{na}$ mEq/L	<20	>30	<20	<20	>30
Other findings	Hypokalemia: Vomiting, diarrhea, diuresis Met Alk: Vomiting			U$_{osm}$ after AVP: Cent: 400-800* Neph: No Δ	
Fluid Rx	Combined water and saline		Water		Water

Abbreviations: ECV, extracellular volume; GI, gastrointestinal; Cent DI, central diabetes insipidus; Neph DI, nephrogenic diabetes insipidus; U$_{osm}$, urine osmolality; U$_{na}$, urine Na; AVP, acqueous vasopressin 5 units subcutaneously; Met Alk, metabolic alkalosis; Rx, therapy.

*Urine osmolality varies with partial vs complete DI.

mental status, seizures, coma, or the most serious complication, central pontine myelinolysis. Therefore, slow correction is the rule for severe degrees of either hypo- or hypernatremia.

For asymptomatic patients with hyponatremia, simple water restriction and observation are adequate. If the patient is hyponatremic and ECV is depleted, isotonic saline can be given. Again, since ADH secretion is volume-sensitive, too rapid a correction can occur as saline is administered; thus, frequent monitoring of serum sodium is required. For patients severely symptomatic with hyponatremia, hypertonic (3%) saline is indicated to increase the serum sodium by no more than 0.5 to 1 mEq/L/hr and no more than 12 mEq/L in a 24-hour period. One can calculate the sodium deficit in these patients as follows: Na deficit = (desired Na − current Na) x 0.6 body weight (kg).

For example, a 70-kg male with a serum sodium of 103 mEq/L would need 504 mEq sodium to increase his serum sodium to 115 mEq/L. This is ~ 3.3 L of isotonic saline (154 mEq/L) or ~ 1 L of 3% saline (513 mEq/L). Again, close observation for too rapid a correction or signs of fluid overload is mandatory in these patients.

For hypernatremia, the water deficit can be calculated as follows: Water deficit = (current Na / target Na) −1 x 0.6 body weight (kg).

For example, a 60-kg male with a serum sodium of 175 mEq/L needs 9 L free water to correct his serum sodium to 140 mEq/L ([175 / 140]) − 1 x 36 L = 9 L). As with hyponatremia, correction should not exceed 0.5 to 1 mEq/L per hour and not more than 12 mEq/L in a 24-hour period in severely hypernatremic patients.

DISORDERS OF SERUM CALCIUM

Calcium, magnesium, and potassium share several features. All are cations with large intracellular stores in dynamic equilibrium with extremely small extracellular fluid (ECF) pools. The amount of each that is absorbed from the GI

Table 5. Differential diagnosis of central andnephrogenic diabetes insipidus (DI)

Central DI	*Nephrogenic DI*
Trauma	Hypercalcemia
Neurosurgery	Hypokalemia
CVA	Tubular Cell Disease
Primary or metastatic tumor	Interstitial nephritis
Granulomata	Sickle cell disease/trait
Familial	Polycystic kidney disease
Drugs	Amyloidosis
Phenytoin	Sarcoidosis
Alcohol	Drugs
	Amphotericin
	Cis platinum
	Demeclocycline
	Glyburide
	Ifosfamide
	Lithium
	Propoxyphene

CVA, cerebrovascular accident.

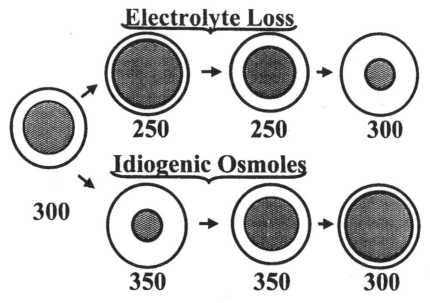

Figure 5. Brain swellilng or shrinkage occurs in response to sudden changes in serum osmolality (represented by the numbers below each diagram). Over time, the brain adapts to hypoosmolarity (top panel) by losing electrolytes; to huperosmolality (bottom panel) by generating osmoles, creating a new steady state at 250 or 350 mOsm/L, respectively. The far right diagram represents the reverse.

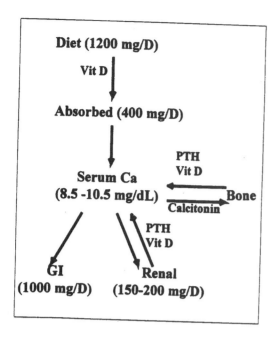

Figure 6. Calcium balance.

tract and excreted by the kidneys daily is a relatively small percentage of total body stores. While the serum concentrations of calcium, magnesium, and potassium may vary with changes in intake and renal excretion, it is primarily the shift into and out of the large intracellular storage pool that accounts for the major clinical derangements of these ions. Therefore, understanding the factors which control this cellular shift is critical to understanding not only the causes, but also the treatment of these electrolyte disorders (3–6).

Calcium balance is depicted in Figure 6 and Table 6. Approximately 400 mg (30% to 35% of an average daily intake of 1200 mg) is absorbed from the intestinal tract. Daily excretion of this amount occurs in the urine and stool (150 to 200 mg/day in each). Vitamin D is the major factor controlling absorption. The fat-soluble vitamin D_3 is absorbed from the diet, 25-hydroxylated in the liver (to calcefediol) and 1-hydroxylated by the kidney to 1,25 dihydroxy vitamin D (calcitriol), the active form of the vitamin. The formation of calcitriol is primarily stimulated by parathyroid hormone (PTH) and hypophosphatemia. Malabsorption, liver disease, and renal disease may cause vitamin D deficiency.

PTH preserves serum calcium by stimulating osteoclast resorption of bone. Vitamin D is a cofactor in this process. PTH also preserves serum calcium by directly increasing renal tubular resorption of filtered calcium. Finally, PTH enhances intestinal calcium absorption by stimulating the production of calcitriol. PTH secretion is stimulated by ionized hypocalcemia and suppressed by hypercalcemia and hypomagnesemia.

Table 6. Parameters of cation balance.

	Ca	Mg	K
Molecular weight	40	24	39
Normal serum:			
mg/dL	8.5-10.5	1.6-2.4	—
m/M	2.1-2.6	0.6-1.0	—
mEq/L	4.2-5.2	1.2-2.0	3.5-5.0
Ionized fraction	45%	55%	
Daily intake	1200 mg	360 mg	100 mEq
GI absorption	400 mg	120 mg	100 mEq
Renal excretion	150-200 mg	120 mg	90 mEq
GI losses	1000 mg	240 mg	10 mEq
Tissue stores (%)	1200 g (99)	25 g (98)	3500 mEq (98)
ECF (%)	0.9 g (1)	0.5 g (2) 7	0 mEq (2)

Ca, calcium; Mg, magnesium; K, potassium; GI, gastrointestinal; ECF, extracellular fluid.

Table 7. Common clinical conditions which dissociate total (T Ca) and ionized (I Ca) calcium (parentheses include the quantitative formula)

Condition	TCa	ICa	Explanation
Hypoalbuminemia	↓ (Δ Alb 1.0 g/dL = Δ Ca 0.8 mg/dL)	N	Decreased binding protein
Hyperalbuminemia	↑ (Δ Alb 1.0 g/dL = Δ Ca 0.8 mg/dL)	N	Increased binding protein
Multiple myeloma	↑	N	Calcium binding to globulin
Respiratory alkalosis	N (Δ H 0.1 = Δ ICa++ 0.16 mg/dL)	↓	Increased albumin binding
Hyperparathyroidism	N	↑	Decreased albumin binding
Hyperphosphatmia	N-↓	↓	Chelation; also true with citrate and lactate

N, No change.

It is primarily the combined action of PTH and vitamin D on bone which controls serum calcium. In the blood, ~ 40% to 50% of calcium is in the ionized or physiologically active form. In critically ill patients, total serum calcium is a poor predictor of ionized calcium (3). Albumin binding, alkalosis, and the presence of chelators such as citrate, phosphate, or lactate can significantly influence the ionized fraction with relatively little alteration of total calcium (Table 7). Pseudohypercalcemia refers to the increase of serum total calcium due to hyperalbuminemia. Similarly, low levels of serum albumin will lower serum total calcium. In neither case will the active or ionized calcium change. This direct relationship of total calcium to albumin can be quantitated: Δalbumin 1 g/dL = Δ total calcium 0.8 g/dL. Direct measurement of ionized calcium by ion-specific electrodes may be necessary in certain cases

Hypercalcemia

Hypercalcemia (Table 8) can occur with excessive GI absorption (milk alkali syndrome, excess vitamin D) or with increased renal resorption of filtered calcium (hyperparathyroidism, thiazides). However, clinically significant hypercalcemia most often occurs with accelerated bone resorption (7). In hyperparathyroidism, direct osteoclast activation by PTH causes hypercalcemia. Various osteolytic factors (PTH or PTH-related peptides

[PTHrP],IL-1, IL-6, TNF, calcitriol) can also be produced by several malignancies (lung, ovary, kidney, bladder) (8). Osteoclast-activating factor, produced by myeloma cells, also causes hypercalcemia. Hypercalcemia caused by direct lytic involvement of bone is seen with breast and prostate cancers. Immobilization can cause hypercalcemia by increasing bone resorption, particularly in young patients or those with

Table 8. Common causes of hypercalcemia.

Increased Gastrointestinal Absorption
    Vitamin D intoxication
    Ectopic Vitamin D
        Sarcoidosis
        Tuberculosis
        Histoplasmosis
        Lymphoma
    Milk alkali syndrome

Increased Bone Absorption
    Hyperparathyroidism
    Ectopic PTH, PTHrP
    Osteolytic metastases
    Multiple myeloma (OAF)
    Immobilization
    Posthypocalcemic (rhabdomyolysis)

Increased Renal Resorption
    Hyperparathyroidism
    Thiazide diuretics

PTH, parathyroid hormone; PTHrP, parathyroid hormone-related peptides; OAF, osteoclast-activating factors.

Table 9. Treatment of hypercalcemia

Therapy	Dose	Onset	Duration	Efficacy[a]	Toxicity
Saline (NS)	3 – 6 L/day	Hrs	Hrs	1 – 2 mg/dL	Volume excess
Furosemide	80 – 160 mg/day	Hrs	Hrs	1 – 2 mg/dL	Volume depletion
Hydrocortisone	200 mg/day × 3 – 5 day	Hrs	Days	Mild[b]	Hypertension, hypokalemia, hyperglycemia
Calcitonin	4 – 8 units/kg SC q 6 – 12 hrs	Hrs	Hrs	1 – 2 mg/dL (40% - 60%)	Nausea, thrombopenia
Mithramycin	25 ìg/kg	12 hrs	Days	1 – 5 mg/dL	Bone marrow, hepatic, renal toxicity
Etidronate	7.5 mg/kg/day × 3 – 7 days	1 –2 days	Days – wks	1 – 5 mg/dL (60% - 100%)	Increase creatinine and phosphorus
Pamidronate	30 – 90 mg iv weekly	Days	2 – 4 wks (90% - 100%)	1 – 5 mg/dL	Fever
Gallium	200 mg/m^2/day	Days	Days – wks (70% - 80%)	1 – 5 mg/dL	Fever

NS, normal saline; SC, subcutaneous; iv, intravenously.

[a]Expected decrease in serum calcium; expected response rate in parenthese; [b]effective for hypercalcemia of vitamin D, sarcoid, myeloma, lymphoma.

Paget's disease. Finally, hypercalcemia is common in the recovery phase of rhabdomyolysis-induced acute renal failure (9).

Severe hypercalcemia (> 14 mg/dL [3.5 mmol/L]) usually requires a combination of factors, including excessive osteoclast-stimulated bone resorption, increased renal tubular calcium resorption (due to PTH, PTHrP, and volume depletion) and immobilization (7). This combination is most often seen in patients with hyperparathyroidism or malignancy in the ICU setting.

The clinical manifestations of hypercalcemia include anorexia, nausea, vomiting, constipation, and abdominal pain. Weakness, lethargy, and obtundation are common. Coma occurs as the serum calcium increases to 16 mg/dL. Polyuria due to nephrogenic DI may produce volume depletion, which in turn stimulates renal tubular calcium resorption and aggravates hypercalcemia. Renal insufficiency is common with acute and/or severe hypercalcemia. A shortened QT interval, bradycardia, and heart block may occur, particularly in patients taking digitalis.

Treatment of mild hypercalcemia (< 12 mg/dL) may only require simple hydration, restricting dietary calcium, and treating the underlying disease (7). As the calcium increases

> 12 mg/dL or the patient becomes symptomatic, specific anticalcemic therapy may be required (Table 9). Intravenous saline (3 to 4 L/day) and furosemide (80 to 160 mg/day) canproduce a modest decrement in serum calcium by enhancing renal calcium excretion (10). When using saline and furosemide, one should achieve a urine output of 150 mL/hr. Corticosteroids (hydrocortisone 200 to 300 mg/day iv or prednisone 40 to 80 mg/day orally) are effective when hypercalcemia is caused by excess vitamin D (vitamin D intoxication, sarcoidosis, lymphomas) or multiple myeloma (11).

More aggressive treatment is required for a serum calcium of > 14 mg/dL. Although relatively weak, calcitonin (4 to 8 U/kg every 6 to 12 hours) can work within hours to lower serum calcium (11). It is also a potent analgesic, and therefore particularly suited to those patients with bone pain. Usually, treatment with mithramycin (25 ìg/kg iv) or the bisphosphonates (etidronate [7.5 mg/kg iv] or pamidronate [30 to 90 mg iv]) will also be necessary. Mithramycin will begin to lower serum calcium within hours; its nadir effect is reached at 48 to 72 hours (12). The effect typically persists for several days, but repeat dosing is often necessary. The effect of etidronate and pamidronate is usually slower but more prolonged with a nadir in serum calcium at 7 days and a duration of several weeks (13). A constant infusion of gallium nitrate (200 mg/m^2/day for 5 days) will normalize serum calcium in 70% to 80% of hypercalcemic patients (14). The onset, however, is relatively slow, and the nadir is usually reached at 8 to 10 days. Use of gallium is limited by its nephrotoxicity. The use of oral (too weak) and intravenous (too dangerous) phosphate is no longer recommended for treatment of hypercalcemia. Hemodialysis or peritoneal dialysis with a zero calcium dialysate is rarely necessary but can be used to treat severe hypercalcemia.

Hypocalcemia

Hypocalcemia (Table 10) can be seen with vitamin D deficiency, PTH deficiency or resistance, or binding by various intravascular or tissue chelators (3). Malabsorption of calcium and vitamin D is most commonly from small-bowel resection or inflammation (e.g., Crohn's disease). Liver disease (decreased synthesis of calcefediol) or renal disease (decreased synthesis of calcitriol) may also cause vitamin D deficiency. Hypoparathyroidism most often occurs post thyroidectomy, but rarely is due to a familial multiglandular condition. Suppression of PTH release is usually due to hypomagnesemia but may accompany severe hypermagnesomia, sepsis, burns, pancreatitis, or rhabdomyolysis. Hypomagnesemia also causes PTH resistance (5). Rapid or massive blood or plasma transfusion may cause calcium chelation by citrate, an effect also seen when citrate is used as an alternative anticoagulant for hemodialysis. The most common calcium chelator, however, is phosphorus; this hypocalcemic syndrome may occur in patients with major tissue damage (burns, rhabdomyolysis), tumor lysis syndrome, or acute and chronic renal failure.

The clinical signs of hypocalcemia include perioral paresthesia, muscular spasms, tetany, and even seizures. Chvostek's and Trousseau's signs do not usually develop unless the serum calcium decreases < 6 mg/dL. Several studies suggest that ionized hypocalcemia and

Table 10. Common causes of hypocalcemia

Decreased GI Absorption
Vitamin D Deficiency
    Malabsorption
    Hepatic failure
    Renal failure
Malabsorption syndromes

Decreased Bone Resorption
    Hypoparathyroidism
        Postthyroidectomy/parathyroidectomy
        Familial
        Hypomagnesemia
        Sepsis
        Burns
        Pacreatitis
        Rhabdomyolysis
    PTH Resistance
        Hypomagnesemia
        Pseudohypoparathyroidism
    Osteoblastic metastases

Intravascular/Tissue Chelation
    Citrate
        Massive transfusion
        Dialysis anticoagulant
    Albumin
    Fatty acids – fat emboli
    Phosphorus
        Burns
        Rhabdomyolysis
    Renal failure
        Tumor lysis

GI, gastrointestinal; PTH, parathyroid hormone.

elevated PTH are associated with an increased mortality (15). Prolongation of the QT interval is common. Bradycardia and hypotension are indications for emergent therapy.

Because treatment of hypocalcemia with calcium alone is only transiently effective, one must identify and correct the underlying cause. Mild or asymptomatic hypocalcemia requires only an increase in dietary calcium. Intravenous calcium (100 to 200 mg iv over 10 minutes followed by 100 mg/hr constant infusion) should be reserved for symptomatic patients or those with serum calcium of < 6 mg/dL. Calcium gluconate (90 mg elemental calcium per 10 mL ampule) is preferred to limit vein irritation and extravasation. Calcium infusion should be avoided in patients with severe hyperphosphatemia. Serum calcium should initially be monitored every 4 hours. Once > 7 mg/dL, the serum calcium usually can be maintained with oral calcium supplements (0.5 to 1.0 g orally 3 times daily). The addition of vitamin D_3 (25,000 to 50,000 U orally 3 times weekly), calcefediol (25-[OH]D3) (50-300 µg/day) or calcitriol (1,25 (OH)2 D3) (0.25 to 1 µg/day) will be necessary in those patients with vitamin D deficiency. Thiazide diuretics, by inducing intravascular volume contraction, increase proximal tubular calcium resorption and can serve as a therapeutic adjunct. Finally, the hypocalcemia of magnesium depletion cannot be corrected until magnesium losses are replaced (16).

DISORDERS OF SERUM MAGNESIUM

One-third of the approximately 360 mg (30 mEq) daily dietary magnesium is absorbed (Table 6; Figure 7). Renal excretion accounts for most of the daily magnesium loss, but some GI secretion occurs as well. Like calcium, magnesium is primarily an intracellular cation stored in bone (60%) and skeletal muscle (40%); < 1% of total body magnesium is in the ECF. Unlike calcium, however, no hormones control magnesium balance, and the serum magnesium is not readily exchangeable with tissue stores. Therefore, loss of magnesium can rather quickly lead to hypomagnesemia, and there is little protection against hypermagnesemia when renal excretion is impaired.

Hypermagnesemia

Hypermagnesemia occurs primarily in patients with renal insufficiency or in those receiving excess magnesium by intravenous (treatment of preeclampsia), rectal (magnesium-containing enemas), or oral (antacids, laxatives) routes. The latter occurs more commonly when absorption is enhanced by GI inflammation (ulcer, gastritis, colitis). Excess dietary magnesium will not cause hypermagnesemia unless renal function is impaired.

The signs and symptoms of hypermagnesemia are related to the plasma level (Table 11). Lethargy and hyporeflexia can occur

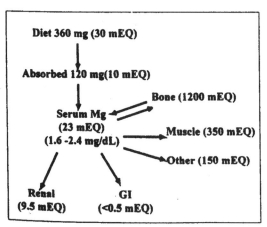

Figure 7. Magnesium balance.

Table 11. Clinical manifestations of hypo/hypermagnesemia.

Serum Level (mg/dL)	
> 12	Muscle paralysis; complete heart block; cardiac arrest
> 7	Somnolence; respiratory depression; hypocalcemia; bradycardia; hypotension
> 4	Lethargy; drowsiness; hyporeflexia
1.6 – 4	Usually asymptomatic
< 2	Normomagnesemic magnesium depletion
< 1.6	Weakness; anorexia; hypokalemia; hypocalcemia
< 1.2	Tetany; Chvostek and Trousseau signs; wide QRS; peaked T wave
< 0.8	Convulsions; prolonged P – R; flat T wave; ventricular tachycardia/ fibrillation

at levels > 4 mg/dL. Respiratory depression, bradycardia, and hypotension are usually seen at levels > 7 mg/dL. A serum magnesium level > 12 mg/dL can cause muscle paralysis, complete heart block, and cardiac arrest. In these cases, intravenous calcium (100 to 200 mg elemental calcium over 5 to 10 minutes) can be lifesaving. Dialysis can also be used when renal function is impaired. Milder symptoms and magnesium levels of < 8 mg/dL require only volume expansion and discontinuing exogenous magnesium.

Hypomagnesemia

Hypomagnesemia occurs in 12% of hospitalized patients, but in 40% to 60% of ICU patients (16). It predicts excess mortality in acutely ill and postoperative adult patients and neonates with ventilatory failure (17). Treatment of hypomagnesemia improves survival in some studies of endotoxic shock (rats), patients with acute myocardial infarction (MI), and postoperative patients with left ventricular dysfunction (18).

GI and renal losses account for most cases of magnesium depletion (Table 12). Extreme diarrhea or malabsorption can readily deplete serum magnesium; prolonged vomiting or gastric secretion more gradually induces hypomagnesemia. Because of obligate daily losses of magnesium in the stool and urine, a 1- to 2-week period of not eating or not receiving magnesium in intravenous fluids will cause hypomagnesemia in most patients (16).

Renal magnesium wasting occurs with excessive diuresis (intravenous fluids, postobstructive, diuretic phase of acute renal failure), diuretic drugs (loop and thiazide diuretics) and with several drugs (Table 12). Renal magnesium loss can easily be distinguished from GI losses by demonstrating an elevated fractional excretion of magnesium (FEMg > 0.5%) in a hypomagnesemic patient.

Hypomagnesemia can result with increased cellular uptake from several causes such as refeeding, insulin therapy, or tissue injury (rhabdomyolysis). Acute pancreatitis can cause hypomagnesemia by saponification.

The clinical manifestations of magnesium depletion are roughly correlated with the plasma level (Table 11). Weakness, anorexia, and neuromuscular irritability can progress to respiratory depression and convulsions in severe cases. The cardiac toxicity is highly dependent on concurrent myocardial perfusion such that severe arrhythmias may occur with seemingly mild hypomagnesemia in the setting of acute MI. Hypokalemia (due to renal potassium wasting) and hypocalcemia (due to altered PTH resistance and release) occur in as many as 40% of magnesium-deficient patients (trication deficiency). Neither the hypokalemia nor hypocalcemia of magnesium deficiency can

Table 12. Causes of hypomagnesemia

Gastrointestinal Losses
    Malabsorption
    Diarrhea
    Gastric suction
    Severe dietary restriction

Renal Losses
    Excessive Urine Volumes
        Intravenous fluids
        Postobstructive diuresis
        Diuretic phase of acute renal failure
    Drugs
        Diuretics
        Aminoglycosides
        Alcohol
        Amphotericin
        Cis platinum
        Cyclosporine
        Ketoacidosis
        Bartter's syndrome
        Renal tubular acidosis

Increased Cellular Uptake
    Refeeding malnourished patients
    Recovery from hypothermia
    Insulin
    Rapid tumor growth
    Rhabdomyolysis
    Pancreatitis

be corrected without magnesium repletion. Hypokalemia and hypocalcemia in the ICU patient often can be corrected with magnesium administration, even in normomagnesemic patients (normomagnesemic magnesium depletion).

Treatment of hypomagnesemia includes correcting the underlying GI or renal cause. Serious complications such as ventricular ectopy, hypokalemia, or hypocalcemic tetany require intravenous magnesium sulfate (1 g [8 mEq] iv stat followed by 6 g over 24 hours). Because serum levels normalize before tissue stores are repleted, renal losses of magnesium usually continue, necessitating daily magnesium replacement (6 to 8 g MgSO$_4$) for 3 to 5 days. Milder cases of hypomagnesemia can be treated by slow-release tablets (Table 13). Amiloride will increase magnesium absorption in the cortical collecting tubule and is an excellent adjunct to magnesium therapy.

Table 13. Treatment of hypomagnesemia

Serum Level (mg/dL)	Symptoms	Treatment	Elemental Magnesium mg	mM	mEq	Comments
≥ 1.6	Chronic depletion	400 mg Mg oxide	241	10	20	Twice daily
≥ 1.6	Prolonged iv fluid	3 – 4 g Mg SO$_4$	300 – 400	12 – 16	24 – 43	Daily
1.2 – 1.6	Minimal	6 – 8 MG SO$_4$	600 – 800	25 – 33	50 – 66	iv over 24 hrs
<1.2	Hyperflexia myoclonus	6 g Mg SO$_4$	600	25	50	iv over 3 – 6 hrs
< 1.2	V arrhythmias	2 – 4 g Mg SO$_4$ or	200 – 400	8 – 16	16 – 32	iv over 15 – 30 mins
		1 g Mg SO$_4$	100	4	8	iv slow push

The use of magnesium to prevent arrhythmias and to improve the survival rate in patients with acute MI remains controversial. It is not recommended routinely. However, in high-risk patients, 16 mEq (8 mmol/L, 192 mg) of magnesium administered intravenously over 5 to 15 minutes prior to reperfusion (thrombolysis or angioplasty) with 128 mEq (64 mM, 1536 mg) over the ensuing 24 hours appears to decrease the incidence of arrhythmia and left ventricular dysfunction and improve the mortality rate (18). It is contraindicated in patients with a greater than first-degree heart block or bradycardia, as magnesium can delay atrioventricular (AV) conduction.

DISORDERS OF SERUM POTASSIUM

Although 2% of total-body potassium is in the ECF, serum potassium is in dynamic equilibrium with intracellular stores (6). Movement into and out of cells is controlled by the adrenergic nervous system, insulin, and alterations in pH. Daily dietary intake (100 mEq) is matched by daily renal (90 mEq) and GI (10 mEq) excretion. Like calcium and magnesium, alterations in serum potassium are best explained by changes in intake, cellular shift, and renal excretion (Figure 8).

Hyperkalemia

The causes of hyperkalemia are outlined in Table 14. Because the kidney is able to substantially increase potassium excretion (up to 300 mEq daily), excess dietary potassium rarely causes hyperkalemia. However, in patients with

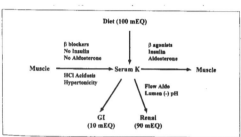

Figure 8. Potassium balance.

mild renal impairment, excessive potassium intake may be an important cause of hyperkalemia. Besides oral potassium supplements, occult sources of potassium include K-penicillin, salt substitutes, stored blood, and oral (chewed) tobacco products.

Hyperkalemia is often due to release of cellular potassium. ß$_2$-blockers (e.g., propranolol) may increase serum potassium levels by this mechanism. Aldosterone deficiency increases serum potassium by causing potassium to move out of cells as well as by decreasing renal excretion (19). Insulin deficiency and hypertonicity (e.g., hyperglycemia) independently cause cellular-to-serum shift of potassium, which explains the hyperkalemia (and the prompt resolution with therapy) so often seen in diabetic ketoacidosis (20). Hyperchloremic acidosis (but not organic acidoses such as ketoacidosis or lactic acidosis) is also associated with hyperkalemia due to cellular shifts. In these cases, the serum potassium increases by an average of 0.5 mEq/L for each 0.1 decrement in pH. Finally, cell lysis can present a potentially huge potassium burden to the ECF (6). Thus, life-threatening hyperkalemia can be seen with rhabdomyolysis, tumor lysis syndrome, massive hemolysis, and

Table 14. Causes of hyperkalemia.

Excess Intake
      Potassium supplements
      Salt substitutes
      Potassium penicillin
      Stored blood
      Oral tobacco products

Cellular Shift
      B_2-blockers
      Aldosterone deficiency
      Insulin deficiency
      Hypertonicity
      Succinylcholine
      Hyperchloremic acidosis
      Cell Lysis
            Rhabdomyolysis
            Hemolysis
            Tumor lysis

Decreased Renal Excretion
      Decreased GFR (< 5 mL/min)
      Decreased Tubular Secretion
            Aldosterone deficiency
            Hypoaldosteronism
            Hyporeninemia
            ACE inhibitors
            Heparin
      Tubulointerstitial Nephritis
            Analgesic nephropathy
            Chronic pyelonephritis
            Sickle cell disease
            Renal allograft
            Obstructive uropathy
      Drugs
            Triamterene
            Amiloride
            Spironolactone
            Cyclosporine
            Trimethoprim
            Pentamidine
            Nonsteroidals

Pseudohyperkalemia

    GFR, glomerular filtration rate; ACE, angiotensin-converting enzyme.

occasionally with succinylcholine, particularly with simultaneous renal insufficiency.

The most common causes of hyperkalemia are due to decreased renal excretion. Since the renal tubules not only resorb nearly all potassium filtered at the glomerulus, but also secrete most of the 90 mEq of potassium excreted daily, hyperkalemia rarely develops from renal failure (low GFR) *per se.* Rather, "renal" hyperkalemia is usually due to some defect in tubular potassium secretion. Tubular secretion of potassium requires aldosterone, good-functioning distal and collecting tubular cells, and an adequate delivery of filtered sodium and water to these nephron segments. Thus, any cause of hypoaldosteronism (hyporeninemia, isolated aldosterone deficiency, angiotensin-converting enzyme [ACE] inhibitors, or heparin) predisposes to hyperkalemia (14). Hyperkalemia frequently accompanies tubulointerstitial renal diseases (particularly chronic pyelonephritis, analgesic nephropathy, sickle cell disease, transplant rejection, and obstructive uropathy) despite relative preservation of renal function (GFR > 20 mL/min). The failure to simultaneously secrete hydrogen ion allows hyperchloremic (nonanion gap) acidosis frequently to accompany hyperkalemia (type IV RTA). Finally, several drugs cause hyperkalemia by inhibiting tubular potassium secretion. In addition to potassium-sparing diuretics (spironolactone, triamterene, and amiloride), cyclosporine, high-dose trimethoprim, pentamidine, nonsteroidals, and ACE inhibitors all share this potential complication.

Pseudohyperkalemia is the release of potassium when blood clots in a test tube. Patients with severe leukocytosis (> 100,000) or thrombocytosis (> 400,000) are particularly prone to this phenomenon. This diagnosis is confirmed by a simultaneously drawn serum (red-top) and plasma (green-top) potassium level.

The toxicity of hyperkalemia is neuromuscular and cardiac. Paresthesias and weakness may progress to flaccid paralysis. Electrocardiographic changes include peaked T waves in the precordial leads followed by decreased R-wave amplitude, widened PR interval, widened QRS complex, and finally, loss of the P wave and the development of the sine wave. Heart block or ventricular standstill may occur at any point.

The treatment of hyperkalemia is outlined in Table 15. With serum potassium of < 6 mEq/L, little therapy is required other than discontinuing the occult sources of dietary

Table 15. Treatment of hyperkalemia

Serum (mEq/L)	ECG	Treatment	Onset/Duration	Mechanism
		Avoid oliguria, nonsteroidals, salt substitutes, potassium-sparing diuretics		
< 6	Normal	Restrict dietary potassium		
> 6	Peaked T	Volume expansion & furosemide, Kayexlate (20 g p.o.)	With diuresis 1 – 2 hrs/6 – 24 hrs	Renal excretion GI excretion
> 7	Prolonged PR, wide QRS	Glucose/insulin Albuterol (10 – 20 mg inhaled) NaHCO$_3$	30 mins/4 – 6 hrs 30 mins/2 – 4 hrs	Redistribution Redistribution Redistribution
> 8	Sine wave	Calcium (10%; 10 – 20 mL iv)	1 – 3 mins/0.5 hr	Membrane antagonism

ECG, electrocardiogram; GI, gastrointestinal; iv, intravenous.

potassium listed in Table 14. As the potassium increases > 6 mEq/L and/or peaked T waves appear, volume expansion (as tolerated), loop diuretics, and oral kayexalate are appropriate. (Kayexalate via rectum is reported to cause colonic necrosis.) Although slow-acting, these treatments actually increase potassium excretion. When more urgent therapy is needed for hyperkalemia (> 7 mEq/L), driving potassium intracellularly with glucose and insulin (25 to 50 g of dextrose with 10 to 20 U of regular insulin) or the β-agonist albuterol (5 to 20 mg [1.0 to 4.0 mL] inhaled) is indicated (21). Albuterol usually works within 30 minutes, will lower the serum potassium by 0.6 to 1.0 mEq/L, and lasts for ≥ 2 hours (22).

Calcium therapy (10 mEq iv over 5 minutes) is reserved for hyperkalemia-induced heart block, the sine wave, or ventricular arrest. Its effect is immediate but short-lived (< 30 minutes). Other maneuvers to remove potassium from the body (such as, diuretics or kayexalate) must be promptly initiated as well. Dialysis (usually hemodialysis) can also be employed to remove potassium.

Hypokalemia

The causes of hypokalemia are listed in Table 16. Significant GI loss of potassium is usually colonic (diarrhea, cathartic abuse) and accompanied by a hyperchloremic acidosis. Although gastric juice contains very little potassium (10 mEq/L), vomiting or gastric suction often cause hypokalemia due to concurrent volume contraction, secondary hyperaldosteronism, and renal potassium wasting. This volume contraction also explains the renal hydrogen ion secretion and the seemingly "paradoxic aciduria" of contraction alkalosis. Renal artery stenosis (secondary hyperaldosteronism) also causes hypokalemia due to urine potassium loss. Renal wastage is also seen when nonresorbable anions (e.g., carbenicillin) are filtered into the urine, increasing distal potassium secretion. Any process that increases tubular flow (diuretics, diuretic phase of acute renal failure, postobstructive diuresis) will enhance tubular potassium secretion (4). RTA (types I and II) and Bartter's syndrome are rare causes of renal hypokalemia. Hypomagnesemia is a more common (although unexplained) cause of hypokalemia due to renal potassium loss.

Hypokalemia caused by the intracellular shift usually accompanies refeeding or treatment of hyperglycemia with insulin. Hypokalemia may cause a wide range of clinical manifestations. Muscle weakness (including respiratory muscles), myalgias, cramps, and even rhabdomyolysis can occur. Gastroparesis, ileus, and constipation are common features.

Table 16. Causes of hypokalemia

Gastrointestinal Losses
    Diarrhea
    Cathartics
    Fistula
    Villous adenoma

Shift into Cells
    Insulin therapy
    Refeeding
    Albuterol
    Periodic paralysis

Renal Losses
    Hypoaldosteronism
        Cushing's syndrome
        Adrenal adenoma
        Volume contraction (vomiting)
        Renal artery stenosis
        Corticosteroid therapy
        Licorice
    Nonabsorbable Anions
        Carbenicillin
        Ticarcillin
        Ketones
    Increased Urine Flow
        Diuretics
        Renal tubular acidosis
        Bartter's syndrome
    Magnesium depletion

Hypokalemia can cause nephrogenic DI, renal phosphate wasting, and acidification defects due to decreased ammonia production. The most serious hypokalemia toxicity, however, is cardiac. Isolated premature ventricular contractions, ventricular tachycardia, delayed conduction, enhancement of digitalis toxicity, and various electrocardiographic changes (U waves, flat T waves, ST-segment depression, and AV block) may all occur.

Treatment of hypokalemia can be enteral or intravenous. Potassium with chloride or other anions (citrate, bicarbonate, phosphate) is effective orally or via a gastric tube and can be given with impunity as long as renal function is normal (6). With more severe degrees of hypokalemia or in patients symptomatic from hypokalemia, rapid correction may be accomplished intravenously (23). When potassium is > 2 mEq/L, and there are no electrocardiographic changes, 10 mEq/hr is sufficient. If the serum potassium is < 2 mEq/L, 40 mEq/hr can be given with cardiac monitoring (24). Peripheral infusions should be concentrated to no more than 60 mEq/L and administered through as large a vein as possible. Central infusions are best administered into the superior vena cava and not the atrium or ventricle.

One must remember the necessity of treating coexistent magnesium depletion in hypokalemic patients.

ANNOTATED REFERENCES

1. Oster JR, Singer I: Hyponatremia, hypoosmolality and hypotonicity: Tables and fables. *Arch Intern Med* 1999; 159:333 –336

2. Rose BD: Hypoosmolal states. *In:* Clinical Physiology of Acid-Base and Electrolyte Disorders. New York, McGraw-Hill, 1994, pp 651 –694
   Excellent review.

3. Zaloga, GP, Kirby RR, Bernards WC, et al: Fluids and electrolytes. *In:* Critical Care. Third Ediction. Civetta JM, Taylor RW, Kirby RR (Eds). Philadelphia, JP Lippincott, 1997, pp 413 –441
   An excellent review with the critical care practitioner in mind.

4. Faber MD, Kupin WL, Heilig CW, et al: Common fluid electrolyte and acid-base problems in the intensive care unit: Selected issues. *Semin Nephrol* 1994; 14: 8–22
   A particularly good review.

5. Alfrey AC: Normal and abnormal magnesium metabolism. *In:* Renal and Electrolyte Disorders. Fourth Edition. Schrier RW (Ed). Boston, Little Brown and Co, 1992, pp 371–404

6. Gabow PA, Peterson LN: Disorders of potassium metabolism. *In:* Renal and Electrolyte Disorders. Fourth Edition. Schrier RW (Ed). Boston, Little Brown and Co, 1992, pp 231–285
   An excellent outline of renal hyperkalemia.

7. Ziegler, R: Hypercalcemic Crisis. *J Am Soc Nephrol* 2001; 12:S3-S9
   Outlines aggressive therapy of hypercalcemia based on pathophysiology.

8. Rosol TJ, Capen CC: Mechanisms of cancer-induced hypercalcemia. *Lab Invest* 1992; 67: 680 –702
   Excellent discussion of hormonal causes of hypercalcemia in cancer patients.

9. Akmal M, Bishop JE, Telfer N, et al: Hypocalcemia and hypercalcemia in patients with rhabdomyolysis with and without acute renal failure. *J Clin Endocrinol Metab* 1986; 63:137–142

10. Suki WN, Yium JJ, Von Minden M, et al: Acute treatment of hypercalcemia with furosemide. *N Engl J Med* 1970; 283:836–840
    Demonstrates the importance of isotonic hydration with furosemide as adjunctive therapy for hypercalcemia.

11. Binstock ML, Mundy GR: Effect of calcitonin and glucocorticoids in combination on the hypercalcemia of malignancy. *Ann Intern Med* 1980; 93:269 –272

12. Perlia CP, Gubisch NJ, Walter J, et al: Mithramycin treatment of hypercalcemia. *Cancer* 1970; 25:389–394

13. Singer FR: Role of biphosphonate etidronate in the therapy of cancer related hypercalcemia. *Semin Oncol* 1990; 17 (Suppl 5):34–39

14. Warrell RP, Israel R, Frisone M, et al: Gallium nitrate for acute treatment of cancer related hypercalcemia; a randomized, double-blind comparison to calcitonin. *Ann Intern Med* 1988; 108:669–674

15. Broner CW, Stidham GL, Westenkirchner DF, et al: Hypermagnesemia and hypocalcemia as predictors of high mortality in critically ill pediatric patients. *Crit Care Med* 1990; 18:921–928
    Emphasizes the importance of electrolyte disorders in critically ill patients.

16. Salem M, Munoz R, Chernow B: Hypomagnesemia in critical illness. *Crit Care* 1991; 7:225–252

17. Rubeiz GJ, Thill-Baharozian M, Hardie D, et al: Association of hypomagnesemia and mortality in acutely ill medical patients. *Crit Care Med* 1983; 21:203–209

18. Woods KL, Fletcher S: Long-term outcome after intravenous magnesium sulfate in inspected acute myocardial infarction: The second Leister intravenous magnesium intervention trial (LIMIT-2). *Lancet* 1994; 343:816–819
    Treatment of acute myocardial infarction with magnesium may improve survival.

19. DeFronzo RA: Hyperkalemia and hyporeninemic hypoaldosteronism. *Kidney Int* 1980; 17: 118 –134
    A complete and excellent review.

20. Fulop M: Serum potassium in lactic acidosis and ketoacidosis. *N Engl J Med* 1979; 300:1087 –1089
    Clarifies the mechanism and therapy of hyperkalemia in patients with metabolic acidosis.

21. Blumberg A, Wiedmann P, Shaw S, et al: Effect of various therapeutic approaches on plasma potassium and major regulating factors in terminal renal failure. *Am J Med* 1988; 85:507–512
    The combination of insulin and glucose is more effective than bicarbonate in treating "renal" hyperkalemia.

22. Montoliu J, Lens XM, Revert L: Potassium-lowering effect of albuterol for hyperkalemia in renal failure. *Arch Intern Med* 1987; 147:713–717
    Albuterol is safe and effective for short-term therapy of hyperkalemia.

23. Hamill RJ, Robinson LM, Wexler HR, et al: Efficacy and safety of potassium infusion therapy in hypokalemic critically ill patients. *Crit Care Med* 1991; 19:694–699

24. Kruse JA, Carlson RW: Rapid correction of hypokalemia using concentrated intravenous potassium chloride infusions. *Arch Intern Med* 1990; 150:613 –617
    The safety and efficacy of high-dose intravenous potassium.

HEMODYNAMIC MONITORING

Jesse B. Hall, MD, FCCM

INTRODUCTION

Hemodynamic monitoring may be defined as the collection and interpretation of various parameters that inform determination of: 1) the etiology of a state of hypoperfusion and/or 2) the response of the cardiopulmonary unit to interventions such as fluid therapy, vasoactive drugs, or adjustments in positive pressure ventilation. This is most often accomplished by placement of an intravascular catheter with transduction of pressures and with right heart catheterization (RHC), determination of vascular flow by thermal dilution. Simultaneous determination of arterial and mixed venous blood gases also permits determination of oxygen contents, oxygen delivery, oxygen consumption, arterio-venous oxygen content difference, and calculation of cardiac output by Fick determination.

Few or no data demonstrate improved patient outcomes from this monitoring approach. Indeed, one recent study suggested that use of the RHC is associated with an independent negative effect on survival. This study has been criticized largely on the basis of design—it was retrospective, and thus even reasonably sophisticated methods of case matching may have failed to control for the inevitable differences in patient status and hence prognosis that might contribute to decisions to perform invasive monitoring. While it is conceivable that RHC carries an independent risk of poor outcome, this writer feels that the absence of consensus on how to act on specific measurements obtained by RHC in diseases such as sepsis or acute hypoxemic respiratory failure, and the well-documented failure of clinicians to accurately interpret RHC data, make this issue unresolvable at present. Accordingly, this presentation is guided to enhance understanding of interpretation of RHC data.

DIFFERENTIAL DIAGNOSIS OF HYPOPERFUSED STATES AND BEDSIDE ASSESSSMENT

A useful and readily applicable bedside algorithm at the time of resuscitation of patients with circulatory inadequacy is—is this low or high output hypotension? If the former, is the heart full or not? And when fluid resuscitation has occurred, is the response definitive or has low output shock now taken on the characteristics of high flow shock (e.g., septic shock with initial hypovolemia, now fluid resuscitated). Often this simple algorithm succeeds in fully resuscitating the patient. If not, further information gathering from invasive monitoring and/or echocardiography is appropriate.

PULMONARY ARTERY CATHETERIZATION

Indications and Complications

Rather than offer a list of many conditions that may require PAC, the reader is guided to the statement above recommending formulation of questions concerning the etiology of hypoperfusion or the response to therapy and answer these questions if possible with clinical data, including volume or drug challenges; when this approach is inadequate, PAC is to be considered. Complications of the procedure are given in Table 2.

Interpretation of Pressure Waveforms

Under most conditions, the waveforms obtained as the pulmonary artery catheter is advanced through the right atrium, right ventricle, and into the pulmonary artery to a wedged position are readily identified as characteristic of each segment of the circulation as it is traversed, as demonstrated in Figure 1.

While waveform recognition is extremely   helpful in positioning the catheter, and often

Table 1. Rapid Formulation of an Early Working Diagnosis of the Etiology of Shock

<u>Defining Features of Shock</u>

Blood pressure	⇓
Heart rate	⇑
Respiratory rate	⇑
Mentation	⇓
Urine output	⇓
Arterial pH	⇓

	High Output Hypotension **Septic Shock**	**Low Cardiac Output** **Cardiogenic and Hypovolemic**
Is Cardiac Output Reduced?	No	Yes
Pulse pressure	⇑	⇓
Diastolic pressure	⇑	⇓
Extremities digits	Warm	Cool
Nailbed return	Rapid	Slow
Heart sounds	Crisp	Muffled
Temperature	⇑ or ⇓	⇔
White cell count	⇑ or ⇓	⇔
Site of infection	++	-

	Reduced Pump Function **Cardiogenic Shock**	**Reduced Venous Return** **Hypovolemic Shock**
Is the Heart Too Full?	Yes	No
Symptoms clinical context	Angina ECG	Hemorrhage dehydration
Jugular venous pressure	⇑	⇓
S$_3$, S$_4$, gallop rhythm	+++	-
Respiratory crepitations	+++	-
Chest radiograph	Large heart ⇑ upper lobe flow Pulmonary edema	Normal

What Does Not Fit?

Overlapping etiologies (septic cardiogenic, septic hypovolemic, cardiogenic hypovolemic)
Short list of other etiologies

High output *hypotension*	*High right atrial* *pressure hypotension*	*Nonresponsive* *hypovolemia*
Liver failure	Pulmonary hypertension	Adrenal insufficiency
Severe Pancreatitis	(most often Pulmonary Embolus)	Anaphylaxis
Trauma with significant	Right ventricular infarction	Spinal shock
SIRS	Cardiac tamponade	
Thyroid storm		
Arteriovenous fistula		
Paget's disease		

Get more information   Echocardiography, right heart catheterization

Table 2. Complications of PA Catheterization

I.   Complications related to central vein cannulation.

II.   Complications related to insertion and use of the PA catheter
   A   Tachyarrhythmias
   B   Right bundle branch block
   C   Complete heart block (pre- existing left bundle branch block)

   D   Cardiac perforation
   E   Thrombosis and embolism
   F   Pulmonary infarction due to persistent wedging
   G   Catheter-related sepsis
   H   Pulmonary artery rupture
   I   Knotting of the catheter
   J   Endocarditis, bland and infective

   K   Pulmonic valve insufficiency
   L   Balloon fragmentation and embolization

makes the use of fluoroscopic techniques unnecessary, it is essential for the measurement and interpretation of waveforms displayed during PAC to be correlated to the EKG tracing so that specific components of the waveform can be identified and various pitfalls in measurement of intravascular pressure can be avoided.

The normal pressure waveform

In sinus rhythm, the atrial pressure waveform is characterized by 2 major positive deflections (A and V waves) and 2 negative deflections (X and Y descents) (See Figure 2). A third positive wave, the C wave, is sometimes seen. The A wave results from atrial systolic contraction and is followed by the X descent as the atria relax following contraction. The C wave results from closure of the atrioventricular valves and interrupts the X descent. After the X descent, the V (ventricular) wave is generated by passive filling of the atria during ventricular systole. Lastly, the Y descent reflects the reduction in atrial pressure as the

atrioventricular valves open. In correlating these waveforms to the EKG, the first positive pressure wave to follow the P wave is the A wave. The right atrial A wave is usually seen at the beginning of the QRS complex, provided that atrioventricular conduction is normal. The peak of the right atrial V wave normally occurs simultaneously with the T wave of the electocardiogram, provided that the Q-T interval is normal.

The pulmonary artery waveform has a systolic pressure wave and a diastolic trough. A dicrotic notch due to closure of the pulmonic valve may be seen on the terminal portion of the systolic pressure wave. Like the right atrial V wave, the PA systolic wave typically coincides with the electrical T wave. The pulmonary artery diastolic pressure (Ppad) is recorded as the pressure just before the beginning of the systolic pressure wave.

The Ppw tracing contains the same sequence of waves and descents as the right atrial tracing. However, when the atrial waveform is referenced to the electrocardiogram, the mechanical events arising in the left atrium (Ppw) will be seen later than those of the right atrium, because the left atrial pressure waves must travel back through the pulmonary vasculature and a longer length of catheter (See Figure 3). Therefore, in the Ppw tracing the A wave usually appears after the QRS complex and the V wave is seen after the T wave. As such, the systolic pressure wave in the PA tracing *precedes* the V wave of the Ppw tracing. An appreciation of the latter relationship is critical when tracings are being analyzed to ensure that balloon inflation has resulted in a transition from an arterial (PA) to atrial (Ppw) waveform, and to detect the presence of a "giant" V wave in the Ppw tracing.

Common problems producing erroneus pressure waveforms

Of the many problems causing artifact or erroneus tracings, the most common encountered are overdamping, catheter whip, overwedging, incomplete wedging, and Zone I catheter conditions.

Overdamping results from air bubbles within the catheter system or kinking, clotting,

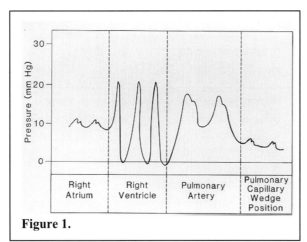

Figure 1.

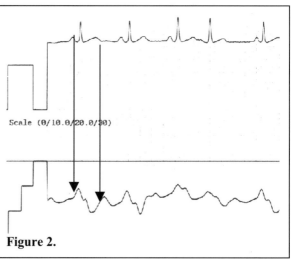

Scale (0/10.0/20.0/30)

Figure 2.

and fibrin deposition along the catheter course. Many times these problems can be resolved by catheter flushing. The main effect of overdamping on the pressure waveform is to artifactually lower the systolic pressure and raise the diastolic pressure with consequent effects on interpretation.

Catheter whip arises from cardiac contractions causing shock transients transmitted to the catheter. The results on the right ventricular or pulmonary arterial waveforms are an exaggerated diastolic pressure in some cycles, highlighting the need to avoid readings obtained by electronic systems:

Overwedging (See Figure 5) is signaled by a rise in recorded pressure with balloon inflation as the balloon herniates over the catheter tip or the tip is pushed into the vessel wall with continued fluid ingress elevating the measured pressure. Over wedging requires repositioning of the catheter.

Incomplete wedging and Zone I positioning of the catheter can be subtle but are important to identify since erroneous and often overestimation of Ppw occur.

Zone I conditions of the lung refer to those segments of the lung in which alveolar pressure exceeds pulmonary vascular pressure and hence there is no flow (See Figure 7).

This phenomenon is uncommon when the catheter is floated into position since this typically results in Zone II or III positioning. It would be more likely to result from forceful positioning of the catheter, hypovolemia emerging after placement, or with large increases in PEEP. This condition should be considered when changes in Ppw track PEEP

changes exactly or when the excursion in pulmonary artery systolic pressures with respiration exceed those Ppw significantly (see Figure 8).

The correlation of pressure to ventricular preload and volume

The use of Ppw as a measure of Plvedp and hence preload depends on the Ppw closely reflecting pulmonary venous, left atrial, and left ventricular pressures, that is, with minimal pressure gradient across the system. One potential confounder to interpretation of intravascular pressures is the fluctuation in intrathoracic pressure related to the respiratory cycle. The effect of varying intrathoracic pressure on the wedge (Ppw) pressure is seen in Figure 9. The top line is a Ppw tracing and the bottom in the intrapleural (Ppl) pressure. In this example the patient is receiving assisted ventilation. Arrows indicate end expiratory pressures. Negative deflections in Ppl and Ppw pressures result from inspiratory muscle activity, and subsequent positive deflections represent lung inflation by the ventilator. At end expiration, the respiratory system has returned to its relaxed state and Ppl is back to baseline (-2 cm H_2O). Transmural wedge pressure remains approximately constant throughout the ventilating cycle. Since Ppl is not usually measured clinically, it is necessary that Ppw be recorded at a point where Ppl can be reliably estimated (i.e., end-exhalation, assuming no expiratory muscle activity).

The correlation of pressure to volume is further complicated by a variety of conditions that cause the ventricle to be effectively stiff (diastolic dysfunction or pericardial disease) or conditions that cause juxta-cardiac pressure to rise related to positive pressure ventilation (PEEP, PEEPi, active expiratory effort) (see Figure 10).

The effects of PEEP in conditions such as ARDS are often blunted, since the stiff lungs of these patients do not distend greatly with high ventilator pressures and hence minimal increases in juxta-cardiac pressure are encountered. However, in cases in which PEEPi exists in COPD/asthma patients undergoing mechanical ventilation, or agitated/obstructed patients have very active expiratory muscle efforts, cardiovascular effects may be large. This effect is shown in Figure 11, where the increase in blood pressure and cardiac output despite a fall in wedge pressure and esophageal pressure is shown during a brief interruption in positive pressure ventilation in a patient with COPD.

This constellation of problems is best avoided by:

1. Awareness of their existence
2. Reading pressure tracings at end expiration
3. Considering measures (sedation, ventilator adjustment, paralysis) that diminish or eliminate PEEPi
4. Considering a ventilator disconnect in patients with severe airflow obstruction and PEEPi to demonstrate limitation to venous return
5. Using a fluid challenge when effective "diastolic" dysfunction may be present, to determine "preload reserve"

In determining the response to a fluid challenge, it is necessary to note that a minimum of 500 cc of crystalloid is required and even then small effects on cardiac output and arterial blood pressure are typically seen. One study has suggested that the use of a drop in the right atrial pressure with respiration is a useful indicator of preload reserve.

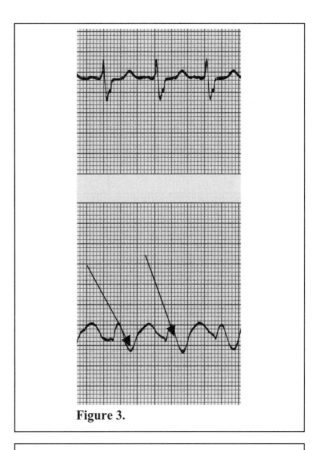

Figure 3.

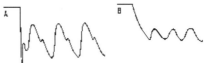

Figure 4. Rapid flush test: a) Appropriately damped system, and b) Over damped system.

Specific disorders

Tricuspid regurgitation is encountered in conditions with direct valvular injury (e.g., endocarditis) and generally in right heart failure. It is characterized by a prominent and broad V wave and a steep Y descent; the latter is often most useful for making this diagnosis. It is useful to note tricuspid regurgitation not only for its implications for underlying disorders but also because it will confound thermal dilution cardiac output determination.

Mitral regurgitation is characterized by a giant V wave that may confound distinction between the PA and Pwp tracings. Significant mitral regurgitation may be present without a giant V wave (ascribed to enlarged and compliant left atrium which does not exhibit a large pressure excursion with the additional volume) and a number of conditions can cause a giant V wave in the absence of mitral regurgitation (hypervolemia, VSD).

Right ventricular infarction is characterized by an elevated RVEDP at initial passage of the catheter with narrow pulse pressures when there is hemodynamic compromise. This same pattern can also be present in conditions causing acute right heart failure secondary to increases in pulmonary vascular resistance (e.g., pulmonary embolus) but in these latter conditions there will be a large PAD-Ppw gradient reflecting the increase in PVR.

Interpretation of flows and parameters of oxygen delivery

In most clinical setting cardiac output is determined by thermal dilution. In addition to a number of technical conditions making the measurement unreliable, tricuspid regurgitation may be present and cause underestimation (usually) or overestimation (rarely) of cardiac output. Under this circumstance, determination of cardiac output by Fick may be useful.

Determination of whether a measured flow is adequate is usually best judged by peripheral parameters of perfusion (e.g., urine volume, presence of lactic acidosis) or by the mixed venous oxygen saturation. Low MVO2 (< 60%) strongly suggests inadequate oxygen delivery and anemia, hypoxemia, or inadequate cardiac output should be sought and corrected. Interpretation of a high MVO2 in high output states is difficult. Accordingly, the greatest utility of modified catheters which permit continuous monitoring of MVO_2 is in circumstances in which there is risk for it to be low and therapy can be directed at early recognition of this phenomenon (e.g., post-op cardiac surgery patients).

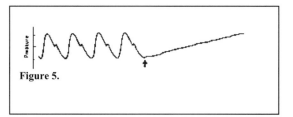

Figure 5.

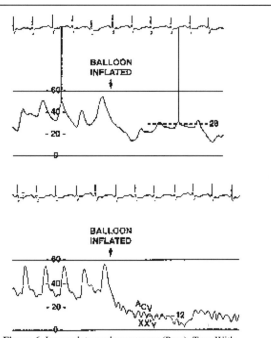

Figure 6. Incomplete wedge pressure (Ppw). Top: With balloon inflation, there is a decrease in pressure to a value that approximates pulmonary artery diastolic pressure (Ppad). The clinical setting (ARDS) is usually associated with a large Ppad-Ppw gradient. Review of the tracings indicates that there is a single positive wave coinciding with the electrocardiographic T wave after balloon inflation, a pattern inconsistent with a left atrial waveform. Bottom: Waveforms after the catheter had been retracted, the balloon inflated, and the catheter floated to a full wedge position. Now, there is a large Ppad-Ppw gradient and the tracing after balloon inflation is consistent with a left atrial waveform. The incomplete wedge tracing yielded an incorrect measurement of the wedge pressure as 28 mm Hg, substantially higher (in a very clinically relevant sense) than the true wedge pressure of approximately 12 mm Hg.

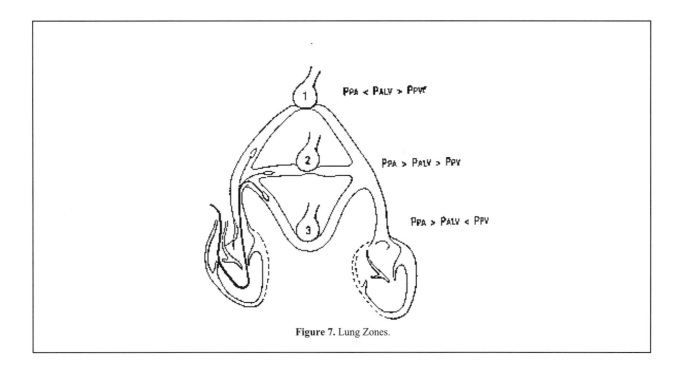

Figure 7. Lung Zones.

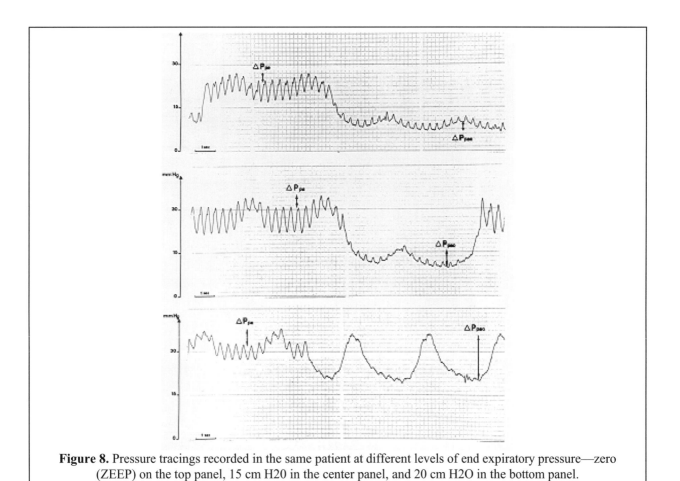

Figure 8. Pressure tracings recorded in the same patient at different levels of end expiratory pressure—zero (ZEEP) on the top panel, 15 cm H20 in the center panel, and 20 cm H2O in the bottom panel.

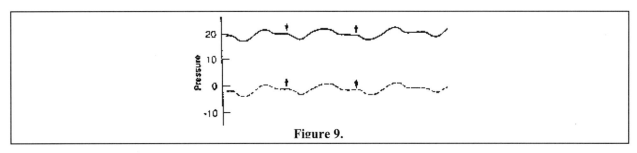

Figure 9.

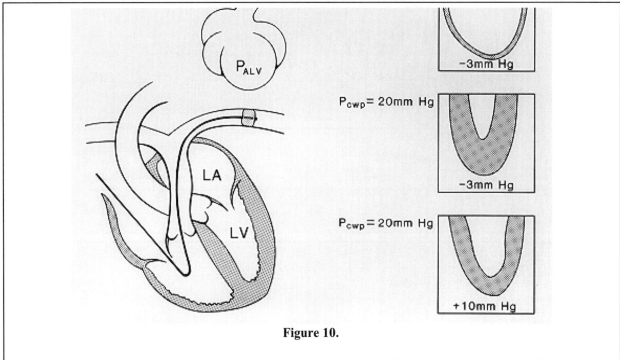

Figure 10.

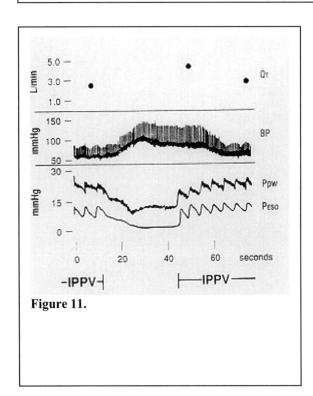

Figure 11.

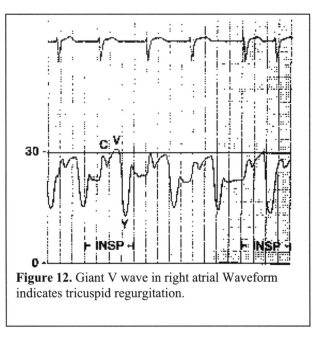

Figure 12. Giant V wave in right atrial Waveform indicates tricuspid regurgitation.

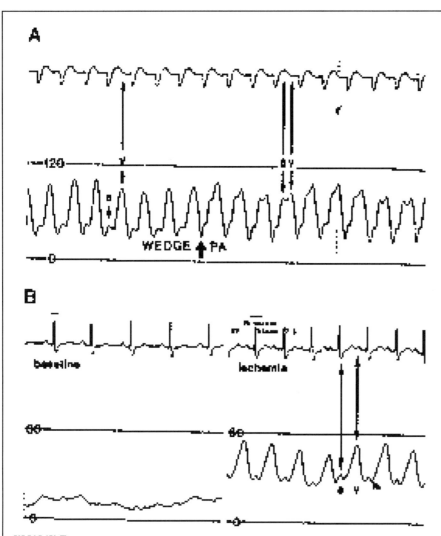

Figure 13. A) Acute mitral regurgitation with giant V wave in pulmonary wedge tracing. The pulmonary artery (PA) tracing has a characteristic bifid appearance due to both a PA systolic wave and the V wave. Note that the V wave occurs later in the cardiac cycle than the PA systolic wave, which is synchronous with the T wave of the electrocardiogram. B) Intermittent giant V wave due to ischemia of the papillary muscle. Wedge tracings are from same patient at baseline and during ischemia. Scale in mm Hg.

Echocardiography

Many of the problems of relating measured pressures to ventricular preload can be addressed by cardiac imaging by echo. In addition this diagnostic tool is useful for identifying a host of structural abnormalities. It should be considered as an adjunct to pulmonary artery catheterization. As technology permits more continuous monitoring by transesophageal route, its use in the ICU is likely to expand

Useful Applications of Echocardiography in the ICU:

1. Identification of ischemia
2. Correlation of pressure to volume and identification of diastolic dysfunction
3. Characterization of valve lesions, VSD, ASD
4. Identification of pericardial disease
5. Identification of right-left heart interactions in acute right heart failure

REFERENCES

1. Leatherman JW, Marini JJ: Clinical use of the pulmonary artery catheter. *In:* Principles of Critical Care. Second Edition. Hall, Schmidt, Wood (Eds). McGraw Hill, 1998. Pp 155-177
   Excellent, concise review of use of PAC.

2. Perret C, Tagan D, Feihl F, Marini JJ: The pulmonary artery catheter in clinical care. *Blackwell Science* 1996; 1-347
   Excellent monograph, includes case studies

3. Connors AF, Speroff T, Dawson NV, Thomas C, Harrell FE, Wagner D, et al: The effectiveness of right heart catheterization in the initial care of critically ill patients. *JAMA* 1996; 276:889-897
   Recent retrospective study employing case-matching methodology, which suggested PAC, is associated with a poor outcome, perhaps apart from patient risk factors.

4. Shah KB, Rao TLK, Laughlin S, et al: A review of pulmonary artery catheterizations in 6,245 patients. *Anesthesiology* 1984; 61:271
   Documents risks and complications.

5. Fuchs RM, Heuser RR, Yin FC, Brinker JA: Limitations of pulmonary wedge V waves in diagnosing mitral regurgitation. *Am J of Cardiology* 1982; 49:849-854

6. Magder S, Georgiadis G, Cheone T; Respiratory variations in right atrial pressure predict the response to fluid challenge. *J Crit Care* 1992; 7:76-85

7. Teboul JL, Besbes M, Andrivet P, Axler O, Douguet D, Zelter M, et al: A bedside index assessing the reliability of pulmonary artery occlusion pressure measurements during mechanical ventilation with positive end-expiratory pressure. *J Crit Care Med* 1992; 7:22-29

8. Russell JA, Phang TP: The oxygen delivery/consumption controversy: Approaches to management of the critically ill. *Am J Respir Crit Care Med* 1994; 149:533-537

THE BLEEDING PATIENT IN THE ICU

Judith A. Luce, MD

Objectives

- To understand the normal components of clotting
- To understand the elements of making the diagnosis of DIC
- To understand the the causes of acquired thrombocytopenia in adults
- To understand the diagnosis of complex coagulopathies in adults
- To understand the remedies available to treat adults with iatrogenic coagulopathy

INTRODUCTION

Elements of Coagulation and Fibrinolysis

Normal clotting is initiated by a variety of factors: exposure of plasma and platelets to nonendothelial surfaces; the response of the endothelium to injury; inflammatory response elements such as cytokines and bradykinins; and miscellaneous procoagulants such as endotoxin. These same factors trigger the proteolytic cascade that results in the cessation of clotting. The initial event in clotting is the formation of an aggregated platelet plug in the vessel and the triggering of the proteolytic cascade that produces thrombin. The final product of clotting is polymers of fibrin, and the key enzyme is thrombin. Plasmin is the proteolytic enzyme that cleaves fibrin clot. Each side of the clotting and unclotting process has direct and indirect inhibitors. The primary inhibitor of thrombin is antithrombin III, of which heparin is a cofactor. The primary inhibitor of plasmin is alpha-2-antiplasmin, which is consumed when plasmin is inactivated.

In order to have normal clotting, patients need 3 elements: intact vessels capable of self repair and vasoconstriction; adequate numbers of normally functioning platelets; and uninhibited normal levels of circulating soluble clotting factors. Clearly, any disorder that involves more than 1 of these elements will produce more severe bleeding than a disorder that involves only 1 of these elements to an equal degree. The term *combined coagulopathy* is used to describe such problems.

History Taking in Evaluating the Bleeding Patient

Familial clotting histories are pertinent but rare. Most families with serious coagulopathies, such as Hemophilia A and B and von Willebrand's disease, are identified in childhood, so that adults with new, severe factor deficiencies have almost always acquired these disorders by virtue of having antibodies to a key factor. Histories of lesser bleeding tendencies may be useful for identifying families with inherited disorders of platelet function. Individual bleeding histories are important: immediate bleeding following a surgical or traumatic incident is usually associated with platelet insufficiency or severe dysfunction; in contrast, factor deficiency bleeding is usually characterized by delayed onset of bleeding. Surface bleeding of the skin or mucosal tissues is most often associated with platelet problems, and deep visceral bleeding with clotting factor deficiencies. Combined coagulopathies will produce both types of bleeding. Bleeding requiring transfusion is significant only if transfusion is rare, such as after elective uncomplicated GI, gynecological, or oral surgery. Histories should also include adult disease associated with bleeding tendencies, including renal disease, diabetes, hematologic conditions, cancer, and liver disease. Drug histories and drug allergies are equally important in evaluating for acquired coagulopathy.

Principles of Therapy

In general, goals of treatment are 2-fold: restoration of the capacity to form adequate clot and abatement of the underlying condition causing the coagulopathy. Prophylaxis is usually

Table 1.

Causes of Acute DIC
Shock, any cause
Infectious
  Gram-negative sepsis
  Severe other bacterial sepsis
  Severe viral, Rickettsial infections
Traumatic
  Crush injury
  Burns
  Severe head injury
  Surgery on prostate
Anaphylaxis
Heatstroke
Snakebite
Obstetric
  Abruptio placentae
  Fetal demise
  Amniotic fluid embolism
  Severe eclampsia
Hemolytic transfusion reaction
Intravascular abnormalities
  Vascular prostheses
  Kasabach-Merritt syndrome
  Extracorporeal circulation

Causes of Chronic DIC
Cancer, most often adenoca
Acute promyelocytic leukemia
Chronic inflammatory diseases

reserved for specific situations: inherited disorders of coagulation such as Hemophilia A and elective surgical events in severe coagulopathy. In order to achieve the first goal, that of restoring normal capacity to clot, targets for transfusion therapy should be set and monitored at a frequency sufficient for the clinical situation. Transfusion therapy should be as selective as possible in order to minimize risk, and simple nursing measures to reduce the risk of bleeding should be employed, such as bedrest, immobilization of affected parts, prevention of erosive gastritis, minimization of invasive procedures, and so forth.

SEVERE, GENERALIZED BLEEDING IN ADULTS

This is the most dreaded clinical situation in the intensive care unit. Bleeding of some type occurs in up to 40% of all patients in the ICU, but diffuse, severe bleeding makes up only a fraction of these cases. This situation arises from only a very limited number of causes:

- Severe, combined coagulopathy: (DIC, et al)
- Severe thrombocytopenia
- Severe single factor deficiencies
- Iatrogenic coagulopathy: heparin, warfarin, and fibrinolysis

Because the aim of this paper is not to discuss pediatric coagulopathies, and because the overwhelming majority of adults with single factor deficiency are identified in childhood as having 1 of a small number of inherited disorders, those will not be considered here. In the critical care unit, patients with congenital coagulopathies such as hemophiliacs must be referred to a skilled hematologist with experience in managing such cases.

SEVERE COMBINED COAGULOPATHY: DIC

Pathophysiology of DIC

Acquired combined coagulopathies are the most complex to diagnose and manage in critically ill adults. The most seminal of these diseases is disseminated intravascular coagulation, or DIC. This disorder is a clinical syndrome with no single diagnostic test and a host of varied manifestations and underlying causes, and thus it is often difficult to diagnose. It may occur in other settings that predispose to combined coagulopathy, and thus be confused with them.

Disseminated intravascular coagulation results when generalized clotting and unclotting take place throughout the vascular tree, usually brought on by some supraphysiologic stress to the clotting system. The diseases with which

DIC is associated are listed in Table 1. Chronic DIC is a term reserved for patients who have low levels of DIC but do not have severe clinical manifestations of bleeding or thrombosis.

The consequences of DIC are notable. Patients who have DIC have a high mortality in the ICU: over 90% in most studies. Whether this is a reflection of the severity of their underlying illness or whether DIC itself causes excess mortality is not clear. Generation of excess thrombin activity results in diffuse clotting, and microscopic clots are found in multiple organs at autopsy in patients who have had DIC. Roger Bone has argued that this is a significant contributor to multi-organ failure in the critically ill patient, although detailed clinical trials of this question have not been done. Intravascular thrombosis results in microangiopathic hemolysis, with the characteristic appearance of schistocytes on the peripheral smear. Ten percent of patients with DIC present with large vessel thrombosis, rather than bleeding, although even this number may be an underestimate.

Diagnosis of DIC

The first step in making a diagnosis of DIC is recognizing that the patient has a *condition that predisposes to DIC*. The second step is using the laboratory to demonstrate the *dynamic changes* that occur during DIC. First, one needs to find *factors that are consumed during the clotting process*, and are therefore falling during DIC, and may have reached abnormal values when the diagnosis is made. *Platelets are consumed* by diffuse intravascular platelet aggregation. Because platelet production by the marrow is relatively slow, it lacks the capacity to replace them promptly, and thrombocytopenia is a hallmark of DIC. *Fibrinogen is being rapidly converted* to fibrin monomers by the action of excess thrombin, and so fibrinogen is similarly depleted. Liver replacement of the entire supply of fibrinogen in the plasma takes over 24 hours in for normally functioning liver, and thus fibrinogen deficiency occurs uniformly in DIC. Also *consumed in clotting are Factors V and VIII*, although we measure them less frequently because the tests are more expensive.

Excess thrombin activity generates fibrinogen deficiency, but it has other effects that may be measured during DIC. The generation of *Fibrinopeptide A*, a fragment that is cleaved away from fibrinogen by thrombin, may be measured. *Fibrin monomers* are normally produced in high local concentrations in physiologic clotting, and they polymerize spontaneously and are thus unmeasurable in the peripheral blood. However, during DIC, fibrin monomers are being generated throughout the vascular tree and become measurable in the peripheral blood.

The *prothrombin time and PTT* both become abnormal during DIC, although the PTT is usually more affected. These 2 measures of intrinsic and extrinsic clotting pathways are affected by the falling supply of fibrinogen and Factors V and VIII. They are also inhibited both by excess circulating fragments of fibrin and activated inhibitors of clotting, so that they are prolonged both because of factor deficiency and inhibitors.

Finally, it is possible to measure the effect of *enhanced plasmin activity* in DIC. This may be done indirectly, by measuring the *loss of plasma alpha-2-antiplasmin*, or directly, by measuring the products of plasmin's cleavage of fibrin molecules. The test that is most often used for this purpose is the *D-dimer* assay, a specific radioimmunoassay for the unique product of cleavage of end-to-end polymers of fibrin. This test is very sensitive for DIC and much more specific than the older "fibrin split products" assay.

The diagnosis of DIC must be made using several of these tests, looking at different aspects of DIC. Platelets, fibrinogen, a PT and PTT, and D-dimers make up the most widely available panel of tests for DIC. The rationale for several tests looking at different aspects of DIC is that only 2 tests may be misleading: when only 2 of 3 tests are suggestive of DIC, the diagnosis is correct only about 65% of the time. Three of 4 tests raises the accuracy to over 75%, and 4 of 4 tests to over 90%. The results of DIC testing may also evolve over time, so that a fibrinogen level that is high at the onset of DIC may not fall into the abnormal level for many hours; but a rapidly falling fibrinogen level in the presence of other indicators of DIC may be a clue to the diagnosis.

Treatment of DIC

The treatment of DIC requires attention to the 2 principles of therapy outlined at the beginning of this article: stopping the cause and treating the hemostatic deficiencies. DIC that has a readily reversible cause, such as hemolytic transfusion reaction or fetal demise, is also readily reversible. It may require no other therapy than the reversal of the underlying condition if the patient is otherwise fairly healthy. But in a critically ill patient, DIC can be protracted because the cause is not readily reversible and the patient is not healthy enough to have the capacity to restore hemostatic factors rapidly. The blood bank is therefore very useful in treating DIC.

Transfusion therapy for DIC usually relies on 2 components: platelets and fibrinogen. Red cells may be necessary in order to replace whole blood loss. Platelets are ordinarily used in groups of 5 or 6 units, and are given with the goal of achieving a platelet count over 50,000/mm3. This may be difficult to sustain when DIC is very brisk, and repeated transfusions over 24 hours may be necessary. Fibrinogen is usually given as cryoprecipitate, since large quantities may be given in small volumes. Plasma is rarely needed, especially since cryoprecipitate also contains Factor VIII. Repeated transfusion may also be needed; the goal of transfusion therapy is a fibrinogen level over 100mg/dL.

DIC treatment aimed at suppressing the coagulation process has been tried in a number of nonrandomized trials. The most frequently used product has been heparin, which has the advantage of acting, with antithrombin III, directly on thrombin. Heparin is always used when DIC is manifested by thrombosis; heparin may be used, with or without other agents, when DIC is protracted or very severe. Heparin may increase bleeding; if this happens, it must be discontinued. Heparin prophylaxis was formerly used for induction therapy of patients with acute promyelocytic leukemia; its routine use in this high-risk setting is now very controversial, since bleeding risk may actually be increased. Heparin is the agent of choice for the treatment of chronic DIC due to cancer. The use of low molecular weight heparin for such purposes has not been standardized, and because low molecular weight heparin is not an antithrombin molecule, the use of this fraction of heparin has theoretical disadvantages. Other newly developed antithrombins have not been subjected to formal clinical trials in DIC.

In patients with DICS, heparin is most commonly given by intravenous continuous infusion at an hourly dose typical for a patient of the same size with thrombosis. Loading doses are usually modified, either greatly reduced or omitted, in order to avoid peak heparin levels which can completely compromise clotting. The PTT target should remain at 2-3 times the normal PTT, not the patient's baseline PTT. The underlying DIC process may be monitored by checking fibrinogen or platelet levels since the PTT will be affected by heparin. Several writers have advocated the simultaneous use of heparin and a plasmin inhibitor such as epsilonamino caproic acid or tranexamic acid. Both drugs are given on multidose or infusion schedules to ensure continuous levels and are stopped when the heparin is stopped.

LIVER FAILURE

This complex coagulopathy may be difficult to distinguish from DIC. Liver failure results in low levels of circulating procoagulants manufactured by the liver. Fibrinogen deficiency may result, for example, although this factor is often present in adequate levels even when multiple others are not. Platelet numbers may be low due to hypersplenism or the effects of alcohol on marrow production. And less specific tests of fibrinolysis may be elevated, such as the old fibrin split products test. Patients having liver failure may also be candidates for DIC, due to clinical circumstances such as shock or sepsis. There are several ways to distinguish DIC from liver failure: D-dimers may be mildly elevated, but usually not to DIC levels, and Factor VIII consumption occurs only in DIC, because it is not made in the liver.

Treatment for liver failure emphasizes platelet and plasma replacement. If DIC supervenes, fibrinogen and platelet requirements will increase. Heparin therapy is not usually considered in this situation, as bleeding risk is very high.

MASSIVE TRANSFUSION

Massive transfusion is a clinical situation that is usually defined as the replacement of at least 1 blood volume by transfusion within a 12-hour period. Trauma and difficult vascular surgery are the usual clinical situations in which massive transfusion occurs, and are often settings in which DIC may also occur. With the use of refrigerated packed red cells as the primary replacement therapy, the clinical situation which may occur with massive transfusion consists of loss of platelets and soluble clotting factors, the so-called "washout syndrome." Patients with massive transfusion without DIC are, like patients with liver failure, unlikely to have significantly elevated D-dimers or depleted Factor VIII levels. Table 2 compares the diagnosis of this situation with liver failure and DIC.

Treatment of massive transfusion requires blood bank supplementation. Several clinical studies clearly show that platelet deficiency occurs earlier during the course of massive transfusion, often at levels of 1.0 to 1.5 blood volumes, than does soluble factor deficiency. Prothrombin times may become elevated to levels of INR greater than 1.5 without symptomatic bleeding occurring. Thus, the hierarchy of replacement consists of empiric (not prophylactic) use of platelets, followed by measurement of prothrombin times and appropriate plasma replacement.

ACQUIRED VITAMIN K DEFICIENCY

Vitamin K is a mixture of compounds primarily found in green and leafy vegetables, is well absorbed, and is important in the carboxylation of glutamate residues on preprocoagulant factors manufactured in the liver. Vitamin K-related substances are also produced by enteric bacteria, so that patients are not often deficient except under the special circumstances of the ICU. Patients at high risk for acquired Vitamin K deficiency include patients who are eating poorly before admission to the hospital, who are made NPO in the hospital, who are not given parenteral nutrition, and who are treated with broad spectrum antibiotic coverage. Because Vitamin K is not stored, these patients may experience rapid depletion of Factors II, VII, IX, and X, and resulting prolongation of the prothrombin time, and to a lesser extent the PTT. If PTs are not rechecked or patients supplemented enterally or parenterally, bleeding may result and be a surprise to clinicians, occurring within a few days of normal admission tests of coagulation. Treatment is also rapidly effective: because of the presence of preprocoagulant proteins, carboxylation may occur within hours, and coagulation be restored within 12 to 24 hours. Slower rates of correction of the PT may be achieved by the use of oral low dose Vitamin K. However, if patients are having active, life-threatening bleeding, plasma repletion may be necessary.

Table 2. Comparison of 3 complex coagulopathies: Laboratory diagnosis

Disorder	PT, PTT	Fibrinogen	Platelets	FDPs	D-dimers	Factor VIII
DIC	High	Low	Low	High	Very high	Normal to low
Liver failure	High	N1 or low	N1 or low	High	Slightly high	Normal to high
Massive transfusion	High	Low	Low	High	Normal	Normal

PT, prothrombin; PTT, partial thromboplastin time; FDPs, fibrin degradation products; N1, normal.

ACQUIRED PLATELET DISORDERS

Introduction

Platelet disorders may be thought of as those of production and those of destruction, although combinations of the 2 are not uncommon. However, the approach to treatment of the 2 situations is different, and thus they are considered separately.

Platelet production by the marrow is normally slower than that of neutrophils: platelets are completely replaced in an average healthy person about every 7-10 days, so daily production of new platelets is about 10-15% of the total number of platelets. Platelet production may be reduced by a variety of diseases and situations, including drugs and marrow toxins, marrow diseases, acute infections, and autoimmune processes. These are summarized in Table 3.

When platelet production is low, platelet counts fall gradually, although not necessarily to zero. Platelet support from the blood bank is indicated when levels fall to below 10,000/mm^3 because of the risk of spontaneous intracerebral hemorrhage. When patients are bleeding or require surgery, platelets may be transfused to achieve levels of more than 50,000/mm^3. Clearly, recovery cannot occur until the underlying cause has been effectively treated.

Platelet destruction is characterized by peripheral loss of platelets produced in presumably adequate numbers by the bone marrow. This consumption may be immune-mediated, as in idiopathic thrombocytopenic purpura or post-transfusion purpura, or nonimmune, as in burns and intravascular devices. Antibodies against platelet membrane antigens may be produced in a variety of settings. Autoimmune disorders may be accompanied by antibody-mediated destruction of platelets; systemic lupus is the most common of these. Platelets may be destroyed as bystanders by the antibodies generated against homologous platelets after transfusion: the resulting thrombocytopenia is transient and resolves spontaneously but may be quite severe, and is called posttransfusion purpura. Neonates

Table 3. Causes of platelet underproduction

Disease:	
	Primary cancers of the marrow (leukemia, myeloma, lymphoma)
	Secondary cancers in the marrow (breast, prostate, GU, GI, melanoma)
	Myelodysplasia
	Inflammatory diseases in the marrow (tuberculosis, histoplasmosis, etc.)
	Immunologic diseases
	Viral infections
Drugs:	
	Anticancer drugs, radiation
	Idiosyncratic reactions:
	Thiazides
	Quinines, related drugs
	Sulfa drugs
	Phenothiazines

GU, genitourinary; GI, gastrointestinal.

may have purpura as a consequence of maternal antibodies.

Clinical Platelet Disorders

Idiopathic thrombocytopenic purpura, or ITP, is a disorder in which the stimulus to platelet antibody formation is unknown. ITP may be transient, as it is most often in children, or chronic and relapsing. Platelets coated with antibodies are destroyed very rapidly in the reticuloendothelial system. Therefore, transfusions result in rapid consumption of homologous platelets and are of little benefit. However, both rapid treatment of the disease process, usually with steroids as the initial therapy, combined with the use of large doses of intravenous immunoglobulin, may permit transfusion of homologous platelets when necessary.

Thrombotic thrombocytopenic purpura (TTP) is a different disorder, caused by the inborn or acquired deficiency of a plasma protease, in which platelet aggregation is the basic mechanism of thrombocytopenia. The normal relationship between platelet and endothelial surface, which does not permit aggregation to occur, is disrupted, and multimers of von Willebrand factor, which appear to mediate this platelet-endothelial interaction, disappear from the circulation. Microvascular platelet aggregation results in intravascular hemolysis. The other attributes of the TTP syndrome include CNS abnormalities, renal dysfunction, and fever. This clinical pentad should not be missed, for the mortality of untreated TTP is high: over 80% in the early series.

It is important to recognize TTP as a clinical entity, for the treatment differs dramatically from DIC, even though the patients may resemble each other clinically. About half of patients presenting with TTP have an underlying autoimmune disease; many develop chronic relapsing TTP after the initial episode. TTP may be caused by drugs, particularly by ticlopidine and clopidogrel. The hemolytic-uremic syndrome has a similar presentation, with the exception of very little CNS involvement; it is more common in children and is thought to be a consequence of exposure to enterobacterial toxins in most cases. Patients with malignant hypertension and other systemic vasculopathy may have platelet consumption and renal insufficiency and be difficult to distinguish from TTP unless an assay for the plasma protease activity can be obtained.

Patients with TTP often appear in the ICU, with the differential diagnosis of sepsis syndrome or other serious illness. Distinguishing their syndrome from DIC is straightforward: fibrinogen consumption is not a feature of TTP. Therefore, the laboratory abnormalities will consist of thrombocytopenia, a microangiopathic hemolytic anemia, and no evidence of excess thrombin activity or fibrinolysis. A DIC screen is usually sufficient to make the distinction. TTP therapy is unique, and consists of plasmapheresis or plasma exchange. The results are occasionally quite dramatic, but are for the most part lifesaving. Chronic TTP may occur after the remission of the acute episode, and may be treated with aspirin, steroids, and other immunosuppressing drugs, and periodic transfusion or pheresis.

Platelet Function Abnormalities

A variety of disorders and drugs may produce platelet function abnormalities. Most of these are accompanied by easy bruisability and mucosal surface bleeding, if they have any clinical manifestations at all. Concerns about platelet function arise in the setting of elective surgical procedures and mild thrombocytopenia, where the severity of bleeding seems greater than the platelet count would predict.

Aspirin and other NSAIDs interfere with platelet cyclooxygenase, and thus with platelet aggregation. Aspirin permanently acetylates the membrane cyclooxygenase, and thus platelets are affected until they are retired from circulation. This results in an approximate doubling of a normal person's bleeding time. However, assuming normal platelet production, most people have normal bleeding times within 24 hours of taking aspirin, and routine elective surgery has not been shown to be compromised by aspirin usage. Arguably, surgery that requires more platelets, such as major vascular surgery, bypass surgery, and surgery on the prostate, require larger pools of fully functioning platelets. Therefore, most clinicians stop aspirin 1 week prior to such surgery.

Inhibitors of the platelet surface receptor IIB/IIIA are a category of platelet function inhibitor widely used following angioplasty for prevention of restenosis. These inhibitors, either the monoclonal antibody or the drugs, are potent inhibitors of platelet function that may occasionally be associated with significant bleeding. Most such bleeding is due to iatrogenic interventions such as the site of the insertion of the angioplasty catheter. The half-life of these agents is generally short, and therefore, only local measures may be needed to arrest bleeding. However, if major bleeding occurs, platelet transfusion may be necessary.

Uremia produces platelet dysfunction that is remediable with more intensive dialysis. Persistent platelet dysfunction in face of adequate dialysis may require treatment: DDAVP may be used to rapidly temporarily raise vonWillebrand Factor levels and improve platelet aggregation; so may cryoprecipitate. Infusions of high doses of conjugated estrogens will produce a similar, more sustained effect.

BLEEDING DUE TO ANTICOAGULATION OR THROMBOLYSIS

Heparin and Bleeding

Anticoagulation is clearly the goal of heparin therapy, but occasionally it is inadvertent due to accidental drug administration or overdose. Bleeding while on therapeutic doses of heparin may occur if continuous infusion is not used, since most bleeding episodes are associated with peak doses and very high PTTs. Making the diagnosis of heparin effect is possible by several tests: a thrombin time is exquisitely sensitive to heparin effect, and unless the patient is known to have a disorder of fibrinogen structure or function, heparin is almost always the cause of a prolonged thrombin time. Where this may be questionable, heparin may be removed from the plasma by filtration on anionic beads, by anti-heparin antibodies, or by the addition of protamine. Heparin-free thrombin times should then be normal. Protamine may be used to reverse the effect of heparin *in vivo*. One milligram of protamine will bind and reverse the effect of about 100 units of heparin. The laboratory may be able to estimate the number of units per cc of plasma by using the PTT; if so, then the calculation of protamine dose requires only an estimate of plasma volume. If this is not available, a half-life for iv heparin and the approximate dose given may be useful for dose calculation.

Heparin-Induced Thrombocytopenia

Heparin therapy is often accompanied by thrombocytopenia, perhaps in as many as 10% of all patients. The majority of such patients have mild thrombocytopenia, generally over 50,000/ul, which occurs in the first 2-5 days of treatment and is self-limited. While this mild syndrome may complicate the assessment of bleeding, it is not necessary to withdraw heparin therapy. The most feared complication of heparin therapy occurs slightly later in the course of therapy, and is caused when antibodies to the heparin-platelet surface complex develop. These cause platelet aggregation, and may cause either severe thrombocytopenia or major vessel thrombosis. HIT, as it is called, is a highly morbid complication, but is without any known predictors except prior heparin sensitivity (in which case it develops more rapidly). Heparin must be discontinued, and low molecular weight heparin is not considered an alternative. If warfarin therapy has been started early, such patients may be adequately anticoagulated, and no further intervention is needed. If such patients require anticoagulation, danaproid or recombinant hirudin (leupiridin) may be used. Thrombolysis of the major clot is an option. If patients have severe thrombocytopenia without thrombosis and require cessation of anticoagulation, at least temporarily, then venous filters are commonly employed. Reexposure to heparin must be avoided.

Bleeding Due to Excess Warfarin or Rat Poison

Bleeding is a common complication of warfarin therapy, although the use of INR to gauge warfarin level has improved the risks of bleeding. Patients who bleed on warfarin may be segregated into 2 groups—those who bleed with therapeutic INRs, and those who bleed with supratherapeutic INRs. Patients who have focal, localized bleeding with therapeutic INRs should probably be evaluated for a cause, since studies of underlying causes of warfarin-associated bleeding suggest that the high-risk patients are mostly distributed within this group. Patients who bleed on supratherapeutic doses of warfarin (above INRs of 3.5) should have their drug discontinued, and may be more acutely treated, but do not necessarily require further evaluation. Serious bleeding should be treated with Vitamin K, and life-threatening bleeding with Vitamin K and fresh frozen plasma (for dose calculation, see Blood Bank section). Rat poison consists of coumarols with extremely long half-lives, usually days to weeks, and thus Vitamin K therapy to reverse the bleeding must be very high dose and sustained for a very long time. Acute, life-threatening bleeding in such patients should also be treated with fresh frozen plasma.

Bleeding Due to Thrombolytic Agents

Thrombolysis may be associated with pathologic bleeding for 2 reasons: the dissolution of existing clots and the inhibition of further clotting. Both streptokinase and alteplase (TPA) produce clot dissolution. This problem is usually seen primarily at recent venipuncture sites, and is treated with local pressure with good results. Both drugs have very short half-lives, and therefore, this effect does not last long. Streptokinase produces hypofibrinogenemia, sometimes to near zero levels, thus further clotting may not occur until fibrinogen is given. The usual source for this is cryoprecipitate, which is empiric, first-line therapy for a patient with life-threatening bleeding due to streptokinase. Both drugs may raise plasma levels of fragments of fibrin clot, which may inhibit further clotting to a slight extent and may inhibit platelet function as well. Therefore, protracted, severe bleeding (after fibrinogen therapy in streptokinase-treated patients) may be further treated by platelet administration or plasma administration, though clinical results are not clear. Administration of heparin following thrombolysis may be accompanied by a further bleeding tendency; the choice to discontinue heparin use depends on the severity and persistence of the bleeding problem.

SUMMARY

DIC is a complex syndrome characterized by excesses of coagulation and thrombolysis, resulting in hemostatic failure in the majority of patients with the disorder. The diagnosis is made by demonstrating the dynamic changes in the coagulation system in an appropriate clinical setting. This entity must be distinguished from several other causes of acute hemostatic failure, which may occur in similar clinical settings: liver failure, massive transfusion, TTP, and acquired Vitamin K deficiency.

Severe thrombocytopenia may be acquired in a variety of ways, but can be categorized generally as disorders in which platelet production fails and platelet support is effective, and as disorders in which platelets are destroyed by immune or nonimmune mechanisms and platelet support may be less effective. Platelet function abnormalities may exacerbate other coagulation problems.

Recognition is key to diagnosing bleeding due to iatrogenic causes. Stopping the offending drug and administering effective local measures to control bleeding are the most important first steps. Use of specific and nonspecific antidotes is necessary when bleeding is profuse or life-threatening.

BIBLIOGRAPHY

1. Bagby GC Jr, ed: Hematologic Aspects of Systemic Disease. *Hematol Oncol Clin N Am* 1987; 1(2):167-349
   A readable summary of many acquiredbleeding and other hematologic problems.
2. Bick RL: Hemostasis defects associated with cardiac surgery, prosthetic devices, and other extracorporeal circuits. *Semin Thromb Hematost* 1985; 11:249
   There are a host of similar articles available. This one is reasonably academic, covers all devices in addition to bypass, and is therefore a good reference.
3. Bick RL: Coagulation abnormalities in malignancy: A review. *Semin Thromb Hemost* 1992;   (4):353-72
   This is another nice academic review by the same author, also a useful reference.
4. Bone RC, Francis PB, Pierce AK: Intravascular coagulation associated with the adult respiratory distress syndrome. *Am J Med* 1976; 61:585
   A now classic article putting forth the idea that microvascular thrombi seen in DIC contribute to organ dysfunction which follows (in this case ARDS). Never proven, this hypothesis nonetheless is important.
5. Bredbacka S, Blomback M, Wiman B, et al: Laboratory methods for detecting disseminated intravascular coagulation (DIC): New aspects. *Acta Anaesth, Scand* 1993; 37:125-30
   A highly speculative article which follows Bone's reasoning that DIC causes multiorgan failure and thus looks for latent DIC in prolonged ventilator patients. Interesting, for aficionados.

6. Brown RB, Klar J, Teres D, et al: Prospective study of clinical bleeding in intensive care unit patients. *Crit Care Med* 1988; I :1 171
    Only study of its kind to examine causes, characteristics, and importance of bleeding in the critically ill, in 1,328 consecutive patients.

7. Buchanan GR: Coagulation disorders in the neonate. *Ped Clin N Am* 1986; 33:203
    Very readable, concise article, just in case you also take care of such individuals.

8. Carvalho AC: Acquired platelet dysfunction in patients with uremia. *Heme Oncol Clin N Amer* 1990; 4:129
    The nature and treatment of the uremic hemorrhagic tendency is reviewed. Most complete recent article on the subject.

9. Colman RWI Robboy SJ, Minna JD: Disseminated intravascular coagulation (DIC): An approach. *Am J Med* 1972; 52:769
    Historically important as strong advocates of the use of heparin in DIC, though with little supporting data.

10. Corrigan JJ Jr, Jordan CM: Heparin therapy in septicemia with disseminated coagulation. *N Engl J Med* 1970; 283:778
    The opposite view of DIC: heparin therapyused with some laboratory but little clinical effect.

11. Klappers-Klunne MC, Boon DM, Hop WC, et al: Heparin-induced thrombocytopenia and thrombosis: A prospective analysis of the incidence in patients with heart and cerebrovascular diseases. *Br J Haematol* 1997; 96:442-6
    Very nice study of unselected patients which shows very low incidence of clinical thrombocytopenia, though much higher incidence of platelet antibodies. Contrast with the Levine and Hirsh trial (Warkentin et al, below).

12. Levi M, ten Cate H, van der Poll I, van Deventer SJ: Pathogenesis of disseminated intravascular coagulation in sepsis. *JAMA* 1993; 270(8):975-9
    Excellent summary of state of the art about how DIC works. Very readable.

13. McKenna, R: Abnormal coagulation in the postoperative period contributing to excessive bleeding. *Med Clin N Am* 2001; 85(5):1277-310

14. Rapaport SI: Blood coagulation and its alterations in hemorrhagic and thrombotic disorders. *Western J Med* 1993; 158:153-61
    This is everything you ever needed to know about clotting in 1 masterful article, which was a grand rounds. His textbook is a bible also.

15. Sane DC, Califf RM, Topol EJ, et al: Bleeding during thrombolytic therapy for acute myocardial infarction: Mechanisms and management. *Ann Intern Med* 1989; 111:1010
    A nice summary of what is known and speculated about why patients bleed. Provides a treatment algorithm.

16. Warkentin TE, Kelton JG: A 14-year study of heparin-induced thrombocytopenia. *Am J Med* 1996; 101(5):502-7
    Their latest summary of the natural history of this entity.

17. Warkentin TE, Levine MN, Hirsh J, et al: Heparin-induced thrombocytopenia in patients treated with low molecular weight heparin or unfractionated heparin. *New Engl J Med* 1995; 332:1330-5
    Prospective randomized trial comparing the 2 (in selected patients for study—see Kappers-Klune above) drugs which shows clearly that low molecular weight heparin is associated with fewer complications.

ACUTE PULMONARY EMBOLISM

R. Phillip Dellinger, MD, FCCP, FCCM

Objectives

- To identify patients at risk for pulmonary embolism
- To know the typical clinical presentations of pulmonary embolism
- To appreciate the role of perfusion lung scanning, leg studies, CT scanning, and D-dimers in the diagnostic approach to pulmonary embolism
- To understand the role of anticoagulation, inferior vena cava filter placement, and thrombolytic therapy in the management of pulmonary embolism

Key Words: thromboembolism; deep-vein thrombosis; pulmonary embolism; ventilation/perfusion lung scanning; compression ultrasound; impedance plethysmography; anticoagulation; thrombolytic therapy

TABLE OF ABBREVIATIONS

CT	computed tomography
CUS	compression ultrasound
DVT	deep-vein thrombosis
INR	international normalized ratio
IPG	impedance plethysmography
IPVC	intermittent pneumatic venous compression
IVC	inferior vena cava
LMWH	low-molecular-weight heparin
MRI	magnetic resonance imaging
PE	pulmonary embolism
PIOPED	Prospective Investigation of Pulmonary Embolism Diagnosis
PT	prothrombin time
PTT	partial thromboplastin time
RAP	right atrial pressure
RV	right ventricular
VTE	venous thromboembolism
V/Q	ventilation/perfusion

Pulmonary embolism (PE) remains a diagnostic challenge. The most common symptoms and signs of PE are nonspecific. Noninvasive tests suffer from less-than-ideal sensitivity and specificity. Each case in question is unique, making a simple algorithm approach unsettling. However, the accumulation of multiple test results to create a more complex algorithm may be useful when combined with pretest clinical suspicion.

RISK FACTORS

Major risk factors for pulmonary emboli are processes that predispose a patient to the development of deep-vein thrombosis (DVT), i.e., any cause of venous stasis, such as venous valvular insufficiency, right-sided heart failure, the postoperative period, and prolonged bed rest, or immobilization. Abdominal operations requiring general anesthesia of $\geq$ 30 minutes place the patient at risk for venous thromboembolism (VTE). Orthopedic surgery of the lower extremity has long been recognized as one of the greatest risk factors for VTE. More than 50% of unprophylaxed patients undergoing elective total hip replacement and knee replacement surgery develop DVT. Over 90% of proximal thrombi occur in hip replacement patients on the operated side. Since the first controlled trials demonstrating a reduced rate of PE mortalities with anticoagulant prophylaxis were carried out in this high-risk group, patients with fractures of the pelvis, hip, or femur are of significant historical relevance.

Trauma to the extremities, advanced malignancy (increasingly recognized as a major risk factor), pregnancy, the postpartum state and, to a lesser degree, birth control pills (current formulations have lowered estrogen content) are significant risk factors. Long distance air travel has also been linked to PE. There is an estimated 40% risk of VTE and a 5% incidence of PE in patients with traumatic spinal cord injury and associated paralysis of lower extremities. The period of greatest risk is during the first 2 weeks post initial injury; death occurs rarely in PE patients after 3 months.

The frequency of VTE increases exponentially between the ages of 20 and 80 years. Although an age of > 40 years has often been used as a break point for age-related increase in VTE, increasing age increases risk beginning with adulthood and continues to increase after the age of 40 years, nearly doubling with each decade. One study demonstrated a 23% incidence of PE in 175,730 tertiary care hospital admissions with linear relation to age. The incidence in women was higher in individuals ≥ 50 years old, but not in those < 50 yrs old (Stein et al, 1999). In patients with a history of thromboembolic disease who undergo hospitalization, there is nearly an 8-fold increase in acute thromboembolism compared with patients without such a history, therefore making acute thromboembolism one of the more important risk factors for VTE.

Patients with a history of VTE who undergo major surgery, periods of immobility, or who are hospitalized for serious medical illnesses must be aggressively targeted for prophylaxis therapy. Although precise estimates of risk increase in malignancy are difficult to ascertain, advanced cancer is associated with a high risk of VTE.

With other risk factors considered equal, surgery for malignant disease results in a 2-to 3-fold increase in thromboembolism compared with surgery for nonmalignant conditions. Hypercoagulable states secondary to deficiencies of antithrombin III, protein C, or protein S, as well as the presence of antiphospholipid antibody or factor V Leiden mutation are predisposing factors for thromboembolic disease. Screening for select hypercoagulable states is appropriate in patients with no obvious risk factors who develop PE. This screening is most appropriate for the 3 coagulopathies that can be measured accurately in the presence of acute clot burden/anticoagulation and have therapeutic implications to include factor V Leiden (most common hypercoagulable state and would warrant more aggressive prophylaxis), antiphospholipid antibody (dictates more

aggressive warfarin therapy), and hyperhomocysteinuria (treatable with B vitamins). Although most pulmonary emboli come from deep veins of the lower extremities, clinically significant emboli also occur from other sites of venous thrombosis to include the axillary/subclavian veins, iliac veins, pelvic veins, and less frequently, the inferior vena cava. Central venous catheters are risk factors for superior vena cava/axillary/subclavian vein thrombosis, as well as femoral vein thrombosis.

SYNDROMES OF ACUTE PULMONARY EMBOLISM

Multiple clinical syndromes are associated with PE. Pulmonary infarction is characterized by a pulmonary infiltrate that is often peripheral and wedge-shaped, pleuritic chest pain, hemoptysis, and not infrequently, a bloody pleural effusion. These findings represent the "textbook" version of PE that is taught to medical students and are seen in only 10% of pulmonary emboli. Pulmonary infarction is rare due to 3 sources of oxygen and 2 sources of nutrient supply to the lung; the bronchial and pulmonary arteries and the airways. In addition, back-perfusion from the pulmonary venous system may also be a potential source of oxygen and nutrient supply. Pulmonary infarction is more likely to occur in the face of pre-existing compromise of nutrient or oxygen supply, such as in intrinsic lung disease or in the presence of reduced cardiac output.

A second clinical syndrome is acute onset of shortness of breath or hypoxemia in the absence of pulmonary infarction, with or without chest pain (often pleuritic when present). Radiographic infiltrates may or may not be present. This is the most common presentation of PE.

A third clinical syndrome is acute massive PE, characterized by a large thromboembolus lodging in the proximal pulmonary circulation, resulting in hypotension and possible syncope. Chest pain may be present and is probably due to right ventricular or left ventricular myocardial ischemia. Infiltrates are usually absent in massive pulmonary embolus unless the embolus has fragmented and moved peripherally. Acute pulmonary hypertension with central dilated pulmonary arteries may also be present. Hypoxemia is almost always present, although hypotension is usually the primary clinical concern.

CLINICAL FINDINGS

The clinical diagnosis of PE is difficult. Clinical acumen falters due to both sensitivity and specificity problems. The most common symptoms/signs of dyspnea, tachypnea, and tachycardia are seen with a myriad of other disorders. Tachypnea and tachycardia may be transient. The physical examination is not typically helpful in considering PE, with the exception of the presence of findings to support acute increases of right-sided pressure such as a right-sided S3, widely split-second heart sound, murmur of tricuspid regurgitation, or an accentuated pulmonary closure sound. Examination of the lower extremity is unreliable for predicting the presence or absence of DVT. Nevertheless, new findings supportive of acute deep-vein obstruction, particularly unilateral leg swelling in the setting of pulmonary symptoms compatible with thromboembolism, should strengthen the possibility of PE. Fever (temperature $\geq 100.0°F$) has been demonstrated to be present in 14% of angiographically documented PE with no other cause of fever. Only 2 of 228 patients had temperatures $\geq 103.0°F$. Leukocytosis may or may not be present.

Tachycardia and nonspecific ST-T changes are the most common electrocardiographic findings in PE. In massive PE, right-heart strain may be indicated by P-wave pulmonale, $S_1Q_3T_3$ pattern, right axis deviation, or right-bundle branch block.

Chest radiographic abnormalities due to PE include pulmonary infiltrate, pleural effusion, elevated hemidiaphragm, and atelectasis. A pleural-based, wedge-shaped infiltrate called a Hampton's hump may be seen in some cases of pulmonary infarction. An unremarkable chest radiograph with significant hypoxemia and no obvious cause, such as asthma or exacerbation of chronic obstructive pulmonary disease, should also raise the concern for PE. Patients who develop PE in the ICU typically have abnormal chest radiographs due to pre-existing pulmonary disease. A recent study found cardiomegaly to be the most common chest radiograph abnormality (Elliott et al).

Analysis of pleural fluid in a patient suspected of having PE is useful only to confirm other diagnoses. There are no pathognomonic pleural effusion findings with PE; the effusion may be a transudate or exudate; it may or may not be bloody. A bloody pleural effusion that accompanies pulmonary embolus usually implies pulmonary infarction. Other potential etiologies of bloody pleural effusions include malignancy and trauma.

Echocardiography is most helpful in delineating other etiologies of clinical findings, such as myocardial ischemia or pericardial tamponade. Findings such as acute right ventricular (RV) dilation and hypokinesis, tricuspid regurgitation, pulmonary hypertension estimated from tricuspid regurgitation jet, pulmonary artery dilation, loss of respiratory variation in IVC diameter, interventricular septum bulge into the left ventricle (LV), and reduced D-shaped LV size may support the diagnosis of PE but are not specific enough to establish the diagnosis. A distinct radiograph pattern has recently been noted in patients with large PE in which regional RV dysfunction is noted but the apex is spared (McConnell et al). Clinically significant PE may also occur in the absence of any abnormal RV findings on echocardiography. Rarely, a clot may be visualized in the right heart and thus allows a specific diagnosis.

Although the older D-dimer assay (latex agglutination) was neither sensitive nor specific for the diagnosis of PE, the enzyme-linked immunosorbent assay (ELISA) D-dimer and other newer non-latex assays may be clinically useful. A D-dimer measured by ELISA was noted to be normal in < 10% of angiographically documented PE in 1 study (Quinn et al). However, a negative D-dimer was rare in any patient with recent surgery, malignancy, or total bilirubin > 2 mg/dL, regardless of the presence or absence of PE. The traditional ELISA assay typically requires 24 hours for results. Newer, second-generation tests, including rapid ELISA, erythrocyte agglutination, turbidometric assay, and immunofiltration may offer reliable and rapid bedside testing. Level-1 data are, however, needed with these tests to establish them as routine care.

A fall in end-tidal CO_2 may also be useful in raising the clinical suspicion of PE, while a decrease in $PaCO_2$ may be a marker of success of thrombolytic therapy in patients with PE (Wiegand et al).

GAS EXCHANGE ABNORMALITIES IN PULMONARY EMBOLISM

Respiratory alkalosis is a common finding in the tachypneic patient with PE. With massive pulmonary embolus, respiratory acidosis may be present due to increased deadspace. Although a room air PaO_2 of > 80 torr (> 10.7 kPa) or a normal alveolar-arterial gradient makes the diagnosis of PE less likely, neither can be relied on to exclude PE. Patients with PE may have a normal alveolar-arterial (A-a) gradient. This finding is more likely to occur in the presence of previous normal cardiopulmonary status. Hypoxemia and an increase in alveolar-arterial gradient may also be transient. Forty-two patients in the Prospective Investigation of Pulmonary Embolism Diagnosis (PIOPED) trial had suspected PE, no prior cardiopulmonary disease, and fulfilled all of the following criteria: $PaO_2 \geq 80$ torr (≥ 10.7 kPa), $PaCO_2 \geq 35$ torr (≥ 4.7 kPa), and normal alveolar-arterial gradient. Sixteen (38%) patients had angiographically documented PE. In patients who had prior cardiopulmonary disease and who met all 3 criteria mentioned above, 14% had PE. Therefore, normal arterial blood gases, in general, and in patients with no prior history of cardiopulmonary disease, in particular, do not allow discontinuation of the pursuit of PE.

Nonmassive PE produces hypoxemia by release of bronchoconstrictors, production of atelectasis (surfactant depletion over hours), and perhaps reperfusion injury to the endothelial-epithelial barrier. Massive PE is almost always associated with hypoxemia and frequently with CO_2 retention. In addition to the same causes of hypoxemia as related above for nonmassive PE, the amputation of pulmonary vascular bed in massive PE produces both a large increase in dead space (as a cause of increased $PaCO_2$) and a large amount of blood flow diverted to noninvolved areas of the lung, causing a low ventilation/perfusion (V/Q) ratio in those areas due to overperfusion. This low V/Q ratio in uninvolved areas of the lung is a likely cause of hypoxemia in massive PE. Other potential causes of hypoxemia in massive PE include low mixed venous oxygen due to low cardiac output, as well as the potential for opening of a propatent foramen ovale due to high right-sided pressures. A propatent foramen ovale is present in a small but significant percentage of the general population. In the presence of very high right-heart pressures, this right-to-left shunt produces hypoxemia unresponsive to oxygen therapy, and also places the patient at risk for embolic cerebral vascular events.

DIAGNOSIS—GENERAL

The treatment of PE or DVT is essentially the same as in patients with suspected PE; therefore, either diagnosis is sufficient for decision-making. Less invasive studies are initially used to pursue the possibility of thromboembolic disease, typically either perfusion lung scanning combined with leg ultrasound or spiral CT scanning. Pulmonary angiography may on occasions be needed.

DIAGNOSIS WITH PERFUSION LUNG SCANNING AND LOWER EXTREMITY ULTRASOUND

Perfusion lung scanning (usually done in combination with ventilation scanning) is typically classified into high probability, intermediate probability, low probability, and normal. Probability of PE increases with size of perfusion defect, number of moderate-to-large size defects, and perfusion defects that are significantly larger than ventilation defects or present in the absence of ventilation defects. Although ventilation scanning is usually performed in combination with perfusion scanning to quantify ventilation defects, chest radiographs can be used in place of ventilation scanning in patients without chronic pulmonary disease or acute bronchospasm. The use of perfusion scanning alone with classification of abnormal scans into those with wedge-shaped defects (PE+) and those without wedge-shaped defects (PE-) has also been demonstrated to be clinically useful in predicting which abnormal scans actually represent PE. In the United States, the PIOPED study is the most frequently utilized reference document for classification of V./Q. lung scanning. The PIOPED study supported the following findings:

- Normal lung scans make PE very unlikely.
- Reliability of a high-probability scan increases with:
  - The degree of clinical suspicion using history, physical examination, and clinical information
  - No underlying cardiopulmonary disease
  - No history of pulmonary emboli
- A minority of patients have high-probability perfusion scans
- A low-probability scan does not exclude PE
- A clinical impression of low likelihood of PE when combined with a low-probability scan increases the predictive value of the low-probability scan
- Intermediate-probability scans cannot be used for definitive decision-making
- The great majority of patients with suspected PE cannot have PE excluded with perfusion scanning
- It is best to call low- and intermediate-probability scans "nondiagnostic," with the classification system becoming high-probability, nondiagnostic, and normal

Nondiagnostic scans require additional testing. Additional testing typically begins with noninvasive leg studies. Subsequent pulmonary angiogram follows if the diagnosis remains in doubt. Spiral (helical) CT scans may be useful in this group as well. No differentiation is made between low and very low probability scans. Other pertinent facts in the consideration of PE include the knowledge that pulmonary emboli rarely predominate in upper lobes and are rarely single. In anticipation of a later question of failure of heparin therapy, a baseline perfusion scan should be considered even when the clinical diagnosis of PE is made, based on the presence of DVT. This will allow repeat scanning for the presence or absence of additional perfusion defects if new symptoms develop or symptoms continue.

Leg ultrasound is typically obtained in the following circumstances:

- A nondiagnostic (low-probability or intermediate-probability) perfusion scan in any patient
- A normal perfusion scan in a high-risk patient
- A high-probability perfusion scan in a low-risk patient

The rationale for combining leg ultrasound with the perfusion scan results is that diagnostic acumen is improved, clinically significant pulmonary emboli are unlikely to occur in the absence of DVT, and morbidity and mortality in PE are due to additional emboli.

CUS combines Doppler venous flow detection with venous imaging and has become the imaging procedure of choice for DVT in most medical centers in the United States. The diagnostic utility of CUS is related to imaging of a venous filling defect that persists with compression of the lesion. Impressive sensitivity and specificity for proximal vein thrombosis are usually obtained with this technique. This technique does not detect isolated thrombosis in the iliac veins or the superficial femoral veins within the adductor canal. It is, however, unlikely that these areas will be involved unless thrombus is also present in the more readily imageable popliteal and deep femoral system. Diagnosis of calf vein thrombosis is more challenging, as these veins are smaller, have slower flow, and have more anatomic variability. CUS, which is more reliable in the calf than IPG, is improving in this area. CUS may also diagnose other etiologies of clinical findings such as Baker's cyst, hematoma, lymphadenopathy, and abscess. Neither IPG nor CUS can be performed if the leg is casted. CUS may also be limited by pain and edema.

Diagnosis of DVT by CUS allows treatment since treatment for PE and DVT are essentially the same. Absence of DVT by CUS, in combination with low-probability perfusion scan and absence of high clinical suspicion, usually allows withholding treatment. One concern in regards to this approach, however, is that the sensitivity of CUS is significantly diminished in high-risk patients without leg symptoms or signs. Clinically evident pulmonary emboli are even more unlikely in the presence of serial negative noninvasive leg studies (typically repeated 2 to 3 times over a period of 10 to 14 days) and may be performed in this group to further enhance clinical acumen. A negative leg ultrasound in a patient with an intermediate-probability scan usually implies the need for an angiogram or spiral CT.

DIAGNOSIS—PREGNANCY

The pursuit of diagnosis of PE in pregnant women is challenging. Ventilation/perfusion scanning is low-risk. Warfarin is an absolute contraindication in the first trimester, and a relative contraindication in the second and third trimesters. Long-term heparin administration in the pregnant woman is a significant risk for osteoporosis. Pulmonary angiographic confirmation of diagnosis may be in the patient's best interest in many cases.

DIAGNOSIS—ANGIOGRAPHY

Pulmonary angiography is the gold standard for diagnosis of PE, and morbidity and mortality are low and acceptable. Angiography is considered positive when a persistent filling defect or cutoff sign is noted. Risk is increased if angiography is followed by thrombolytic therapy. In most cases, the risk/benefit ratio of pulmonary angiography is acceptable, and the risk to the patient is usually greater from anticoagulation in the absence of PE or failure to treat PE, which is present. The death rate from pulmonary angiogram in the PIOPED study was 0.5%, with a low incidence of major nonfatal complications. Major nonfatal complications were 4 times more likely to occur in ICU patients. Despite early studies that suggested a higher incidence of mortality due to pulmonary angiogram in patients with high pulmonary artery pressures, this was not found to be true in the PIOPED study. A pulmonary angiogram done within 1 week of acute symptoms should reliably detect pulmonary emboli even in the presence of anticoagulation. In patients with

angiographically proven pulmonary embolism, perfusion defects persist for at least 7 days without resolution, and in the majority at 14 days (Dalen et al). This is an important consideration since patients may be referred to a tertiary care center with uncertain diagnosis of PE, having received therapy for a considerable period of time.

COMPUTED TOMOGRAPHY

Spiral (helical) computed tomography (CT) is of significant value in detecting pulmonary emboli. A negative spiral CT makes pulmonary emboli unlikely when using the most recent CT imaging with digital reconstruction. A positive study assuming this same technology and an experienced, well-trained reader allows diagnosis and treatment.

The primary concern with the use of spiral CT in the evaluation for PE is sensitivity and whether, as a single test, if a negative study rules out PE. Although specificity (the chance of a positive test being a true positive) is very good, sensitivity in some studies has ranged from 53% to 67%. A meta-analysis of 15 identified prospective studies revealed only 2 series of consecutive patients, 1 study that included a broad spectrum of patients, and 8 studies that independently interpreted angiogram and CT. The authors concluded that there has been no prospective study of CT diagnosis of PE in which anticoagulant therapy has been withheld without additional testing for PE in consecutive patients with suspected PE and negative spiral CT.

A recent study (Lorut et al) developed a protocol approach in which all patients with suspected PE received a perfusion lung scan, spiral CT, and D-dimer (Figure 1). Patients with positive spiral CTs were treated as PE. Those with negative spiral CTs and high probability perfusion scans received angiography. Those with negative spiral CTs and either normal/unchanged Q scans or non-elevated D-dimer or other diagnosis on CT were judged to have no PE. All other patients had a leg ultrasound to dictate decision on no PE (negative ultrasound) or PE (positive ultrasound).

One sensitivity issue with the spiral CT diagnosis of PE is the decreased ability to detect vessels beyond the segmental arteries. This may be of less clinical significance, since the natural history of pulmonary emboli limited to subsegmental arteries may have a benign course, especially in patients with self-limited risk factors.

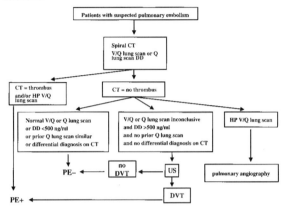

Figure 1. Demonstrated is flow of patients through PE diagnosis protocol based on results of CT, Q scan, and D-dimer. Ultrasound was used with indeterminate scenario.

ANTICOAGULATION

Heparin therapy is discontinued after a minimum of 4 to 5 days of therapy, at least 48 hours of warfarin therapy, and a warfarin-induced prolongation of international normalized ratio (INR) for prothrombin time (PT) of > 2.0. The partial thromboplastin time (PTT) should be maintained at 1.5 to 2 times control with heparin therapy. Although subtherapeutic aPTT is strongly correlated with thromboembolic recurrence, a supratherapeutic aPTT does not appear to correlate with important bleeding complication. Instead, bleeding complications correlate with concurrent illness such as renal disease, heavy ethanol consumption, aspirin use, and peptic ulcer disease. Based on this information, targeting an aPTT of 2.0 normal rather than 1.5 normal may be ideal. Adequate heparinization prevents additional clot formation, but the body's own fibrinolytic system must clear the clot that is already present so that patients who are hemodynamically unstable or who have poor cardiopulmonary reserve may remain at risk during early anticoagulation therapy. In patients without a contraindication for anticoagulation, heparin therapy should be instituted as soon as thromboembolic disease is considered. A

loading dose of 5,000 to 10,000 units of heparin is indicated for PE (Table 1).

Failure to achieve adequate heparinization in the first 24 hours of treatment has been demonstrated to increase the risk of recurrent emboli. Additionally, less heparin is typically required to maintain adequate anticoagulation after the first 48 hours of therapy.

Low-molecular-weight heparin (LMWH) is an effective subcutaneous therapy for DVT, and with a longer plasma half-life, LMWH may potentially be given once a day, although twice-daily therapy is recommended by some for treatment of symptomatic thromboembolism. It is as effective as standard heparin therapy in patient populations thus far tested. Although many studies have suggested either equal therapeutic effect with less bleeding or increased efficacy with the same bleeding complications when treating PE, large randomized, controlled trials have not been able to prove any statistically significant difference in clinical outcome. However, trends favor equal benefit with less bleeding with LMWH. Studies of higher power would be necessary to prove or disprove this benefit. Advantages of LMWH over unfractionated heparin for treatment of PE are, nevertheless, capability for outpatient treatment of DVT and decreased incidence of heparin-induced thrombocytopenia. Its disadvantages are greater cost of the heparin and in the critically ill patient in need of frequent invasive procedures, the longer half-life may be problematic. However, decreased administration costs and no need for monitoring coagulation in most patients may make LMWH cost efficacious. LMWH is approved for inpatient and outpatient DVT treatment, but it is not yet approved by the Food and Drug Administration for the outpatient treatment of PE. The outpatient administration of LMWH for DVT is cost-saving. Thrombocytopenia is uncommon enough that no more than 1 platelet count is recommended during a treatment period of 5 to 7 days. If therapy is prolonged > 7 days, subsequent platelet counts should be done. LMWH does not prolong PTT. Factor Xa levels reflect LMWH activity but are not routinely available or thought to be necessary in most patients treated. Factor Xa levels are

Table 1. Weight-based heparin dosing for pulmonary embolism[a]

Make calculations using total body weight in kilograms
Administer heparin, 80 units/kg, as an intravenous bolus
Intravenous heparin infusion, 18 units/kg/hr (20,000 units of heparin
       in 500 mL of D5W = 40 units/mL)
Stat activated partial thromboplastin time (aPTT) 6 hrs after heparin bolus.
Adjust heparin infusion based on sliding scale below:

aPTT (sec)	Dose Change
aPTT < 35	80-units/kg bolus, increase infusion rate
aPTT 35–45	40-units/kg bolus, increase infusion rate
aPTT 46–70	No change
aPTT 71–90	Reduce infusion rate by 2 units/kg/hr
aPTT > 90	Hold heparin for 1 hr, reduce infusion

Order aPTT 6 hours after dosage change, adjusting heparin infusion by the sliding scale until aPTT is
   therapeutic (46 to 70 seconds). When 2 consecutive aPTTs are therapeutic, order aPTT (and
   readjust heparin drip as needed) every 24 hours.
Make changes as promptly as possible and round off doses to the nearest mL/hr (nearest 40 units/hr)

   Adapted with permission from Raschke RA, Reilly BM, Guidry JR, et al: The weight-based heparin dosing nomogram compared with a "standard care" nomogram: A randomized controlled trial. *Ann Intern Med* 1993; 119:874

recommended when LMWH treatment is rendered to patients with renal failure (creatinine clearance of < 30 mL/min), or to very large persons or very small persons. When bleeding occurs after recent administration of LMWH, protamine is recommended for reversal, but degree of effectiveness in this circumstance is somewhat cloudy.

It is important to remember that warfarin therapy is contraindicated in pregnancy, and anticoagulation should be maintained with heparin. In addition, heparin dosage requirements are increased in pregnancy. Decreases in platelet count (heparin-induced thrombocytopenia or HIT) may occur with heparin therapy. A nonimmunologically mediated decrease in heparin (HIT-1) may occur, and is usually mild without dramatic drops in platelet count, occurs early in treatment, and does not usually require discontinuation of heparin. A more dramatic and clinically significant decrease in platelet count (HIT-2)

may rarely occur later in heparin therapy (day 3-4), is immunologically mediated, and does require immediate discontinuation of heparin therapy. Arterial thrombosis (white clot) may be a part of this more severe syndrome. When the platelet count falls precipitously or in a sustained fashion, heparin therapy should be stopped. When the platelet count falls to < 100,000, heparin therapy should be stopped. With HIT-2, warfarin should not be instituted for 2 days because of the possibility of increased clot formation. In addition, there is a chance for cross reactivity with LMWH, and that is not advisable as a therapeutic option. Therefore, although LMWH might be chosen as a better option than unfractionated heparin in patients with thrombocytopenia at baseline, once thrombocytopenia occurs on unfractionated heparin, switching to LMWH is not a good option. Since 4 to 5 days may be required to achieve anticoagulation with warfarin in that circumstance, hirudin or heparinoid therapy is recommended to protect in the interim.

THROMBOLYTIC THERAPY

Streptokinase, urokinase, and recombinant plasminogen activator (rTPA) are all thrombolytic agents for consideration of treatment of PE. Urokinase is not currently available. Indications for thrombolytic therapy are controversial since thrombolytic therapy has not been proven to alter clinical end points, such as mortality. Thrombolytic therapy followed by heparin has, however, been shown to provide more rapid improvement in RV function than heparin alone; therefore, its utility in the face of hemodynamic instability is its primary potential utilization. Severe hypoxemia despite maximum oxygen supplementation is also a generally accepted indication. All other uses are controversial (see discussion to follow). Traditional contraindications for thrombolytic therapy are active internal bleeding, recent acute cerebrovascular event (2 months), or recent cerebrovascular procedure (2 months). Severi et al, however, reported the successful use of urokinase thrombolytic therapy of pulmonary embolism in 9 neurosurgical patients (mean 19 days after surgery) with no intracranial hemorrhage (1 subgaleal hematoma). Intracranial bleeding, a primary concern, occurs in 1% - 2% of patients with PE who are treated with thrombolytic therapy. Retroperitoneal hemorrhage can also be life-threatening, and most frequently occurs as a sequela of previous femoral vein access for pulmonary angiography or other associated femoral lines. Relative contraindications to thrombolytic therapy include any history of cerebrovascular event, a ≤ 10-day postpartum period, recent organ biopsy or puncture of a noncompressible vessel, recent serious internal trauma, surgery within the last 7 days, uncontrolled coagulation defects, pregnancy, cardiopulmonary resuscitation with rib fracture, thoracentesis, paracentesis, lumbar puncture, and any other conditions which place the patient at risk for bleeding. In general, angiographic documentation of PE should be obtained before thrombolytic therapy. Spiral CT diagnosis is sufficient. Occasionally, thrombolytic therapy may be considered in hemodynamically unstable patients with a high-probability perfusion scan who cannot be moved to receive pulmonary angiography. Bedside echocardiography, if immediately available, is also a consideration to offer additional support for diagnosis. When neither angiography nor perfusion scanning is possible, the patient is at risk for death, and the clinical scenario is strongly suggestive, echocardiography supporting PE may be adequate diagnosis. No coagulation tests are typically necessary during thrombolysis. Blood samples should be limited during the thrombolytic agent infusion period. Heparin should not be administered during thrombolysis, but heparin therapy should be resumed without a bolus when the PTT is 1.5 to 2 times control. If bleeding should occur during thrombolytic therapy, this therapy should be discontinued to control hemorrhage due to the short half-life of the thrombolytic agent. If bleeding should persist, cryoprecipitate infusion or fresh-frozen plasma should be considered.

Although no study has demonstrated thrombolytic therapy-induced improvement in survival or decrease in recurrent thromboembolic events, its use is advocated by some in the presence of large clot burden or especially with echocardiographic evidence of acute RV dilation. This latter argument is based on the fact that RV dysfunction strongly correlates with mortality in patients with PE. Those who argue against thrombolytic use in this circumstance point to the low mortality rate once PE is diagnosed (8% - 9%), the absence of studies demonstrating clinical outcome benefit in this group, and the low but potentially catastrophic incidence of intracranial hemorrhage with thrombolytic therapy. A recently published case series of 7 consecutive patients with massive PE associated with RV thrombi used continuous transthoracic echocardiography to demonstrate complete clot lysis at 45 to 60 minutes with r-TPA (Greco et al). A recent study (Grifoni et al) evaluated 200 consecutive patients with documented PE (diagnosis made by high probability V./Q., spiral CT, or angiography) who had echocardiography to document the presence on absence of acute RV dysfunction. Of the 65 normotensive patients with acute RV dysfunction (31% of patients), 6 developed PE-related shock after admission and 3 died. A contrasting study comes to a contrasting opinion (Hamel et al). Using a retrospective cohort analysis of 2 matched groups of 64 patients, the study concluded that although thrombolytic therapy improved lung scan more rapidly, there were no differences in recurrences or death rate from PE but increased death rate from bleeding.

The management of free-floating RV thrombi remains controversial. Echocardiography usually demonstrates evidence of right ventricular overload (> 90%), paradoxical interventricular septal motion (75%), and pulmonary hypertension (86%) (Chastin et al). The clots are usually worm-like, mortality is high (45%), and thrombolytic therapy, if not contraindicated, is recommended as the treatment of choice by some investigators (Chartier et al). Infusion of a thrombolytic agent directly onto a pulmonary thrombus via the pulmonary artery has never been convincingly shown to be superior to infusion of the agent through a peripheral vein. There is some data in the radiology literature to suggest this may be useful for deep vein thrombus. The use of thrombolytic agents in PE remains controversial. The ACCP Consensus Statement of Thromboembolism states that the use of thrombolytic agents continues to be highly individualized, and clinicians should have latitude in their use. They are, however, recommended in general for hemodynamic instability and massive ileofemoral thrombosis.

In the United States, the most frequently used thrombolytic agent for the treatment of PE is rTPA. FDA-approved dosing is 100 mg over 2 hours. In the patient with massive PE in whom death appears imminent without thrombolytic intervention, more rapid administration may be appropriate. One proposed alternative, which seems reasonable in that circumstance is 40 mg over minutes followed by 60 mg over the remainder of the 2-hour period. One study of pulmonary embolism as the cause of arrest noted a clinical diagnosis of pulmonary embolism made in 70% of patients (30% were not suspected until autopsy) (Kurkcigan et al). In 21 of these 24 patients, r-TPA was administered; 2 of these patients survived to hospital discharge.

USE OF INFERIOR VENA CAVA FILTER

Traditional indications for IVC filter placement include contraindication to anticoagulation, onset of bleeding with anticoagulation, and failure of anticoagulation to abate thromboembolic events. In hemodynamically unstable patients who will not be given thrombolytic therapy, IVC filters have been used as a bridge to warfarin therapy. Hirudin and heparinoids, if available, are less invasive and more appropriate alternatives in this situation. The empiric use of IVC filter in patients with a large clot burden or poor cardiopulmonary reserve is more controversial. Filter placement may also be considered in patients with high risk for DVT and relative or absolute contraindications for anticoagulation prophylaxis of DVT. The decision to anticoagulate patients who have had an IVC filter placed is controversial, but the use of anticoagulation may prevent further clot formation and increase the patency rate of the filter over time and, therefore, facilitate venous drainage. Patency can be maintained, however, without concomitant heparin therapy. Documentation of deep venous thrombotic disease is usually required before placement of an IVC filter. A filter may also benefit patients at high risk for chronic anticoagulation, such as poorly compliant patients or patients at risk for falls. Complications of filter placement include vessel injury at the time of insertion, subsequent venous thrombosis at the insertion site, filter migration, and embolization into the heart, filter erosion through the IVC, and IVC obstruction.

PULMONARY EMBOLISM INDUCED HYPOPERFUSION STATE

The right ventricle cannot increase stroke volume in response to sudden increases in afterload. Instead, the right ventricle dilates as ejection fraction decreases. Failure of the right ventricle to compensate for the increased afterload produces hypotension and, if severe, syncope. Studies of hemodynamic profiles in patients with acute PE have demonstrated mean pulmonary artery pressures > 40 mm Hg only in patients with pre-existing cardiopulmonary disease, suggesting that the normal right ventricle is incapable of generating pressures > 40 mm Hg in the setting of acute pulmonary vascular bed obstruction.

Pulmonary artery catheterization may be useful to optimize therapy in the hypotensive patient, but the catheters may be difficult to pass due to high pulmonary artery resistance and low flow state. A right atrial pressure (RAP) of ~ 15 to 20 mm Hg is probably optimal. Overdistention of the right ventricle (more likely when mean RAP is > 20 mm Hg) may be problematic for several reasons. First, the right ventricle may be made ischemic due to decreased coronary perfusion related to the high RV pressure since perfusion pressure of the right ventricle is approximated by aortic diastolic pressure minus mean RV pressure. With high right-sided pressures, left ventricular compliance may also be decreased as the interventricular septum shifts into the left ventricle.

Based on the above, volume therapy is typically ineffective and may be deleterious with resultant overdistension of the right ventricle. RV ischemia may be a primary cause or a major contributing factor to hypotension. Therapy should be targeted toward reducing RV afterload (RV work) by reducing pulmonary clot burden, avoiding volume-induced RV overdistension (RAP > 20 mm Hg), and maintaining adequate aortic diastolic pressure (upstream filling pressure for the left ventricle).

RV contractility may be improved by the use of inotropic drugs. Dopamine at doses beginning at 5 µg/kg/min is the recommended inotrope in the presence of hypotension. Dobutamine or milrinone may be preferred in the presence of hypoperfusion but absence of hypotension. Isoproterenol alone should be avoided. Vasopressors may also be beneficial by increasing aortic diastolic pressure when it is critically low. Norepinephrine is an appropriate choice. Combination inotrope/vasoconstrictor is recommended in the hypotensive patient. Vasoconstriction of systemic vascular bed with selective vasodilation of pulmonary vascular bed would be ideal. Inhaled nitric oxide has anecdotally been demonstrated to improve hemodynamics in PE by this mechanism. Benefit could only occur through vasodilation of PE-released humorally mediated vasoconstriction.

Surgical thrombectomy may be considered in situations of severe hemodynamic instability with a contraindication to thrombolytic therapy and close proximity to the operating room. Bypass capability is necessary, and the clinical scenario should indicate a certain or almost certain clinical diagnosis of massive PE. It should also be considered when hemodynamic instability persists despite thrombolytic therapy.

PREVENTION OF PULMONARY EMBOLISM

The most powerful statement that can be made for prophylaxis is that, of the patients who die of pulmonary emboli, most patients survive < 30 minutes after the event, which is not long for most forms of treatment to be effective. Without prophylaxis, the frequency of fatal PE is ~ 7% for emergency hip surgery, 2% after elective hip surgery, and 1% after elective surgery. Length of surgery, age, and type of surgery (hip, pelvis, knee, prostate) are important considerations for risk of emboli. Autopsy findings demonstrate that PE causes 5% of deaths in mechanically ventilated patients. The frequency of PE after myocardial infarction in the absence of prophylaxis may be ≤ 5%. The great majority of patients in the ICU should receive heparin prophylaxis for thromboembolic disease. The dose for general surgical patients or in medical patients is typically 5,000 units of unfractionated heparin subcutaneously twice daily or 3 times daily or LMWH once daily. Hemorrhagic side effects of low-dose heparin are rare (< 2%) in patients without hemorrhagic diathesis. High-risk patients or those who have contraindications for heparin should receive intermittent pneumatic venous compression (IPVC), additively or as a replacement, respectively. Low-dose LMWH is the heparin of choice in knee surgery patients, hip surgery patients, and central nervous system trauma patients. Recent reports of epidural hematoma after LMWH use in patients who have had epidural puncture should alert the physician to this potential complication with any anticoagulation in place, independent of type. IPVC is a nonpharmacologic prophylaxis alternative for knee surgery. IPVC is contraindicated in the face of arterial compromise of extremity. IPVC can be added to heparin prophylaxis in patients with additive risk factors. In high-risk patients such as those undergoing elective hip surgery, the use of either LMWH, adjusted-dose unfractionated heparin targeting heparin to prolong PTT 4 to 5 seconds at the mid-dose interval, or low-dose warfarin is recommended. Low-dose warfarin can be instituted at 1 mg/day, beginning 21 days before elective surgery and continuing through the postoperative hospitalization. For hip fracture surgery, LMWH or full-dose warfarin (INR 2.0 to 3.0) is recommended.

Clinically significant DVT develops in many trauma cases. Risk factors include advanced age, prolonged immobilization, severe head trauma, paralysis, pelvic and lower extremity fractures, direct venous trauma, shock, and multiple transfusions. Low-dose heparin or IPVC may not be effective in the highest-risk patient. In trauma patients at high risk for bleeding and those at high risk for pulmonary emboli, prophylactic IVC filter placement has been recommended by some investigators, especially if leg injury prevents application of pneumatic compression devices. Similar rationale has been offered when PE is diagnosed in advanced malignancy. Neither of these uses has been validated.

SUMMARY

PE is a treatable condition with a nonspecific clinical presentation that makes diagnosis difficult. Although pulmonary angiography remains the gold standard appropriate use of a combination of clinical suspicion, Q lung scanning, leg studies, D-dimer, and CT scanning may negate the necessity of pulmonary angiography. A positive spiral CT should be considered as diagnostic of PE in most patients. More important than diagnosis of PE is the prevention of this condition. Physicians should consider prophylactic measures for all patients at risk.

SUGGESTED READINGS

1. ACCP Consensus Committee on Pulmonary Embolism: Antithrombotic therapy for venous thromboembolic disease. *Chest* 2001; 119:176S-193S
   Most recent ACCP consensus statement on therapy of PE.

2. ACCP Consensus Committee on Pulmonary Embolism: Opinions regarding the diagnosis and management of venous thromboembolic disease. *Chest* 1996; 190:233–237
   Question and answer format for controversial areas of VTE management.

3. ACCP Consensus Committee on Pulmonary Embolism: Opinions regarding the diagnosis and management of venous thromboembolic disease. *Chest* 1998; 113:499–504
   More question and answer format for controversial areas of VTE management.

4. American Thoracic Society: The diagnostic approach to acute venous thromboembolism—Clinical practice guidelines. *Am J Respir Crit Care Med* 1999; 160:1043-1066
   Comprehensive clinical practice guideline for the diagnosis and treatment of DVT and PE. Extensive discussion of DVT diagnostic strategy. Also very good review on utility and risk of pulmonary angiogram.

5. Baile EM, King GG, Müller NL, et al: Spiral computed tomography is comparable to angiography for the diagnosis of pulmonary embolism. *Am J Respir Crit Care Med* 2000; 161:1010-1015
   Pig model using colored methacrylate beads and post-mortem methacrylate casting showing no difference in diagnosis of subsegmental clot between angiography and spiral CT.

6. Bergin CJ: Chronic thromboembolic pulmonary hypertension: The disease, the diagnosis, and the treatment. *Ultrasound* 1997; 18:383–391
   A general review of diagnostic and treatment considerations in chronic thromboembolism induced pulmonary hypertension.

7. Bode FR, Dellinger RP: Deep vein thrombosis, pulmonary embolism. *In:* Postoperative Care of the Critically Ill Patient. Gallagher TJ (Ed). Baltimore, Williams & Wilkins, 1995, pp 445–472
   Although this review is targeted toward the surgery patient, the basic principles are

applicable to evaluation and management of thromboembolic disease in general in the critically ill patient.

8. Bounameaux H, de Moerloose P, Perrier A, et al: D-dimer testing in suspected venous thromboembolism: An update. *QJM* 1997; 90:437–442
Discusses potential use of D-dimer thresholds for refining diagnostic acumen in pulmonary embolism and the potential to use D-dimer to decrease invasive testing.

9. Chartier L, Béra J, Delomez M, et al: Free-floating thrombi in the right heart: Diagnosis, management, and prognostic indexes in 38 consecutive patients. *Circulation* 1999; 99:2779-2783
Argues that thrombolytic therapy is faster and more readily available for free-floating thrombi in the right heart and can be used as only therapy or as bridge to surgery.

10. Dalen JE, Banas JS, Brooks HL, et al: Resolution rate of acute pulmonary embolism in man. *N Engl J Med* 1969; 280:1194-1199
No resolution of PE by angiogram before day 14.

11. Dellinger RP: Pulmonary embolism. *In:* Current Therapy in Critical Care Medicine. Third Edition. Parrillo JE (Ed). Philadelphia, Mosby, 1997, pp 216–223
General review targeted toward diagnosis and treatment.

12. Dellinger RP: Pulmonary embolism. *In:* Yearbook of Intensive Care and Emergency Medicine. Vincent J-L (Ed). Berlin, Springer-Verlag, 1997, pp 317–326
General review targeted toward diagnosis and treatment.

13. Dellinger RP: Prophylaxis of venous thromboembolism. *In:* Critical Care Symposium—1997. Anaheim, CA, Society of Critical Care Medicine, 1997, pp 51–76
An in-depth view of specific risk factors for development of deep vein thrombosis as well as recommended prophylactic regimens; significant literature review on surgical prophylaxis studies.

14. Elliott CG, Goldhaber SZ, Visani L, DeRosa M: Chest radiographs in acute pulmonary embolism. *Chest* 2000; 118:33-28
Review of chest radiographs in 2,454 patients with diagnosis of PE. Cardiomegaly (27%) was most common abnormal finding, as well as the most common finding. Twenty-four percent were normal.

15. Erdman WA, Clarke GD: Magnetic resonance imaging of pulmonary embolism. *Ultrasound* 1997; 18:338–348
Review of the potential value of magnetic resonance imaging of pulmonary embolism to exclude proximal clot. Discusses potential advantages as well as limitations.

16. Fennerty T: The diagnosis of pulmonary embolism. *BJM* 1997; 314:425–429
Concise, general review article on pulmonary embolism diagnosis.

17. Goldhaber SZ: Pulmonary embolism. *N Engl J Med* 1998; 339:93–104
Recent medical intelligence review article of pulmonary embolism management.

18. Greco F, Bisignani G, Serafini O, et al: Successful treatment of right heart thromboemboli with IV recombinant tissue-type plasminogen activator during continuous echocardiographic monitoring. *Chest* 1999; 116:78-82
Study demonstrated complete resolution of all right heart clots studied when continuous echocardiography was employed after r-TPA.

19. Grifoni S, Olivotto I, Cecchini P, et al: Short-term clinical outcome of patients with acute pulmonary embolism, normal blood pressure, and echocardiographic right ventricular dysfunction. *JAMA* 2000; 101:2817-2822
Demonstrated significant morbidity and mortality developing in patients with PE, acute RV dysfunction, and initial hemodynamic stability.

20. Hamel E, Pacouret G, Vincentelli D, et al. Thrombolysis or heparin therapy in massive pulmonary embolism with right ventricular dilation: results from a 128-patient monocenter registry. *Chest* 2001; 120:6-8
Two retrospective cohort massive PE groups were matched with the exception of thrombolytic therapy. Although lung scan improved more rapidly in the thrombolytic group, there were no differences in

recurrent PE with increased bleeding deaths in the thrombolytic group.

21. Hansell DM: Spiral computed tomography and pulmonary embolism: Current state. *Clin Radiol* 1997; 52:575–581
   General review of literature relevant to use of CT scanning in patients with suspected pulmonary embolism.

22. Hull RD, Raskob GE, Rosenbloom DR, et al: Optimum therapeutic level of heparin therapy in patients with venous thromboembolism. *Arch Intern Med* 1992; 152:1589-1595
   Subtherapeutic aPTT correlated well with thromboembolic recurrence but supratherapeutic aPTT correlates poorly with important bleeding complications.

23. Hyers TM, Hull RD, Weg JG, et al: Antithrombotic therapy for venous thromboembolic (VTE) disease. *Chest* 1998; 114:561S–578S
   Most recent recommendation by ACCP Consensus Committee for treatment and prophylaxis of venous thromboembolic disease.

24. Hyers TM: Venous thromboembolism. *Am J Respir Crit Care Med* 1999; 159:1–14
   Recent concise general review of diagnosis and prevention of pulmonary embolism.

25. Jerges-Sanchez C, Ramirez-Rivera A, Garcia M, et al: Streptokinase and heparin versus heparin alone in massive pulmonary embolism: A randomized control trial. *J Thromb Thrombolysis* 1995; 2:227-229
   Paper frequently used to justify utility of thrombolytic therapy in massive PE and value of streptokinase in particular. However, only 4 patients in each group. Furthermore, all 4 patients in thrombolytic therapy group diagnosed in ED of hospital performing study, while all 4 patients in heparin-only group transferred to that institution from other hosptials with recurrent PE on heparin.

26. Kelly MA, Abbuhl S: Massive pulmonary embolism. *Respiratory Emergencies II* 1994; 13:547–560
   This article deals primarily with the ICU-type pulmonary embolism (PE) issue, i.e., massive PE; good discussion of hemodynamic issues as well as inferior vena cava filter placement, and addresses thrombolytic therapy and even acute embolectomy.

27. Kürkciyan I, Meron G, Sterz F, et al: Pulmonary embolism as cause of cardiac arrest: Presentation and outcome. *Arch Internal Med* 2000; 160:1529-1535
   10% salvage rate when r-TPA is given to patients with either confirmed PE or those highly likely to have PE.

28. Lorut C, Ghossains M, Horellou MH, et al: A noninvasive diagnostic strategy including spiral computed tomography in patients with suspected pulmonary embolism. *Am J Respir Crit Care Med* 2000; 162:1413-1418
   A protocol was used for evaluation and decision as to presence or absence of PE using CT, Q scan, and D-dimer. Ultrasound was used in middle-ground situation as a final decision maker. Only 1.7% of untreated patients had PE over next 3 months.

29. Lund O, Nielsen TT, Schifter S, et al: Treatment of pulmoary embolism with full-dose heparin, streptokinase, or embolectomy. *Thorac Cardiovasc Surg* 1986; 32:240-246
   Compared thrombolytic therapy with embolectomy for massive PE. Hospital mortality equal (21% and 22%), but 5-year survival better in embolectomy group. Nonrandomized study of 28 and 25 patients, respectively, but severity of illness score greater in embolectomy group at baseline.

30. McConnell MV, Solomon SD, Fayan ME, et al: Regional right ventricular dysfunction detected by echocardiography in acute pulmonary embolism. *Am J Cardiol* 1996; 78:469-473
   The finding of abnormal wall motion in RV mid-free wall and normal motion in apex was very predictive of PE among patients with acute symptoms and evidence of pulmonary artery hypertension.

31. Miniati M, Pistolesi M, Maseri C, et al: Value of perfusion lung scan in the diagnosis of pulmonary embolism: Results of the Prospective Investigative Study of Adult Pulmonary Embolism Diagnosis (PISA-PED). *Am J Respir Crit Care Med* 1996; 154:1387-1393

Studied the use of perfusion scanning/chest radiograph analysis without ventilation scanning in 890 consecutive patients with suspected pulmonary embolism. Abnormal scans were considered PE+ if scans demonstrated 1 or more wedge-shaped perfusion defect and PE- if it did not. Sensitivity was 92% (most patients with angiographically proven PE had PE+ scans) and specificity was 87% (most patients without angiographically proven PE had PE- scans). The addition of pretest clinical probability further heightened predictive capability.

32. Molina JE, Hunter DW, Yedlicka JW, et al: Thrombolytic therapy for postoperative pulmonary embolism. *Am J Surg* 1992; 163:375-380

   Thirteen patients within 2 weeks of surgery (mean 9.6 days). Used modified urokinase regimen to demonstrate complete lysis of PE with no bleeding complications.

33. Pandey AS, Rakowski H, Mickleborough LL, et al: Right heart pulmonary embolism in transit: A review of therapeutic considerations. *Can J Cardiol* 1997; 13:397–402

   This article presents the challenges of reacting to the presence of right-heart clot on ultrasound as it is pertinent to decision-making in patients with pulmonary embolism. This finding is particularly problematic in the unstable patient and the patient with contraindication to thrombolytic therapy.

34. The PIOPED Investigators: Value of the ventilation/perfusion scan in acute pulmonary embolism: Results of the prospective investigation of pulmonary embolism diagnosis (PIOPED). *JAMA* 1990; 263:2753–2759

   The article includes a discussion of the use of Bayes theorem, as well as the role of the previous cardiopulmonary disease and previous pulmonary embolism in reliability of scanning.

35. Quinn DA, Fogel RB, Smith CD, et al: D-dimers in the diagnosis of pulmonary embolism. *Am J Respir Crit Care Med* 1999; 159:1445-1449

   Non-elevated D-dimers make PE very unlikely, while elevated D-dimers were not useful.

36. Rathbun SW, Raskob GE, Whitwett TL: Sensitivity and specificity of helical computed tomography in the diagnosis of pulmonary embolism: A systematic review. *Ann Intern Med* 2000; 132:227-232.

   A review of the 15 prospective English-language studies of use of helical (spiral) CT in the diagnosis of PE. Found that only 2 studies had consecutive patients, 8 studies had independently interpreted angiogram and CT, and only 1 study included a broad spectrum of patients. Concluded that there is not currently enough data to support withholding of heparin after negative spiral CT without additional testing. Large prospective trials are needed.

37. Raschke RA, Reilly BM, Guidry JR, et al: The weight-based heparin dosing nomogram compared with a '"standard care"' nomogram: A randomized controlled trial. *Ann Intern Med* 1993; 119:874–881

   Valuable discussion and helpful summary of weight-based heparin anticoagulation therapy

38. Rosenow EC: Venous and pulmonary thromboembolism: An algorithmic approach to diagnosis and management. *Mayo Clin Proc* 1995; 70:45–49

   An algorithm is presented based on clinical suspicion that includes diagnostic choices as well as anticoagulation decisions.

39. Severi P, LoPinto G, Doggio R, et al: Urokinase thrombolytic therapy of pulmonary embolism in neurosurgical patients. *Surg Neurol* 1994; 42:469-470

   Nine neurosurgery patients (mean 19 days following surgery) received urokinase. All survived, no intracranial hemorrhage, one subgaleal hemorrhage.

40. Stein PD, Afzal A, Henry JW, et al: Fever in pulmonary embolism. *Chest* 2000; 117:39-42

   Demonstrated no source of fever (temp $\geq$ 100.0°F) other than PE in 14% of patients with angiographically documented PE. Fever correlated with DVT but not with infarction. Only 2 of 268 patients had temperatures $\geq 103.0°F$.

41. Stein PD, Athanasoulis C, Alavi A, et al: Complications and validity of pulmonary angiography in acute pulmonary embolism. *Circulation* 1992; 85:462-468

    Interobserver radiologist agreement on angiographic diagnosis of pulmonary embolism: lobar 98%, segmental 90%, subsegmental 66%.

42. Stein PD, Huang H, Afzal A, Noor HA: Incidence of acute pulmonary embolism in a general hospital. *Chest* 1999; 116:909-913

    Women ≥ 50 years old, but not women < 50 years old, have greater incidence of PE than men.

43. Turkstra F, Koopman MM, Buller HR: The treatment of deep vein thrombosis and pulmonary embolism. *Thromb Haemost* 1997; 78:489–496

    Concise, general review article on treatment of deep-vein thrombosis and pulmonary embolism.

44. Verstraete M, Miller GAH, Bounameaus H, et al: Intravenous and intrapulmonary recombinant tissue-type plasminogen activator in the treatment of acute massive pulmonary embolism. *Circulation* 1988; 77:353-360

    Demonstrated no beneficial effect of thrombolytic therapy infused into pulmonary artery versus peripheral administration.

45. Weinmann EE, Salzman EW: Deep-vein thrombosis. *N Engl J Med* 1994; 331:1630–1641

    Review of deep-vein thrombosis; very comprehensive and clinically oriented to cover diagnoses, clinical epidemiology, and treatment. Surgical and thrombolytic therapy are covered.

    Very good, concise review of prophylactic therapy, as well as venous interruption.

46. Wiegand UKH, Kurowski V, Giannitsis E, et al: Effectiveness of end-tidal carbon dioxide tension for monitoring of thrombolytic therapy in acute pulmonary embolism. *Crit Care Med* 2000; 28:3588-3592

    End-tidal CO_2 decreases as thrombolytic therapy improves hemodynamics as indicator of decreased dead space.

USE OF BLOOD AND BLOOD PRODUCTS IN CRITICAL CARE

Judith A. Luce, MD

Objectives

- To define the blood products currently available for use in the ICU
- To refine the criteria for red cell transfusion
- To understand the indication for platelet and plasma transfusions
- To evaluate the infectious risks of transfusions
- To understand other risks associated with transfusions

GENERAL PRINCIPLES

Component therapy has arisen because of the need of blood banks to provide special portions of whole blood, such as platelets, cryoprecipitate, and plasma for patients with unique replacement needs. However, most transfusions are now components, and whole blood transfusion is ordinarily reserved for equally special circumstances, such as trauma and massive transfusion. Precision in the use of components is an important principle in transfusion therapy: directed use of blood products for specific disorders and situations, rather than a "shotgun" approach.

Risk management has become an important part of the use of blood products, since physicians and the public are not only more aware of the hazards of transfusion, but also less willing to accept them. Risk management requires not only judicious use of blood products, but also the use of laboratory and clinical assessment of the efficacy of the blood product in order to document the benefit to the patient. Wise physicians have been using blood products this way for years, and most transfusion services in hospitals now make some effort to enforce proper and appropriate use of blood products in order to reduce hospitals' risk.

Reevaluation of the effect of transfusion after each episode is an essential part of monitoring the effectiveness of therapy. The appropriate laboratory tests and appropriate intervals for reevaluation are dictated by the disease process requiring transfusion and by the pace of the patient's disease. In the critical care setting, this may mean evaluating coagulation parameters or blood counts every few hours.

Understanding the underlying disease process and the natural history of the disease process are integral to effective use of the blood bank.

Components Available from the Blood Bank

Whole Blood

Whole blood, generally stored in an acid-citrate-dextrose medium, is most often available only for replacement during acute hemorrhage where transfusion requirements are likely to be large. Because of the increasing use of components rather than whole blood, whole blood has become less available. Fresh whole blood that has been removed from donors within a few hours of its use has not been shown to be more effective than stored whole blood, and is only rarely available. Whole blood from autologous predeposit or from designated donors is stored in similar fashion and tested in similar fashion to volunteer donor-banked blood.

Packed Red Blood Cells

Packed red blood cells are essentially all of the red cells in a unit of blood, with platelets and plasma largely removed, so that the resulting cells are at a hematocrit of about 70%. They are customarily stored for up to 72-90 days; during that time, they gradually become deficient in 2,3-DPG, in spite of our best efforts to prevent this. A fraction of stored cells also gradually lyse, releasing potassium, hemoglobin, and red cell stroma into the pack. Usage beyond the storage period can result in higher risks of bacterial transmission.

Heat and mechanical fragmentation both can disrupt stored red cells. Blood warmers must be checked for temperature accuracy, since exposure to temperatures over 42° C can result in significant hemolysis of red cells. Attempts to restore the 2,3-DPG levels of stored red cells are not necessary, as the cells rapidly replete when transfused.

Specialized Red Cells

Red blood cells store well when frozen, usually in glycerol or DMSO. Their shelf life is vastly extended, and they can be shipped with little risk of loss. Packed red cell units donated by persons with rare blood types may be stored and shipped to institutions with an acute need and no available donors. Frozen red cells are no less likely to transmit most diseases than refrigerated stored red cells. "Washed" red cells are produced by recentrifugation in saline solution in order to remove plasma and contaminating white blood cells. They must be used rapidly after washing, and because of the risk of contamination of the opened unit. Because of the cost of the washing procedure, most institutions use white blood cell filters to prevent febrile transfusion reactions prior to considering the "washing" procedure. Irradiation of blood products renders the lymphocytes nonviable, and is used to prevent graft-versus-host disease (see below).

Plasma and Plasma Fractions

Plasma may be stored whole, usually as fresh, frozen, whole plasma. Each bag of plasma from the blood bank is about 200-250 cc. Fresh frozen plasma has a long shelf life, but the coagulation factors transfused from this product have a shorter half life than the native coagulation factors. Commercial pooled plasma products manufactured from a larger donor pool carry a much higher disease transmission risk, and should not be used unless they have been heat treated or processed by the manufacturer to enhance safety. Such products often also have the immunoglobulins removed in order to prevent anaphylaxis.

Cryoprecipitate is prepared from fresh plasma by freezing, then slow thawing to 60° F. What precipitates is Factor VIII (including Von Willebrand moiety), fibrinogen (about one-third of that in the unit of blood), and fibronectin. When made into cryoprecipitate, a unit of plasma yields about 80-100U Factor VIII$_C$/VWF, and about 200-300 mg of fibrinogen. Cryoprecipitate can be reconstituted in extremely small volumes, making it useful when volume overload is a concern. It is an excellent source of fibrinogen.

Specific coagulation factors, mainly VIII and IX, are available as factor manufactured from pooled plasma or as recombinant DNA products. The latter are more expensive but have fewer complications, including sensitization and disease transmission.

Platelets

Platelets are removed from fresh whole blood by sedimentation, then stored at 22° C under continuous agitation. They may also be obtained by pheresis of a single donor, a procedure that harvests about the same amount as 5 to 6 units of platelets. Stored platelets may be good for up to a week, although older units have a shorter survival: transfused platelets last up to 72 hours in normal recipients. Because of short storage time, blood bank supplies of platelets are more tenuous than red cell supplies. Transfusion of 1 unit of platelets raises the recipient's platelet count by 6,000-10,000/mm^3, assuming average body size and no consumption.

Platelets pheresed from a single donor may be used to reduce the risk of immunization of recipients who are repeatedly exposed to platelet transfusions. The routine use of single donor platelets in such individuals does reduce the risk of platelet sensitization and resultant immune destruction. Platelets may be crossmatched to specific platelet antigens, and HLA haplotype matching of donor to recipient may also be used to reduce the likelihood of sensitization. Both techniques may be used to successfully give platelet transfusions to recipients who have already become sensitized to random donor platelets.

Granulocytes

Granulocytes are obtained by pheresis of single donors, and collected either by centrifugation or by nylon filtration; donors are often treated with steroids to increase the peripheral WBC numbers or with hydroxyethyl starch to promote rapid red cell sedimentation. Granulocytes must be promptly administered, both because of the risk of contamination and because of spontaneous aggregation and degranulation. The ONLY defined role for granulocyte transfusion is in the neutropenic patient with documented bacteremic infection who is failing appropriate antibiotic therapy; this includes immunosuppressed patients and neonates. The use of granulocyte transfusions is now largely supplanted by use of G-CSF or GM-CSF.

White blood cells from specific donors are used in the bone marrow transplant setting to augment the engraftment process, and increasingly, to obtain graft-versus leukemia effects in the event of recurrence. The collection technique is similar, but the product may be subjected to procedures to remove granulocytes in order to avoid leukoagglutination reactions.

Indications for Transfusion of Blood Components

Indications for Red Blood Cell Transfusion

Red cell transfusion is a common event in the ICU. Published reports suggest that bleeding is a common problem in critically ill patients, and that phlebotomy for diagnostic tests an additional significant source of red cell loss. The frequency of red cell transfusion is reported at 0.2 to 0.4 units per day.

Controversy has emerged over the appropriate use of red cell transfusions in the critically ill. Prior to 1999, hemoglobin levels above 10 were universally regarded as tolerable unless proven otherwise in individuals with severe arterial hypoxemia. Hemoglobin levels below 5 are clearly associated with mortality due to tissue hypoxia alone. Most chronically anemic individuals tolerate lower hemoglobin levels than acutely anemic individuals; the decision to transfuse a chronically anemic individual must be more carefully thought out because of the risks of chronic red cell transfusion.

Symptoms of tissue hypoxia that are standard indications for red cell transfusion of anemic individuals include angina, confusion, ECG changes, syncope, CHF, and arrhythmias. Many clinicians also regard headaches, lightheadedness or dizziness, and marked fatigue as standard indications for transfusion.

One of the physiologic manifestations of inadequate supply of oxygen to tissues is a higher rate of peripheral extraction of oxygen from red cells. In the ICU setting, in the absence of reported symptoms, the following may be used as indicative of tissue hypoxia:

a) a mixed venous pO_2 less than 25 mm Hg;

b) oxygen consumption falling to less than 50% of the patient's baseline value, assuming this isknown;

c) oxygen extraction ratio greater than 50%, to wit:

$$\frac{O_2 \text{ consumed}}{O_2 \text{ delivered}} \geq 50\%$$

or

$$\frac{C_aO_2 - C_vO_2}{C_aO_2} \geq 0.5$$

The Canadian Trial (*NEJM*, 1999) was a prospective randomized study of red cell tranfusion in the ICU setting, wherein target hemoglobin levels were set as the goal for a "liberal" (hemoglobin 10-12) versus "conservative" (hemoglobin 7-9) transfusion strategy. The study demonstrated no major outcome differences between the 2 groups, and indeed there was suggestive evidence that for younger patients and perhaps those with significant vascular disease, clinical outcomes may be superior using a conservative transfusion strategy. This trial has not been replicated elsewhere, but the American Association of Blood Banks' recommendation for audit of red cell transfusions includes all patients who are not actively bleeding who receive a red cell transfusion when their hemoglobin is 8 or greater. Ultimately, judgments about the utility of an individual red blood cell transfusion are clinical choices. However, the clinician who has made the judgment to transfuse is obligated to document the effect of that transfusion and to assess whether the goal of transfusion has been met.

Indications for Platelet Transfusion

Platelet transfusions are also subject to some controversy. The purpose of platelet transfusion is to either aid in correcting a coagulopathy *when the patient is actively bleeding* or to prevent spontaneous hemorrhage in a patient with profound thrombocytopenia. Platelet transfusion as surgical prophylaxis is indicated in a very limited number of patients: platelet counts over 50,000 are adequate for general surgical procedures and closed medical procedures.

Guidelines may be outlined as follows:

1. *Failure of Platelet Production, With Bleeding or Surgical Intervention.* The goal is to maintain platelets at a level which will either stop bleeding or at > 50,000/mm^3.
2. *Failure of Production, No Bleeding.* The risk of spontaneous life-threatening CNS hemorrhage becomes increased at platelet counts around 10,000-20,000/mm^3. If the patient has other risk factors for hemorrhage, transfuse at 20,000/mm^3; if the patient has none, transfuse at 10,000/mm^3. Even this guideline is subject to controversy in the area of management of patients with hematologic disorders. However, most critically ill patients have multiple risk factors for bleeding, and the more conservative guideline listed here is still considered reasonable for the ICU.
3. *Failure of Production, With Platelet Dysfunction.* The goal is to make the threshold slightly higher, since platelets are not as effective. Removal of any offending agents (aspirin, other drugs, renal failure) is desirable. A bleeding time is one way to measure function, but does become prolonged as the platelet count falls. One formula for estimating whether platelet function is a problem is as follows:

$$\text{Bleeding time} = 30.5 - \frac{\text{platelet count/mm}^3}{3,850}$$

A bleeding time less than twice the upper limit of normal (usually upper limit of normal is 8 to 10 minutes) probably does not mandate platelet transfusion, unless there are other disorders of coagulation. Whether some newer commercial whole blood platelet aggregation tests can supplant the imperfect technology of the bleeding time is not yet clear. However, good prospective data does suggest that these devices are fairly sensitive for detecting platelet dysfunction, though not specific for its etiology.

4. *Platelet Consumption.* Platelet transfusion may be performed in disorders where platelet consumption is the rule. Disorders of platelet consumption may be divided into immune and nonimmune mediated processes, and platelet transfusion practice differs in the 2 situations. Nonimmune consumption occurs in massive trauma, burns, and in consumptive disease states such as DIC and TTP. Transfused platelets' survival may be greatly shortened, but transfusions are useful. When the underlying process is arrested, platelet replacement may be necessary in order to make up for poor marrow production in sick patients. The 1-hour post-transfusion platelet count will usually indicate an increment from transfusion, even in DIC. In immune-mediated thrombocytopenia, e.g., ITP, drugs (still around), platelet transfusions alone are generally useless, since they usually do not produce even a short-lived increment in platelet count. In cases of life-threatening bleeding, it may be possible to raise the platelet count by pre-treating with high-dose iv IgG and then giving random donor platelets with better efficacy.

Fresh Frozen Plasma

The specific indications for plasma transfusion are narrowly defined. They include *replacement of isolated factor deficiencies: factors II, V, VII, IX, X, XI.* Clinicians need to be aware of the amount of plasma required to replace a given factor (for example, very little for X). Plasma may be used for *reversal of warfarin anticoagulation in patients with life-threatening bleeding.* Plasma is used to *replace Antithrombin III when the commercial preparation is not available* for patients who require surgery or must have heparin for treatment of acute thrombosis. Plasma is important in the *treatment of thrombotic thrombocytopenic purpura*, usually along with pheresis. Plasma may be used in the course of treating *coagulopathy due to massive blood transfusion*, where whole blood is not available and bleeding is demonstrably due to factor deficiency. Rarely, plasma is used for treatment of *certain immunodeficiencies*, for example, protein-losing enteropathy in infants not responding to parenteral nutrition. There are no other "routine" or prophylactic situations in which FFP should be used. It is not an appropriate volume expander or source of nutrition or albumin.

Fresh frozen plasma must be thawed carefully, so it takes time to prepare after it is ordered. "Stat" orders are not realistic unless the blood bank has provisions for always having some thawed. The object of using fresh frozen plasma is to attain plasma levels of the desired factors rapidly so that hemostasis can occur. The half-lives of frozen plasma clotting factors are less than they are *in vivo*, so the effect will wear off over hours after administration. It makes little sense to give fresh frozen plasma as a continuous infusion, a popular trend in surgical ICUs. This loses the benefit of fairly rapid infusion of a bolus dose of clotting factors, and ensures that the levels achieved never reach the appropriate level. Both fresh frozen plasma and cryoprecipitate may be administered rapidly, as fast as the patient will tolerate the infusion. Speed has no apparent effect on the incidence of febrile or urticarial reactions. The biggest problem with fresh frozen plasma is the large volumes required.

Calculating the approximate dose required to achieve hemostasis is a common problem with fresh frozen plasma. Most adults have a plasma volume between 30 and 35 cc/kg, although this can fluctuate when fluid shifts are occurring between the vascular space and tissues. In addition, approximating the factor deficit may be difficult also, depending on the particular methods used to measure clotting times in the laboratory. However, most prothrombin times at an INR of 2 or greater represent factor levels at 10% or less. Therefore, in order to bring a 70 kg person's plasma to a factor level of 50% (roughly adequate for hemostasis), one would need to transfuse 35cc/kg x 70kg x 0.50, or more than 1200 cc of plasma. Most clinicians underdose fresh frozen plasma.

Cryoprecipitate

Because it is a source of all components of the complex Factor VIII molecule, cryoprecipitate may be used in replacement of VWF in patients with deficiency; it is also useful for Hemophilia A, although more potentially hazardous than new monoclonal products. It is a low volume, easily infused source of fibrinogen, and is the product of choice in treatment of patients with afibrinogenemia or dysfibrinogenemia. Replacement dose calculations are similar to those for fresh frozen plasma, based on assumed plasma volume, body size, and a target plasma level of fibrinogen of greater than 100 mg/dL. Cryoprecipitate is the product of choice for replacement of fibrinogen in consumption states, such as DIC.

Specialized Clotting Factors

The use of prepared prothrombin extracts and activated tissue factor extracts has been advocated for the treatment of a variety of coagulopathies, including acquired factor deficiencies due to antibody formation. There are no routine indications for the use of these specialized factors, and consultation with an expert in coagulopathy is recommended. The use of Factors VIIIc and IX for treatment of hemophilia A and B should also be done in consultation with an expert in the care of hemophilaic patients.

Hazards of Blood Product Administration

Crossmatching and Sensitization

Red cells are matched by reacting recipient serum with type-specific (ABO and Rh) donor cells at 2 different temperatures (major crossmatch). This takes *time*, and only under desperate circumstances should it not be done. Crossmatching may be difficult due to a variety of problems. Nonspecific cold agglutinins are seen in a host of medical conditions, and they cause difficulty matching at room temperature and sometimes at 37° C. Cold agglutinins are usually not associated with hemolytic reactions *in vivo* unless complement is fixed in the cold (hence cold agglutinin disease). Not only do nonspecific cold agglutinins make crossmatching difficult but also they may mask the presence of other antibodies. Warm antibodies are usually IgG, are associated with autoimmune disease and certain malignancies, and make conventional crossmatching of red cells almost impossible. Blood banks have techniques for eluting out the warm antibodies so that a crossmatch may be performed, but this specialized service is not widespread. If antibody elution is not available, the consensus is that one arrives at the best possible match of type-specific blood and uses it, knowing that hemolysis may be no greater than it is endogenously. Surface antigens are weakly expressed in neonates, extremely elderly, and massively transfused patients, making crossmatching difficult. Larger volumes of blood will be needed to crossmatch these persons.

Platelets and plasma are not routinely crossmatched. Because the plasma they contain may have antibodies to the recipient's cells, they are generally type-specific, but in an emergency even this is not necessary.

In spite of crossmatching, sensitization to homologous blood transfusion occurs, and may become a clinical problem for repetitively transfused individuals, especially those who have rare blood types. The risk of sensitization to red cells is estimated at 1% per transfusion episode; the risk of platelet sensitization is 5 to 10 percent per pooled random donor transfusion episode. Platelet crossmatching, either by HLA haplotype or by platelet antigens, is available when multiple platelet transfusions are likely to occur—usually in the course of treatment of acute leukemia and other hematologic disorders. Sensitization to leukocyte antigens occurs and may be the basis for some febrile reactions, but is otherwise usually of little clinical significance.

Hemolytic Transfusion Reactions

Intravascular hemolysis of transfused red blood cells is caused by ABO or Rh incompatibility, or by a strong, high-titer antibody such as anti-Kell. Binding of high titer antibodies results in complement fixation and rapid intravascular destruction. The syndrome that results from massive intravascular hemolysis is due to the release of red cell stroma, which causes cytokine, bradykinin, and granulocyte mediator release. Hypotension, capillary leak, and oliguria are manifestations that follow very rapidly after the onset of intense intravascular hemolysis; the most feared complications are DIC, acute renal failure, and ARDS. The majority of acute hemolytic transfusion reactions are caused by clerical or nursing error; fatal hemolytic transfusion reactions occur at a rate of approximately 1 in 100,000 red cell transfusion episodes.

The treatment of hemolytic transfusion reactions is supportive. Recognizing the syndrome and stopping the offending transfusion are critical. Most clinicians believe that supporting high urine output is important, but diuretics should be used only if the patient shows intravascular volume overload. The use of mannitol is controversial. There is no role for steroids, antihistamines, heparin, colloid, or other specific pharmacological

intervention. Treatment of the complications should be vigorous, as the majority of patients survive the event.

Delayed Transfusion Reactions

Red cell sensitization may result in an antibody response that is initially weak and does not persist. The next exposure of a patient to that red cell antigen will arouse an anamnestic immune response, however, and higher titers of antibody may occur fairly rapidly after transfusion. If this happens rapidly and produces a response capable of fixing complement, patients may have intravascular hemolysis of the transfused cells within a few days of transfusion. These delayed transfusion reactions usually produce jaundice, elevated LDH, and low haptoglobin levels, but may occasionally be severe and result in oliguria. If the antibody does not fix complement, extravascular hemolysis of the transfused red cells will occur. This type of delayed transfusion reaction is often subtle, but results in elevations in LDH and indirect bilirubin, occasionally the appearance of spherocytes in the peripheral blood smear, a positive Coomb's test, and falling hemoglobin levels. Documentation of such a reaction is important so that future transfusions are more carefully screened.

Other Types of Transfusion Reaction

Febrile transfusion reactions are most often attributed to the presence of granulocytes in transfused blood, although they may also be caused by plasma factors such as exogenous immunoglobulins. They may be distinguished from the fever associated with hemolytic transfusion reactions by the lack of hypotension or other signs of hemolysis and by the generally delayed onset of fever compared to hemolytic transfusion reactions. These reactions are usually treated with acetaminophen or aspirin; use of these drugs for prophylaxis is also common. Patients who are repetitively transfused and who have febrile reactions should receive WBC filtered blood.

Urticarial transfusion reactions are probably induced by plasma components. One rare subset of patients with congenital IgA deficiency may have anaphylaxis due to plasma exposure, but in general, urticarial reactions are not accompanied by a risk of anaphylaxis. They are usually treated with antihistamines and may be treated prophylactically. Patients who have repetitive urticarial reactions in spite of prophylaxis may need to receive related donor blood products.

Leukoagglutination and pooling of granulocytes in the lungs may occur, although it is rare in settings other than granulocyte transfusions. Most of the time, leukoagglutination results in mild dyspnea and pulmonary infiltrates and spontaneously resolves, but occasionally lung injury occurs as a result of this phenomenon and ARDS results.

Graft versus host disease (GVHD) occurs when viable immunocompetent lymphocytes are transfused into an immunoincompetent recipient and proliferate and respond to recipient HLA antigens. The syndrome develops as fever, skin rash, and liver function abnormalities occurring 2 to 6 weeks after transfusion. Graft versus host disease is highly lethal in reported cases outside of the transplantation situation; it is very morbid in transplant settings as well. It primarily occurs in transplant, leukemia, and other forms of severely immunosuppressed patients, but it has been reported in cardiac surgery and neonates. GVHD has not been reported in AIDS. Recognizing the syndrome and obtaining a skin biopsy makes the correct diagnosis. Prevention in the nonbone marrow transplant setting is to irradiate the blood product before use: whole blood, packed cells, platelets. Treatment of active graft-versus-host disease involves further immunosuppression with cyclosporine, antithymocyte globulin, steroids, and cytotoxic drugs. Critically ill patients in the ICU who are receiving family member blood transfusions should have those related donor products irradiated.

Risks of Disease Transmission

Hepatitis transmission due to blood transfusion is rapidly becoming an historical event. Screening for Hepatitis B is universal. The current generation screening test for Hepatitis C provides good protection: it detects more than 90% of potentially infectious units of blood, and is thought to have reduced the rate of posttransfusion hepatitis to about 1% nationwide. Individuals who have an acute hepatitis-like illness after transfusion should be tested for Hepatitis C, however, since the screen is not perfect. The vast majority of individuals infected do develop antibodies within the first 6 months after transmission. Many of those people do lose their antibodies later on, hence the less than perfect screening test. Other as yet poorly characterized hepatitis viruses may cause posttransfusion hepatitis, but it is an uncommon event when donor screening by questionnaire and serology is performed.

AIDS transmission is also an unusual event. Elisa testing is an effective way to screen donor blood, since both viral culture and RNA based tests performed in both endemic and nonendemic areas have failed to detect potentially infectious units of blood that are Elisa negative. The risk of AIDS transmission is currently estimated to occur at a rate of 1:400,000 to 1,000,000 transfusions. The combination of an effective donor questionnaire and serologic screening is critical to ending transfusion-related cases of AIDS.

Cytomegalovirus transmission remains a clinical problem. Clinical studies have estimated transmission to occur in 3-12 recipients/100 units of blood transfused. Rises in antibody titers or seroconversion have been shown in up to 30% of transfused surgical patients. Chronic infection is often asymptomatic. More than 90% of seroconverters/titer increases are asymptomatic. Neonates, premature, or low birth weight infants are at highest risk: 25-30% get CMV, up to 1 in 4 dies of it. Bone marrow transplant recipients have a high rate of early deaths due to CMV pneumonitis, although most of this is thought to represent endogenous reactivation of virus replication. Seronegative bone marrow transplant recipients who receive marrow from a seropositive donor are at the highest risk, however. Other vulnerable patients include cancer patients, AIDS patients, and splenectomy patients. Adler has estimated that 20% of all transfused patients in the U.S. fall into the category of immunosuppressed, and that estimate excludes patients with HIV infection. Symptomatic acute cytomegalovirus infection results in a clinical syndrome which is infectious mononucleosis-like. Chronic infection is usually asymptomatic. Treatment of cytomegalovirus diseases is marginally effective: ganciclovir and foscarnet are useful in treating retinitis in AIDS, but not very effective in the bone marrow transplant setting.

Chemoprophylaxis appears to work better in the bone marrow transplant setting, and transmission is prevented in neonates by the use of seronegative donor blood products. Seropositive transplant recipients can be prophylaxed with acyclovir and/or ganciclovir.

Other transfusion transmissible diseases include EB virus, malaria, brucellosis, trypanosomiasis, syphilis, and Toxoplasmosis. These events are rare in the U.S.

Alternatives to Use of Blood Bank Products

Presurgical storage of patient blood is allowed in most blood banks nationally. Recent studies suggest that autologous donation is underused. Generally, practice has been to have patient donate a unit every 2 to 3 weeks prior to surgery while taking oral iron supplementation. There is some evidence that more units may be predeposited with the concomitant use of erythropoietin, although the ultimate clinical impact of such use is unknown. Autologous donors are anemic at the time of surgery. The FDA permits the use of autologous units that are hepatitis or AIDS-infected; individual institutions may not wish to assume the risk of handling such units and may reject such autologous donors. Autologous donation of platelet-rich plasma has not been shown to significantly reduce blood loss or blood utilization following cardiac surgery.

Designated donors, usually members of a patient's family, are often requested by physicians and patients as sources of blood products, usually with the idea that designated donors are less likely to have infectious diseases. Unfortunately, the data in the literature suggest that in comparison to regular volunteer donors who have been screened, designated donor blood is more likely to test positive for infectious diseases. Designated donor blood is not necessarily safer than volunteer donor banked blood.

Artificial blood substitutes are still in development. Perfluorocarbon products are chemically inert polyfluorinated hydrocarbons, insoluble in plasma, but in which oxygen is soluble. They are produced as emulsions with surfactants and added hydroxyethyl starch and need to be stored frozen. The oxygen delivery capability of these products is good, but the use of perfluorocarbons is limited by less efficient oxygen uptake, which require 100% inspired oxygen delivery. In addition, the total dose and carrying capacity are limited, so that at the maximum dose, the contribution to the total hematocrit by perfluorocarbon, or "fluorocrit," is very low. Finally, the drug is short acting, with a half-life of only about 24 hours.

Hemodilution and intraoperative autologous transfusion are occasionally used to avoid transfusion. Hemodilution lowers blood viscosity, thought to be an advantage by some. While there are no formal data that this process is useful, studies in cardiac bypass surgery, orthopedic surgery, and Jehovah's witness patients suggest that hemodilution techniques are safe and can result in saving blood transfusions.

Intraoperative scavenging and reuse of red cells using cell saver technology has become widespread practice in major blood loss surgeries such as cardiac and vascular procedures. It remains controversial in trauma or "dirty" operative fields, however. Washing of red cells as part of the process is thought to be the safest procedure in terms of contamination, hemolysis, and coagulopathy. However, techniques using sedimentation without washing have never been formally compared to washing devices (the latter are clearly more expensive and require full-time, dedicated technician). A great deal of unrandomized, selected case reports attest to the relative safety of most "washing" cell savers now in use. The use of heparin, antibiotics, filters, and other adjuncts is not standardized.

ANNOTATED BIBLIOGRAPHY

1. Crosby E: Perioperative haemotherapy: I. Indications for blood component transfusion. *Can J Anaesth* 1992; 39:695-707
2. Crosby E: Perioperative haemotherapy: II. Risks and complications of blood transfusion. *Can J Anaesth* 1992; 39:822-37
3. Dodd, RY: The risk of transfusion-transmitted infection. *N Engl J Med* 1992; 327:419-213
4. Ereth MH, Oliver WC, Santrach PJ: Perioperative interventions to decrease transfusion of allogeneic blood products. *Mayo Clin Proc* 1994; 69:575-5864
5. Giblett ER: Blood group alloantibodies. *Transfusion* 1977; 17:2795

6. Gould SA, Rice CL, Moss GS: The physiologic basis of the use of blood and blood products. *Surg Annu* 1984; 16:136

7. Gould SA, Rosen AL, Sehgal, LR, et al: Fluosol-DA as a red-cell substitute in acute anemia. *N Engl J Med* 1986; 314:16537

8. Hallett JW, Popovsky M and Ilstrup D: Minimizing blood transfusions during abdominal aortic surgery: Recent advances in rapid autotransfusion. *J Vasc Surg* 1987; 5:601 8

9. Kahn RA, Allen RW, Baldessare J: Alternate sources and substitutes for therapeutic blood components. *Blood* 1985; 66:1 9

10. Lostumbo MM, Holland PV, Schmidt PJ: Isoimmunization after multiple transfusions. *N Engl J Med* 1966; 275:141
    Nothing much has changed since this very fine article was written.

11. McCullough J, Steeper TA, Connelly DP, et al: Platelet utilization in a university hospital. *JAMA* 1988; 259:241411

12. Menitove JE, Abrams RA: Granulocyte transfusions in neutropenic patients. *CRC Crit Rev Oncol Hematol* 1987; 7:89
    A couple of old pros review the field comprehensively and come to the conclusion that there are few, if any, solidly accepted reasons for granulocyte transfusions.

13. NHLBI Consensus Panel: Transfusion Alert: Indications for the Use of Red Blood cells, Platelets, and Fresh Frozen Plasma. http://www.nhlbi.nih.gov/health/prof/blood/transfusion/transfin.htm

14. Office of Medical Applications of Research, National Institutes of Health: Fresh frozen plasma: Indications and risks. *JAMA* 1985; 253:551-5314

15. Office of Medical Applications of Research, National Institutes of Health: Platelet transfusion therapy. *JAMA* 1987; 257:1777-8015

16. Office of Medical Applications of Research, National Institutes of Health: Perioperative Red Cell Transfusion. *JAMA* 1988; 260:2700-2703

17. Pineda AA, Taswell HF, Brzica SM: Delayed hemolytic transfusion reactions. *Transfusion* 1978; 18:1, 1978
    A solid summary of an often-missed problem in transfusion medicine.

18. Rossi EC: Red cell transfusion therapy in chronic anemia. *Hematol Oncol Clin N Amer* 1994; 8:1045-1051
    Useful review of the short list of indications for transfusion therapy in chronic anemia. Emphasizes the compensatory mechanisms and physiology of chronic anemia. Cautions a conservative approach.

19. Selik, RM, Ward JW, Buehler, JW: Trends in transfusion-associated acquired immune deficiency syndrome in the United States, 1982 through 1991. *Transfusion* 1993; 33:890-9319

20. Toy, PT, et al: NHLBI Consensus Panel. Transfusion Alert: Use of Autologous Blood. http://www.nhlbi.nih.gov./health/prof/transfusion/logo.htm

21. Toy PT, Strauss RG, Stehling LC, et al: Predeposited autologous blood for elective surgery. A national multicenter study. *N Engl J Med* 1987; 316:517

22. Widmann FK: Untoward effects of blood transfusions. *Postgrad Med* 1981; 69:40
    An older, housestaff-oriented summary of problems, but a good teaching tool.

UPPER GASTROINTESTINAL BLEEDING, LOWER GASTROINTESTINAL BLEEDING, AND HEPATIC FAILURE

Gregory T. Everson, MD

Objectives

- Use clinical clues to differentiate between upper and lower gastrointestinal hemorrhage
- Examine results of vital signs, blood tests, and NG aspirate to assess severity of gastrointestinal hemorrhage and define immediate resuscitative measures
- Define the common causes of gastrointestinal hemorrhage in the intensive care unit
- Develop a diagnostic strategy and plan of management
- Discuss the advantages and disadvantages of therapeutic options for treatment of gastrointestinal hemorrhage
- Distinguish between acute hepatitis, acute liver failure, fulminant hepatitic failure, and an acute flare of chronic liver disease
- Assess the clinical features that define poor outcome and need for emergent transplantation
- Define that main causes of acute liver failure in patients presenting to the intensive care unit
- Initiate an appropriate plan for diagnosis and management
- Understand the indications, complications, and utility of ICP monitoring
- Describe advantages, disadvantages, and outcome of a wide array of treatments, including hepatocyte transplantation, bioartificial liver support, and transplantation (conventional and living donor liver transplantation using the right lobe)

Key Words: Gastrointestinal hemorrhage, Resuscitation, Nonsteroidal Anti-inflammatory Drugs (NSAIDs), Hematochezia, Melena, Hematemesis, Varices, Diverticulosis coli, Peptic Ulcer Disease, Endoscopy, Angiography, Acute Hepatitis, Hepatic Failure, Encephalopathy, Cerebral edema, Hepatocyte Transplantation, Liver Transplantation, Living Donor Liver Transplantation, Bioartificial Liver, N-acetyl cysteine, Acetaminophen

UPPER GASTROINTESTINAL HEMORRHAGE

Upper gastrointestinal hemorrhage accounts for 0.1% of all admissions to the hospital, occurs twice as frequently in men, is more common in the elderly, and remains a significant cause of ICU morbidity and mortality. For unknown reasons, UGI bleeding from peptic ulcer disease is more common in winter months. Current mortality from transfusion-requiring hemorrhage ranges from 5 to 15%. Mortality increases with age, hemodynamic instability, volume of transfusion requirement ($\geq$ 6 U pRBCs), evidence of organ dysfunction, underlying cardiopulmonary disease, and underlying liver disease. Risk of death increases 3-fold if the patient is already hospitalized at the time of the initial bleed. Three principals underline management: volume and blood product resuscitation, emergent endoscopy for diagnosis, and prompt definition and institution of therapy targeted to the underlying etiology. Surgical consultation should be obtained in the early stages of resuscitation and evaluation.

Case Presentation 1

A 42-year-old woman experienced sudden hematemesis at work while performing her usual secretarial duties. She was noted by co-workers to be pale, diaphoretic, and faint. Emergency medical technicians started peripheral intravenous lines and administered saline. On arrival at the emergency room, she was alert and oriented, pale, with BP 95/55, P 120, RR 22, T 37 C. She passed a melenic stool and examination revealed only a few scattered spider telangiectasia with mild hepatosplenomegaly. Two units of pRBCs were infused, a nasogastric tube was placed revealing dark blood with clots in the stomach, and she was admitted to the medical ICU. She described recent use of ibuprofen for headaches but denied alcohol or any knowledge of underlying liver disease. Past medical history was unremarkable except for receipt of blood transfusion at age 23 for postpartum hemorrhage.

Resuscitation

Initial assessment of severity of bleeding requires critical evaluation of vital signs. Hematocrit is not a reliable indicator of the degree of hemorrhage because it does not decrease immediately with acute bleeding. The decrease in hematocrit that occurs with bleeding is due to re-equilibration of body fluid and may take 24 to 72 hours to manifest. The patient who has sustained an upper gastrointestinal hemorrhage typically exhibits features of hypovolemia or hypovolemic shock. Immediate measures are focused at restoring intravascular volume and maintaining tissue oxygenation. Two large bore indwelling intravenous catheters should be placed early in the resuscitation effort and blood pressure immediately corrected with bolus infusion of normal saline. The ideal hematocrit guiding transfusion of blood or packed-RBCs is somewhat controversial, although most recommend a target hematocrit of 25 to 30% (this latter hematocrit is recommended for elderly patients, age > 60, or in those with underlying ischemic cardiovascular disease). Oxygen delivery to tissues is insured by volume replacement to restore blood pressure, maintenance of RBC volume to restore oxygen-carrying capacity, and administration of nasal O2 to saturate the carrying capacity of blood. Coagulopathic patients may require platelets, fresh frozen plasma, or cryoprecipitate (to replace fibrinogen). Calcium infusion may be required in those receiving massive units of citrate-treated stored blood since citrate may chelate calcium and lower its plasma concentration.

During resuscitative efforts the patient should be evaluated for underlying organ dysfunction due to the hemorrhage and examined for the presence of chronic liver disease. Lactic acidosis, renal failure, myocardial ischemia and infarction, bowel ischemia, cerebral ischemia, and limb ischemia may all complicate hemorrhagic shock. UGI hemorrhage in the setting of chronic liver disease is related to portal hypertension in approximately 50% of cases (varices or portal hypertensive gastropathy). Management is influenced significantly by the presence of underlying chronic liver disease and its etiology.

Etiology

The causes of UGI bleeding are given in Table 1. Endoscopy or radiologic imaging is required to establish the cause of bleeding. The most common etiology is duodenal ulcer disease, representing 30 to 35% of all cases of UGI bleeding. Bleeding from gastric ulcer is the next most common diagnosis, followed by Mallory-Weiss lesions, portal hypertensive gastropathy, and varices. However, a wide array of conditions may present with UGI hemorrhage (Table 1).

NSAIDs and Risk of Bleeding

The risk of bleeding with use of nonselective NSAIDs is approximately 0.5% after 6 months of ongoing treatment. Risk increases with age, history of ulcer disease, history of cardiovascular disease, and is related to dose of NSAID. Risk is reduced, but not eliminated, by use of the more selective COX-2 inhibitors (celecoxib, rofecoxib). Co-administration of nonselective NSAIDs to patients taking steroids or anticoagulation therapy (heparin or warfarin) increases the relative risk of bleeding up to 12-fold. H. pylori, although proven to increase the risk for ulcer disease, is not an independent risk factor for UGI bleeding.

Diagnosis

Initial findings at physical examination may be useful in providing clues as to the location of the bleeding lesion in the gastrointestinal tract. Evaluation of vital signs,

Table 1. Causes of Upper Gastrointestinal Hemorrhage

Esophageal	**As % of All UGI Bleeds**
Varices	10%
Erosive Esophagitis	2%
Mallory-Weiss lesion	5 to 15%
Medication-induced ulceration	$\leq 1\%$
Caustic ingestion	$\leq 1\%$
Infectious Esophagitis	$\leq 1\%$
Herpes	
CMV	
HIV	
Candida	
Carcinoma	$\leq 1\%$
Gastric	
Peptic Lesions	15 to 20%
Gastric ulcer	
Gastritis	
NSAID ulcers	
Dieulafoy's lesion	$\leq 1\%$
Varices	1 to 3%
Portal Hypertensive Gastropathy	10 to 15%
Vascular malformations	$\leq 1\%$
Neoplastic Lesions	$\leq 1\%$
Carcinoma	
Lymphoma	
Leiomyoma	
Duodenum	
Peptic ulcer	30 to 35%
Vascular malformation	$\leq 1\%$
Aorto-enteric fistula	$\leq 1\%$
Hemobilia	$\leq 1\%$
Hemosuccus pancreatitis	$\leq 1\%$

abdominal examination, and appearance of the bowel movement may localize the bleeding site. A patient passing bright red blood per rectum with stable vital signs and a benign abdomen is most likely bleeding from a lower, left-sided colonic lesion. A hemodynamically stable patient passing purplish clots and darker blood may be bleeding from the right colon or small bowel. Mild to moderate UGI bleeding is characterized by loose, black bowel movements (melena). Development of melena requires a minimum bleed of ≥ 100 ml and prolonged residence in the gut (≥ 12 hours). Massive bleeding from varices or an artery in an ulcer base is often characterized by hemodynamic instability or shock, and hematemesis. With

brisk bleeding from an upper GI source (≥ 1000 ml), one may observe passage of red blood per rectum; almost always mixed with darker blood or clots and characterized by hypotension. Approximately 5 to 15% of cases, initially thought to be bleeding from a LGI source, are actually bleeding from an UGI source.

Nasogastric tubes can be helpful diagnostically in some cases, but hemoccult testing of aspirates is not useful and not recommended. If the aspirate lacks blood and contains bile, an upper GI source for ongoing active bleeding is less likely. However, 16% of UGI bleeds from duodenal ulcer disease are associated with a clear NG aspirate. The major role for nasogastric tubes is to allow lavage and clearance of blood from the stomach for the purpose of performing endoscopy or other diagnostic studies. Other clues to an UGI source are elevation of BUN, hyperactive bowel sounds, and physical findings (spider telangiectasia, jaundice, hepatosplenomegaly, acanthosis nigricans, pigmented lip lesions, palpable purpura). Some gastroenterologists use the nasogastric tube to also assess the patient for activity of ongoing bleeding and to determine prognosis. A patient admitted for melena, who has a clear NG aspirate, has a predicted mortality of ≤ 5%. In contrast, a patient admitted with hematochezia, who has a red NG aspirate, has a predicted mortality of ~ 30%.

Emergent endoscopy, after resuscitation of the patient and clearance of blood and clots from the stomach, is indicated for nearly all acute UGI bleeders. Not only is endoscopy diagnostic in over 90% of cases it can also be used to provide definitive therapy (variceal ligation or sclerotherapy, electocautery, alcohol or sclerosant injection, biopsy for H. pylori in some cases may lead to antibiotic treatment). In addition, endoscopy is useful in identifying patients at high risk of rebleeding who may benefit from early surgical intervention (visible vessel failing endoscopic management, giant ulcer, diffuse hemorrhagic gastritis, miscellaneous lesions) (Table 2).

Case 1 (continued)

Our patient underwent endoscopy, which revealed esophageal varices with stigmata of recent hemorrhage (cherry red spot over varix) and minimal erosive gastritis. She was treated with endoscopic ligation of varices, had no further bleeding, and was discharged from the hospital 72 hours after admission. Subsequent evaluation revealed cirrhosis due to chronic hepatitis C. Varices were eradicated by repeated ligation treatments and she underwent evaluation for liver transplantation.

Imaging studies may also be useful in localizing a bleeding source. If endoscopic studies are nondiagnostic and bleeding persists, a nuclear medicine Tc99m-RBC scan may indicate the site of bleeding. This scan is more sensitive than angiography and when sequential scans are performed the bleeding site may be localized in 60 to 80% of case. Although the scan can localize bleeding to a site in the bowel, etiology is rarely, if ever, defined from this study. Angiography is used in patients with higher bleeding rates and may be therapeutic if embolization the bleeding site is performed. Angiography can be diagnostic for vascular lesions of the bowel. Meckel's scan (Technetium pertechnetate) are usually performed only after all other studies have failed to provide a diagnosis. Barium studies are not recommended in the initial evaluation of UGI bleeding.

Table 2. Prediction of Outcome after UGI Bleed from Peptic Lesions

Increased Risk of Mortality is Associated with
    Age > 60 years
    Hemodynamic instability with initial bleed
    Onset of bleeding during hospitalization for unrelated co-mordid condition
    History of cancer
    Underlying comorbid conditions
    Endoscopic finding of giant ulcer
    Endoscopic finding of visible vessel in base of ulcer

Endoscopic Features Predictive of Rebleeding
    Spurting artery (actively bleeding)
    Nonbleeding but elevated visible vessel
    Adherent clot
    Flat cherry red or black spot with oozing

Specific Therapeutic Approaches.

Bleeding from *peptic lesions* of the upper GI tract are treated by:

1. Gastric acid suppression (PPIs are favored over H2-blockers but are not effective in the setting of active bleeding)
2. Octreotide, 50 ug bolus followed by 50 ug/h infusion. Use of octreotide for this indication is controversial but some studies suggest that rebleeding rate is reduced by 30 to 50%
3. Correction of coagulopathy
4. Therapeutic endoscopy (electocautery, injection of sclerosant). Effectiveness of endoscopic therapy is limited by arterial size. Arterial bleeders with diameter ≥ 2 mm usually do not respond and require surgery. Rebleeding after initial control with endoscopic treatment is best managed by repeat endoscopic therapy or radiologic intervention. Surgery is only necessary in ~10% of rebleeds
5. Surgery, for those who fail endoscopic management
6. After resolution of the acute bleed, all patients with duodenal ulcer should be treated with triple therapy against helicobacter pylori. Other peptic lesions may also require this therapy if the patient is H. pylori positive.

Varices

Risk of bleeding from esophageal varices are directly related to portal pressure ($\geq$ 12 mm Hg), variceal size and appearance on endoscopy, advanced Child-Pugh score (Table 3), and coincident gastric varices. Mortality from UGI hemorrhage from varices ranges from 30 to 50%. The treatment of bleeding from esophageal varices is aimed at control of portal hypertension using pharmacological agents and direct application of endoscopic treatment to the bleeding variceal channels. A number of pharmacologic agents can lower portal hypertension: beta-blockers, nitroglycerin, vasopressin, and somatostatin. We currently favor use of octreotide or vapreotide since they are effective, well-tolerated, and have few side effects. A loading dose of 50 ug is administered initially, and followed by continuous infusion at 50 ug/h. The majority of patients bleeding from esophageal varices can be controlled by endoscopic ligation, especially if done with co-administration of long-acting somatostatin analogue. Endoscopic ligation treatment ("banding") is associated with fewer complications than endoscopic sclerotherapy and is currently the preferred modality. Patients bleeding from gastric varices or who rebleed from esophageal varices despite endoscopic treatment may require placement of a Sengstaken-Blakemore tube and performance of either transjugular intrahepatic portal-systemic shunt (TIPS) or surgical shunt (Table 4). TIPS placement is successful in 90 to 95% of cases but TIPS may thrombose or stenose and require repeated radiological interventions. In addition, TIPS is costly and 15 of 30% of patients undergoing TIPS suffer from post-TIPS encephalopathy. Mortality rates from bleeding varices are directly related to Childs-Pugh score, ongoing alcohol use, and comorbid illness. Mortality is over 50% in Childs class C cirrhotics (Table 5).

Table 3. Child-Pugh Criteria

	1 point	2 points	3 points
Bilirubin (mg/dl)	<2	2-3	>3
Albumin (g/dl)	>3.5	2.8-3.5	<2.8
PT (sec prolonged)	1-3	4-6	>6
Ascites	None	slight	moderate
Encephalopathy	None	1-2	3-4

Grades: A = 4-6 points; B = 7-9 points; C = 10-15 points

Pugh's modification of the Child-Turcotte prognostic classification (Pugh RN, Murray-Lyon IM, Dawson JL, et al: Transection of the esophagus for bleeding of esophageal varices. *Br J Surg* 1973; 60:646

LOWER GASTROINTESTINAL HEMORRHAGE

The principals of management for LGI bleeding are similar to those mentioned above for UGI bleeding: resuscitation, diagnosis, and planning for specific therapy. One initial consideration in evaluating the LGI bleeder is to exclude an UGI source. A negative nasogastric lavage may obviate the need for upper endoscopy but nearly 5 to 15% of patients thought to have LGI bleeding are actually diagnosed with an UGI source and about 5% are from the small bowel. The average age of LGI bleeders is 65 year. Causes of LGI bleeding include: hemorrhoids, angiodysplasia, diverticular disease, neoplastic lesions, inflammatory bowel disease, and other vascular lesions or tumors of the lower GI tract (Table 6).

Colonoscopy

The primary diagnostic test in LGI bleeding is colonoscopy after purgation of the bowel by use of Colyte. Studies comparing colonoscopy to air-contrast barium enema (ACBE) indicate that colonoscopy is far superior, identifying the source in ~ 70% of cases compared to only ~30% for ACBE. Another advantage of colonoscopy is the ability to provide treatment (cautery, polypectomy, sclerotherapy). However, there is a 2% risk of perforation with endoscopic treatments when administered in the setting of acute bleeding. Sigmoidoscopy should be reserved for the evaluation of minor LGI bleeding in relatively young patients (≤ 40 year).

Angiography

Angiography can be diagnostic in up to 75% of cases if the rate of bleeding is ≥ 0.5 ml/min. This diagnostic and therapeutic modality is usually restricted to cases where endoscopy is not possible due to large amounts of blood in the gut lumen or when certain treatments are planned (vasopressin infusion, embolization). Angiography is particularly useful in the diagnosis and management of isolated vascular malformation.

Table 4. Indications for and Contraindications to TIPS

Indications	Contraindications
Accepted:	**Absolute:**
Gastroesophageal variceal hemorrhage	Heart failure with elevated CVP
-refractory acute variceal bleeding	Polycystic liver disease
-refractory recurrent variceal bleeding	Severe hepatic failure
-bleeding from intestinal varices	**Relative:**
Cirrhotic Hydrothorax	Active intrahepatic or systemic infection
Promising:	Portal vein occlusion
Refractory Ascites	Hypervascular hepatic neoplasms
Hepatorenal Syndrome	Poorly-controlled hepatic encephalopathy
Budd-Chiari Syndrome	Stenosis of celiac trunk

Table 5. Risk of Death from Variceal Hemorrhage According to Severity of Liver Disease

Child-Pugh Class A	≤ 5%
Child-Pugh Class B	≤ 25%
Child-Pugh Class C	> 50%

Others

Technetium-labelled RBC scans are often ordered because of the ease of performance of the test and the perception that valuable information is gained. However, these scans rarely provide definitive information regarding cause or localization of bleeding and cannot provide therapy. The usefulness of RBC scans is quite limited.

Diverticular Disease

Diverticuli are the cause of LGI bleeding in 0% of all cases and 50% of those with active hemorrhage undergoing angiography. However, diverticuli are very common and prevalence increases with advancing age. Overall, only 3% of patients with diverticulosis coli ever experience LGI bleeding. When bleeding occurs, it is usually sudden, painless, and often from the right colon (in up to 70% of cases). Eighty percent of acute bleeds stop spontaneously but 20 to 25% rebleed. Localization of the site of bleeding is essential to plan appropriately for treatment, which may include segmental colonic resection or even subtotal colectomy.

The list of other relatively common causes of LGI bleeding is given in Table 6. Additional rare causes of LGI bleeding include infectious colitis, NSAID ulcers, rectal varices, vasculitis, and juvenile polyps. As with other causes of GI bleeding, treatment is directed at the underlying etiology.

ACUTE HEPATIC FAILURE

Definitions

Acute Hepatitis

The standard definition of acute hepatitis is the development of acute liver parenchymal injury from exposure to hepatotoxins or infectious agents, such as viral hepatitis, toxins, or medications. Typical patients with self-limited disease exhibit variable elevations in transaminases (AST & ALT 100 to 1000 IU/L), limited elevations in bilirubin (< 5 mg/dl), have normal serum albumin, and no coagulopathy (prothrombin time or INR is normal). Most patients with acute hepatitis recover uneventfully, but approximately 1% will experience severe injury with evidence of liver failure. Patients with chronic liver disease, such as chronic hepatitis C, who experience intercurrent acute hepatitis, such as acute hepatitis A, may experience hepatic decompensation and signs of liver failure.

Acute Liver Failure

Acute liver failure is defined by the development of coagulopathy (prothrombin time > 2 sec prolonged, INR > 1.5) in a patient with acute hepatitis who lacks underlying chronic liver disease. Patients with acute liver failure usually have greater elevations of AST & ALT with the initial injury (1000 to 5000 IU/L), often are jaundiced, and exhibit more constitutional symptoms. These patients are at risk for fulminant hepatic failure, although most recover uneventfully.

Table 6. Causes of Significant Acute Lower GI Bleeding

Diverticulosis		30%
Post-polypectomy		7%
Ischemic colitis	6%	
Colonic ulcerations		6%
Neoplasm (cancer and polyps)	5%	
Angiodysplasia	4%	
Radiation Proctitis		2%
Inflammatory bowel Disease	2%	
Miscellaneous Lesions	12%	
Undiagnosed LGI Bleeding		26%

Table 7. Causes of Acute Liver Failure	
Acetaminophen	20%
Cryptogenic	15%
Nonacetaminophen drug toxicity	12%
Hepatitis B	10%
Hepatitis A	7%
Autoimmune Hepatitis	6%
Wilson's Disease	6%
Miscellaneous*	24%

*Budd-Chiari syndrome, herpes simplex, paramyxovirus, Epstein-Barr virus, amanita poisoning, ischemia, malignant infiltration

Adapted from Schiodt FV, Atillasoy E, Shakil O, et al: Etiologic factors and outcome for 295 patients with acute liver failure in the United States. *Liver Transplant Surg* 1999; 5:29-34

Fulminant Hepatic Failure

The classification of fulminant liver failure requires evidence of hepatic encephalopathy within 8 weeks of the onset of jaundice related to acute liver injury. One criterion for this diagnosis is the absence of underlying chronic liver disease, the only exception being Wilson's disease. There are approximately 2000 cases of fulminant hepatic failure in the U.S. each year.

Case Presentation 2

A 38-year-old businessman presents with a 3-day history of progressive malaise, myalgia, and anorexia. In the last 24 hours he has noted dark urine and jaundice. His wife reports that the patient has been mildly confused. He and his family deny a past history of underlying medical illness, intravenous drug use, or other exposure to blood or blood products. He described his usual alcohol intake as 2 to 4 mixed drinks each day. In the week prior to the onset of his illness he drank from 5 to 8 mixed drinks each day and frequently skipped meals. In addition, he described taking eight to ten 500 mg tablets of acetaminophen per day for the last 10 days for headaches. Physical examination revealed jaundice, mild hepatomegaly with tenderness to palpation, with no other features of cirrhosis. He was an icteric man who was unaware of the date and had mild asterixis. Laboratory: ALT 6250 IU/L, AST 9,765 IU/L, total bilirubin 6.5 mg/dl, albumin

3.8 g/dl, prothrombin time 21.5 seconds (INR 2.3), creatinine 2.2 mg/dl, and arterial pH 7.25.

Etiology

The main causes of acute hepatitis are viral hepatitis, drug-induced liver injury, and alcoholic hepatitis. Fulminant liver failure, defined by severe hepatocellular injury, coagulopathy and hepatic encephalopathy, is most often due, in order, to acetaminophen, drug toxicity, hepatitis B, and hepatitis A. However, the second leading diagnostic category for fulminant hepatic failure is cryptogenic, cause unknown (Table 7). Recent data, since 1998, indicate that over 50% of cases of FHF in the U.S. are due to acetaminophen (38%) or other idiosyncratic drug reactions (~14%). Sporadic cases of FHF due to both cocaine and Ecstacy have recently been described. FHF from mushroom poisoning occasionally occurs with inexperienced amateur mushroom fanciers. Infiltration of the liver with rapid progression of tumor growth can lead to FHF and has been described for breast carcinoma, lymphoma, and melanoma. Biopsy of the liver is required to establish the latter diagnoses. FHF may also occur in the third trimester of pregnancy related to acute fatty liver of pregnancy, HELLP syndrome, or disseminated Herpes infection.

Acetaminophen-induced acute liver failure occurs in the setting of intentional overdose (majority of cases), but a substantial portion occurs as a "therapeutic misadventure." In these cases injury occurs despite taking doses

Table 8. Labeling of Acetaminophen
Alcohol Warning • If you drink 3 or more alcoholic beverages every day, ask your doctor if you should take TYLENOL® or other pain relievers. Chronic heavy alcohol users may be at increased risk of liver damage when taking more than the recommended dose (overdose) of TYLENOL®.
Directions: • Adults and children 12 years of age and older: Take 2 geltabs (500mg/geltab) every 4 to 6 hours as needed. Do not take more than 8 geltabs in 24 hours, or as directed by a doctor. • Do not use: -with any other product containing acetaminophen -for more than 10 days for pain unless directed by a doctor -for more than 3 days for fever unless directed by a doctor

of acetaminophen within the recommended therapeutic range, as little as 4 gm/day for several days, in the setting of moderate alcohol intake and fasting. Enhanced toxicity is due to induction of metabolizing enzymes by alcohol, which increase formation of the toxic intermediate of acetaminophen and lead to depletion of hepatic glutathione. Liver injury in this circumstance is associated with towering AST levels, often > 5,000 IU/dl, and mortality may exceed 20%. This high mortality rate contrasts with mortality of <1% after acetaminophen overdose among nonalcoholics. Recognition of the association of alcohol use with higher risk of fulminant hepatic failure and death after acetaminophen use has led to labeling changes of over-the-counter acetaminophen preparations (Table 8).

Prognosis

A major determinant of prognosis is the level of encephalopathy (Table 9). Patients with fulminant hepatic failure who have progressed to higher stages of encephalopathy (Stage III or IV) have the worst prognosis. Additional clinical features that indicate a poor prognosis include: metabolic acidosis, renal failure, severe jaundice, or markedly prolonged prothrombin time. The likelihood of survival varies with the cause of acute liver injury. Patients with acetaminophen overdose have a relatively favorable outcome—over 50% survive. Patients with fulminant HAV and HBV infection have an intermediate prognosis in the range of 30% to 50%. In contrast, patients with a fulminant presentation of Wilson's disease or severe

sporadic non-A, non-B, non-C hepatitis have a survival of less than 10%.

Clinical Management

Once recognized, patients with fulminant liver failure should be transferred to a center with expertise in managing fulminant hepatic failure and who can offer liver transplantation.

Case 2 *(continued)*

The patient described above had acute liver failure with encephalopathy and was transferred to a liver transplantation center. After transfer, the patient's neurological status, coagulation profile, and liver chemistries were carefully monitored. He underwent evaluation for liver transplantation, including living donation, but concern was raised about his chronic excessive alcohol use. Over the next 48 hours, his mental status deteriorated, and his INR increased, despite a precipitous decline in aminotransferases. He was listed at status 1 and received a cadaveric liver transplant and his clinical state, including neurologic condition completely resolved.

General Measures

Indications for hospitalization include nausea and vomiting severe enough to result in dehydration, or severe impairment of liver function resulting in encephalopathy, ascites, gastrointestinal (GI) bleed, or rising prothrombin time. All admitted patients should be placed on needle (HB, NANB) and stool (HA) precautions but not in isolation. Gloves should be worn when handling biological specimens and specimens should be clearly labeled (Hepatitis patient). All used instruments should be autoclaved or appropriately disposed. No effective antiviral therapy exists for acute viral hepatitis or fulminant hepatic failure; corticosteroids are contraindicated as they may increase the risk of developing chronic hepatitis. Removal of the offending drug, toxin, or alcohol is the mainstay of therapy of drug-induced and alcoholic hepatitis, respectively. N-acetyl cysteine is an effective primary intervention for hepatic injury related to acetaminophen and is currently under investigation in the treatment of fulminant hepatic failure due to other etiologies (Table 10).

Upper GI Bleed

By definition, patients with fulminant hepatic failure have acute liver disease and, therefore, lack manifestations of cirrhosis, such as esophageal varices. Upper gastrointestinal bleeding in the setting of fulminant hepatic failure is typically not due to varices or portal hypertension. UGI bleeding in this setting is usually mild, controlled by correction of coagulopathy, and is usually due to either erosive gastritis or peptic ulcer disease. Emergent endoscopy is indicated to identify the bleeding lesion, plan management, and possibly to apply therapy. The key management issue is prevention of UGI bleeding by acid suppression with either H2-blockers (intravenously or orally) or proton pump inhibitors (orally) or by use of sucralfate via the nasogastric tube in patients who cannot take oral medications and in whom an adverse effect of H2 blockers (thrombocytopenia) is to be avoided. Doses of the first 2 agents are adjusted to achieve maximum acid suppression and optimum prophylaxis by monitoring gastric pH (target is pH $\geq$ 5) via a nasogastric tube. Sucralfate is dosed at 1 g q6h, irrespective of gastric pH.

Table 9. Grades of Encephalopathy in Patients with Fulminant Hepatic Failure

Grade 0:   No alteration of mental status

Grade I: Awake and responsive
Mild confusion and disorientation
Altered personality
Asterixis may or may not be present

Grade II: Awake, but agitated
Increasingly confused and disoriented
Hallucinations

Grade III: Increasing suppression of mental status
Stuporous but arousable to vocal or tactile stimuli
May require endotracheal tube for airway protection

Grade IV: Unresponsive to vocal or tactile stimulation
Essentially comatose but with intact pupillary reflexes
Usually still withdraw to painful stimuli

Irreversible Brain Injury (Guidelines only):

1. Cerebral edema on brain imaging (CT or MRI) with ischemic necrosis, hemorrhage, and compromised perfusion.
2. Sustained elevation of intracranial pressure by ICP monitoring with cerebral perfusion pressure (MAP – ICP) of < 40 mmHg for more than 4 hours.
3. Lack of brainstem function on neurologic examination (absent pupillary response, corneal reflex, gag reflex, and lack of any physiologic response or withdrawal to painful stimuli).

Table 10. Use of N-Acetyl Cysteine in Treatment of Acetaminophen Overdose

Oral Dosing Schedule
1. Avoid use of activated charcoal since it will bind N-acetyl cysteine, reducing its efficacy
2. Place nasogastric tube for administration of N-acetyl cysteine. N-acetyl cysteine is highly unpalatable; most patients cannot tolerate its oral administration. The NG tube is necessary to insure dosing of the medication.
3. Dosage: 140 mg/kg initially, followed by 70 mg/kg q 4 hours, to a total of 17 doses of N-acetyl cysteine.
4. Toxicity: nausea, vomiting

Intravenous Dosing Schedule (Limited availability in Research Centers)
1. Intravenous access for administration
2. Obtain informed consent
3. Dosage: Dilute in crystalloid solution to final concentration of 3%. Doses are infused over one hour through a 0.22 micron filter. Loading dose is 140 mg/kg initially, followed by 70 mg/kg q 4 hours, to a total of 12 doses of N-acetyl cysteine
4. Adverse reactions occur in approximately 15%: flushing and transient skin rash (usually responds to diphenhydramine), wheezing, nausea, vomiting. Patient should be monitored for anaphlyaxis (Rx with epinephrine, H1 and H2 blockers, supportive care)

Encephalopathy

Encephalopathy is a hallmark of fulminant hepatic failure and is also observed in patients with underlying chronic liver disease who sustain a superimposed acute liver injury. The mechanisms of encephalopathy differ but share some common features. Encephalopathy in the setting of chronic liver disease is linked to ammonia production (and several other factors) and responds to measures that effectively reduce blood ammonia levels: protein restriction, lactulose, and nonabsorbable oral antibiotics, such as neomycin.

In contrast, the encephalopathy of acute hepatic failure is usually related to cerebral edema. The exact mechanisms causing cerebral edema are unknown but experiments with animal models suggest a role for brain ammonia, production of glutamine, retention of glutamine in astrocytes, and astrocyte swelling. Progressively worsening encephalopathy in patients with acute liver failure is an ominous clincal feature; development of grade III or IV encephalopathy may herald the death of the patient due to central herniation of the brain. Efforts to control the encephalopathy of acute liver failure are directed at preventing or resolving cerebral edema (Table 11). Because emerging evidence suggests that ammonia may play a role in the development of cerebral edema we recommend limited use of protein (< 40 g/d) and lactulose to purge the bowel. However, one must exercise caution in using lactulose in the setting of fulminant hepatic failure; dosing should be monitored carefully and adjusted to avoid alterations in electrolytes and volume depletion. If lactulose (PO) is given simultaneously with IV mannitol, marked loss of free water may occur, inducing severe hypernatremia. Rapid shifts in sodium concentration have been associated with central pontine myelinolysis.

Table 11. Measures used to Monitor and Control Cerebral Edema due to Fulminant Hepatic Failure

1. **Correction of metabolic abnormalities**
- Electrolytes (Na, K, Cl, HCO3)
- Acid-Base (If patient is on mechanical ventilation, induce mild respiratory alkalosis)
- Glucose (maintenance intravenous glucose infusion)

2. **Avoid over-transfusion or over-hydration**
- Carefully match Intake and Output once patient is euvolemic
- Daily Weights
- Avoid use of blood products unless indicated for ongoing bleeding and correction of coagulopathy or to maintain hemostasis when intracranial monitor has been placed. In the latter circumstance you may need to diurese the patient to avoid an excess intravascular volume, especially from plasma.

3. **Institute Dialysis in Patients in Renal Failure**
- Continuous arterio-venous or veno-venous hemodialysis is preferred over standard hemodialysis
- Avoid severe volume shifts, stabilize blood pressure, maintain euvolemia, correct electrolyte and acid-base abnormalities

4. **Mechanical Ventilation (worsening encephalopathy, ≥ Grade II)**
- Main indication in liver failure is airway protection to prevent aspiration pneumonia
- Induce mild respiratory alkalosis (pH 7.45 to 7.50, pCO2 20 to 30 mmHg)
- Elevate the head of the bed 15 to 30 degrees
- Use sedation to avoid having the patient "fight the ET tube"

5. **Consider Placement of Intracranial Pressure (ICP) Monitor in the Epidural Space**
- Should be considered when patients evolve from stage II (agitated confusion) to stage III (stuporous) encephalopathy.
- Maintain adequate platelet count (> 60,000) with platelet transfusions and INR ≤ 1.5 with fresh frozen plasma, if necessary.
- Mannitol is used to control ICP in patients with intact renal function or in those on dialysis. Mannitol is given in 0.5 to 1.0 g/kg doses. Serum electrolytes, glucose, and osmolarity should be checked every 4 to 6 hours. If ICP elevated, osmolarity < 310, and Na <145, then give mannitol. Mannitol should be held if the patient has excessive serum osmolarity or significant hypernatremia.

Coagulopathy

In general, the coagulopathy of acute liver failure is due to depletion of clotting factors related to inadequate hepatic production. Some patients exhibit features of disseminated intravascular coagulation or primary fibrinolysis. Once the patient is diagnosed with severe acute liver failure or fulminant hepatic failure, we recommend administration of mephyton (Vitamin K) 10 mg/d SQ. Prophylactic infusions of clotting factors are not of proven benefit. Use of clotting factors, such as blood, fresh frozen plasma and fresh platelets, should be restricted to ongoing bleeding, such as GI hemorrhage.

Sepsis

Prophylactic antibiotics are not recommended. Blood, urine and sputum should be cultured frequently (even in absence of fever or other signs of infection) and antibiotic therapy directed towards specific organisms. Development of fever usually signifies intercurrent infection and should not be attributed to the liver injury, per se. Febrile patients should be fully cultured and treated empirically with antibiotics. The most common sources of infection are respiratory, urinary, and line sepsis. Currently we use vancomycin with a fluroquinolone in initial treatment and then tailor antibiotic use once results of cultures are known.

Glucose

Glycogen in the liver represents a main storage supply of glucose during periods of stress or fasting. Hepatic failure impairs glycogenolysis, and depletes the liver of its glycogen stores, resulting in severe, potentially life-threatening hypoglycemia. It is imperative that all patients with acute liver failure or fulminant hepatic failure be treated with glucose infusions and that blood glucose is checked every 4 to 6 hours.

Liver Support Systems

Several methods have been used in FHF: Exchange blood transfusion, plasmapheresis, cross circulation with human and baboon donors, hemoperfusion through isolated human or animal liver, hemodialysis (conventional and polyacrylonitrate), and column hemoperfusion (microencapsulated charcoal, albumin-covered amberlite XAD-7 Resin). Only exchange transfusion and charcoal hemoperfusion have been evaluated by controlled trial, and the mortality was either similar or greater in the treated group. Since none of these techniques has been demonstrated to improve survival, their use in FHF is not currently recommended (unless under IRB-approved protocols in major liver centers).

Bioartificial Liver

Extracorporeal liver assist devices (ELAD) or bioartificial liver machines (BAL) have recently emerged as potential therapeutic interventions in the treatment of fulminant hepatic failure. However, their use currently is experimental and none have yet been conclusively shown, in randomized controlled trials, to improve outcome for patients with FHF. The major principal behind these devices is the use of a "bioreactor" which contains liver cells in a dialysis cartridge, external to the capillary luminae through which blood or plasma flows. The liver cells used in these reactors vary from primary porcine hepatocytes to transformed cells (subclones of HepG2 cells). "Toxins" or metabolites diffuse across the capillary membrane where the liver cells can remove, metabolize, or inactivate them. Experimental models suggest that removal of toxins and metabolites may reduce the neurotoxicity of fulminant hepatic failure by inhibiting the formation of cerebral edema. In clinical terms, the goal is stabilization of neurological function to allow for hepatic regeneration or to bridge the patient to liver transplantation. Randomized controlled trials in the US are currently examining the efficacy of 2 different bioartificial livers in treatment of fulminant hepatic failure.

Stange, and colleagues, recently reported use of a bioartificial liver (MARS) in 26 patients with chronic liver disease who had either acute or chronic liver failure. The treatments lowered plasma bilirubin and bile acids but effect on clinical outcome was unclear: 9 patients with advanced liver disease (equivalent to UNOS 2A) died within an average of 15 days but the remainder survived and were thought to have benefited. Further studies will be needed to define benefit and overall utility.

Hepatocyte Transplantation

The prinipals guiding use of hepatocyte transplantation are similar to those of the bioartificial liver: provide support during a period of critical need so that the patient can be bridged to recovery or transplantation. One potential advantage of hepatocyte transplantation is the ability of liver stem cells to regenerate raising the potential for repopulation of a dying or dead liver by allogeneic donor hepatocytes. The latter theoretical consideration has not been proven. Experience with hepatocyte transplantation in fulminant hepatic failure is limited. We have used this technique in 6 patients, who were not candidates for liver transplantation due to active substance abuse or who had prohibitive underlying medical illness and 1 patient, listed for transplantation, who had disseminated herpes infection. Despite a suggestion of improvement in neurologic status after hepatocyte transplantation, all 7 died. Difficulties with this approach include: inadequacy of the supply of human hepatocytes, need for arterial puncture in a coagulopathic patient to access either splenic artery for intrasplenic infusion of hepatocytes or hepatic artery for intrahepatic infusion, need for transjugular approach to portal vein if intraportal infusion of hepatocytes is to be performed, compromise of arterial circulation to spleen or liver during infusion, and use of immunosuppression to prevent hepatocyte rejection in setting of severe hepatic failure. Clearly, at this point hepatocyte transplantation for FHF should be viewed as unproven and experimental.

Liver Transplantation

Liver transplantation is the only treatment that has been proven to improve survival in patients with fulminant hepatic failure and grade III or IV encephalopathy. Survival of this group of patients without transplantation is 10 to 20%. Survival increases to 60 to 80% with liver transplantation. Patients with FHF are listed at status 1 and given top priority for transplantation. The major limitation in performance of liver transplantation is inadequate availability of donor organs. As of May 1, 2001, there were greater than 18,000 patients on the U.S. waiting list for liver transplantation. In the last 4 years, the number of liver transplants performed has ranged from 4000 to 4500 annually. Although, most UNOS regions in the U.S. currently "share" livers between organ procurement organizations (OPO) within each region for status 1 patients, this practice does not increase total donor organ availability. Available organs from patients with more stable chronic liver disease are simply shifted to those with acute liver failure and in greatest immediate need. Expansion of the donor pool is essential to resolve the donor—recipient mismatch.

Adult Living Donor Liver Transplantation using the Right Lobe

There are currently 2 major approaches to expanding the donor pool: splitting cadaveric donor livers and use of living donors. Split livers are used primarily in the setting of an adult and pediatric recipient, simultaneously in need of urgent transplantation. The left lateral segment is transplanted into the child and the remaining liver is used for the adult. Splitting livers into right and left hemi-livers for implantation into 2 adult recipients is under investigation.

Living-donor liver transplantation has been performed successfully in approximately 1500 pediatric cases, typically from parent to child using the lateral segment of the left lobe, and in over 800 adults, typically using either full left lobe or, more recently the right lobe. Donor safety is a major concern in the performance of LDLT. Current statistics suggest that donor mortality is approximately 0.13% for adult-to-pediatric cases and 0.25% for adult-to-adult cases. Recent surveys indicate that donors have been satisfied with their decision to donate and in 1 survey from our institution all indicated a willingness to donate again, if they could.

In adults with fulminant hepatic failure, survival is dependent upon an adequate functional hepatic mass. The left lateral segment is not thought to have sufficient hepatocellular mass to support an adult patient. For this reason, living-donation of the left lateral segment for adults with fulminant hepatic failure has not been actively pursued. In contrast, an increasing number of liver transplant centers have begun to use the right lobe from living donors to perform hepatic transplantation. Experience with this approach in fulminant hepatic failure, however, is limited. At a recent NIH-sponsored workshop (December 2000), outcome after LDLT for FHF was reviewed. Fourteen patients had undergone LDLT for FHF, of these all survived the surgical procedure and the 1-year survival was 90%. These favorable results are encouraging, since results with cadaveric transplantation have yielded 1-year survivals of 60 to 80%.

Examination of a single case is instructive. We used LDLT in a young woman with fulminant hepatitis who was in coma, on mechanical ventilation and dialysis, with CT evidence of cerebral edema. There was no cadaveric donor available in our region and her brother inquired into the feasibility of performing living donor transplantation It should be noted that our center was already experienced with adult-to-adult, right lobe, living donor transplantation in patients with chronic liver disease. The patient sustained complete clinical and neurological recovery following the living-donor transplant. The donor was discharged from the hospital within 1 week of surgery. Liver volume in both recipient and donor regenerates rapidly after resection and implantation. Within 2 to 12 weeks liver volume normalized. Increasing availability of surgical expertise to perform this procedure may allow more widespread application and timely transplantation of patients with fulminant hepatic failure.

REFERENCES

Portal Hypertension

1. Grace ND, Bhattacharya K: Pharmacologic therapy of portal hypertension and variceal hemorrhage. *Clin in Liver Dis* 1997; 1:59-75
2. Pagliaro L, D'Amico G, Sorrenson TA, et al: Prevention of first bleeding in cirrhosis: A meta-analysis of randomized trials of nonsurgical treatment. *Ann Intern Med* 1992; 117:59
3. Grace ND: Diagnosis and treatment of gastrointestinal bleeding secondary to portal hypertension. *Am J Gastroenterol* 1997; 92(7):1081-1091
4. Corley DA, Cello JP, Adkisson W, Ko WF, Kerlikowski K: Octeotide for Acute Esophageal Variceal Bleeding: A Meta-Analysis. *Gastroenterology* 2001; 120:946-954
5. Cales P, Masliah C, Bernard B, Garnier PP, Silvain C, Szostak-Talbodec N, Bronowicki JP, Ribard D, Botta-Fridlund D, Hillon P, Besseghir K, Lebrec D, for the French Club for the Study of Portal Hypertension: Early Administration of Vapreotide for Variceal Bleeding in Patients with Cirrhosis. *N Engl J Med* 2001; 344:23-28

Upper GI Bleed

6. Lau JYW, Sung JJY, Lam YH, Chan ACW, Ng EKW, Lee DWH, Chan FKL, Suen RCY, Chung SCS: Endoscopic Retreatment Compared with Surgery in Patients with Recurrent Bleeding after Initial Endoscopic Control of Bleeding Ulcers. *N Engl J Med* 1999; 340:751-756

7. Rockall TA, Logan RF, Devlin HB, Northfield TC: Selection of Patients for Early Discharge or Outpatient Care after Acute Upper Gastrointestinal Haemorrhage: National Audit of Acute Upper Gastrointestinal Haemorrhage. *Lancet* 1996; 347:1138-1140
8. Rockey DC, Koch J, Cello JP, Sanders LL, McQuaid K: Relative Frequency of Upper Gastrointestinal and Colonic Lesions in Patients with Positive Fecal Occult-Blood Tests. *N Engl J Med* 1998; 339: 153-159
9. Gostout CJ, Wang KK, Ahlquist DA: Acute Gastrointestinal Bleeding: Experience of a Specialized Management Team. *J Clin Gastroenterol* 1992; 14:260-267
10. Rockall TA, Logan RFA, Devlin HB, Northfield TC: Incidence and mortality from acute gastrointestinal hemorrhage in the United Kingdom. *Br Med J* 1995; 311:222-226
11. Zimmerman J, Siguencia J, Tsvang E: Predictors of Mortality in Patients Admitted to Hospital for Acute Gastrointestinal Hemorrhage. *Scand J Gastroenterol* 1995; 30:327-331

Lower GI Bleed

12. Bokhari M, Vernava AM, Ure T, Longo WE. Diverticular hemorrhage in the Elderly—Is it well-tolerated? *Dis Colon Rectum* 1996; 39:191-195
13. Richter JM, Christensen MR, Kaplan LM, Nishioka NS: Effectiveness of current technology in the diagnosis and management of lower gastrointestinal hemorrhage. *Gastrointest Endosc* 1994; 41:93–98

Acute Liver Failure

14. Schiodt FV, Atillasoy E, Shakil AO, et al: Etiology and outcome for 295 patients with acute liver failure in the United States. *Liver Transplant Surg* 1999; 5:29-34 *Results of retrospective survey which, reviews the cause and course of fulminant hepatic failure among patients, recently admitted to U.S. 12 liver transplantation centers. Drug induced liver injury,*

specifically acetaminophen toxicity, is the most prevalent single cause of fulminant hepatic failure in this survey.

15. Lee WM: Medical progress: Acute liver failure. *N Engl J Med* 1993; 329;1862-1872
    A thorough review of fulminant hepatic failure.

16. Hoofnagle JH, Carithers RL, Shapiro C, Ascher N: Fulminant hepatic failure: Summary of a workshop. *Hepatology* 1995; 21:240-252
    Review of topics discussed at a recent NIH consensus conference on fulminant hepatic failure.

17. Strom SC, Chowdhury JR, Fox IJ: Hepatocyte Transplantation for the Treatment of Human Disease. *Seminars in Liver Disease* 1999; 19:39-48

18. Clemmesen JO, Larsen FS, Kondrup J, Hansen BA, Ott P: Cerebral Herniation in Patients with Acute Liver Failure is Correlated with Arterial Ammonia Concentration. *Hepatology* 1999; 29:648-653

19. Belay ED, Bresee JS, Holman RC, Khan AS, Shahriari A, Schonberger LB: Reye's Syndrome in the United States from 1981 through 1997. *N Engl J Med* 1999; 340:1377-1382

20. Schiodt FV, Rochling FA, Casey DL, Lee WM: Acetaminophen Toxicity in an Urban County Hospital. *N Engl J Med* 1997; 337:1112-1117

21. Charlton M, Adjei P, Poterucha J, Zein N, Moore B, Therneau T, Krom R, Wiesner R: TT-Virus Infection in North American Blood Donors, Patients with Fulminant Hepatic Failure, and Cryptogenic Cirrhosis. *Hepatology* 1998; 28:839-842

22. Lee WM, Williams R: Acute Liver Failure. Cambridge, UK, 1997, Cambridge University Press

23. Lee WM: Acute Liver Failure. *Clin Perspectives in Gastroenterol* 2001; March/April:pp 101 – 110

24. Riordan SM, Williams R: Use and Validation of Selection Criteria for Liver Transplantation in Acute Liver Failure. *Liver Transplantation* 2000; 6:170-173

25. Shakil AO, Kramer D, Mazariegos GV, Fung JJ, Rakela J: Acute Liver Failure: Clinical Features, Outcome Analysis, and Applicability of Prognostic Criteria. *Liver Transplantation* 2000; 6:163-169

26. Stange J, Mitzner SR, Klammt S, Freytag J, Peszynski P, Loock J, Hickstein H, Korten G, Schmidt R, Hentschel J, Schulz M, Lohr M, Liebe S, Schareck W, Hopt UT: Liver Support by Extracorporeal Blood Purification: A Clinical Observation. *Liver Transplantation* 2000; 6:603-613

27. Tsiaoussis J, Newsome PN, Nelson LJ, Hayes PC, Plevris JN: Which Hepatocyte will it be? Hepatocyte Choice for Bioartificial Liver Support Systems. *Liver Transplantation* 2001; 7:2-10

28. Trotter J, Wachs M, Everson GT, Kam I: Adult-to-adult right hepatic lobe living donor liver transplantation. *N Engl J Med* 2002; 346:1074-1082

MECHANICAL VENTILATION

Gregory A. Schmidt, MD, FCCP

Objectives

- To describe the role of the ventilator in determining respiratory mechanics
- To recommend disease-specific ventilator strategies aimed at reducing the adverse consequences of mechanical ventilation
- To review new information regarding ventilation in ARDS
- To address the role of noninvasive ventilation
- To discuss the complications of mechanical ventilation

Key Words: Mechanical ventilation; ARDS; COPD; status asthmaticus; tidal volume; noninvasive ventilation; assist-control; pressure support; pressure control; SIMV; inverse ratio ventilation

TABLE OF ABBREVIATIONS

ACRF	acute-on-chronic respiratory failure
ACV	assist-control ventilation
ARDS	acute respiratory distress syndrome
COPD	chronic obstructive pulmonary disease
Crs	compliance of the respiratory system
f	respiratory rate
I:E	inspiratory to expiratory rate
IRV	inverse ratio ventilation
NIV	noninvasive ventilation
PCV	pressure-control ventilation
PEEP	positive end-expiratory pressure
Pinsp	inspiratory pressure
Ppeak	peak airway opening pressure
Pplat	plateau airway pressure
PSV	pressure-support ventilation
SIMV	synchronized intermittent mandatory ventilation
Ti	inspiratory time
Te	expiratory time
Vt	tidal volume

TRAUMA

This lecture offers an approach in which the ventilator is used as a probe of the patient's respiratory system mechanical derangements following which the ventilator settings are tailored to the patient's mechanical and gas exchange abnormalities. This facilitates early stabilization of the patient on the ventilator in such a way as to optimize carbon dioxide removal and oxygen delivery within the limits of abnormal neuromuscular function, lung mechanics, and gas exchange.

The fundamental purpose of mechanical ventilation is to assist in elimination of carbon dioxide and uptake of adequate oxygen while the patient is unable to do so or should not be allowed to do so. Such patients fall into 2 main groups: 1) those in whom full rest of the respiratory muscles is indicated (such as during shock; severe, acute pulmonary derangement; or deep sedation or anesthesia), and 2) those in whom some degree of respiratory muscle use is desired (e.g., to strengthen or improve the coordination of the respiratory muscles; to assess the ability of the patient to sustain the work of breathing; or to begin spontaneous ventilation). It is important for the intensivist to be explicit about whether the respiratory muscles should be rested or exercised, since the details of ventilation (mode, settings) usually follow logically from this fundamental point.

If full rest of the respiratory muscles is desired, it is incumbent on the physician to assure that this is indeed achieved. Although some patients are fully passive while being ventilated (those with deep sedation, some forms of coma, metabolic alkalosis, sleep disordered breathing), most patients will make active respiratory efforts, even on assist control ventilation, at times performing extraordinary amounts of work. Unintended patient effort can be difficult to recognize, but, aside from obvious patient effort, may be signaled by an inspiratory fall in intrathoracic pressure (as noted on a central venous or pulmonary artery pressure tracing, or with an esophageal balloon) or by triggering of the ventilator. Recognizing patient effort has been greatly aided by the provision of real-time displays of flow and pressure waveforms, now commonly available on modern ventilators.

Choosing a ventilatory mode and settings appropriate for each individual patient depends, not only on the physician's goals (rest versus exercise), but also on knowledge of the mechanical properties of the patient's respiratory system. Most ventilators now have the capability of displaying waveforms of pressure, flow, and volume versus time, as well as flow versus volume. Using waveforms, it is easiest to gather information regarding the patient-ventilator interaction when patients are ventilated with a volume-preset mode [assist-control (ACV) or synchronized intermittent mandatory ventilation (SIMV)]. Still, some useful information can be gleaned from waveforms during pressure-preset ventilation [pressure-support ventilation (PSV) and pressure-control ventilation (PCV)].

The first step is to seek signs of inspiratory effort in the pressure tracing. Respiratory muscle contraction does not cease in most patients receiving mechanical ventilation, even in the ACV mode. Thus it is possible that a weak patient will remain weak, through continued breathing effort, despite the institution of mechanical support. In volume-preset modes, the signs of persistent effort include the presence of triggering, concavity during inspiration, and a variable Ppeak. When the goal of ventilation is to rest the respiratory muscles, ventilator adjustments, psychological measures, pharmacologic sedation, and therapeutic paralysis can be useful. Ventilator strategies to reduce the patient's work of breathing include increasing the minute ventilation to reduce PCO_2 (although this may run counter to other goals of ventilation, especially in patients with ARDS or severe obstruction), increasing the inspiratory flow rate, and changing the mode to pressure-support ventilation (PSV).

The next step is to determine whether the patient has significant airflow obstruction. This can be inferred by inserting a brief end-inspiratory pause, then determining the difference between Ppeak and Pplat. Alternatively, one can examine the expiratory flow waveform, seeking low flow and prolonged expiration, signs that are present regardless of the mode of ventilation (ACV, SIMV, PSV, PCV). Bronchodilator therapy can be assessed by noting whether expiratory flow increases, the expiratory time shortens, or there is a reduction in Ppeak, Pplat, or autoPEEP.

Finally, one should assure that the patient and ventilator are synchronized, that is, that each attempt by the patient to trigger the ventilator generates a breath. The most common situation in which the patient fails to trigger breaths occurs in severe obstruction when autoPEEP is present. This is recognized at the bedside when the patient makes obvious efforts that fail to produce a breath. Using waveforms, these ineffective efforts cause a temporary slowing of expiratory flow, sometimes halting it completely.

MODES OF MECHANICAL VENTILATION

Technological innovations have provided a plethora of differing modes by which a patient can be mechanically ventilated (8). Various modes have been developed with the hope of improving gas exchange, patient comfort, or speed of return to spontaneous ventilation. Aside from minor subtleties, however, nearly all modes allow full rest of the patient, on the one hand, or substantial exercise on the other. Thus in the great majority of patients, choice of mode is merely a matter of patient or physician preference. Noninvasive ventilation should be considered before intubation and ventilation in many patients who are hemodynamically stable and do not require an artificial airway, especially those with acute-on-chronic respiratory failure, postoperative respiratory failure, and cardiogenic pulmonary edema.

During volume-preset ventilation (and assuming a passive patient), Pplat is determined by the Vt and the static compliance of the respiratory system (Crs) where

$$Pplat = Vt/Crs + PEEP$$

where PEEP also includes autoPEEP. On the other hand, in pressure-preset modes, a fixed inspiratory pressure (Pinsp) is applied to the respiratory system, whatever the resulting Vt. However, the Vt is predictable (again, passive patient) when the Crs is known:

$$(Vt = [Pinsp - PEEP] \times Crs)$$

assuming time for equilibration between Pinsp and alveolar pressure. Thus a patient with static Crs of 50 ml/cm H_2O ventilated on assist-control at a tidal volume of 500cc with no PEEP (or autoPEEP) will have a Pplat of about 10cm H_2O, while the same patient ventilated on pressure control at 10cm H_2O will have a tidal volume of about 500cc. Thus while physicians' comfort level with volume-preset and pressure-preset modes may be very different, the modes can be similar since they are tied to each other through the patient's Crs.

A potential advantage of pressure-preset ventilation is greater physician control over the peak airway pressure (Ppeak) (since Ppeak = Pinsp) and the peak alveolar pressure, which could lessen the incidence of ventilator-induced lung injury. However, this same reduction in volutrauma risk should be attainable during volume-preset ventilation if tidal volumes appropriate to the lung derangement are chosen. Indeed, the ARDSNet trial, which demonstrated a mortality reduction in the low Vt group, used ACV and tidal volumes of 6cc/kg (9). Nevertheless, pressure-preset modes make such a lung protection strategy easier to carry out by dispensing with the need to repeatedly determine Pplat and periodically adjust the Vt. During pressure-preset modes the patient also has greater control over inspiratory flow rate, and therefore potentially increased comfort. A disadvantage of pressure-preset modes is that changes in respiratory system mechanics (e.g., increased airflow resistance or lung stiffness) or patient effort may decrease the minute ventilation, necessitating alarms for adequate

ventilation. Also, the mechanics cannot be readily determined.

In the following descriptions, each mode is first illustrated for a passive patient, such as following muscle paralysis, then for the more common situation in which the patient plays an active role in ventilation. On some ventilators, tidal volume (Vt) can be selected by the physician or respiratory therapist, while on others a minute ventilation and respiratory rate (f) are chosen, secondarily determining the Vt. Similarly, on some machines an inspiratory flow rate is selected, while on others flow depends on the ratio of inspiratory time to total respiratory cycle time and f, or an inspiratory:expiratory (I:E) ratio and f.

Conventional Modes of Ventilation

Assist Control Ventilation (ACV)

Passive Patient

The set parameters of the assist-control mode are the inspiratory flow rate, frequency (f), and tidal volume (Vt). The ventilator delivers f equal breaths per minute, each of Vt volume. Vt and flow determine the inspiratory time (Ti), expiratory time (Te), and the inspiratory:expiratory (I:E) ratio. Pplat is related to the Vt and the compliance of the respiratory system, while the difference between Ppeak and Pplat includes contributions from flow and inspiratory resistance.

Active Patient

The patient has the ability to trigger extra breaths by exerting an inspiratory effort exceeding the pre-set trigger sensitivity, each at the set Vt and flow, and to thereby change Ti, Te, I:E ratio, and to potentially create or increase autoPEEP. Typically, each patient will display a preferred rate for a given Vt and will trigger all breaths when the controlled ventilator frequency is set a few breaths/min below the patient's rate; in this way, the control rate serves as an adequate support should the patient stop initiating breaths. When high inspiratory effort continues during the ventilator-delivered breath, the patient may trigger a second, superimposed ("stacked") breath (rarely a third as well). Patient effort can be increased (if the goal is to exercise the patient) by increasing the magnitude of the trigger or by lowering Vt (which increases the rate of assisting). Lowering f at the same Vt generally has no effect on work of breathing when the patient is initiating all breaths.

Synchronized Intermittent Mandatory Ventilation (SIMV)

In the passive patient, SIMV cannot be distinguished from controlled ventilation in the ACV mode. Ventilation is determined by the mandatory f and Vt. However, if the patient is not truly passive, he may perform respiratory work during the mandatory breaths. More to the point of the SIMV mode, he can trigger additional breaths by lowering the airway opening pressure below the trigger threshold. If this triggering effort comes in a brief, defined interval before the next mandatory breath is due, the ventilator will deliver the mandatory breath ahead of schedule in order to synchronize (SIMV) with the patient's inspiratory effort. If a breath is initiated outside of the synchronization window, Vt, flow, and I:E are determined by patient effort and respiratory system mechanics, not by ventilator settings. The spontaneous breaths tend to be of small volume and are highly variable from breath to breath. The SIMV mode is often used to gradually augment the patient's work of breathing by lowering the mandatory breath f (or Vt), driving the patient to breath more rapidly in order to maintain adequate ventilation, but this approach appears to prolong "weaning" (2, 4). Although this mode continues to be used widely, there is little rationale for it and SIMV is falling out of favor.

Pressure Control Ventilation (PCV)

In the passive patient, ventilation is determined by f, the inspiratory pressure increment (Pinsp - PEEP), I:E ratio, and the time constant of the patient's respiratory system. In patients without severe obstruction (i.e., time constant not elevated) given a sufficiently long Ti, there is equilibration between the ventilator determined Pinsp and Palv so that inspiratory flow ceases. In this situation, tidal volume is highly predictable, based on Pinsp (=Palv), and the mechanical properties of the respiratory system (Crs). In the presence of severe obstruction or if Ti is too short to allow equilibration between ventilator and alveoli, Vt will fall below that predicted based on Pinsp and Crs.

The active patient can trigger additional breaths by reducing the Pao below the triggering threshold, raising the I:E ratio. The inspiratory reduction in pleural pressure combines with the ventilator Pinsp to augment the transpulmonary pressure and the tidal volume. Because Ti is generally set by the physician, care must be taken to discern the patients neural Ti (from the waveforms display) and adjust the ventilator accordingly, otherwise additional sedation might be necessary.

Pressure Support Ventilation (PSV)

The patient must trigger the ventilator in order to activate this mode, so pressure support is not applied to passive patients. Ventilation is determined by Pinsp, patient determined f, and patient effort. Once a breath is triggered, the ventilator attempts to maintain Pao at the physician-determined Pinsp, using whatever flow is necessary to achieve this. Eventually flow begins to fall due to cessation of the patient's inspiratory effort or to increasing elastic recoil of the respiratory system as Vt rises. The ventilator will maintain a constant Pinsp until inspiratory flow falls an arbitrary amount (e.g., to 20% of initial flow) or below an absolute flow rate. The patient's work of breathing can be increased by lowering Pinsp or making the trigger less sensitive, and can inadvertently increase if respiratory system mechanics change, despite no change in ventilator settings. Respiratory system mechanical parameters cannot be determined readily on this mode since the ventilator and patient contributions to Vt and flow are not represented by Pao; accordingly, these important measurements of Pplat, Ppeak-Pplat, and autoPEEP are measured during a brief, daily switch from pressure support to volume-preset ventilation. A potential advantage of pressure support ventilation is improved patient comfort.

Mixed Modes

Some ventilators allow combinations of modes, most commonly SIMV plus PSV. There is little reason to use such a hybrid mode, although some physicians use the SIMV as a means to add sighs to PSV, an option not otherwise generally available. Since SIMV plus PSV guarantees some backup minute ventilation (which PSV does not), this mode combination may have value in occasional patients at high risk for abrupt deterioration in central drive.

Triggered Sensitivity

In the assist-control, SIMV, and pressure support modes, the patient must lower the Pao below a preset threshold in order to "trigger" the ventilator. In most situations this is straightforward, with the more negative the sensitivity, the greater effort demanded of the patient. This can be used intentionally to increase the work of breathing when the goal is to strengthen the inspiratory muscles. When autoPEEP is present, however, the patient must lower Palv by the autoPEEP amount in order to have any impact on Pao, then further by the trigger amount to initiate a breath. This can dramatically increase the required effort for breath initiation.

Flow-triggering systems ("flow-by") have been used to further reduce the work of triggering the ventilator. In contrast to the usual approach in which the patient must open a demand valve in order to receive ventilatory assistance, continuous flow systems maintain a continuous high flow, then further augment flow when the patient initiates a breath. These systems can reduce the work of breathing slightly below that using conventional demand valves but do not solve the problem of triggering when autoPEEP is present.

Unconventional Ventilatory Modes

Inverse Ratio Ventilation (IRV)

IRV is defined as a mode in which the I:E ratio is greater than 1. There are 2 general ways to apply IRV: pressure-controlled IRV (PC-IRV) in which a preset airway pressure is delivered for a fixed period of time at an I:E ratio greater than 1, or volume-controlled IRV (VC-IRV) in which a tidal volume is delivered at a slow (or decelerating) inspiratory flow rate (or an end-inspiratory pause is inserted) to yield an I:E greater than 1. For PC-IRV, the physician must specify the inspiratory airway pressure, f, and I:E ratio, while Vt and flow profile are determined by respiratory system impedance as discussed for PCV above. Commonly, the initial Pinsp is 20-40 cm H_2O (or 10-30 cmH_2O above the PEEP), f is 20/min, and the I:E is 2:1 to 4:1. For VC-IRV, the operator selects a tidal volume, f, flow (typically a low value), flow profile, and, possibly, an end-inspiratory pause). The chosen values result in an I:E greater than 1:1 and as high as 5:1.

Compared to conventional modes of ventilation, lung oxygen exchange is often improved on IRV, owing to increased mean alveolar pressure and volume consequent to the longer time above functional residual capacity, or due to creation of autoPEEP. It is remotely possible that IRV causes better ventilation of lung units with long time constants, but these are so short in normal lungs (and shorter in AHRF) that such redistribution is unlikely to occur with slower flow, and could not reduce shunt even if it did. Because autoPEEP is a common consequence of IRV, serial determination of its magnitude is essential for safe use of this mode. Both PC-IRV and VC-IRV generally require heavy sedation with or without muscle paralysis.

Airway Pressure Release Ventilation

Airway pressure release ventilation (APRV) consists of continuous positive airway pressure (CPAP), which is intermittently released to allow a brief expiratory interval. Conceptually, this mode is pressure-controlled IRV during which the patient is allowed to initiate spontaneous breaths. A potential advantage of APRV is that mean alveolar pressure is lower than it would be during positive-pressure ventilation from the same amount of CPAP, possibly reducing the risks of barotrauma and hemodynamic compromise. Whether this mode provides any benefit over modern low tidal volume ventilation remains to be shown.

Proportional-Assist Ventilation

Proportional-assist ventilation is intended only for spontaneously breathing patients. The goal of this novel mode is to attempt to normalize the relationship between patient effort and the resulting ventilatory consequences (13, 14). The ventilator adjusts Pinsp in proportion to patient effort both throughout any given breath and from breath to breath. This allows the patient to modulate his breathing pattern and total ventilation. This is implemented by monitoring instantaneous flow and volume (V) of gas from the ventilator to the patient and varying the Pinsp as follows:

$$Pinsp = f1 \times V + f2 \times flow,$$

where f1 and f2 are selectable functions of volume (elastic assist) and flow (resistive assist), values for which can be estimated from the patient's respiratory mechanics. Potential advantages of this method are greater patient comfort, lower Ppeak, and enhancement of the patient's reflex and behavioral respiratory control mechanisms.

High Frequency Ventilation (HFV)

Several modes of ventilation have in common the use of tidal volumes smaller than the dead space volume (3). Gas exchange does not occur through convection as during conventional ventilation, but through bulk flow, Taylor diffusion, molecular diffusion, nonconvective mixing, and possibly other mechanisms. These modes include high frequency oscillatory ventilation (HFOV) and high frequency jet ventilation (HFJV). Theoretical benefits of HFV include lower risk of barotrauma due to smaller tidal excursions, improved gas exchange through a more uniform distribution of ventilation, and improved healing of bronchopleural fistulas. A substantial risk is that dynamic hyperinflation is the rule and alveolar pressure is greatly underestimated by monitoring pressure at the airway opening. Controlled trials of HFV have failed to demonstrate any clinically relevant benefit and

complications (especially barotrauma and tracheal injury) are seen frequently.

Noninvasive Ventilation

Mechanical ventilation for acute respiratory failure carries a high morbidity and mortality due, in part, to violation of the glottis by the endotracheal tube. In patients with acute-on-chronic respiratory failure, numerous studies have demonstrated that noninvasive ventilation (NIV) effectively relieves symptoms, improves gas exchange, reduces the work of breathing, lessens complications, shortens the ICU length of stay, and improves survival.

Both nasal and oronasal masks have been used successfully. Nasal masks are especially difficult to use in edentulous patients who are unable to control mouth leak. Careful attention to mask leaks and adjusting air flow and pressure-support levels are important considerations. Inflatable cuffs, nasal bridge protection, and the availability of a range of mask sizes to ensure proper fit can minimize mask complications. I find it useful to initiate ventilation by briefly holding the mask (already connected to the ventilator) onto the patient's face, rather than first strapping the mask on and then initiating ventilatory assistance. Sedative medications are occasionally appropriate and can improve tolerance of NIV, but carry some risk of respiratory depression and aspiration.

Patient-ventilator asynchrony describes a patient's breathing efforts which do not trigger the ventilator. During NIV, 2 mechanisms of PVA are common. The first is failure of the patient to lower sufficiently the proximal airway pressure (mask pressure) due to the presence of autoPEEP. As during invasive ventilation, counterbalancing the autoPEEP with externally-applied PEEP provides a means by which to lower the work of triggering. The second common mechanism for PVA is failure of the ventilator to detect end-inspiration because the patient's subsiding effort is cloaked by a mask leak. Most pressure-support ventilators terminate inspiration when inspiratory flow falls to a pre-set threshold, often at an arbitrary low value of flow or at a fixed percent of the peak inspiratory flow. Mask leaks prevent the flow from falling to this threshold, so the ventilator fails to switch off the inspiratory pressure, even while the patient is making active expiratory efforts. This serves to increase patient discomfort and the work of breathing. Using other methods for terminating inspiration, such as time-cycled pressure-support or volume assist-control, could minimize this problem.

Either conventional ICU ventilators or one of many portable bilevel pressure-targeted ventilators, initially designed for home ventilation, can be used. Limitations of portable pressure-targeted ventilators include the lack of waveform displays, the inability to deliver high FiO_2 (greater than about 40%; some new machines allow an FiO2 as high as 1.0), and the potential for rebreathing of exhaled gas. Whether volume-preset ventilation (such as assist-control) or pressure-preset ventilation is superior for NIV remains debated. Both modes have been used successfully, but direct comparisons between modes are few.

I believe the following points will minimize the chances that NIV will fail:

1. Develop an individual and institutional commitment to NIV.
2. Select patients carefully, excluding those with hemodynamic instability, inadequate airway protective reflexes, or little prospect of improvement within the next several days;
3. Have available a selection of oronasal and nasal masks to increase the probability of a good fit;
4. Use the pressure-support mode, beginning with modest settings, such as PEEP = 3 cm H_2O, PSV = 5 cm H_2O, and the most sensitive trigger, periodically removing the mask to allow the patient to sense its effect;
5. Education, reassurance, and modest sedation (when required) may improve tolerance to the mask and ventilator;
6. Increase the PEEP to ease the work of triggering with a goal of (typically) 4-8 cm H_2O; raise the level of PSV until the patient is subjectively improved, the tidal volume is sufficient, and the rate begins to fall, with goal of 10-15 cm H_2O;
7. Detect and correct mask leaks by repositioning, achieving a better fit, changing the type of mask, removing nasogastric tubes (gastric decompression in not recommended

during NIV), or adjusting the ventilator to reduce peak airway pressure.
8. Pay particular attention in the first 1h to patient-ventilator synchrony, using waveform displays as a guide.

MANAGEMENT OF THE PATIENT

Initial Ventilator Settings

Initial ventilator settings depend on the goals of ventilation (e.g., full respiratory muscle rest versus partial exercise), the patient's respiratory system mechanics, and minute ventilation needs. Although each critically ill patient presents myriad challenges, it is possible to identify 5 subsets of ventilated patients: 1) the patient with normal lung mechanics and gas exchange; 2) the patient with severe airflow obstruction; 3) the patient with acute-on-chronic respiratory failure; 4) the patient with acute hypoxemic respiratory failure, and 5) the patient with restrictive lung or chest wall disease.

In all patients the initial FiO_2 should usually be 0.5 to 1.0 to assure adequate oxygenation, although it can usually be lowered within minutes when guided by pulse oximetry and, in the appropriate setting, applying PEEP. In the first minutes following institution of mechanical ventilation, the physician should remain alert for several common problems. These include, most notably, airway malposition, aspiration, and hypotension. Positive-pressure ventilation may reduce venous return and so cardiac output, especially in patients with a low mean systemic pressure (e.g., hypovolemia, venodilating drugs, decreased sympathetic tone from sedating drugs, neuromuscular disease) or a very high ventilation-related pleural pressure (e.g., chest wall restriction, large amounts of PEEP, or obstruction causing autoPEEP). If hypotension occurs, intravascular volume should be rapidly expanded while steps are taken to lower the pleural pressure (smaller tidal volumes, less minute ventilation).

The Patient with Normal Respiratory Mechanics and Gas Exchange

Patients with normal lung mechanics and gas exchange can require mechanical ventilation: 1) because of loss of central drive to breathe (e.g., drug overdose or structural injury to the brainstem); 2) because of neuromuscular weakness (e.g., high cervical cord injury, acute idiopathic myelitis, myasthenia gravis); 3) as an adjunctive therapy in the treatment of shock; or 4) in order to achieve hyperventilation (e.g., in the treatment of elevated intracranial pressure following head trauma). Following intubation, initial ventilator orders should be an FiO_2 of 0.5 to 1.0, tidal volume of 8-15 cc/kg, rate of 8 - 12, and inspiratory flow rate of 40-60 L/min. Alternatively, if the patient has sufficient drive and is not profoundly weak, PSV can be used. The level of pressure support is adjusted (usually to the range of 10 to 20 cm H_2O above PEEP) to bring the respiratory rate down into the low 20s, usually corresponding to tidal volumes of about 400cc. If gas exchange is entirely normal, the FiO_2 can likely be lowered further based upon pulse oximetry or arterial blood gas determinations.

Soon after the initiation of ventilation, airway pressure and flow waveforms should be inspected for evidence of patient-ventilator dyssynchrony or undesired patient effort. If the goal of ventilation if full rest, the patient's drive can often be suppressed by increasing the inspiratory flow rate, frequency, or tidal volume; of course, the latter 2 changes may induce respiratory alkalemia. If such adjustments do not diminish breathing effort, despite normal blood gases, to an undetectable level, sedation may be necessary. If this does not abolish inspiratory efforts and full rest is essential (as in shock), muscle paralysis should be considered. Measures to prevent atelectasis should include sighs (6-12/hour at 1.5-2 times the Vt) or small amounts of PEEP (5-7.5 cm H_2O).

Patients with Severe Airflow Obstruction

Severe obstruction is seen most commonly in patients with status asthmaticus, but also rarely in those with inhalation injury or central airway lesions, such as tumor or foreign body, that are not bypassed with the endotracheal tube. Some of these patients may benefit from NIV, but most will require invasive ventilation. These patients are usually extremely anxious and distressed. Deep sedation should be provided in such instances, supplemented in some patients by therapeutic paralysis, although the use of paralytic drugs occasionally causes long-lasting weakness. These interventions help to reduce oxygen consumption (and hence carbon dioxide production), to lower airway pressures, and to reduce the risk of self-extubation.

Because the gas exchange abnormalities of airflow obstruction are largely limited to ventilation perfusion mismatch, an FiO_2 of 0.5 suffices in the vast majority of patients. Ventilation should be initiated using the ACV mode (or SIMV), the tidal volume should be small (5 to 7 mL kg), and the respiratory rate 12 to 15 breaths per minute. A peak flow of 60 L/min is recommended and higher flow rates do little to increase expiratory time. For example, if the Vt is 500, the rate 15, and the flow is 60L/min, the expiratory time is 3.5 seconds. Raising flow (dramatically) to 120L/min increases the expiratory time to only 3.75 seconds, a trivial improvement. In contrast, a small reduction in respiratory rate to 14/min increases the expiratory time to 3.8 seconds. This example serves to emphasize not only the relative lack of benefit of raising the flow rate but also the importance of minimizing minute ventilation when the goal is to reduce autoPEEP. Finally, if the patient is triggering the ventilator, some PEEP should be added to reduce the work of triggering (6). Although this occasionally compounds the dynamic hyperinflation, potentially compromising cardiac output, usually autoPEEP increases little as long as PEEP is not set higher than about 85% of the autoPEEP. The goals are (1) to minimize alveolar overdistention (Pplat < 30) and (2) to minimize dynamic hyperinflation (autoPEEP below 10 cm H_2O or end-inspiratory lung volume < 20ml/kg), a strategy which largely prevents barotrauma (11, 12). Reducing minute ventilation to achieve these goals generally causes the PCO_2 to rise above 40 mm Hg, often to 70 mm Hg or higher.

Although this requires sedation, such permissive hypercapnia is quite well-tolerated except in patients with increased intracranial pressure, and perhaps in those with ventricular dysfunction or critical pulmonary hypertension (5).

Patients with Acute-On-Chronic Respiratory Failure

Acute-on-chronic respiratory failure (ACRF) is a term used to describe the exacerbations of chronic ventilatory failure, often requiring ICU admission, usually occurring in patients with COPD. Unlike patients with status asthmaticus, patients in this population tend to have relatively smaller increases in inspiratory resistance, their expiratory flow-limitation arising largely from loss of elastic recoil. As a consequence, in the patient with COPD and minimally reversible airway disease, peak airway pressures on the ventilator tend not to be extraordinarily high, yet autoPEEP and its consequences are common. At the time of intubation, hypoperfusion is common, as manifested by tachycardia and relative hypotension, and typically responds to briefly ceasing ventilation combined with fluid loading.

Since the majority of these patients are ventilated after days to weeks of progressive deterioration, the goal is to rest the patient (and respiratory muscles) for 36 to 72 hours. Also, since the patient typically has an underlying compensated respiratory acidosis, excessive ventilation risks severe respiratory alkalosis and, over time, bicarbonate wasting by the kidney. Many such patients can be ventilated effectively with NIV, as described above. For those who require intubation, the goals of rest and appropriate hypoventilation can usually be achieved with initial ventilator settings of a tidal volume of 5 to 7 mL/kg and a respiratory rate of 24 to 28 breaths per min, with either an SIMV or an ACV mode set on minimal sensitivity. Since gas exchange abnormalities are primarily those of ventilation-perfusion mismatch, supplemental oxygen in the range of an FiO_2 of 0.4 should achieve better than 90% saturation of arterial hemoglobin.

The majority of patients with COPD will appear exhausted at the time when mechanical support is instituted and will sleep with minimal sedation. To the extent that muscle fatigue has played a role in a patient's functional decline, rest and sleep are desirable. Two to 3 days of such rest presumably will restore biochemical and functional changes associated with muscle fatigue, but 24 hours is probably not sufficient. Small numbers of patients are difficult to rest on the ventilator, continuing to demonstrate a high work of breathing. Examination of airway pressure and flow waveforms can be very helpful in identifying this extra work, and in suggesting strategies for improving the ventilator settings. In many patients, this is the result of autoPEEP-induced triggering difficulty. Adding extrinsic PEEP to nearly counterbalance the autoPEEP dramatically improves the patient's comfort.

Patients with Acute Hypoxemic Respiratory Failure

Acute hypoxemic respiratory failure is caused by alveolar filling with blood, pus, or edema, the end results of which are impaired lung mechanics and gas exchange. The gas exchange impairment results from intrapulmonary shunt, which is largely refractory to oxygen therapy. In ARDS, the significantly reduced FRC due to alveolar flooding and collapse leaves many fewer alveoli to accept the tidal volume, making the lung appear stiff, and dramatically increasing the work of breathing. The ARDS lung should be viewed as a small lung, however, rather than a stiff lung. In line with this current conception of ARDS, it is now clearly established that excessive distention of the ARDS lung compounds lung injury and may induce systemic inflammation (7, 10). Ventilatory strategies have evolved markedly in the past decade, changing clinical practice and generating tremendous excitement.

The goals of ventilation are to reduce shunt, avoid toxic concentrations of oxygen, and choose ventilator settings, which do not amplify lung damage. The initial FiO_2 should be 1.0 in view of the typically extreme hypoxemia. PEEP is indicated in patients with diffuse lung lesions, but may not be helpful in patients with focal infiltrates, such as lobar pneumonia. In patients with ARDS, PEEP should be instituted immediately, then rapidly adjusted to the least PEEP necessary to produce an arterial saturation of 90% on an FiO_2 no higher than 0.6 ("least PEEP approach"). An alternative approach is to set the PEEP at a value 2 cm H_2O higher than the lower inflection point of the inflation PV curve ("open-lung approach[1]" (1)), but this approach has not been validated, is rather complex, and is not recommended. Recruitment maneuvers have not been shown to be useful or necessary. The tidal volume should be 6 mL/kg on ACV, higher tidal volumes being associated with higher mortality. Alternatively, pressure-control ventilation (PCV) can be used, with an inspiratory pressure (PEEP plus the pressure increment) of 30 cm H_2O. This will generally drive tidal volumes of 350-550 ml. In either mode the respiratory rate should be set at 24-28 as long as there is no autoPEEP. The combination of high levels of PEEP (especially when the open-lung approach is used) and low end-inspiratory pressures leaves only a small range for tidal ventilation. An occasional consequence is hypercapnia. This approach of preferring hypercapnia to alveolar overdistention, is termed "permissive hypercapnia."

The Patient with Restriction of the Lungs or Chest Wall

Small tidal volumes (5-7 cc/kg) and rapid rates (18-24/minute) are especially important in order to minimize the hemodynamic consequences of positive-pressure ventilation and to reduce the likelihood of barotrauma. The FiO_2 is usually determined by the degree of alveolar filling or collapse, if any. When the restrictive abnormality involves the chest wall (including the abdomen), the large ventilation-induced rise in pleural pressure has the potential to compromise cardiac output. This in turn will lower the mixed venous PO_2 and, in the setting of VQ mismatch or shunt, the PaO_2 as well. If the physician responds to this falling PaO_2 by augmenting PEEP or increasing the minute ventilation, further circulatory compromise ensues. A potentially catastrophic cycle of worsening gas exchange, increasing ventilator settings, and progressive shock is begun. This circumstance must be recognized, since the treatment is to reduce dead space (e.g., by lowering minute ventilation or correcting hypovolemia).

THE AIRWAY DURING SPLIT-LUNG VENTILATION

The lungs may be separated for purposes of differential ventilation by 2 major means: a) blocking the bronchus of a lobe or whole lung while ventilating with a standard endotracheal tube, or b) passing a double-lumen tube (DLT). A number of different devices have been used to obstruct a bronchus, but experience is largest with the Fogarty embolectomy catheter. DLTs carry the advantages of allowing each lung to be ventilated, collapsed, reexpanded, or inspected independently.

Split-lung ventilation is only rarely useful in the critical care unit, but occasionally its benefits are dramatic. Large bronchopleural fistulas severely compromise ventilation and may not respond to HFV. A DLT will maintain ventilation of the healthy lung while facilitating closure of the BPF. During massive hemoptysis, lung separation may be lifesaving by minimizing blood aspiration, maintaining airway patency, and tamponading the bleeding site while awaiting definitive therapy. Finally, patients with focal causes of acute hypoxemic respiratory failure such as lobar pneumonia or acute total atelectasis may benefit from differential ventilation and application of PEEP.

REFERENCES

1. Amato MBP, Barbas CSV, Medeiros DM, et al: Beneficial effects of the "open lung approach" with low distending pressures in acute respiratory distress syndrome: A prospective randomized study on mechanical ventilation. *Am J Respir Crit Care Med* 1995; 152:1835-1846

2. Brochard L, Rauss A, Benito S, et al: Comparison of three methods of gradual withdrawal from ventilatory support during weaning from mechanical ventilation. *Am J Respir Crit Care Med* 1994; 150:896-903

3. Drazen JM, Kamm RD, Slutsky AS, et al: High-frequency ventilation. *Physiol Rev* 1984; 64:505-543

4. Esteban A, Alía I, Gordo F, et al: Extubation outcome after spontaneous breathing trials with T-tube or pressure support ventilation. *Am J Respir Crit Care Med* 1997; 156:459-465

5. Feihl F, Perret C: Permissive hypercapnia: How permissive should we be? *Am J Respir Crit Care Med* 1994; 150:1722-1737

6. Ranieri VM, Giuliani R, Cinnella G, et al : Physiologic effects of positive end-expiratory pressure in patients with chronic obstructive pulmonary disease during acute ventilatory failure and controlled mechanical ventilation. *Am Rev Respir Dis* 1993; 147:5-13

7. Ranieri VM, Suter PM, Tortoella C, et al: Effects of mechanical ventilation on inflammatory mediators in patients with acute respiratory distress syndrome: A randomized controlled trial. *JAMA* 1999; 282:54-61

8. Slutsky A: Mechanical ventilation. *Chest* 1993; 104:1833-1859

9. The Acute Respiratory Distress Syndrome Network. Ventilation with lower tidal volumes as compared with traditional tidal volumes for acute lung injury and the acute respiratory distress syndrome. *N Engl J Med* 2000; 342:1301-8

10. Tremblay L, Valenza F, Ribeiro SP, et al: Injurious ventilatory strategies increase cytokines and c-fos m-RNA expression in an isolated rat lung model. *J Clin Invest* 1997; 99:944-952

11. Tuxen DV, Lane S: The effects of ventilatory pattern on hyperinflation, airway pressures, and circulation in mechanical ventilation of patients with severe air-flow obstruction. *Am Rev Respir Dis* 1987; 136:872-879

12. Tuxen DV, Williams TJ, Scheinkestel CD et al. Use of a measurement of pulmonary hyperinflation to control the level of mechanical ventilation in patients with acute severe asthma. *Am Rev Respir Dis* 1992; 146:1136-1142

13. Younes M: Proportional assist ventilation, a new approach to ventilatory support: Theory. *Am Rev Respir Dis* 1992; 145:114-120

14. Younes M, Puddy A, Roberts D, et al : Proportional assist ventilation: results of an initial clinical trial. *Am Rev Respir Dis* 1992; 145:121-129

WEANING FROM MECHANICAL VENTILATION

James K. Stoller, MD, MS, FCCP

Objectives

- To review the frequency of weaning failure
- To discuss the logic of weaning, i.e., questions to ask when approaching the ventilated patient
- To assess available predictors of weaning success and failure
- To describe the techniques of weaning and the evidence supporting their use
- To understand special considerations in weaning, e.g., auto-positive end-expiratory pressure, imposed work of breathing, cardiac ischemia, the importance of psychological factors, routine interruption of sedation, and of a systematic approach to weaning

Key Words: Weaning; mechanical ventilation; work of breathing; auto-positive end-expiratory pressure; pressure support; T-piece

TABLE OF ABBREVIATIONS

COPD	chronic obstructive pulmonary disease
CPAP	continuous positive airway pressure
f/VT	frequency to tidal volume ratio
IMV	intermittent mandatory ventilation
PEEP	positive end-expiratory pressure
WOB	work of breathing

INTRODUCTION

Weaning from mechanical ventilation is the process of freeing the patient from dependence on mechanical ventilatory assistance. The use of the term "weaning" must be distinguished from the term "extubation," which is the removal of the endotracheal tube.

As is obvious at the bedside, but sometimes vague in studies that describe the outcomes of ventilated patients, the criteria for weaning differ from those of extubation, as some patients may be able to support normal ventilation, but still require an endotracheal tube to provide airway protection.

This chapter will first review the frequency with which weaning fails, and will then discuss the weaning process, beginning with the logic of weaning. A discussion of weaning predictors follows, with emphasis on predictors of weaning success and of weaning failure. Available weaning predictors are assessed critically with specific attention to their diagnostic performance. Techniques of weaning are reviewed, followed by an analysis of available studies regarding the preferred approach to weaning patients from mechanical ventilation. Finally, special considerations in weaning, such as work of breathing measurements, the role of auto-positive end-expiratory pressure (PEEP), and psychological factors, and management of sedation are addressed.

Recent evidence-based guidelines for weaning and discontinuing ventilatory support have been issued by a collective task force of the American College of Chest Physicians, the American Association for Respiratory Care, and the American College of Critical Care Medicine (1). These guidelines are presented (Table 1) and cited where appropriate.

Table 1. Recommendations from the Task Force for Evidence-Based Guidelines for Weaning and Discontinuing Ventilatory Support

Recommendation 1 In patients requiring mechanical ventilation for > 24 hours, a search for all the causes that may be contributing to ventilatory dependence should be undertaken. This is particularly true in the patient who has failed attempts at withdrawing the mechanical ventilatory. Reversing, all possible ventilatory and nonventilatory issues should be an integral part of the ventilatory discontinuation process.

Recommendation 2 Patients receiving mechanical ventilation for respiratory failure should undergo a formal assessment of discontinuation potential if the following criteria are satisfied:

- Evidence for some reversal of the underlying cause for respiratory failure.
- Adequate oxygenation (e.g., PaO_2/FiO_2 ratio > 150 to 200; requiring positive end-expiratory pressure [PEEP] $\leq$ 5 to 8 cm H_2O; $Fio_2 \leq$ 0.4 to 0.5); and pH (e.g., $\geq$ 7.25);
- Hemodynamic stability, as defined by the absence of active myocardial ischemia and the absence of clinically significant hypotension (i.e., a condition requiring no vasopressor therapy or therapy with only low-dose vasopressors such as dopamine or dobutamine, < 5 mcg/kg/min); and the capability to initiate an inspiratory effort.

The decision to use these criteria must be individualized. Some patients not satisfying all of the above criteria (e.g., patients with chronic hypoxemia values below the thresholds cited) may be ready for attempts at the discontinuation of mechanical ventilation.

Recommendation 3 Formal discontinuation assessments for patients receiving mechanical ventilation for respiratory failure should be performed during spontaneous breathing rather than while the patient is still receiving substantial ventilatory support. An initial brief period of spontaneous breathing can be used to assess the capability of continuing onto a formal spontaneous breathing trial. The criteria with which to assess patient tolerance during SBTs are the respiratory pattern, the adequacy of gas exchange, hemodynamic stability, and subjective comfort. The tolerance of SBTs lasting 30 to 120 minutes should prompt consideration for permanent ventilator discontinuation.

Recommendation 4 The removal of the artificial airway from a patient who has successfully been discontinued from the ventilatory support should be based on assessments of airway patency and the ability of the patient to protect the airway.

Recommendation 5 Patients receiving mechanical ventilation for respiratory failure who fail an SBT should have the cause for the failed SBT determined. Once reversible causes for failure are corrected, and if the patient still meets the criteria listed in Table 3, subsequent SBTs should be performed every 24 hours.

Recommendation 6 Patients receiving mechanical ventilation for respiratory failure who fail an SBT should receive a stable, nonfatiguing, comfortable form of ventilatory support.

Recommendation 7 Anesthesia/sedation strategies and ventilator management aimed at early extubation should be used in postsurgical patients.

Recommendation 8 Weaning/discontinuation protocols that are designed for nonphysican healthcare professionals (HCPs) should be developed and implemented by ICUs. Protocols aimed at optimizing sedation also should be developed and implemented.

Recommendation 9 Tracheotomy should be considered after an initial period of stabilization on the ventilator when it becomes apparent that the patient will require prolonged ventilator assistance. Tracheotomy then should be performed when the patient appears likely to gain one or more of the benefits ascribed to the procedure. Patients who may derive particular benefit from early tracheotomy are the following:

- Those requiring high levels of sedation to tolerate translaryngeal tubes;
- Those with marginal respiratory mechanics (often manifested as tachypnea) in whom a tracheostomy tube having lower resistance might reduce the risk of muscle overload;
- Those who may derive psychological benefit from the ability to eat orally, communicate by articulated speech, and experience enhanced mobility; and
- Those it whom enhanced mobility may assist physical therapy efforts.

Recommendation 10 Unless there is evidence for clearly irreversible disease (e.g., high spinal cord injury or advanced amyotrophic lateral sclerosis), a patient requiring prolonged mechanical ventilatory support for respiratory failure should not be considered permanently ventilator-dependent until 3 months of weaning attempts have failed.

Recommendation 11 Critical care practitioners should familiarize themselves with facilities in their communities, or units in hospitals they staff, that specialize in managing patients who require prolonged dependence on mechanical ventilation. Such familiarization should include reviewing published peer-reviewed data from those units, if available. When medically stable for transfer, patients who have failed ventilator discontinuation attempts in the ICU should be transferred to those facilities that have demonstrated success and safety in accomplishing ventilator discontinuation.

Recommendation 12 Weaning strategies in the prolonged mechanical ventilation patient should be slow-paced and should include gradually lengthening self-breathing trials.

LOGIC OF WEANING: QUESTIONS TO ASK

The process of weaning proceeds by addressing two sequential questions: a) Is the patient a candidate to begin weaning? b) If the patient is deemed a candidate to wean, is weaning likely to succeed? This logic is reflected in Recommendations 1 and 2 of the available evidence-based guidelines on weaning (Table 1). In this context, to initiate weaning, the following conditions must be satisfied:

Recommendations

- Improvement in the underlying process causing respiratory failure
- Adequacy of mental status and muscular strength, including:
  -Resolution of the effects of sedating and paralyzing medications
  -Wakefulness sufficient to allow cooperation in weaning and to allow subsequent extubation, as well as ability to clear and handle secretions
- Hemodynamic stability, generally considered to be resolution of sepsis or the need for pressor support
- Normality of acid-base and electrolyte status, with special attention given to assuring restoration of baseline acid-base balance (i.e., allowing hypercapnia if chronically present and avoiding new metabolic alkalosis) and to assuring the normality of electrolytes that affect muscle function (e.g., phosphate, calcium, and potassium)
- To understand special considerations in weaning, e.g., auto-positive end-expiratory pressure, imposed work of breathing, cardiac ischemia, the importance of psychological factors, routine interruption of

sedation, and of a systematic approach to weaning
- Nutritional repletion
- Adequacy of oxygenation, e.g., PaO2 exceeding 60 torr (8.0 kPa) with FIO_2 of <0.5 and PEEP of <5 cm H_2O.

When the aforementioned conditions are satisfied, it is reasonable to proceed with weaning. Attention then turns to assessing the likelihood that the weaning effort will succeed. In this regard, many different predictors of weaning have been proposed (2, 3).

Table 2. Proposed univariate predictors of weanability

Lung Mechanics and Work
    VC > 10 mL/kg
    VT > 300 mL
    Maximal inspiratory force < - 30 cm H_2O
    $P_{0.1}$ < 6 cm H_2O
    Dynamic compliance > 25 mL cm H_2O
    Respiratory rate < 25 breaths/min
    Minute ventilation < 10 L/min
    MVV > 2 times minute ventilation
    Respiratory frequency/VT < 105 breaths/min/L
    Oxygen cost of breathing < 15%
    VD/VT < 0.60

Gas Exchange and Perfusion
    $P(A-a)O_2$ < 350 torr (46.7 kPa) on FIO_2 of 1.0
    PaO_2/FIO_2 > 238
    PaO_2/PaO_2 > 0.47
    Gastric pH > 7.30 and/or ↓ by < 0.09 during weaning

VC, vital capacity; VT, tidal volume; $P_{0.1}$, airway occlusion pressure; VD/VT, dead space volume to tidal volume; MVV, maximum ventilatory ventilation; $P(A-a)O_2$, alveolar-arterial oxygen tension difference.

PREDICTORS OF WEANING

Weaning prediction is the process of estimating the likelihood that weaning and/or extubation efforts will succeed or fail in a specific patient at a specific time. As with decision-making in clinical medicine in general, weaning success or failure is a dichotomous outcome (i.e., the patient either does or does not wean) and the process of predicting weaning outcome involves applying a weaning predictor to estimate the probability of weaning or extubation failure or success (2).

Many different weaning predictors have been proposed (Table 2) (2, 3). Available univariate (single variable) predictors include measures of lung mechanics and work of breathing (e.g., forced vital capacity, maximal inspiratory pressure), measures of gas exchange adequacy (e.g., ratios of PaO_2/FIO_2 and PaO_2/PAO_2), and measures of the adequacy of systemic perfusion (i.e., gastric intramural pH). Tables 3 through 5 review the statistical performance of several commonly used univariate weaning predictors (i.e., the minute ventilation of <10 L/min [Table 3], the forced vital capacity [Table 4], and the maximal inspiratory force of <–30 cm H_2O [Table 5]) and show that the positive predictive values of univariate weaning predictors generally exceed their negative predictive values. Remembering that the positive predictive value estimates the likelihood that the patient will wean if the predictor indicates success and that the negative predictive value estimates the likelihood of

weaning failure if the predictor indicates failure, it can be concluded that univariate predictors are more reliable indicators of weaning success than they are of weaning failure. That is, the failure to satisfy the univariate weaning predictor does not confidently predict failure to wean; as shown by Krieger et al (4), slavish attention to deferring weaning when a univariate weaning predictor is not met could unduly delay weaning (i.e., in up to 41% of patients using the maximal inspiratory force of <–30 cm H_2O as the criterion).

To improve the capability to predict weaning success and failure, a number of multivariate weaning predictors have been developed and evaluated (2, 3, 5). As reviewed in Table 6 (2, 6–16), these multivariate predictors vary in content from simple combinations of univariate predictors (e.g., maximal minute ventilation > twice minute ventilation, maximal inspiratory force of <–30 cm H_2O, and minute ventilation of <10 L/min) to more complex scoring systems that assess dozens of clinical variables and provide an overall score that is used to predict weanability (e.g., the Adverse Factor and Ventilator Score [7] and the Burns Weaning Assessment Program [13]). In general, these multivariate indices demonstrate higher positive and negative predictive values than the univariate predictors;

Table 3. Minute ventilation <10 L/min as a univariate weaning predictor

Study (date)	N	Sensitivity (%)	Specificity (%)	Prediction Performance	
				Positive Value	Negative Value
Sahn & Lakshminarayan (1973)[a]	100	92	100	100	71
Tahvanainen et al (1983)[b]	47	45	78	89	25
Krieger et al (1989)	269	NS	NS	93	15
Yang & Tobin (1989)	41	24	69	55	37

NS, not stated.

Minute ventilation <10 L/min; maximal inspiratory pressure (MIP) <–30 cm H_2O; and maximal voluntary ventilation (MVV) >2 times minute ventilation; *b*minute ventilation <10 L/min; MIP <–30 cm H_2O; and MVV >2 times minute ventilation.

Reproduced with permission from Stoller JK: Establishing clinical unweanability. *Respir Care* 1991; 36:186–198 they are, therefore, more useful and reliable predictors, although their general failure to achieve perfect predictive capability should cause the astute clinician to regard them with circumspection in completely assuring or excluding weanability.

As a specific example of a widely used multivariate weaning predictor, the rapid shallow breathing index (otherwise known as the frequency to tidal volume ratio [f/VT]) calculates the patient's spontaneous breathing frequency divided by the patient's spontaneous tidal volume in liters, both determined with the patient who does not receive mechanical ventilatory assistance (i.e., breathing through an endotracheal tube connected to a respirometer). As first proposed by Yang and Tobin (10), an f/VT value of <105 was found to best discriminate between patients who were successfully weaned (defined as maintaining spontaneous breathing for >24 hours after extubation) and who were not successfully weaned. This threshold value was developed from a "hypothesis-generating" set of 36 patients and subsequently validated in a "hypothesis-testing" set of 64 patients, in whom an f/VT of >105 had an overall negative predictive value (the chance that a patient would fail to wean if f/Vt exceeded 105) of 0.95 and a

positive predictive value of 0.78. In the subset of 20 patients who received mechanical ventilation for >8 days, the negative and positive predictive values were slightly lower (0.89 and 0.64, respectively), emphasizing the increased difficulty of establishing unweanability in long-term, mechanically ventilated patients. Subsequent studies (1, 15) have largely confirmed the usefulness of the rapid shallow breathing index, while also emphasizing its shortcomings in predicting weaning outcome when nonrespiratory factors are at play (e.g., congestive heart failure or upper airway obstruction as causes).

At the same time, Vallverdu et al (17) have emphasized that the diagnostic accuracy of different weaning parameters differs according to the underlying cause of respiratory failure. Specifically, in a series of 217 consecutive patients with respiratory failure of various etiologies, the rapid shallow breathing index demonstrated highest diagnostic accuracy in predicting weaning success in patients with chronic obstructive pulmonary disease (COPD) (0.76), but lower accuracy in patients with neurologic disease (0.65) or miscellaneous causes of acute respiratory failure (0.66). In contrast, values of maximal inspiratory pressure and maximal expiratory pressure best

Table 4. Vital capacity (measured in mL/kg) as a univariate weaning predictor

Study (Date)	Criterion	N	Sensitivity (%)	Specificity (%)	*Prediction Performance*	
					Positive Value	Negative Value
Milbern et al (1978) [a]	>15	33	25	0	58	0
Tahvanainen et al (1983)	>10	47	97	13	83	50
Pardee et al (1984)	>17	133	90	60	88	NS

NS, not stated.
[a] Vital capacity > 15 mL/kg and maximal inspiratory pressure <-25 cm H_2O.
Reproduced with permission from Stoller JK: Establishing clinical unweanability. *Respir Care* 1991; 36: 186-198.

distinguished patients who were successfully intubated versus those patients who failed extubation when the cause of respiratory failure was neurologic disease. Overall, the recent evidence-based guidelines report (1) concludes that "judging by areas under the receiving operator curves for all variables, none of these variables demonstrate more than modest accuracy in predicting weaning outcome." The putative reason is that in available studies, clinicians making weaning decisions have already considered the results of weaning predictors when choosing patients for weaning.

TECHNIQUES OF WEANING

A variety of techniques for weaning patients from mechanical ventilation have been described (3, 18–21), including T-piece trials of increasing duration that interrupt periods of completely supported breaths, intermittent mandatory ventilation (IMV) weaning in which the IMV rate is decreased progressively, pressure support weaning in which the level of pressure support is decreased progressively, and combinations of the above (e.g., pressure support weaning with an IMV back-up rate).

Strategies in use have changed as available ventilatory modes have evolved. For example, a survey of technical directors of respiratory care departments conducted by Venus et al (22) in 1987 indicated that IMV was the primary mode of weaning employed by 72% of the respondents. A survey of practices in 47 Spanish ICUs by Esteban et al (19) showed that in 195 patients who were being weaned, T-piece trials of increasing duration were used most commonly (24%), followed by synchronized IMV weaning (18%), pressure support weaning (15%), and combined pressure support with an IMV back-up rate (9%). Other combinations applied concurrently or in succession were used in 33%. Finally, in a randomized trial (21) of daily observation of spontaneous (T-piece) breathing versus "routine" weaning practice, the most common routine weaning mode was pressure-support with IMV (43%), followed by IMV alone (31%), pressure support alone (15%), continuous positive airway pressure (CPAP, 5%), and other (6%).

Recent attention has focused on comparing available techniques of weaning. Three important studies have provided important insights. Each of the weaning techniques is described below, followed by a summary of the evidence supporting specific techniques of weaning.

T-Piece Trials

Also known as Briggs trials, T-piece trials allow the patient to breathe spontaneously through the endotracheal tube (or tracheostomy) connected to a T-piece set-up. CPAP can be applied to the T-piece circuit, although PEEP levels >5 cm H_2O would be unlikely during weaning trials, because adequate oxygenation on acceptably low levels of PEEP is considered a criterion for beginning weaning.

Intermittent Mandatory Ventilation Weaning

IMV weaning was first proposed in 1973 as a new and preferred weaning strategy (23). With IMV weaning, a volume and frequency of breaths are set, and the frequency is decreased gradually until the patient has assumed most of the minute ventilation.

Pressure Support Ventilation

Unlike IMV, which is a volume-cycled mode of mechanical ventilation, pressure support ventilation (24) delivers gas at a set pressure level for a duration determined by the patient's inspiratory flow demands (i.e., flow-cycled). Pressure support weaning involves the gradual diminution of the pressure level, allowing the patient gradually to assume more of the work of breathing (WOB).

STUDIES COMPARING WEANING MODES

Three controlled trials (18, 21, 25) have contributed important insights and comparisons of available weaning strategies. Brochard et al (18) conducted a randomized, controlled trial in which 109 patients who failed initial weaning attempts were randomized to 1 of 3 weaning strategies: a) T-piece trials, in which progressively increasing intervals of spontaneous breathing through a T-piece were undertaken until the patient tolerated up to 3 T-piece trials lasting 120 mins (n = 35 patients); b) synchronized IMV weaning, in which the IMV rate was decreased by 2 to 4 breaths/min twice daily, until the patient tolerated 24 hours at an IMV rate of <4 (n = 43 patients); or c) pressure-support weaning, in which the level of pressure was decreased by 2 or 4 cm H_2O twice daily until the patient could tolerate breathing at pressure-support of <8 cm H_2O for 24 hours (n = 31 patients). The study concluded that pressure support was the preferred weaning mode (Fig. 1) based on the following: a) Fewer patients failed to wean with pressure-support than with the other modes (23% versus 43% [T-piece] and 42% [IMV], $p < 0.05$); b) time-to-event analysis showed that the probability of requiring continued ventilatory support was lower with pressure support than with the other modes ($p = 0.03$); and c) weaning duration was shorter with pressure support (mean 5.7 ± 3.7 days) than for the other modes pooled (mean 9.3 ± 8.2 days, p <0.05).

In a second randomized trial of weaning modes, Esteban et al (25) randomized 130 patients who had failed initial weaning attempts to one of four weaning modes: a) IMV weaning, in which the rate was decreased by 2 to 4 breaths/min at least twice daily until the patient tolerated an IMV rate of <5 for 2 hours (n = 29 patients); b) pressure support weaning, in which the pressure was decreased by 2 to 4 cm H_2O at least twice daily until a pressure support level of 5 cm H_2O was tolerated for 2 hours (n = 37 patients); c) intermittent trials of spontaneous breathing, in which T-piece trials of increasing length were undertaken at least twice daily until the patient could tolerate 2 hours of spontaneous breathing (n = 33 patients); and d) once-daily T-piece trials, in which a single T-piece trial was undertaken daily until 2 hours of spontaneous breathing were tolerated without distress (n = 31 patients). Unlike the study by Brochard et al (18), this study concluded that a once-daily T-piece trial was the preferred strategy (Fig. 2), based on the following findings: a) The rate of successful weaning was higher with this technique than with IMV or pressure support weaning; and b) weaning was more rapid with

once daily T-piece trials than with pressure support or IMV modes.

Finally, the most recent controlled trial of different weaning strategies by Ely et al (21) randomized patients to a once-daily respiratory assessment and trial of spontaneous breathing for up to 2 hours with physician notification of a successful trial (n = 149 patients) versus usual care by the managing physicians (pulmonologist, cardiologist, or intensivist; n = 151 patients). As shown in Figure 3, this study shows that a strategy of conducting daily trials of spontaneous breathing is preferred because this approach was associated with shorter weaning time (median 1 versus 3 days, $p <$ 0.001), shorter duration of mechanical ventilation (median 4.5 versus 6 days, $p <$ 0.003), fewer total complications (20% versus 41%, $p < 0.001$), a lower rate of reintubation (4% versus 10%, $p = 0.04$), and lower ICU costs (median \$15,740 versus \$20,890, $p < 0.03$). Overall, these three studies show that contrary to early views and practices (22), IMV weaning is the least likely to effect successful extubation and requires longer weaning than other available strategies, and that daily assessment of respiratory status and spontaneous breathing trials was associated with shorter weaning duration than usual practice. Attempts (26) to reconcile the discordant conclusions from the studies of Brochard et al and Esteban et al have attributed the differing results to differing definitions of weaning failure in the two studies (14 days on mechanical ventilation [Esteban et al] versus 21 days), and to different constraining conditions for attempting extubation with the compared weaning modes (i.e., Brochard et al permitted extubation from 8 cm H_2O of pressure support versus 5 cm H_2O by Esteban et al and Brochard et al required IMV breathing on <4 breaths for 24 hours before attempting extubation versus an IMV rate of <5 for 2 hours by Esteban et al).

Table 5. Maximal inspiratory pressure ≤ -30 cm H_2O as a univariate weaning predictor

| Study (date) | N | Patient Type | Sensitivity (%) | Specificity (%) | *Prediction Performance* | |
					Positive Predictive Value	Negative Predictive Value
Sahn & Lakshmin-arayan (1973) [a]	100	Mean MV duration 37 hrs	92	100	100	71
Milburn et al (1978) [b]	33	Mean MV 3.1 hrs	25	0	58	0
Tahvanainen et al (1973)	47	Mean MV 5 days	68	0	74	0
DeHaven et al (1986)	48	Mean MV 55 hrs	49	100	100	12
Krieger et al (1989)	269	Mean age >70 yrs, MV 71 hrs	NS	NS	92	21
Yang & Tobin (1989)	41	NS	76	25	61	40

MV, mechanical ventilation; NS, not stated.

Maximal inspiratory pressure <–30 cm H_2O, minute ventilation <10 L/min, and maximal voluntary ventilation ≥2 minute ventilation; bmaximal inspiratory pressure <–30 cm H_2O and vital capacity ≥15 mL/kg.

Reproduced with permission from Stoller JK: Establishing clinical unweanability. *Respir Care* 1991; 36:186–198

Table 6. Summary of selected multivariate indices for weaning prediction

Study (Date) (Ref)	N	Index	Patient Type	Positive Predictive	Negative Predictive
Hilberman et al (1976) (6)	124	Nurse assessments	Open-heart surgery	82%	67%
Krieger et al (1984) (4)	269	NIF <-30 cm H_2O, VE >10 L/min	>70 yrs old, on MV mean 71 hrs	93%	15%
Morganroth et al (1984) (7)	11	Adverse factor and vent score	COPD, on MV >30 days	73%	97% [a]
Higgins et al (1988) (8)	29	Vent dependence score	Post-OHS on MV >48 hrs	NS	NS
Yang & Tobin (1989) (9)	41	CROP score	NS (abstract)	87%	72%
Yang & Tobin (1991) (10)	100	CROP >13, Freq/VT Æ105	On MV 8.2 ± 1.1 days	711%	70% [b]
Jabour et al (1991) (11)	38	Weaning index <4	MICU on MV <3 days	96%	95%
Ashutosh et al (1991) (12)	24	Neural network discriminant function	On MV 12.7 days	100% [b]	100% [b]
Burns et al (1991) (13)	37	BWAP	Stable on MV >1 wk, felt ready to wean	—	97%
Scheinhorn et al (1995) (14)	565	P(A-a)O2, BUN, gender	On MV >6 wks	71%	67%
Epstein (1995) (15)	184	Freq/VT >100	MICU on MV, f/VT measured within 8 hrs of wean onset	83%	40%
Gluck et al (1995) (16)	55	Score (5 variables), points >3	On MV ≥3 wks	83%	100%

NIF, negative inspiratory force; MV, mechanical ventilation; VE, minute ventilation; COPD, chronic pulmonary obstructive disease; OHS, open-heart surgery; NS, not stated; BWAP, Burns Weaning Assessment Program; BUN, blood urea nitrogen; MICU, medical intensive care unit; VT, tidal volume.

[a]Hypothesis-generating study, not confirmed in a separate data set; [b]hypothesis-testing data set included.

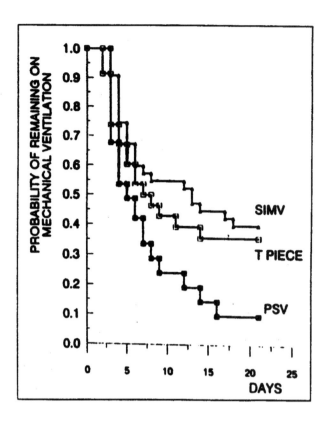

Figure 1. Probability of remaining on mechanical ventilation in patients with prolonged difficulties in tolerating spontaneous breathing. This probability was significantly lower for pressure-support ventilation (*PSV*) than for T-piece of synchronized intermittent ventilation (*SIMV*) (cumulative probability for 21 days, $p < 0.03$ with the log-rank test). Reproduced with permission from Brochard et al (18).

More recently, Esteban et al (27) examined whether a spontaneous breathing trial should last ≤2 hours (i.e., 30 mins) before extubation In a multicenter trial in which 526 patients were allocated randomly to 30- versus 120-minute trials of spontaneous breathing, these investigators found no differences between the two durations in rates of extubation failure or ICU or hospital mortality, but a longer length of hospital stay in the group undergoing a 2-hour trial. These findings endorse use of the shorter, 30-minute period of spontaneous breathing before an extubation decision.

Finally, recent attention has turned to the value of noninvasive ventilation in accelerating extubation. Nava et al (28) conducted a randomized, controlled trial in which patients intubated because of acute ventilatory failure complicating COPD were randomized to a traditional pressure-support

weaning approach versus a new strategy (in which patients were extubated after 48 hours and managed thereafter with noninvasive ventilation). Patients managed with noninvasive ventilation experienced several advantages: a) fewer days on mechanical ventilation; b) fewer days in the ICU; c) a higher weaning success rate on day 21; d) a lower rate of nosocomial pneumonia; and e) a higher survival rate at 60 days (92% versus 72%, $p = 0.0009$). These and other, more recent confirmatory results from Girault et al (29) suggest that early extubation with subsequent noninvasive ventilatory support may be a beneficial weaning strategy in patients with respiratory failure due to COPD.

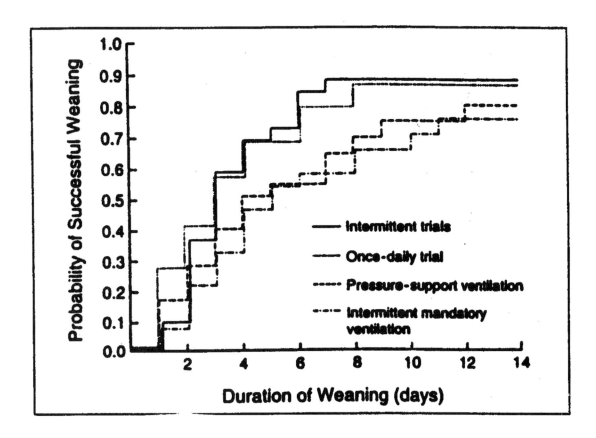

Figure 2. Kaplan-Meier curves of the probability of successful weaning with intermittent mandatory ventilation (IMV), pressure support ventilation (PSV), intermittent trials of spontaneous breathing (SB), and a once-daily trial of SB. After adjustment for baseline characteristics in a Cox proportional hazards model, the rate of successful weaning with a once-daily trial of SB was 2.83 times higher than that with IMV ($p < 0.006$) and 2.05 times higher than that with PSV ($p < 0.04$). Reproduced with permission from Esteban et al (20).

Special Considerations in Weaning

To optimize the possibility of weaning, attention to several special considerations can be helpful in some clinical circumstances. These special considerations include: a) the possibility of unsuspectedly high imposed WOB and the contribution of the endotracheal tube, b) auto-PEEP as a source of increased inspiratory work in circumstances where dynamic hyperinflation accompanies airflow limitation, c) occult cardiac ischemia as an impediment to weaning, d) the importance of psychological readiness and motivation to wean, e) the importance of routine daily cessation of sedative medications in patients receiving mechanical ventilation, and f) the importance of implementing protocols by respiratory therapists and/or nurses to accelerate

liberation from mechanical ventilation. Each of these special considerations is discussed below.

Work of Breathing and Role of the Endotracheal Tube

Measuring the inspiratory WOB by integrating the area under a pressure-volume curve has been advocated because elevated WOB predicts inspiratory muscle fatigue with subsequent weaning failure as an expected consequence. Various threshold values of WOB have been proposed (Table 7) (30-34), but few of these threshold values have been validated prospectively or compared head-to-head with other available weaning parameters. In a small,

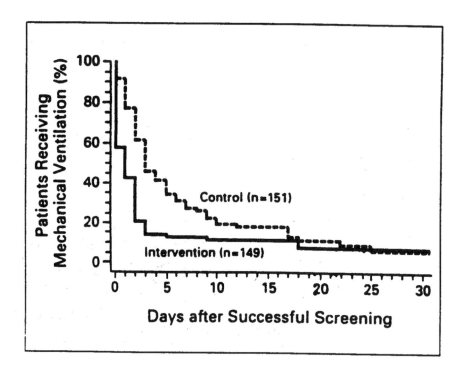

Figure 3. Kaplan-Meier analysis of the duration of mechanical ventilation after a successful screening test. After adjustment for the severity of illness at baseline (as measured by the APACHE II score), age, gender, race, location of the ICU, and duration of intubation before enrollment, a Cox proportional hazards analysis showed that mechanical ventilation was discontinued more rapidly in the intervention group than in the control group (relative risk of successful extubation, 2.13; 95% confidence interval, 1.55 to 2.92; $p < 0.001$). Reproduced with permission from Ely et al (21).

hypothesis-generating study of 17 patients, Fiastro et al (33) compared WOB with vital capacity, negative inspiratory force, tidal volume, and minute ventilation as weaning predictors and showed that as WOB values decreased <1.60 kg•m/min (16 joules/min), WOB better discriminated between patients with weaning success versus weaning failure than did the other more conventional measures. Until recently, the persisting uncertainty about a useful threshold value for WOB and the lack of methods for easy and widespread clinical measurement precluded adoption of WOB measurement for clinical practice outside of an investigative context. More recently, commercial devices that permit straightforward measurement of WOB have become available and have fostered enthusiasm for using WOB measurements in guiding weaning decisions. For example, Gluck et al (16) compared a weaning protocol using measurements of WOB and f/V$_T$ with a clinical approach using conventional weaning criteria (e.g., minute ventilation,

negative inspiratory force, tidal volume, and static compliance) in 23 ventilated patients. This study showed that the protocol incorporating WOB measurements would hasten weaning in at least 41% of instances and that the projected duration of weaning was shortened in these patients by 1.68 days.

Apart from appreciating the potential value of measuring WOB to enhance decision-making about weaning, clinicians should be attentive to sources of imposed WOB that can hamper weaning. That the endotracheal tube can contribute importantly to imposed WOB has been shown by Shapiro et al (35). In a study of 3 normal volunteers breathing through endotracheal tubes of various caliber (6- to 10-mm inner diameter), these investigators showed

Table 7. Proposed work of breathing (transpulmonary) as a weaning predictor[a]

First Author (Date) (Ref)	No. of Patients	Threshold Value (kg • m/min)	Comment
Peters (1972) (30)	55	1.80	—
Proctor (1973) (31)	168	1.35	13.7% false-positive and false-negative rate with value
Henning (1977) (32)	28	1.70	—
Fiastro (1988) (33)	17	1.60	Better discriminator than vital capacity, tidal volume, minute ventilation, negative inspiratory force
Brochard (1989) (34)	8	0.8	—

that WOB rose precipitously as the caliber decreased and as minute ventilation rose. For subjects breathing through 6- and 7-mm inner diameter tubes at levels of minute ventilation routinely achieved clinically (15 to 25 L/min), the tension-time index approached values of 0.15 at which respiratory muscle fatigue is expected. Thus, use of larger caliber (i.e., >7.5-mm inner diameter) endotracheal tubes and avoidance of nasotracheal intubation in patients experiencing weaning difficulty are advised. More recently, WOB measurements have been shown to be useful in helping to identify patients whose weaning difficulty is attributable to unsuspectedly high imposed WOB (36). From a group of 116 surgical ICU patients on mechanical ventilation for >48 hours, Kirton et al (36) identified 28 patients (24%) with oral endotracheal tubes of >8-mm inner diameter who developed marked tachypnea during a CPAP trial despite satisfying simple weaning criteria. WOB measurements in these 28 patients were performed and included a measurement of the work imposed by the endotracheal tube. Using a value of <0.8 joules/L as a WOB threshold, the investigators identified six patients with total WOB below this value, all of whom were successfully extubated. Of the remaining 22 patients whose total WOB

measurements exceeded this threshold (mean WOB 1.6 ± 0.83 joules/L), 21 patients were found to have a major component of their total WOB imposed by the endotracheal tube, leaving their "physiologic" work of breathing below the threshold value. Extubation was successfully undertaken in all 21 (with subsequent reintubation for unrelated and unpredictable reasons in two patients), leading to the conclusion that high imposed WOB can unsuspectedly contribute to weaning failure and that WOB measurements directed at identifying the components of "imposed" and "physiologic" WOB can enhance decision-making in a subset of difficult-to-wean patients.

Auto-PEEP as a Source of Imposed Work of Breathing

Auto-PEEP is defined as PEEP that is present in the alveoli but not measured at the mouthpiece without special maneuvers (37), e.g., an end-expiratory hold. Synonyms for auto-PEEP include intrinsic PEEP, occult PEEP, endogenous PEEP, and unidentified PEEP. As shown by Brown and Pierson (38), auto-PEEP occurs commonly among mechanically ventilated patients (39% of 62 patients assessed) and may produce high alveolar pressures at end-expiration (i.e., up to 15 cm H_2O). Three varieties of auto-PEEP can be considered (38), each of which may occur under distinct physiologic circumstances even though several types may coexist. The first type is auto-PEEP with dynamic hyperinflation and airflow limitation, which commonly accompanies COPD, both in spontaneously breathing and mechanically ventilated patients. Other types include auto-PEEP with dynamic hyperinflation but no airflow limitation (e.g., during high minute ventilation or with a small endotracheal tube that hampers lung emptying) and auto-PEEP without dynamic hyperinflation (e.g., due to expiratory muscle recruitment).

In considering weaning, the first type of auto-PEEP—auto-PEEP with dynamic hyperinflation and air flow limitation—is most significant because such auto-PEEP imposes an inspiratory threshold load that must be overcome by the inspiratory muscles before inspiration can begin (37, 39, 40). Such auto-PEEP arises when lung emptying is impaired due to expiratory airflow resistance and expiratory flow limitation; end-expiratory lung volume then exceeds resting functional residual capacity; air is trapped at end-expiration and alveolar pressure exceeds downstream pressure (at the mouth) with resulting auto-PEEP. By imposing an inspiratory load, such auto-PEEP can be the source of imposed WOB. As shown by Petrof et al (39) and Smith and Marini (40), application of external PEEP can decrease the inspiratory WOB by offsetting the inspiratory load imposed by the auto-PEEP. Levels of external PEEP, up to ~85% of the auto-PEEP, can lessen imposed WOB without increasing end-expiratory lung volume or lessening cardiac output. On this basis, clinicians should be attentive to the possibility of auto-PEEP in managing patients on mechanical ventilation. If found in a clinical circumstance favoring dynamic hyperinflation with airflow limitation (i.e., in patients with COPD), careful application of external PEEP to levels not exceeding the level of auto-PEEP may be helpful to lessen imposed WOB and enhance weaning.

Other Special Considerations in Weaning

Besides giving attention to WOB imposed by the endotracheal tube and by auto-

PEEP, clinicians should appreciate other potential impediments to weaning, including unsuspected cardiac ischemia (41), the patient's anxiety and lack of psychologic readiness to wean (42), and the lack of a systematic weaning routine in the ICU. Recent studies suggest that weaning can be accelerated by detection and treatment of cardiac ischemia, by providing biofeedback to lessen anxiety and to assure ventilatory targets, and by implementing a team to conduct regular weaning (43) and/or weaning protocols supervised by respiratory therapists and nurses (44, 45). Also, use of a collaborative, multidisciplinary weaning approach using a bedside "weaning board" and flow sheet was associated with a shortened ICU length of stay and a trend toward shortened time on mechanical ventilation (46). Finally, a recent randomized controlled trial (47) has shown that daily interruption of sedative medications to reassess neurologic status and weaning readiness is associated with a shortened duration of mechanical ventilation.

SUGGESTED READINGS

1. The collective task force facilitated by the American College of Chest Physicians; the American Association for Respiratory Care, and the American College of Critical Care Medicine. Evidence-based guidelines for weaning and discontinuing ventilatory support. *Chest* 2001; 120 (Suppl): 375S–484S
   This supplement presents a systematic review of available literature and recommendations regarding weaning.

2. Stoller JK: Establishing clinical unweanability. *Respir Care* 1991; 36:186–198
   This comprehensive review paper considers the diagnostic performance of various weaning predictors and considers whether predictors perform sufficiently well to assure weaning failure.

3. Lessard MR, Brochard LJ: Weaning from ventilatory support. *Clin Chest Med* 1996; 17:475–489
   This is an excellent recent review of weaning principles and techniques.

4. Krieger BP, Ershowsky PF, Becker DA, et al: Evaluation of conventional criteria for

predicting successful weaning from mechanical ventilatory support in elderly patients. *Crit Care Med* 1989; 17:858–861

5. Tobin MJ, Yang K: Weaning from mechanical ventilation. *Crit Care Clin* 1990; 6:725–747

6. Hilberman M, Kamm B, Lamy M, et al: An analysis of potential physiological predictors of respiratory adequacy following cardiac surgery. *J Thorac Cardiovasc Surg* 1976; 71:711–720

7. Morganroth ML, Morganroth JL, Nett LM, et al: Criteria for weaning from prolonged mechanical ventilation. *Arch Intern Med* 1984; 144:1012–1016

8. Higgins TL, Kraenzler EJ, Blum JM: Evaluation of criteria for discontinuing mechanical ventilation following open heart surgery. Abstr. *Chest* 1988; 94 (Suppl 1):40S

9. Yang KL, Tobin MJ: Decision analysis of parameters used to predict outcome of a trial of weaning from mechanical ventilation. Abstr. *Am Rev Respir Dis* 1989; 139:A98

10. Yang KL, Tobin MJ: A prospective study of indexes predicting the outcome of trials of weaning from mechanical ventilation. *N Engl J Med* 1991; 324:1445–1450
This study reports the diagnostic performance of various indices of weaning in 100 patients who were clinically stable and deemed ready for a weaning trial. The frequency to tidal volume ratio (f/Vt) was found to be most discriminative, with values exceeding 105, indicating rapid shallow breathing and predicting weaning failure.

11. Jabour ER, Rabil DM, Truwit JD, et al: Evaluation of a new weaning index based on ventilatory endurance and the efficiency of gas exchange. *Am Rev Respir Dis* 1991; 144:531–537

12. Ashutosh K, Lee H, Mohan C, et al: Prediction criteria for successful weaning from respiratory support: Statistical and connectionist analyses. *Crit Care Med* 1992; 20:1295–1301

13. Burns SM, Fahey SA, Barton DM, et al: Weaning from mechanical ventilation: A method for assessment and planning. *AACN Clin Issues Crit Care Nurs* 1991; 2:372–389.

14. Scheinhorn D, Hassenpflug, Artinian BM, et al: Predictors of weaning after six weeks of mechanical ventilation. *Chest* 1995; 107:500–505.

15. Epstein SK: Etiology of extubation failure and the predictive value of the rapid shallow breathing index. *Am J Respir Crit Care Med* 1995; 152:545–549.

16. Gluck EH, Barkoviak MJ, Balk RA, et al: Medical effectiveness of esophageal balloon pressure manometry in weaning patients from mechanical ventilation. *Crit Care Med* 1995; 23:504–509.

17. Vallverdu I, Calaf N, Subirana M, et al: Clinical characteristics respiratory functional parameters, and outcomes of a two-hour T-piece trial in patients weaning from mechanical ventilation. *Am J Respir Crit Care Med* 1998; 158:1855–1862.

18. Brochard L, Rauss A, Benito S, et al: Comparison of three methods of gradual withdrawal from ventilatory support during weaning from mechanical ventilation. *Am J Respir Crit Care Med* 1994; 150:896–903.

19. Esteban A, Alia I, Ibanez J, et al: Modes of mechanical ventilation and weaning: A national survey of Spanish hospitals. *Chest* 1994; 106:1188–1193.
This study reports a survey of 47 Spanish intensive care units in which 195 patients were weaning. T-piece trials were the most common weaning mode used (24%), followed by synchronized intermittent mandatory ventilation(18%), and pressure-support (15%), with other combinations in the remainder.

20. Esteban A, Frutos F, Tobin MJ, et al: A comparison of four methods of weaning patients from mechanical ventilation. *N Engl J Med* 1995; 332:345–350.
This is one of the three large, randomized, controlled trials of various strategies for weaning. The study concludes that once-daily trials of spontaneous breathing is preferred to intermittent mandatory ventilation and slightly better than pressure-support weaning.

21. Ely EW, Baker AM, Dunagan DP, et al: Effect on the duration of mechanical ventilation of identifying patients capable of breathing spontaneously. *N Engl J Med* 1996; 335:1864–1869.

This is a large, randomized, controlled trial of weaning strategies and shows that daily trials of spontaneous breathing with reporting of results to managing clinicians can accelerate weaning compared with standard practice.

22. Venus B, Smith RA, Mathru M: National survey of methods and criteria used for weaning from mechanical ventilation. *Crit Care Med* 1987; 15:530–533.

23. Downs JB, Klein EF, Desautels D, et al: Intermittent mandatory ventilation: A new approach to weaning patients from mechanical ventilation. *Chest* 1973; 64:331–335.
This is one of the original descriptions of intermittent mandatory ventilation.

24. MacIntyre NR: Respiratory function during pressure support ventilation. *Chest* 1986; 89:677–682.

25. Esteban A, Frutos F, Tobin MJ, et al: A comparison of four methods of weaning patients from mechanical ventilation. *N Engl J Med* 1995; 332:345–350.
This is one of the three large randomized trials of weaning strategies. The investigators conclude that once-daily trials of spontaneous breathing is the preferred mode of weaning.

26. Tobin MJ: Problematic weaning. *In:* Critical Care Medicine: A Concise Review. Northbrook, IL, ACCP, 1995, pp 202–206.

27. Esteban A, Alia I, Tobin MJ, et al: Effect of spontaneous breathing trial duration on outcome of attempts to discontinue mechanical ventilation. *Am J Respir Crit Care Med* 1999; 159:512–518.

28. Nava S, Ambrosino N, Clini E, et al: Noninvasive mechanical ventilation in the weaning of patients with respiratory failure due to chronic obstructive pulmonary disease. *Ann Intern Med* 1998; 128:721–728.

29. Girault C, Daudenthum I, Chevron V, et al: Noninvasive ventilation as a systematic extubation and weaning technique in acute-on-chronic respiratory failure: A prospective, randomized controlled study. *Am J Respir Crit Care Med* 1999; 160: 86-92.

30. Peters RM, Hilberman M, Hogan JS, et al: Objective indications for respiratory therapy in posttrauma and postoperative patients. *Am J Surg* 1972; 124:262–269.

31. Proctor HJ, Woolson R: Prediction of respiratory muscle fatigue by measurements of the work of breathing. *Surg Gynecol Obstet* 1973; 136:367–370.

32. Henning RJ, Shubin H, Weil MH: The measurement of the work of breathing for the clinical assessment of ventilator dependence. *Crit Care Med* 1977; 5:264–268.

33. Fiastro JF, Habib MP, Shon BY, et al: Comparison of standard weaning parameters and the mechanical work of breathing in mechanically ventilated patients. *Chest* 1988; 94:232–238.

34. Brochard L, Harf A, Lorino H, et al: Inspiratory pressure support prevents diaphragmatic fatigue during weaning from mechanical ventilation. *Am Rev Respir Dis* 1989; 139:513–521.

35. Shapiro M, Wilson RK, Cesar G, et al: Work of breathing through different sized endotracheal tubes. *Crit Care Med* 1986; 14:1028–1031.

36. Kirton OC, DeHaven CB, Morgan JP, et al: Elevated imposed work of breathing masquerading as ventilator weaning intolerance. *Chest* 1995; 108:1021–1025.

37. Ranieri VM, Grasso S, Fiore T, et al: Auto-positive end-expiratory pressure and dynamic hyperinflation. *Clin Chest Med* 1996; 17:379–394.

38. Brown DG, Pierson DJ: Auto-PEEP is common in mechanically ventilated patients: A study of incidence, severity, and detection. *Respir Care* 1986; 31:1069–1074.

39. Petrof BJ, Legaré M, Goldberg P, et al: Continuous positive airway pressure reduces work of breathing and dyspnea during weaning from mechanical ventilation in severe chronic obstructive pulmonary disease. *Am Rev Respir Dis* 1990; 141:281–289.

40. Smith TC, Marini JJ: Impact of PEEP on lung mechanics and work of breathing in severe airflow obstruction. *J Appl Physiol* 1988; 65:1488–1499.

41. Chatila W, Ani S, Guaglianone D, et al: Cardiac ischemia during weaning from mechanical ventilation. *Chest* 1996; 109:1577–1583.

42. Holliday JE, Hyers TM: The reduction of weaning time from mechanical ventilation using tidal volume and relaxation biofeedback. *Am Rev Respir Dis* 1990; 141:1214–1220.
    This paper describes a randomized, controlled trial showing that formal biofeedback (i.e., by providing feedback on tidal volume and on relaxation [with an electromyogram of the frontalis muscle]) was associated with a shortened duration of mechanical ventilation compared with usual visits and reassurance.

43. Cohen IL, Bari N, Strosberg MA, et al: Reduction of duration and cost of mechanical ventilation in an intensive care unit by use of a ventilatory management team. *Crit Care Med* 1991; 19:1278–1284.

44. Kollef MH, Shapiro SD, Silver P, et al: A randomized controlled trial of protocol-directed versus physician-directed weaning from mechanical ventilation. *Crit Care Med* 1997; 25:567–574.

45. Marelich GP, Murin S, Battistella F, et al: Protocol weaning of mechanical ventilation in medical and surgical patients by respiratory care practitioners and nurses: Effect on weaning time and incidence of ventilator-associated pneumonia. *Chest* 2000; 118:459-467.

46. Hennemann E, Dracup K, Ganz T, et al: Effect of a collaborative weaning plan on patient outcome in the critical care setting. *Crit Care Med* 2001; 29:297-303.

47. Kress JP, Pohlman AS, O'Connor MF, Hall JB. Daily interruption of sedative infusions in critically ill patients undergoing mechanical ventilation. *New Engl J Med* 2000; 342: 1471-1477

HYPOTHERMIA, HYPERTHERMIA, AND RHABDOMYOLYSIS

Janice L. Zimmerman, MD, FCCP, FCCM

Objectives

- To understand the physiologic changes associated with hypothermia
- To outline supportive measures and rewarming techniques appropriate for the severity of hypothermia
- To describe predisposing factors and cooling methods for heat stroke
- To discuss the clinical manifestations and management of malignant hyperthermia and neuroleptic malignant syndrome
- To describe etiologies, clinical presentation, and treatment of rhabdomyolysis

Key Words: hypothermia; hyperthermia; heat stroke; malignant hyperthermia; neuroleptic malignant syndrome; rhabdomyolysis

TABLE OF ABBREVIATIONS

ACR   active core rewarming
AER   active external rewarming
CNS   central nervous system
DIC   disseminated intravascular coagulation
ECG   electrocardiogram
MH   malignant hyperthermia
NMS   neuroleptic malignant syndrome
PER   passive external rewarming
VF   ventricular fibrillation

TEMPERATURE REGULATION

The balance between heat production and heat loss normally maintains the core body temperature at 36.6 ± 0.38°C (97.9 ± 0.7°F). Heat is produced from the dissolution of high-energy bonds during metabolism. At rest, the trunk viscera supply 56% of heat; during exercise, muscle activity may account for 90% of generated heat. Heat production may increase two- to four-fold with shivering and more than six-fold with exercise. Most heat loss (50% to 70%) normally occurs through radiation in neutral environments. Conduction of heat through direct contact with cooler objects or loss of heat due to convection accounts for a smaller percentage of heat loss. Evaporation of sweat from the skin is the major mechanism of heat loss in a warm environment.

The anterior hypothalamus is responsible for the perception of temperature and initiation of physiologic responses. Information is received from temperature-sensitive receptors in the skin, viscera, and great vessels, as well as receptors located in the hypothalamus. When a temperature increase is perceived, hypothalamic modulation results in increased sweating, cutaneous vasodilation, and decreased muscle tone. Conversely, a decrease in temperature results in decreased sweating, cutaneous vasoconstriction, and increased muscle tone and shivering. These homeostatic mechanisms deteriorate with age.

HYPOTHERMIA

Definition and Etiologies

Hypothermia is defined as a core body temperature (tympanic, esophageal, or rectal) of <35°C (<95°F). Multiple factors may lead to increased heat loss, decreased heat production, or impaired thermoregulation (Table 1). Hypothermia may be characterized as primary (accidental), due to exposure to cold temperatures, or secondary, resulting from a disease process such as myxedema or sepsis. However, exposure along with underlying disease processes is found frequently in hypothermic patients, especially the elderly. Immersion hypothermia is often distinguished from nonimmersion hypothermia because it occurs more rapidly and is more often accompanied by asphyxia. Hypothermia is frequently noted in trauma patients and is associated with increased mortality rates.

To facilitate management, hypothermia can be classified by the degree of temperature reduction. Mild hypothermia refers to core temperatures of 32° to 35°C (90° to 95°F); moderate hypothermia 28° to 32°C (82° to 90°F); and severe hypothermia <28°C (<82°F).

Pathophysiology

General Metabolic Changes. Hypothermia produces multisystemic involvement that varies with core temperature (Table 2). The initial response to cold is cutaneous vasoconstriction, which results in shunting of blood from colder extremities to the body core. Vasodilation secondary to ethanol can prevent this normal compensatory vasoconstriction. Vasoconstriction fails at temperatures <24°C (<75°F), and the rate of heat loss increases due to relative vasodilation. Heat production is increased by the onset of shivering with core temperatures of 30° to 35°C (86° to 95°F). Shivering lasts only until glycogen stores are depleted, which usually occurs when the body temperature reaches 30°C (86°F).

Cardiovascular System. An initial tachycardia is followed by progressive bradycardia. The pulse rate decreases by 50% when core temperature reaches 28°C (82°F). Bradycardia is secondary to alterations in conductivity and automaticity that are generally refractory to standard treatment (e.g., atropine). Cardiac function and blood pressure also decline proportionately as the core temperature decreases. Systemic vascular resistance predictably increases.

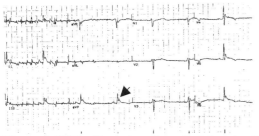

Figure 1. EKG of hypothermic patient showing J wave (arrow).

Hypothermia produces a variety of myocardial conduction abnormalities. Atrial fibrillation is common and usually converts to sinus rhythm spontaneously during rewarming.

At temperatures of <29°C (<84°F), ventricular fibrillation (VF) can occur spontaneously or be induced by movement or invasive procedures (e.g., central line, nasogastric tube). Asystole occurs at temperatures <20°C (<68°F). Ventricular fibrillation and other arrhythmias are extremely refractory to defibrillation and drug treatment until the core temperature increases to ~30°C (~86°F).

Although many electrocardiogram (ECG) abnormalities have been described, the most characteristic of hypothermia is the J wave (also called the Osborn wave) at the junction of the QRS complex and ST segment (Figure 1). The J wave can occur in patients with core temperatures of <32°C (<90°F) and is almost always present at temperatures of <25°C (<77°F). The presence of this wave is neither pathognomonic for hypothermia nor does it have prognostic value. Prolongation of the PR, QRS, and QT intervals may be noted.

Other Organ Systems. As temperature decreases, tidal volume and respiratory rate will decrease. The cough reflex may be blunted and cold-induced bronchorrhea may contribute to atelectasis. Hypoxemia may develop early depending on the circumstances (e.g., water immersion, aspiration). Although renal blood flow and glomerular filtration rate decrease in hypothermia, there is an initial cold-induced diuresis due to the relative central hypervolemia resulting from peripheral vasoconstriction. Additional contributory factors include the inhibition of antidiuretic hormone release and renal tubular concentrating defects. Ethanol exacerbates the diuresis. With warming, volume depletion may become evident.

With mild hypothermia, victims may exhibit confusion, lethargy, or combativeness. Below a core temperature of 32°C (<90°F), the patient is usually unconscious with diminished brainstem function. Pupils dilate below a core temperature of 30°C (<86°F). Intestinal motility decreases at <34°C (<93°F), resulting in the common finding of ileus. Hepatic dysfunction affects the generation of glucose as well as drug metabolism.

Table 1. Factors predisposing to hypothermia

Increased Heat Loss	Impaired Thermoregulation
Environmental exposure	Peripheral Dysfunction
Skin Disorders	Neuropathies
Burns	Spinal cord transaction
Dermatitis	Diabetes
Psoriasis	Central Dysfunction
Vasodilation	CNS hemorrhage/trauma
Alcohol	CVA
Drugs (phenothiazines)	Drugs
Iatrogenic	Sedatives
Heat stroke treatment	Alcohols
Environmental cold (operating suite)	Cyclic antidepressants
	Narcotics
Decreased Heat Production	Neoplasm
Endocrine Disorders	Parkinson's disease
Hypopituitarism	Anorexia nervosa
Hypothyroidism	
Hypoadrenalism	Miscellaneous States
Insufficient Fuel	Sepsis
Hypoglycemia	Pancreatitis
Anorexia nervosa	Carcinomatosis
Malnutrition	Uremia
Extreme exertion	Giant cell arteritis
Neuromuscular Inefficiency	Sarcoidosis
Extremes of age	
Inactivity	
Impaired shivering	

CNS, central nervous system; CVA, cerebrovascular accident.

Laboratory Findings. The physiologic changes described are reflected by clinical laboratory tests. An increased hematocrit is usually found, with platelet and white blood cell counts being normal or low. The increase in hematocrit is due to hemoconcentration and splenic contraction. However, restoration of intravascular volume and warming often result in a mild anemia. Platelet and white blood cell counts may drop as temperatures decrease. Platelet dysfunction occurs with hypothermia and may compromise hemostasis. Although disseminated intravascular coagulation (DIC) may develop, initial coagulation studies (prothrombin time, partial thromboplastin time) are often normal since these laboratory measurements are performed on warmed blood. Electrolytes are variable and no consistent changes are predictable. Increased values of blood urea nitrogen and creatinine result from hypovolemia. Hyperglycemia is common due to catecholamine release and inhibition of insulin transport. The acid-base status is difficult to predict in hypothermia, but factors such as respiratory acidosis, lactate generation from shivering, decreased acid excretion, and decreased tissue perfusion contribute to acidemia. There is general agreement that arterial blood gas values do not need to be corrected for temperature. However, the Pao2 should be corrected to evaluate oxygen delivery and the alveolar-arterial gradient.

Diagnosis

The clinical manifestations of hypothermia vary with the etiology, severity,

Table 2. Manifestations of hypothermia.

Core Temp (°C)	Musculoskeletal	Neurologic	Other
MILD			
38			
36	Shivering begins	Slurred speech	
34	Maximal shivering	Increased confusion	
33	Decreased shivering	Stupor	Decreasing BP; respiratory alkalosis; cold diuresis
MODERATE			
32	Shivering nearly absent; onset muscle rigidity	Pupils dilated	Arrhythmias; J waves on ECG
30 hypoventilation		DTRs absent	Severe
			VF possible
28	Extreme muscle rigidity	No voluntary movement	Shock; inaudible heart sounds
SEVERE			
26			
24	Patient appears dead		Severe risk of VF; minimal cardiac activity
22			
20		Isoelectric EEG	Asystole
18		Isoelectric EEG	Asystole

BP, blood pressure; ECG, electrocardiogram; DTR, deep tendon reflexes; VF, ventricular fibrillation; EEG, electroencephalogram.

To convert Celsius temperature to Fahrenheit temperature, multiply by 9/5, then add 32.

and duration. It is most imperative to recognize early signs of mild hypothermia, especially in the elderly. These patients may present with confusion, lethargy, impaired judgment, and the unusual manifestation of "paradoxical undressing." More severe hypothermia results in manifestations that are easily recognizable: muscle rigidity, decreased reflexes, decreased respiratory rate, bradycardia, hypotension, and even the appearance of death. The clinical suspicion of hypothermia should be confirmed with an accurate core temperature measurement. Any low temperature (35°C; 95°F) should be checked with a thermometer capable of registering lower temperatures. A rectal probe is most practical even though it may lag behind core changes. The probe should be inserted to an adequate depth avoiding cold fecal material. An esophageal probe is an alternative, but readings may be falsely elevated in the intubated patient who receives heated inhalation. Reliability of tympanic temperature devices has not been established in hypothermia.

Management

Hospital Management. The severity of hypothermia, clinical findings, and comorbid conditions of the patient determine the aggressiveness of resuscitation techniques. The following measures should be instituted as indicated.

- *Airway Management.* Intubation is often necessary for airway protection and/or delivery of supplemental oxygen. The orotracheal route is preferred due to the risk of traumatic bleeding with the nasal route. However, muscle rigidity may preclude orotracheal intubation. Endotracheal tube cuff pressures should be monitored after rewarming because volume and pressure will increase.
- *Supplemental Oxygen*
- *Cardiopulmonary Resuscitation.* Cardiopulmonary resuscitation should be initiated if the patient is pulseless(assess for 30-45 seconds) or has a nonperfusing rhythm such as asystole or ventricular fibrillation. Chest wall compression is often difficult.
- *ECG Monitoring*
  - Bradycardia: Avoid pharmacologic manipulation and pacing.
  - VF: Initial defibrillation should be attempted even if the temperature is <30° to 32°C (<86° to 90°F). If unsuccessful, institute rewarming. Avoid intravenous drugs until the temperature increases to ~30°C (~86°F) and then utilize the lowest effective dose. Dosing intervals should be increased in hypothermic patients. Epinephrine and vasopressin have improved coronary artery perfusion pressure in hypothermic animals. The efficacy of amiodarone has not been established in hypothermia, but it is a reasonable initial antiarrhythmic drug. Magnesium sulfate has also been used successfully. Lidocaine has limited efficacy and procainamide may increase the incidence of VF.
  - Asystole: Follow advanced cardiac life support guidelines and administer pharmacologic agents when the temperature approaches 30°C (86°F).
  - *Core Temperature Monitoring*

- *Rewarming* (See below)
- *Intravenous Fluids.* All patients require fluids for hypovolemia. Warm normal saline solution containing glucose is a reasonable choice. Increased fluid requirements are often necessary during rewarming to prevent or treat hypotension. Lactated Ringer's solution should be avoided due to impaired hepatic metabolism of lactate.
- *Vasopressor Drugs.* Hemodynamic instability should first be addressed with volume replacement. Vasopressor drugs have a minimal effect on constricted vessels and increase the risk of dysrhythmias.
- *Nasogastric or Orogastric Tube:* to relieve gastric distention.
- *Urinary Catheter*
- *Venous Access.* Peripheral venous catheters are preferred. Central venous lines (subclavian, internal jugular) are not routinely recommended because they may precipitate dysrhythmias.
- *Laboratory Studies.* Studies should include complete blood count, prothrombin time, partial thromboplastin time, electrolytes, creatine kinase level, and arterial blood gases. Thyroid function evaluation, toxicology screen, and blood cultures as warranted.
- *Search for associated conditions* requiring urgent intervention, such as hypoglycemia, sepsis, and hypothyroidism.

Rewarming Methods: Choices and Controversies. Although warming is the primary treatment for hypothermia, controversy exists as to the optimal method, duration, and rate of rewarming. No controlled studies comparing rewarming methods exist and rigid treatment protocols cannot be recommended. Three types of rewarming procedures exist: passive external rewarming (PER), active external rewarming (AER), and active core rewarming (ACR).

PER is the least invasive and the slowest method. It involves placing the patient in a warm environment, providing warm clothing or blankets, and allowing the body to regain heat. This technique should be applied as the sole method only in patients with mild hypothermia. The patient must be able to generate heat for PER to be effective. Rewarming rates with PER in mild hypothermia vary between 0.5° and 2.0°C/hr (1° and 3.6°F/hr).

AER involves the external application of heat, such as warming blankets, heating pads, radiant heat lamps, or immersion in warm water. Currently, forced air warming devices are the most effective and practical means of applying AER, particularly in the perioperative period. A potential disadvantage of this method is the theoretical concern of "after-drop." When a heat source is applied, peripheral vasodilation occurs and colder peripheral blood is transported to the relatively warmer core, thereby reducing the core temperature. After-drop has been hypothesized to increase the incidence of VF. In response to this concern, it has been suggested that heat be applied only to the thorax, leaving the extremities vasoconstricted. The advantages of AER are its ease of institution, ready availability, low cost, and noninvasiveness. Earlier studies showing high mortality when AER was utilized have not been supported by more recent experience.

ACR is the most rapid and most invasive method, and involves the application of heat to the body core. ACR is indicated in patients with a core temperature of <28°C (<82°F) or with an arrested cardiac rhythm. Techniques for ACR include heated humidified oxygen, heated intravenous fluids, thoracic lavage, peritoneal lavage, gastric/rectal lavage, hemodialysis, continuous arteriovenous/venovenous rewarming, and cardiopulmonary bypass.

One of the simplest methods to institute is warm, humidified, inhaled oxygen (42° to 45°C) (107.6° to 113°F), which prevents further respiratory heat loss and may result in a modest heat gain. A rewarming rate of 1° to 2.5°C/hr (2° to 4.5°F/hr) can be expected. This technique should be utilized routinely on most victims of moderate-to-severe hypothermia. Heated intravenous fluids (40° to 42°C) (104° to 107.6°F) are also easy to institute. Although gastric, bladder, or rectal lavage with warm

fluids is a simple procedure, there is little information regarding the efficacy of this method. It should generally be used only as an adjunct until more invasive rewarming methods can be initiated.

For patients with severe hypothermia, more invasive ACR is preferred: peritoneal lavage, thoracic lavage, hemodialysis, continuous arteriovenous/venovenous rewarming, and cardiopulmonary bypass. These procedures require specialized equipment and intensive care. However, they are very efficient at rewarming and, in the case of cardiopulmonary bypass, may provide for hemodynamic stabilization of the patient. Peritoneal lavage can be instituted through a peritoneal dialysis catheter, using dialysate heated to 40° to 45°C (104° to 113°F). Closed thoracic lavage involves placement of anterior and posterior chest tubes, infusion of heated saline (40° to 42°C) (104° to 107.6°F) through the anterior tube, and gravity drainage from the posterior tube. Hemodialysis, utilizing a two-way-flow catheter, may be best suited for the patient who does not have hemodynamic instability. Continuous arteriovenous/venovenous rewarming utilizes a modified fluid warmer with 40°C (104°F) water infused through the inner chamber. Cardiopulmonary bypass is the most invasive and labor-intensive technique for rewarming. It has the advantage of providing complete hemodynamic support and rapid rewarming rates (1-2°C every 3-5 minutes).

The choice of rewarming methods may combine techniques, such as truncal AER with ACR, using heated oxygen and intravenous fluids. Availability of resources may be a decisive factor in choosing the method of rewarming. In all cases, complications of rewarming such as DIC, pulmonary edema, compartment syndromes, rhabdomyolysis, and acute tubular necrosis must be anticipated.

Outcome from Hypothermia

There are currently no strong predictors of death or permanent neurologic dysfunction in severe hypothermia. Therefore, there are no definitive indicators to suggest which patients can or cannot be resuscitated successfully.

Severe hyperkalemia (>10 mEq/L) may be a marker of death. In general, resuscitative efforts should continue until the core temperature is 32°C (90°F). However, the decision to terminate resuscitation must be individualized based on the circumstances.

HYPERTHERMIA

Heat Stroke

Definition. Heat stroke is a life-threatening medical emergency that occurs when homeostatic thermoregulatory mechanisms fail. This failure usually results in elevation of body temperature to >41°C (>105.8°F), producing multiple system tissue damage and organ dysfunction. Two syndromes of heat stroke occur: classic heat stroke (nonexertional) and exertional heat stroke. Classic heat stroke typically affects infants and elderly individuals with underlying chronic illness. The occurrence

Table 3. Predisposing factors for heat stroke

Increased Heat Production
    Exercise
    Fever
    Thyrotoxicosis
    Hypothalamic dysfunction
    Drugs (sympathomimetics)
    Environmental heat stress

Decreased Heat Loss
    Environmental heat stress
    Cardiac disease
    Peripheral vascular disease
    Dehydration
    Obesity
    Skin disease
    Anticholinergic drugs
    Ethanol
    B-blockers

---

of classic heat stroke is often predictable when heat waves occur. The syndrome develops over several days and results in significant dehydration and absence of sweating. Exertional heat stroke typically occurs in young individuals such as athletes and military recruits exercising in hot weather. These individuals usually have no chronic illness, and this syndrome occurs sporadically and often unpredictably. Dehydration is mild and ~50% of individuals will have profuse sweating.

Predisposing Factors. Heat stroke results from increased heat production and/or decreased heat loss (Table 3). Environmental factors of high heat and humidity contribute to heat production as well as limiting heat loss. Sympathomimetic drugs, such as cocaine and amphetamines, increase muscle activity and may also disrupt hypothalamic regulatory mechanisms. Numerous drugs interfere with the ability to dissipate heat. Drugs with anticholinergic effects, such as cyclic antidepressants, antihistamines, and antipsychotics, inhibit sweating and disrupt hypothalamic function. Ethanol may contribute to heat stroke by several mechanisms - vasodilation resulting in heat gain, impaired perception of the environment, and diuresis. β-adrenergic blockers may impair cardiovascular compensation and decrease cutaneous blood flow. Factors that increase the risk of death, as identified in the July 1995 heat wave in Chicago, include being confined to bed due to medical problems and living alone.

Diagnosis. The diagnosis of heat stroke requires a history of exposure to a heat load (either internal or external), severe central nervous system (CNS) dysfunction, and elevated temperature (usually >40°C [>104°F]). The absolute temperature may not be critical since cooling measures often have been instituted before the patient is admitted to a healthcare facility. Sweating may or may not be present.

Clinical Manifestations. Profound CNS dysfunction characterizes heat stroke. Dysfunction may range from bizarre behavior, delirium, and confusion, to decerebrate rigidity, cerebellar dysfunction, seizures, and coma. These changes are potentially reversible, although permanent deficits can occur. Lumbar puncture results may show increased protein, xanthochromia, and lymphocytic pleocytosis.

Tachycardia, an almost universal cardiovascular finding in heat stroke, occurs in response to peripheral vasodilation and the need for increased cardiac output. The peripheral vascular resistance is usually low unless severe hypovolemia is present. If the patient is unable to increase cardiac output, hypotension develops. A variety of ECG changes have been described in heat stroke, including conduction defects, increased Q-T interval, and nonspecific ST-T changes.

Tachypnea may result in a significant respiratory alkalosis. However, victims of exertional heat stroke usually have lactic acidosis. Rhabdomyolysis and renal failure occur more commonly with exertional heat stroke and may be due to myoglobinuria, thermal parenchymal damage, or decreased renal blood flow due to hypotension. Hematologic effects include hypocoagulability, which may progress to DIC.

An inflammatory response may cause or contribute to the clinical manifestations of heat stroke. Increased concentrations of endotoxin, tumor necrosis factor, soluble tumor necrosis factor receptor, and interleukin-1 have been demonstrated in heat stroke victims. Interleukin-6 and nitric oxide metabolite concentrations correlate with the severity of illness. Endothelial cell activation/injury is suggested by findings of increased concentrations of circulating intercellular adhesion molecule-1, endothelin, and von Willebrand factor-antigen.

Electrolyte concentrations are variable in heat stroke. Hyperkalemia can result from rhabdomyolysis, but hypokalemia occurs more commonly. Hypocalcemia can occur, particularly with rhabdomyolysis, but usually does not require therapy.

Differential Diagnosis. The history and physical findings usually indicate the diagnosis of heat stroke. In the absence of adequate history, other processes to be considered include CNS infection, hypothalamic lesions, thyroid storm, and other hyperthermic syndromes such as neuroleptic malignant syndrome.

Treatment. Along with resuscitative measures, immediate cooling should be instituted for any patient with a temperature of >41°C (>105.8°F). Two methods of cooling have been utilized: conductive cooling and evaporative cooling. Because definitive human studies are lacking, the optimal cooling method remains controversial.

Direct cooling by enhancing conduction of heat from the body is accomplished by immersion of the patient in cold water. Skin massage to counteract cutaneous vasoconstriction in the limbs has been recommended. This method requires considerable staff time and makes it difficult to treat seizures and perform other resuscitative measures. Ice water soaks are a variant of this method and entail application of ice packs to the axillae, groin, and neck.

Evaporative cooling is a more practical cooling method. The patient is placed nude on a stretcher and sprayed with warm (not cold) water. Air flow is created with use of fans to enhance evaporative cooling. This method allows personnel to institute other resuscitative measures while cooling occurs. Other cooling methods, such as peritoneal lavage, iced gastric lavage, or cardiopulmonary bypass have not been effectively tested in humans. Antipyretics are not indicated and dantrolene is ineffective.

In addition to cooling, most patients will require intubation for airway protection. Supplemental oxygen should be instituted for all patients. The type and quantity of intravenous fluids should be individualized based on assessment of electrolytes and volume status. Overaggressive hydration may result in cardiac decompensation, especially in the elderly. Hypotension often responds to cooling as peripheral vasodilation decreases. A thermistor probe should be used for monitoring of core temperature during cooling efforts. Cooling should be stopped at 38.0° to 38.8°C (100.4° to 102°F) to prevent hypothermic overshoot.

Outcome. With appropriate management, the survival rate from heat stroke approaches 90%. However, morbidity is related to the duration of hyperthermia and to underlying conditions. Advanced age, hypotension, coagulopathy, hyperkalemia, acute renal failure, and prolonged coma are associated with a poor prognosis. In retrospective studies, rapid cooling (<1 hour) was associated with a decreased mortality.

Malignant Hyperthermia

Table 4. Diagnostic criteria for NMS*

Major Criteria
        Fever
        Muscle rigidity
        ↑ Creatinine kinase

Minor Criteria
        Tachycardia
        Abnormal blood pressure
        Tachypnea
        Altered consciousness
        Diaphoresis
        Leukocytes

---

*Diagnosis of NMS is suggested by the presence of all 3 major criteria or by the presence of 2 major and 4 minor criteria.

Definition. Malignant hyperthermia (MH) is a drug- or stress-induced hypermetabolic syndrome characterized by hyperthermia, muscle contractures, and cardiovascular instability. It results from a genetic defect of calcium transport in skeletal muscle. The primary defects are postulated to be impaired reuptake of calcium into the sarcoplasmic reticulum, increased release of calcium from the sarcoplasmic reticulum, and a defect in the calcium-mediated coupling contraction mechanism. It is genetically transmitted as an autosomal dominant trait and occurs in 1 in 50 to 1 in 150,000 adults who receive anesthesia.

Triggers. Halothane and succinylcholine have been involved in the majority of reported cases of MH. Additional potentiating drugs include muscle relaxants, inhalational anesthetic agents, and drugs such as ethanol, caffeine, sympathomimetics, parasympathomimetics, cardiac glycosides, and quinidine analogs. Less commonly, MH can be precipitated by infection, physical or emotional stress, anoxia, or high ambient temperature.

Clinical Manifestations. Manifestations of MH usually occur within 30 minutes of anesthesia in 90% of cases. Muscle rigidity begins in the muscles of the extremities or the chest. In patients receiving succinylcholine, the stiffness most commonly begins in the jaw. The development of masseter spasm after administration of a paralyzing agent must be considered an early sign of MH. Tachycardia is another early, although nonspecific, sign. Monitoring of arterial blood gases or end-tidal CO_2 may detect an early increase in CO_2. Hypertension and mottling of the skin also occur. The increase in temperature usually occurs later but is followed rapidly by acidosis, ventricular arrhythmias, and hypotension. Laboratory abnormalities include increased sodium, calcium, magnesium, potassium, phosphate, creatine kinase, and lactate dehydrogenase.

Lactate levels are increased and arterial blood gases indicate hypoxemia and an increase in $Paco_2$.

Treatment. Once the diagnosis of MH is entertained, the inciting drug should be discontinued immediately. The most effective and safe therapy is dantrolene. It acts by uncoupling the excitation contraction mechanism in skeletal muscle to decrease thermogenesis. Dantrolene should be administered by rapid intravenous push beginning at a dose of 1 to 2.5 mg/kg and continuing until the symptoms subside or the maximum dose of 10 mg/kg has been reached. Decreasing muscle rigidity should be evident within minutes. Subsequent doses of 4 to 8 mg/kg every 6 hours should be continued for 24 to 48 hours. If dantrolene is ineffective or slowly effective, evaporative cooling methods can also be utilized.

Neuroleptic Malignant Syndrome

Definition. Neuroleptic malignant syndrome (NMS) is an idiosyncratic reaction, usually to neuroleptic drugs, characterized by hyperthermia, muscle rigidity, alterations in mental status, autonomic dysfunction, and rhabdomyolysis. It may occur in up to 1% of all patients on neuroleptic agents and affects males more than females and the young more than the old. The pathogenesis is unknown but is thought to be related to CNS dopamine antagonism.

Triggers. Although the majority of cases have been associated with haloperidol, the following agents have been associated with NMS: butyrophenones (e.g., haloperidol);

phenothiazines (e.g., chlorpromazine, fluphenazine); thioxanthenes (e.g., thiothixene); dopamine-depleting agents (e.g., tetrabenazine); dibenzoxazepines (e.g., loxapine); and withdrawal of levodopa/carbidopa or amantadine. Rechallenge with an inciting drug may not result in recurrence of NMS.

Clinical Manifestations. NMS usually occurs 1 to 3 days after initiating a neuroleptic agent or changing the dose, and the syndrome may last for a period of 1 to 3 weeks. Hyperthermia is universally present and the average maximal temperature is 39.9°C (103.8°F). Autonomic dysfunction includes tachycardia, diaphoresis, blood pressure instability, and arrhythmias. Autonomic dysfunction may precede changes in muscle tone. A general increase in muscle tone or tremors occurs in >90% of patients. Early manifestations of changes in muscle tone include dysphagia, dysarthria, or dystonia. Altered mental status occurs in 75% and can range from agitation to coma. Rhabdomyolysis occurs frequently with elevations of creatine kinase. Various diagnostic criteria have been proposed (Table 4), but NMS remains a clinical diagnosis based on exposure to neuroleptic agents or other dopamine antagonists in association with characteristic manifestations.

Treatment. Dantrolene is the most effective agent for reducing muscle rigidity and decreasing temperature. It is given in the same doses as described for MH. In addition, dopamine agonists have been reported to have beneficial effects in NMS. These drugs include bromocriptine (2.5 to 10 mg three times daily), amantadine (100 mg twice daily), and levodopa/carbidopa. Supportive therapies must also be instituted as indicated. Complications may include respiratory failure, cardiovascular collapse, renal failure, arrhythmias, or thromboembolism.

RHABDOMYOLYSIS

Definition. Rhabdomyolysis is a clinical and laboratory syndrome resulting from skeletal muscle injury with release of cell contents into the plasma. Rhabdomyolysis occurs when demands for oxygen and metabolic substrate exceed availability. This syndrome may result from primary muscle injury or secondary injury due to infection, vascular occlusion, electrolyte disorders, or toxins. Table 5 provides an overview of causes of rhabdomyolysis.

Manifestations. Clinical manifestations of rhabdomyolysis consist of myalgias, muscle swelling and tenderness, discoloration of the urine, and features of the underlying disease. However, overt symptoms or physical findings may not be present. Laboratory evaluation reflects muscle cell lysis with elevation of muscle enzyme levels (creatine kinase, lactate dehydrogenase, aldolase, and aspartate aminotransferase), hyperkalemia, hyperphosphatemia, and hypocalcemia. Coagulation abnormalities consistent with DIC may occur. Renal failure may result secondary to release of myoglobin and other toxic muscle components. A urine dipstick positive for blood and an absence of red blood cells on microscopic examination suggest the presence of myoglobinuria.

Treatment. The treatment of

Table 5. Causes of rhabdomyolysis			
Traumatic	Infections	Toxins/Drugs	Metabolic Disorders
Crush syndrome	Coxsackie	Alcohol	Enzyme deficiencies
Muscle compression	Gas gangrene	Amphetamines	Hyperosmolar states
Hyperthermic syndromes	Hepatitis	Carbon monoxide	Hypokalemia
Burns	Influenza B	Cocaine	Hypomagnesemia
Electrical injury	Legionella	Phencyclidine	Hypophosphatemia
Exertion	Salmonella	Snake/spider venom	Inflammatory muscle disease
Seizures	Shigella	Steroids	Thyroid disease
Vascular occlusion	Tetanus		Vasculitis

rhabdomyolysis is aimed at treating the underlying disease and preventing complications. Maintenance of intravascular volume and renal perfusion is the most important aspect of preventing renal failure. Volume resuscitation should target a urine output of 2 to 3 mL/kg/hr. Although increased urine output is beneficial, other interventions to prevent renal failure are more controversial. Alkalinization of the urine may be helpful, but clinical relevance has not been established. The greatest benefit of administering sodium bicarbonate may be restoration of intravascular volume rather than a change in pH. Treatment with bicarbonate should be individualized, based on the patient's ability to tolerate the sodium and fluid load. Loop diuretics and osmotic diuretics have been advocated to be protective of the kidneys, but convincing clinical data are lacking. Loop diuretics theoretically can worsen renal tubular acidosis, which is thought to potentiate myoglobin-induced nephropathy. Diuresis should not be attempted without adequate volume replacement.

Electrolyte abnormalities should be anticipated and treated expeditiously. The most life-threatening abnormality is hyperkalemia. Hypocalcemia does not usually require treatment and empiric administration of calcium may exacerbate muscle injury.

The patient must be closely observed for the development of a compartment syndrome. Monitoring of intracompartmental pressures may be required. Fasciotomy is often recommended for intracompartmental pressures of >30 to 35 mm Hg.

SUGGESTED READINGS

Hypothermia

1. Bartley B, Crnkovich DJ, Usman AR, et al: Techniques for managing severe hypothermia. *J Crit Illness* 1996; 11:123-127
2. Danzl DF, Pozos RS: Accidental hypothermia. *N Engl J Med* 1994; 331:1756-1760
3. Delaney KA, Howland MA, Vassallo S, et al: Assessment of acid-base disturbances in hypothermia and their physiologic consequences. *Ann Emerg Med* 1989; 18:72-82
4. Gentilello LM: Advances in the management of hypothermia. *Surg Clin North Am* 1995; 75:243-256
5. Gentilello LM, Cobean RA, Offner PJ, et al: Continuous arteriovenous rewarming: Rapid reversal of hypothermia in critically ill patients. *J Trauma* 1992; 32:316-327
6. Hanania NA, Zimmerman JL: Accidental hypothermia. *Crit Care Clin* 1999; 15:35-49
7. Kornberger E, Schwarz B, Linder KH, et al: Forced air surface rewarming in patients with severe accidental hypothermia. *Resuscitation* 1999; 41:105-11
8. Krismer AC, Lindner KH, Kornberger R, et al: Cardiopulmonary resuscitation during severe hypothermia in pigs: Does epinephrine or vasopressin increase coronary perfusion pressure? *Anesth Analg* 2000; 90:69-73
9. Schaller MD, Fischer AP, Perret CH: Hyperkalemia, a prognostic factor during acute severe hypothermia. *JAMA* 1990; 264:1842-1845
10. Thornton D, Farmer JC: Hypothermia and hyperthermia. *In*: Critical Care Medicine. Second Edition. Parrillo JE, Dellinger RP (Eds). Mosby Inc, St. Louis, 2000, pp 1525-38

Hyperthermia

11. Aiyer MK, Crnkovich DJ, Carlson RW: Techniques for managing severe hyperthermia. *J Crit Illness* 1995; 10:643-646
12. Balzan MV: The neuroleptic malignant syndrome: a logical approach to the patient with temperature and rigidity. *Postgrad Med J* 1998; 74:72-6
13. Bouchama A, De Vol EB: Acid-base alterations in heatstroke. *Inten Care Med* 2001; 27:680-85

14. Carbone JR: The neuroleptic malignant and serotonin syndromes. *Emerg Med Clin North Am* 2000; 18:317-25

15. Caroff SN, Mann SC: Neuroleptic malignant syndrome. *Med Clin North Am* 1993; 77:185-202

16. Chan TC, Evans SD, Clark RF: Drug-induced hyperthermia. *Crit Care Clin* 1997; 13:785-808

17. Denborough M: Malignant hyperthermia. *Lancet* 1998; 352:1131-36

18. Hubbard RW, Gaffin SL, Squire DL: Heat-related illness. *In:* Wilderness Medicine: Management of Wilderness and Environmental Emergencies. Fourth Edition. Auerbach PS (Ed). St Louis, CV Mosby, 2001, pp 195

19. Tomarken JL: Malignant hyperthermia. *Ann Emerg Med* 1987; 16:1253-1265

20. Weiner JS, Khogali M: A physiological body-cooling unit for treatment of heat stroke. *Lancet* 1980; 1:507-509

21. Yarbrough B, Vicario S: Heat illness. *In:* Emergency Medicine: Concepts and Clinical Practice. Fifth Edition. Marx JA, Hockberger RS, Walls RM (Eds). St Louis, Mosby, 2002, pp 1997-09

Rhabdomyolysis

22. Farmer JC: Rhabdomyolysis. *In:* Critical Care. Third Edition. Civetta JM, Taylor RW, Kirby RR (Eds). Philadelphia, Lippincott-Raven, 1997, pp 2195-2202

23. Reilly KM, Salluzzo R: Rhabdomyolysis and its complications. *Res Staff Phys* 1990; 36:45-52

24. Holt SG, Moore KP: Pathogenesis and treatment of renal dysfunction in rhabdomyolysis. *Int Care Med* 2001; 27:803-11

LIFE-THREATENING AIRFLOW LIMITATION

Richard K. Albert, MD

Objectives

- Describe the physiologic abnormalities of asthma and COPD leading to auto-PEEP, its measurement and consequences (particularly with regard to work of breathing), and the interventions available to reduces these consequences
- Describe the approaches to ventilatory support of patients with asthma and COPD, specifically the new information pertaining to noninvasive positive pressure ventilation
- Review the appropriate pharmacological interventions for acute exacerbations of asthma and COPD

Auto-PEEP, Work of Breathing and Respiratory Muscle Fatigue

The primary pathophysiologic cause of airflow obstruction in patients with asthma is bronchospasm and/or mucosal inflammation. The primary abnormality in emphysema is loss of elastic recoil. Both, in turn, reduce expiratory airflow. Patients with emphysema also have a loss of the distending effects of parenchymal tethering. In both conditions airway closure is premature, air trapping and an increase in lung volume. Although the increase in lung volume has the beneficial compensatory effect of augmenting elastic recoil and distending airways, the reduced airflow and premature airway closure cause alveolar pressure (P_A) to exceed atmospheric pressure (Patm) at end-exhalation (i.e., auto-PEEP, or intrinsic PEEP) when, in normal subjects P_A = Patm at end-exhalation (i.e., at FRC). Although auto-PEEP may exist under chronic, steady-state conditions, it is of particular concern when any acute airway infection, bronchospasm, or other abnormality causing airway narrowing abruptly increases the degree of air-trapping as this markedly increases the work of breathing in patients whose respiratory muscles are already working at considerable disadvantage (i.e., diaphragms are flat, and at near maximum length, both of which decrease the maximum tension that can be generated, and the chest wall pressure-volume curve generates an inward recoil because of marked expansion, as opposed to the outward recoil that exists at more normal lung volumes). Auto-PEEP is also increased if expiratory time is shortened, as will occur with hyperventilation from any cause. Accordingly, the problem may be encountered in conditions in which shunt, low ventilation-perfusion ratios, high dead space or any metabolic acidosis mandates a high minute ventilation in order to maintain normal CO_2 elimination and/or acid-base balance.

The development of, or the abrupt increase in, the level of auto-PEEP is the primary cause for acute ventilatory failure in patients with asthma and COPD, as the increased work of breathing needed to decrease pleural pressure (Ppl) to the extent that P_A falls below Patm, allowing air to be inhaled, increases CO_2 production beyond the capacity of the compromised respiratory muscles to increase alveolar ventilation (Fig. 1). In addition, since patients with asthma and COPD have a very limited ability to increase their minute ventilation (as their tidal volume approaches their FEV_1's during an acute exacerbation), any increase predisposes them to respiratory muscle fatigue (Fig. 2).

Auto-PEEP also has the effect of increasing mean intrathoracic pressure, thereby restricting right heart filling and limiting venous return, both of which will decrease cardiac output.

Measurement of Auto-PEEP

In mechanically ventilated patients auto-PEEP can be measured by occluding the expiratory circuit of the ventilator just prior to inhalation, and noting the resulting airway pressure (which reflects P_A since the above maneuver will produce a condition of no flow and the pressure measured at the mouth will equal the pressure in the alveolus). It is important to note that any expiratory muscle activity (e.g., rectus abdominus, extensor obliques) will increase both Ppl and P_A such that the P_A measured will over-estimate the true value of auto-PEEP. Accordingly, accurate measurement of auto-PEEP can only be accomplished in paralyzed patients (but certainly, patients should *never* be paralyzed simply to make this measurement).

In spontaneously breathing patients, the degree of paradoxical pulse reflects the degree to which Ppl is decreasing with each breath.

Auto-PEEP can also be evaluated by recording the change in pressure that is required to initiate lung inflation. The degree of auto-PEEP measured in this fashion is thought to reflect the *least* amount of auto-PEEP existing in any region of the lung and, accordingly, the values measured should be *less* than recorded by airway occlusion at end-exhalation as the latter should reflect an *average*, or overall value of auto-PEEP existing in the *entire* lung.

Treating the Effects of Auto-PEEP

There are a number of ways to go about treating the effects of auto-PEEP. Since it is abruptly increased by reductions in expiratory time, auto-PEEP can be reduced in patients who are spontaneously breathing by encouraging them to adopt a breathing pattern that emphasizes slow exhalations (which will decrease the respiratory rate). Exhaling through pursed lips has been suggested by some to stent the airways open, but others propose that the major effect of pursed-lip breathing is simply to slow the expiratory time. Slowing the expiratory time also limits the degree to which Ppl becomes positive during exhalation, and any positive Ppl, in the setting of loss of parenchymal tethering, augments airway closure.

Although CPAP or PEEP have no ability to decrease the amount of auto-PEEP, they both reduce the work of breathing resulting from auto-PEEP. Every cm H_2O of CPAP or PEEP added at the mouth translates to a cm H_2O reduction in the degree to which Ppl must be lowered to initiate inhalation. By reducing work of breathing CPAP or PEEP immediately reduce CO_2 production and this will be associated with an immediately obvious improvement in patient comfort. It is not necessary to titrate the level of CPAP or PEEP to the point that it exactly equals

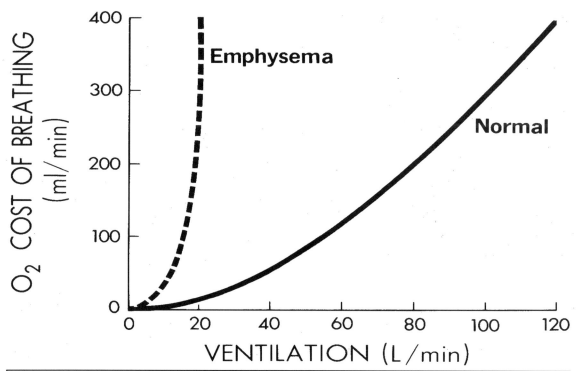

Figure 1. Oxygen Cost of Breathing in Normal Subjects and Patients with Emphysema.

the level of auto-PEEP. *Any* reduction in the degree to which Ppl must be lowered to trigger inhalation will translate into an improvement in work of breathing. On the other hand, if the level of CPAP or PEEP exceeds the level of auto-PEEP, further lung expansion will result with marked patient discomfort. The degree of auto-PEEP can change rapidly (i.e., within minutes or hours) during the course of treating an acute exacerbation of COPD. Accordingly, one should expect to frequently reduce the level of CPAP or PEEP added at the mouth. Initially, clinically apparent improvement can generally be seen with CPAP or PEEP levels < 15 cm H$_2$O.

Auto-PEEP is perhaps the most common cause of patients "fighting the ventilator" as the sensation of dyspnea must be enormous when patients lower their Ppl in an attempt to take a breath, but find that no air enters (since P$_A$ has not dropped below Patm and the ventilator is not triggered).

Ventilatory Support

The large majority of patients with acute exacerbations of asthma or COPD can be successfully managed without intubation or mechanical ventilation. Recently, noninvasive positive pressure ventilation (NIPPV) has been employed with increasing frequency on the basis of numerous studies suggesting that it reduces mortality and the need for intubation (at least in COPD patients).

The conclusions of a recent international consensus conference on NIPPV have recently been published. From this extensive review of the published literature and discussion with investigators working in the field, the jury concluded that (1) there is a sound physiologic rationale for treating acute hypercapnic respiratory failure with NIPPV, (2) that there was a sound rationale for using both expiratory and inspiratory pressure when using NIPPV for

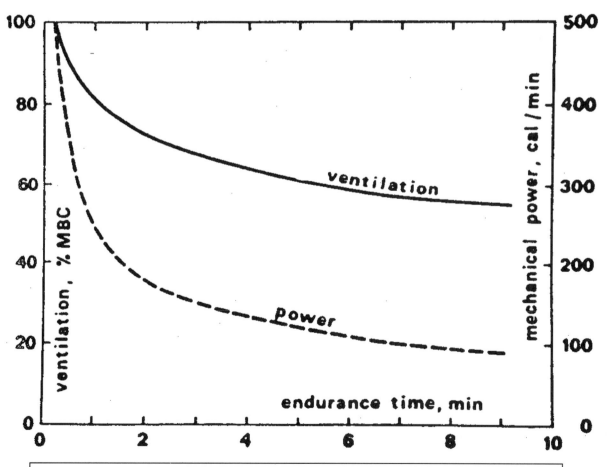

Figure 2. Development of Respiratory Muscle Fatigue at High Minute Ventilation.

acute exacerbations of COPD, (3) that if adequate alveolar ventilation is provided NIPPV may reduce the morbidity and mortality associated with these exacerbations, (4) that there is no evidence supporting the use of any specific interface (although the clinical impression of many investigators working in the field is that full face masks may provide better support), (5) that centers choosing to provide NIPPV must have a variety of interfaces readily available,(6) that the inspiratory pressure support component of NIPPV should be titrated to the lowest value that improves dyspnea, (7) that NIPPV can be delivered outside the ICU but that the venue where it is delivered depends on the training and experience of the nurses, therapists and physicians at each specific center, and (8) that NIPPV does not appear to increase the workload. The group also concluded that NIPPV may shorten weaning time, it may reduce the need to reintubate, it is clearly beneficial for patients with obstructive sleep apnea and the obesity hypoventilation syndrome, it may have a use in treating postoperative atelectasis, and that the expiratory pressure component can increase the PaO_2 in many pulmonary conditions. Although the modality has been used to support patients who are on record as not wanting to be intubated or resuscitated the consensus panel had difficulties with the ethics of this approach.

Oxygen Therapy

The physiologic cause of the hypoxemia that occurs during acute exacerbations of asthma or COPD is a combination of reduced alveolar ventilation and ventilation-perfusion heterogeneity. Accordingly, small increases in alveolar oxygen tension will markedly improve the PaO_2. If F_IO_2's greater than 0.4 are needed to achieve this result, alternate causes of hypoxemia should be considered (e.g., pulmonary embolus, pneumonia, congestive heart failure).

The amount of oxygen administered should be limited to that which increases the PaO_2 to 55 or 60 torr as higher levels have been associated increased $PaCO_2$'s and worsening respiratory failure. Standard teaching has

attributed this effect to suppression of the hypoxic drive (in the setting of a blunted hypercarbic drive). More recent studies suggest that it results from relaxation of hypoxic vasoconstriction which, in turn, results in increasing flow to alveoli with limited alveolar ventilation, in a patients whose overall minute ventilation is also limited by the pre-existing loss of elastic recoil and/or by the acute exacerbation itself.

If mechanical ventilation is judged to be necessary it should be provided without hesitation. The only reason for not doing so would be patient preferences regarding this form of support. Concerns about being left with a ventilator-dependent patient are rarely appropriate as there is nothing about an episode of acute respiratory failure that is precipitated by acute bronchitis which should not be completely reversible. This may not be the case in patients who have necrotizing pneumonia, but this is a rare cause of acute exacerbations.

Pharmacological Intervention

Inhaled β-2 agonists should be preferably administered via metered dose inhalers (MDI) as opposed to nebulizer as correct MDI use will include the patient taking breaths to full inspiratory capacity, as opposed to the tidal breathing most commonly used when patients use nebulizers. Larger inspiratory volumes will result in better deposition of the medication in smaller airways.

β-2 agonists have an abrupt onset of action and the bronchodilating effects gradually abate over 2-6 hours. Accordingly, there is little rational for continuous administration, and some laboratory studies suggest that continuous occupation of the β-2 receptor by its agonist may be deleterious. Most studies indicate that continuous nebulization only result in a higher incidence of side-effects. A recent randomized, controlled trial demonstrates that intermittent nebulization of β-2 agonists via heliox allows better deposition of the medication on the airways and greater bronchodilation. There is no role for oral or subcutaneous β-2 agonists administration in older adult patients as they the b-1 side-effects are well-recognized to cause coronary vasospasm and tachycardia, and can even precipitate myocardial infarction.

Inhaled anticholinergics are also generally recommended. Studies indicate better bronchodilation with anticholinergics in patients with COPD, presumably on the basis of either down-regulation or drop-out of β-2 receptors with chronic β-2 agonist use and/or or with aging. Anticholinergics have a more gradual onset of action (30-60 minutes) but last longer (3-6 hours) such that they should not be administered more frequently than every 4 hours.

Four randomized controlled trials have demonstrated that systemic corticosteroids result in more rapid improvement in airflow than placebo in patients with COPD. Systemic corticosteroids are a mandatory element of treatment of patients with life-threatening asthma. It is important to note that a dose of 0.5 mg/kg intravenously every 6 hours seems to be sufficient to cause this improvement, that greater doses do not seem to have a more beneficial effect, and that, in COPD patients, the medication can be abruptly discontinued after 72 hours of therapy (except in those who take systemic doses chronically and, accordingly, would be expected to have at least some degree of adrenal suppression). Although less-well studies several reports indicate that a similar response to corticosteroids will be obtained regardless of whether the medication is given orally or intravenously.

Inhaled corticosteroids seem to be effective in treating stable COPD patients but not as effective as when they are given systemically.

Several reviews of the literature have concluded that theophylline, mucolytics, subcutaneous epinephrine and intravenous β-2 agonists cannot be recommended.

Antibiotics directed at H. influenza, S. pneumonia and M. cataralis are also almost universally prescribed and their use can be somewhat supported by a large, randomized study in nonhospitalized patients which found that patients who had increased cough, shortness of breath and increased sputum purulence improved faster when receiving antibiotics than those who received a placebo.

If patients with COPD have pedal edema and/or ascites, the use of diuretics should be considered. Although diuretics have not been assessed in clinical trials, physiologic studies suggest that even small amounts of fluid accumulation in the abdomen (e.g., ascites, bowel wall edema) can increase the work of breathing by having adverse effects on abdominal compliance. The diaphragm is part of the chest wall and any decrease in abdominal compliance will increase the work required of the diaphragm.

REFERENCES

1. ATS Statement. Standards for diagnosis and care of patients with chronic obstructive pulmonary disease. *Am J Respir Crit Care Med* 1995; 152:S77-S120

2. Banner MJ, Jaeger MJ, Kirby RR: Components of the work of breathing and implications for monitoring ventilator-dependent patients. *Crit Care Med* 1994; 22:515-23

3. Marini JJ: Should PEEP be used in airflow obstruction? *Am Rev Respir Dis* 1989; 140:1-3

4. Ranieri VM, Grasso S, Fiore T, et al: Auto positive end-expiratory pressure and dynamic hyperinflation. *Clin Chest Med* 1996; 17:379-94

5. Tobin MJ: Mechanical ventilation. *N Eng J Med* 1994; 330:1056-61

6. Jubran A, Van de Graaff WB, Tobin MJ: Variability of patient-ventilator interaction with pressure support ventilation in patients with chronic obstructive pulmonary disease. *Am J Respir Crit Care Med* 1995; 152:129-36

7. Appendini L, Purro A, Patessio A, et al: Partitioning of inspiratory muscle workload and pressure assistance in ventilator-dependent COPD patients. *Am J Respir Crit Care Med* 1996; 154:1301-9

8. Lessard MR, Lofaso F, Brochard L: Expiratory muscle activity increases intrinsic positive end-expiratory pressure independently of dynamic hyperinflation in mechanically ventilated patients. *Am J Respir Crit Care Med* 1995; 151:562-9

9. Maltais F, Reissmann H, Navalesi P, et al: Comparison of static and dynamic measurements of intrinsic PEEP in mechanically ventilated patients. *Am J Respir Crit Care Med* 1994; 150:1318-24

10. Appendini L, Patessio A, Zanaboni S, et al: Physiologic effects of positive end-expiratory pressure and mask pressure support during exacerbations of chronic obstructive pulmonary disease. *Am J Respir Crit Care Med* 1994; 149:1069-76

11. Evans TW, Albert RK, Angus DC, Bion JF, Ciche J-D, Epstein SK, Fagon JY, Ranieri M, Sznajder JI, Torres Aaa, Walley KR: International consensus conferences in intensive care medicine: Noninvasive positive pressure ventilation in acute respiratory failure. *Am J Respir Crit Care Med* 2001; 163:283-91

ISSUES IN SEDATION, PARALYTIC AGENTS, AND AIRWAY MANAGEMENT

Jeanine P. Wiener-Kronish, MD, FCCP

Objectives

- To review the issues concerning the quantity and methods of administration of sedation in the ICU
- To review pharmacokinetics of sedation agents
- To review issues of airway management

Key Words: sedation, assessment, morphine, propofol, ketamine, etomidate, fentanyl, vecuronium, rocuronium, cisatracurium

ISSUES REGARDING SEDATION IN THE ICU

Publications from the late 1980s suggested that approximately half of the patients in the ICU described their period of mechanical ventilation as unpleasant and stressful, and that their time requiring mechanical ventilation was associated with fear, agony, and panic. In the late 1990s and more recently, publications have suggested that there is an association between the administration of large quantities of sedation in the ICU and the development of posttraumatic stress disorders and memory problems in the recipients (1). Furthermore, there have now been investigations that have documented undesirable outcomes associated with the administration of large quantities of sedation. These outcomes include significantly prolonged length of stays in the ICU and in the hospital (2, 3), significantly increased acquisition of CT scans for patients because of depressed mental function (3), and an increased incidence of nosocomial pneumonia in patients receiving sedation and paralytic agents (4). Therefore, the present-day conundrum is how much to sedate patients in the ICU to prevent their fear and anxiety, and which drugs to utilize.

Assessment of Sedation

There is no consensus as to what level of sedation is optimal for patients in the ICU; most likely, the optimal level of sedation will vary depending on the underlying physical and mental problems of each patient and the level of movement that is safe for the patient. A recent investigation documented that the more severely ill a patient is in the ICU, the less the patients remember about their ICU experience (5). The more severely ill patients tend to receive more sedation, as they require mechanical ventilation for more prolonged periods, and there is some question whether their illness and their medicines may affect short-term memory (5). More is being discovered about the effects of sedatives on cognition, memory, and learning; precise goals may eventually be possible (i.e., anxiolysis without decreased cognition). Furthermore, we may be able to achieve some anxiolysis with nonpharmacologic interventions; relaxation tapes, warm milk, and herbal tea were shown to be useful in the treatment of hospitalized elderly patients as the administration of these adjunctive "therapies" decreased the need for sedation and decreased the incidence of delirium (6).

Despite the lack of consensus and our incomplete knowledge, sedation should only be administered after an assessment of the patient is done. Thus, some quantitative assessment of a patient's anxiety should be made before the administration of medication; the patient then should be reassessed after receiving the drug. The most common assessment tool utilized is the Ramsay scale (Table 1). The Ramsay scale is a 6-point scale that describes the patient as anxious and agitated (+3) to unresponsive (level -3). The scale includes an assessment of movement; thus, that the administration of

Table 1. Sedation-Agitation Scale

Score	Description
1	Patient anxious and agitated, or restless, or both
2	Patient cooperative, oriented, and tranquil
3	Patient responds to commands only
4	Brisk response to a light glabellar tap or loud auditory stimulus
5	Sluggish response to a light glabellar tap or loud auditory stimulus
6	No response to a light glabellar tap or loud auditory stimulus

neuromuscular blockade would preclude the use of this assessment tool.

NARCOTICS AND SEDATIVE-HYPNOTIC AGENTS

All the sedative-hypnotic agents utilized for sedation or to optimize airway management have a depressant effect on blood pressure and cardiac function. The effects vary depending on the patient's age (7), underlying medical problems, and cardiovascular stability. Furthermore, when drugs are used in combination, their effects are more than additive. This potentiation of effects can be beneficial, as when analgesic effects are intensified; however, combinations of drugs may also potentiate respiratory depression and cardiovascular instability. Therefore, the decision to administer a sedative-hypnotic agent must first address whether the patient is stable enough to tolerate such a medication and if so, what dose the patient will tolerate.

Patients who do not tolerate the cardiac depressant effects of sedative-hypnotics include patients who are in shock, bleeding, severely volume-depleted, or who have inadequate cardiac function. Patients who have suffered a cardiac arrest or are very hypotensive should not be given normal doses of sedative-hypnotic agents, as the drugs will hinder cardiac function. Aging affects the pharmacokinetic and pharmacodynamics of the sedative-hypnotics; furthermore, the sensitivity of the elderly brain to sedative-hypnotic agents appears to be increased (7). Sedative-hypnotics are also associated with confusion and delirium in the elderly (see the chapter titled "Pain, Delirium, and Ischemia in the Perioperative Period").

Liver disease affects the metabolism of drugs in many ways, and is hard to predict. In severe cirrhosis (associated with altered clotting times and encephalopathy), elimination half-lives of drugs are increased and drug clearance is reduced. These results suggest that smaller doses of drugs should be administered, and should be administered less frequently (7-9). Metabolism of drugs that undergo glucuronidation (i.e., lorazepam, oxazepam) appear to be relatively unaffected by liver disease. Drugs that are metabolized by phase I oxidative pathways (i.e., diazepam and chlordiazepoxide) are affected by acute and chronic liver disease (8). Nonetheless, morphine, which undergoes glucuronidation, is associated with an increased half-life and decreased clearance in patients with end-stage, decompensated liver disease (8).

A retrospective examination of the medical records of 28 patients who required more than 7 days of intensive care documented the occurrence of withdrawal symptoms and signs (restlessness, irritability, nausea, cramps, muscle aches, dysphoria, insomnia, myoclonus, delirium, sweating, tachycardia, vomiting, diarrhea, hypertension, fever, seizure, or tachypnea) in 9 of these patients (10). The patients had to have 3 or more signs, or 3 or more symptoms, to be considered as having withdrawal. These patients received several-fold higher doses of analgesic and sedative hypnotic medications than the patients who did not experience withdrawal symptoms (10). The patients who did *not* experience withdrawal received an average daily dose of fentanyl equivalent to 1.4 mg/day and lorazepam equivalent to 11.1 mg/day. The patients who experienced withdrawal were significantly more likely to have received neuromuscular blocking agents. Increased doses of narcotics and sedatives might have been given to ensure that patients were not paralyzed and awake. The patients who experienced withdrawal symptoms were also significantly younger than those that did not experience the symptoms; the younger patients may be more prone to tolerance of opioids and sedatives, or the younger patients may have been more likely to survive. The authors recommended: a) weaning the doses of the drugs by 5% to 10% per day, b) that drugs might be weaned even more slowly if both opioids and benzodiazepines are being weaned, and c) that long-acting oral agents could be given, which can be weaned outside the ICU (10).

Continuous Infusions

The clearance of a sedative drug is affected by the duration of the infusion of the drug. Both midazolam and lorazepam become longer-acting drugs when they are administered as continuous infusions (11). Patients also rapidly become tolerant to benzodiazepines when these agents are administered frequently (11).

Assessment of Pain

The treatment of pain is not only compassionate, but it is now mandated by the JACHO. Pain associated with procedures should be treated with analgesia. Chronic pain may require therapy other than opioids, as most patients who have been treated for chronic pain are tolerant to narcotics. Patients with chronic pain may benefit from a multidisciplinary approach to their pain treatment.

A patient's pain should be quantified prior to and after treatment. The typical assessment tool is a visual analog scale (VAS), which has been validated and shown to have good interobserver reproducibility.

Morphine Sulfate

Morphine has a rapid initial redistribution phase of 1-1.5 minutes and an initial half-life of 10-20 minutes; the terminal elimination half-life is between 2 to 4.5 hours (8, 9). Compared to fentanyl, morphine has low lipid solubility; this is important in that morphine slowly penetrates the blood-brain barrier. Therefore, morphine's peak effect is after 20 to 30 minutes, whereas the peak effect of the highly lipid-soluble fentanyl is within a few minutes. Fentanyl rapidly redistributes away from the brain and hence is short-acting; in contrast, morphine's low lipid solubility prevents rapid redistribution and causes a longer duration of action (Table 2). The liver primarily metabolizes morphine; however, the kidneys metabolize 40% of the drug. A major metabolite of morphine (morphine-3-glucuronide) has opiate activity and persists in the circulation of patients with renal failure, and can cause prolonged sedation (3, 8, 9).

The sensitivity to pain decreases with age, opiate receptor density is decreased in the elderly, and there is evidence for reduced activity within the opiate receptor system with increasing age (7, 8). Elderly patients are found to develop increased concentrations of morphine when compared to younger patients given the same dose, and the morphine concentration persists for longer intervals, suggesting decreased clearance. Therefore, smaller doses of morphine should be utilized in elderly patients.

Morphine administration is associated with hypotension; doses of 1-4 mg/kg iv are commonly associated with hypotension, but hypotension has been reported with doses of 5 mg iv (9). The faster the rate of administration, the more pronounced the hypotension seen; morphine can also be associated with histamine release, and morphine causes arterial and venous dilation that potentiates hypotension. Finally, morphine can slow the heart rate, probably by its stimulation of the vagus nerve and its depressant effects on the sinoatrial node.

Table 2. Pharmacokinetics and pharmacodynamics of opioid agents[a]

Drug	Lipid Solubility	Half-Life (hr)	Onset of Action (min)	Peak Effect (min)	Duration of Action (hr)
Morphine	Low	2–3	5	20–30	2–7
Fentanyl	High	4–10	1–2	5–15	0.5–1
Meperidine	Moderate	5–8	5	20–60	2–4
Hydromorphone	Low	2.5–3	10–15	15–30	2–4

Pharmacokinetic and pharmacodynamic parameters are based on single intravenous dosing in normal patients. Reproduced with permission from Volles DF, McGory R: Pharmacokinetic consideration. *Crit Care Clin* 1999; 15:64.

Fentanyl

Fentanyl is 50 to 100 times more potent than morphine (fentanyl has greater affinity for the mu opiate receptor), so that the usual intravenous doses are 50 to 100 mcg, depending on the condition of the patient. As fentanyl is very lipid-soluble (40 times more lipid-soluble than morphine), it penetrates the central nervous system quickly and leaves it quickly, and therefore has a very rapid onset of action and a short duration of action (Table 2). The onset of action of fentanyl is within 30 seconds, and its peak effect is within 5-15 minutes (9, 12). The liver metabolizes fentanyl and the kidney eliminates inactive metabolites. Decreased liver perfusion can decrease the clearance of fentanyl. When fentanyl is administered as a continuous infusion, the terminal half-life of the drug is 16 hours; prolonged effects seen after infusions or repeated bolus injections of fentanyl occur due to the large amounts of the drug, which accumulate in the fatty tissues and then have to be metabolized by the liver.

Fentanyl is similar to morphine in that fentanyl concentrations are higher in elderly patients, apparently due to decreased clearance of the drug. Fentanyl is more potent in the elderly in that loss of consciousness occurs with smaller doses and chest wall rigidity occurs more often (7, 12, 13).

Fentanyl administration infrequently causes hypotension; it can cause hypotension by causing bradycardia and decreased sympathetic tone (12, 13). Patients who are maintaining their blood pressure by an increase in sympathetic tone can become hypotensive with the administration of fentanyl (12, 13, 14). The rate of administration appears to affect the development of bradycardia; when fentanyl is administered rapidly, bradycardia more frequently develops (12, 14).

Remifentanil

Remifentanil is an ultrashort-acting narcotic with a potency that is similar to fentanyl. Remifentanil penetrates the blood-brain barrier within 1 minute, and its blood concentration decreases 50% by 6 minutes after a 1-minute infusion and 80% by 15 minutes (15). The novel aspect of remifentanil is its rapid hydrolysis by circulating and tissue nonspecific esterases (the beta adrenergic blocker esmolol is metabolized by similar enzymatic machinery). Unlike fentanyl, there does *not* appear to be a cumulative effect seen with longer infusions because of this unique metabolism. Organ dysfunction does not appear to alter the metabolism of this drug (15). The clearance of remifentanil is reduced by about 25% in the elderly, according to the product information.

This drug produces respiratory depression, hypotension, bradycardia, and hypertonus of skeletal muscle; the rigidity produced by this drug can make ventilation by mask difficult or impossible. The administration of propofol or a paralytic agent prior to the administration of remifentanil can attenuate the skeletal rigidity seen with the drug. In studies where fentanyl, 1 mcg/kg iv was compared to 0.5-1 mcg/kg iv of remifentanil, hypotension occurred somewhat more often with fentanyl (14-16). Peak hemodynamic effects of remifentanil are seen within 3 to 5 minutes after the administration of a single bolus, and hemodynamic effects are dose-dependent.

It has been shown that when large doses of remifentanil are administered intraoperatively, patients develop acute opioid tolerance. Tolerance occurs more quickly in response to shorter-acting narcotics such as remifentanil and alfentanil. In fact, profound tolerance can be documented after 90 minutes of remifentanil administration to volunteers. However, it also appears that the administration of large doses of opioids can also produce delayed hyperalgesia, suggesting a central sensitization that reduces the threshold to receptive fields. In support of this, the administration of NMDA receptor antagonists before the administration of large doses of opioids can block the hyperalgesia that can be induced by heroin or fentanyl.

Etomidate

Etomidate exists as 2 isomers, but only the + isomer is active; etomidate is R- (+)-ethyl-1-(α-methylbenzyl)-1H-imidazole-5-carboxylate. It is formulated as a 2-mg/mL solution in 35% propylene glycol. The propylene glycol is irritating to veins, and etomidate should not be mixed with other intravenous solutions. Etomidate had been utilized in critical care units throughout the world because of its characteristics, including its minimal hemodynamic effects, minimal respiratory depression ,and cerebral protective effects. However, etomidate causes a dose-dependent, temporary, and reversible inhibition of steroid synthesis after a single dose or after an infusion (16). Other side effects that discourage its use include nausea and vomiting due to activation of the nausea center (concurrent administration of fentanyl increases the incidence), pain on injection, superficial thrombophlebitis 48-72

hours after injection, and myoclonus. Etomidate appears to enhance the neuromuscular blockade of nondepolarizing paralytic agents (17). Nonetheless, etomidate continues to be utilized as it causes minimal hemodynamic perturbations when small doses are administered.

The liver metabolizes etomidate, and its main metabolites are inactive. Doses of etomidate that have been utilized are 0.2-0.6 mg/kg; this dose can be decreased if narcotics and/or benzodiazepines are also administered. After 0.3 mg/kg, the effect is seen within the time that it takes the drug to circulate to the brain; redistribution is the mechanism that terminates the effects of a bolus of etomidate. Hepatic dysfunction does not appear to alter the rapid recovery from the hypnotic effects of etomidate (17-18). The elimination half-life of the drug is 2.9-5.3 hours (17). In the elderly, the elimination clearance and volume of the central compartment are both decreased, causing a higher blood concentration from a given dose (18).

Etomidate affects transmission at $GABA_A$ receptors and may increase the number of $GABA_A$ receptors (12). Etomidate causes hypnosis and does not have analgesic activity. Etomidate has minimal effects on ventilation; in fact, etomidate can produce a brief period of hyperventilation, which can be followed by apnea (17-18). Hiccups and coughing may also be seen after etomidate administration. After the administration of 0.3 mg/kg to patients, there is almost no change in heart rate, mean arterial pressure, mean pulmonary artery pressure, central venous pressure, stroke volume, or cardiac index (17-18). Etomidate does not affect the sympathetic nervous system or baroreceptor function.

Propofol

Propofol, 2,6,-diisopropylphenol, is formulated as a 1% aqueous emulsion, containing 10% soybean oil, 2.25% glycerol, and 1.2% egg phosphatide (19). EDTA has recently been added to propofol in an attempt to discourage bacterial growth; propofol has been found to be the drug most frequently contaminated by bacteria. An ampule of the drug should only be utilized for 1 patient; great care should be taken when the drug is used for infusions so that bacterial contamination does not occur.

The effects of propofol 2.5 mg/kg are seen within the time it takes for the drug to circulate to the brain. The duration of the hypnosis is 5-10 minutes after a bolus injection; redistribution and elimination terminate the effects of propofol. Propofol has no analgesic activity but has some antiemetic properties. The clearance of propofol cannot be explained by hepatic clearance alone; there appears to be extrahepatic sites of elimination. The clearance of propofol is extremely rapid, and the recovery from propofol remains rapid even after prolonged infusions (17). The pharmacokinetics of propofol in patients age 65 years and older reveal that the elimination clearance is slower, but that plasma concentrations appeared similar to those of younger patients (18).

Propofol causes a dose-dependent hypotension that is very similar or somewhat greater than the hypotension produced by the administration of thiopental. Propofol causes vasodilation and myocardial depression (19). The hypotensive effects of this drug can be more exaggerated in elderly patients and in patients who have poor cardiac function (17-19). Propofol causes respiratory depression; initially, an increase in respiratory rate is seen for about 30 seconds and then apnea occurs. Airway reflexes are depressed, and propofol prophylactically attenuates induced bronchoconstriction by depression of neurally induced bronchoconstriction (17, 20). Propofol does not affect resting airway tone, nor has it been utilized in asthmatics to treat acute bronchoconstriction (19, 20).

Side effects produced by propofol include intense dreams and disinhibition, dystonic or choreoform movements, pain at the injection site, phlebitis, hyperlipidemia, and pancreatitis.

Ketamine

Ketamine, a phencyclidine derivative, is unique among the intravenous agents in that it causes analgesia as well as amnesia. The drug does not necessarily cause a loss of consciousness, but the patient is not aware; the drug appears to cause a dissociative state by electrophysiologic inhibition of the thalamocortical pathways and stimulation of the limbic system (20-22). The drug is a racemic mixture of 2 optical enantiomers; the S(+) ketamine has approximately 4-fold greater affinity at phencyclidine binding sites on the NMDA receptor than does the R(-) ketamine. The S(+) ketamine appears to allow the use of significantly smaller doses, faster recovery, and possibly fewer side effects. The compound will be in use in Europe (20-22).

Doses of 0.1-0.5 mg/kg of ketamine have analgesic action and can be utilized before the onset of pain for effective preemptive analgesia. Ketamine has an elimination half-life of 3 hours. Recovery from an induction dose (0.5-1.5 mg/kg) is from redistribution from its receptor. Ketamine causes amnesia, altered short-term memory, decreased ability to concentrate, altered cognitive performance, nightmares, nausea, and vomiting. Thus, it is common practice to administer small doses of benzodiazepine with ketamine; this practice does prolong recovery from ketamine.

Ketamine directly stimulates the autonomic nervous system, releases catecholamines and steroids, and causes tachycardia and increases blood pressure. If a patient cannot release catecholamines (i.e., is critically ill or has autonomic nervous system blockade), then ketamine administration can cause vasodilation and myocardial depression (20-22). Data regarding ketamine in the elderly are lacking; the emergence phenomena and dysphoria ketamine causes may be difficult for the elderly, particularly if the baseline mental status is not normal (20-22).

Ketamine is a useful agent for patients with airway diseases in that it attenuates neurally-induced bronchoconstriction (20). It also has a small direct effect on smooth muscle activation; however, it is unclear whether it can be utilized to improve asthma attacks. Ketamine administration will decrease the neurally-induced bronchoconstriction that occurs with airway manipulation during intubation.

Table 3. Properties of muscle relaxants used in the ICU

Drug	Initial Dose[a] (mg/kg)	Duration[b] (min)	Cost Factor[c]	Advantages	Complications
Pancuronium	0.07–0.1	60–120	1	Inexpensive	Tachycardia; active metabolite
Pipecuronium	0.05–0.07	60–120	5	CVS stability	Active metabolite
Doxacurium	0.04–0.05	60–120	5	CVS stability	None
Vecuronium	0.1	30–45	20	CVS stability	Active metabolite
Atracurium	0.05	30–45	20	Reliable recovery	Histamine release; active metabolite
Rocuronium	0.6–1.2	30–90	20	Rapid onset	None
Cisatracurium	0.1–0.2	30–90	10	Reliable recovery	Slow onset; active metabolite
Mivacurium	0.2	10–20	N/A	Short duration	Histamine release; metabolites
Succinylcholine	1–2	5–10	N/A	Fast onset; fast recovery	Hyperkalemia; dysrhythmia

CVS, cardiovascular system; N/A, not recommended for long-term use.

For tracheal intubation; [b]time from intubation dose until first Train-of-Four response might return; [c]numbers are multiples of the cost of pancuronium, which is ~ $10/day.

Reproduced with permission from Caldwell JE, Miller RD: Muscle relaxants in the intensive care unit. *Hospital Physician* 1996; 32:14

Midazolam

Midazolam is a water-soluble benzodiazepine that has the notable property of causing antegrade amnesia in conscious patients. Midazolam has an elimination half-life of 2.7 hours (compared to 46.6 hours for diazepam) (17-18). In the elderly, the elimination half-life is longer and elimination clearance decreases (17-18). Drug effects are terminated by redistribution, suggesting that pharmacodynamic changes in the elderly cause the prolonged effects seen in this age group (17-18).

After doses of 0.05-0.2 mg/kg of midazolam iv, tidal volumes will decrease by 40%, but minute ventilation remains unchanged (17-18). However, after slightly larger doses, apnea is seen. When opioids and midazolam are administered together, respiratory depression is assured, as midazolam decreases the tidal volume and the opioids will decrease the respiratory rate. In patients with chronic obstructive airways disease and in patients with altered respiratory drives, more prolonged and more profound respiratory depression has been noted (17-18).

Midazolam causes more hypotension than etomidate; when given to patients with normal cardiovascular function, small decreases in blood pressure and increases in heart rate are seen. When midazolam was given to patients who had valvular heart disease, some impairment of cardiac function was seen; when it was utilized for cardiac catheterization in patients with coronary artery disease, these patients experienced approximately a 15% decrease in their mean arterial pressures (17-18). When patients have significant cardiac dysfunction or are hypovolemic, midazolam will depress cardiovascular function and has been associated with fatalities.

Unlike propofol, ketamine, or etomidate, midazolam will take longer for its peak effect on the central nervous system. The drug takes approximately 5 minutes to achieve its peak effect; recovery of normal central nervous function takes about 20 minutes after 1 dose (17-18). However, in the elderly, prolonged amnesia even during the recovery period may occur (17-18).

Midazolam and the other benzodiazepines, except for lorazepam (ativan) or temazepam (restoril), have been noted to interact with protease inhibitors including ritonavir (Norvir™), indinavir (Crixivan™), nelfinavir (Viracept™), and saquinavir (Invirase™). The interaction involves the inhibition of P-450 –3A enzyme that metabolizes many of the benzodiazepines. Therefore, the levels of the benzodiazepines can be increased and cause prolonged amnesia and sedation (23). There is now a warning on the protease inhibitors to avoid the administration of the above benzodiazepines to patients who are taking protease inhibitors. The warning also exists for meperidine, fentanyl, codeine, and hydromorphone, levels of which are also increased by the protease inhibitors (23).

INTRODUCTION TO MUSCLE RELAXANTS

Muscle relaxants are utilized for several reasons, including to: facilitate endotracheal intubation, facilitate mechanical ventilation, reduce elevated intracranial pressure, reduce work of breathing, reduce spasms associated with tetanus, and to reduce movement associated with status epilepticus (24). Short-term use is considered < 2 days, because complications have not been reported with administration for < 2 days (24). Complications associated with muscle relaxants include anaphylaxis, hyperkalemia associated with succinylcholine administration (seen in patients with burns, neurologic injury, muscle trauma, long-term immobilization, or elevated serum potassium), inadequate ventilation of paralyzed patients, inadequate analgesia and sedation of paralyzed patients, and persistent weakness after long-term use (24-25). Persistent weakness occurs in about 20% of patients who receive muscle relaxants for > 6 days and in up to 70% of patients who are receiving steroids as well as receiving muscle relaxants (24). Risk factors for prolonged weakness include vecuronium in female patients who have renal failure, high-dose steroids, and > 2-day duration of relaxant administration and administration of high doses of muscle relaxants.

There appear to be several etiologies to the persistent weakness. The persistent weakness may be due to persistent paralysis. Vecuronium has an active metabolite, 3-desacetyl vecuronium, which persists particularly in female patients with renal failure. Pancuronium and pipecuronium also form these metabolites. Therefore, these drugs should not chronically be administered to patients who are in renal failure.

Patients on corticosteroids who receive long-term muscle relaxants appear to develop a myopathic syndrome characterized by flaccid paralysis, increased creatine kinase, and myonecrosis; these patients recover after many months. Plasma creatine kinase concentrations appear to increase when the myopathy develops; therefore, serum creatine kinase should be monitored in patients on corticosteroids who are receiving muscle relaxants. All muscle relaxants have been associated with this syndrome.

A motor neuropathy has been reported after the administration of vecuronium, pancuronium, or atracurium. The neuropathy affects all extremities, is associated with absent tendon reflexes, and can be accompanied by muscle wasting. This syndrome also takes months to resolve. Another syndrome consisting of persistent motor weakness but with preservation of sensory sensation has been reported in patients receiving pancuronium, vecuronium, or metocurine. These patients do not have normal neuromuscular transmission, and their symptoms also took months to resolve.

Patients do become tolerant to the effects of the muscle relaxants. The tolerance can develop within 24–48 hours and appears to be due to upregulation of acetylcholine receptors secondary to chronic denervation. One method to decrease the incidence of tolerance is to minimize the amount of muscle relaxant given; the drug should only be given for a defined clinical outcome. The only reason to monitor the Train-of-Four method is to document that complete block is not obtained, as the presence of a Train-of-Four response does not ensure that persistent weakness will not occur.

Comparison of Muscle Relaxants

For rapid tracheal intubations, either succinylcholine or rocuronium (Table 3) should

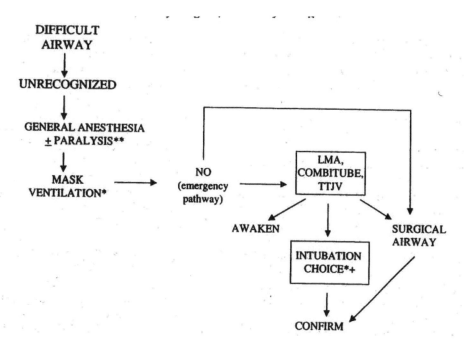

*Always <u>consider</u> calling for help (e.g., technical, medical, surgical, etc.) when difficulty with mask ventilation and/or tracheal intubation is encountered
**Consider the need to preserve spontaneous ventilation
+ Nonsurgical tracheal intubation choices of laryngoscopy with a rigid laryngoscope blade (many types), blind orotracheal or nasotracheal technique, fiberoptic/stylet technique, retrograde technique, illuminating stylet, rigid bronchoscope, percutaneous dilational tracheal entry. See Reference 3 for a complete discussion of these TI choices.

Figure 1. Difficult airway algorithm. Reproduced with permission from Benumof JL: Laryngeal mask airway and the ASA Difficult airway algorithm. *Anesthesiology* 1996; 84:687

be administered. Succinylcholine only lasts for 5-10 minutes, which can be helpful if there is concern that the patient's trachea cannot be intubated. Succinylcholine has several significant side effects, including bradycardia, junctional arrhythmias, ventricular arrhythmias, masseter spasm, and muscle pains. Rocuronium is the first nondepolarizing muscle relaxant that has a fast onset similar to succinylcholine; however, paralysis will persist for up to 90 minutes, thus mask ventilation and/or tracheal intubation must be successful.

Vecuronium has active metabolites that have been associated with persistent weakness, particularly in female patients with renal failure. Rocuronium does not have active metabolites. Atracurium and cisatracurium are utilized because their duration of action is not affected by liver or kidney disease. Cisatracurium's duration of action is as long, if not longer than,

that of rocuronium. All muscle relaxants have been associated with allergic reactions. In fact, muscle relaxants are the leading cause of perioperative anaphylaxis (succinylcholine is associated with 48% of the cases) (25). A recent report of cisatracurium-induced anaphylaxis documented that cardiovascular collapse can be the only sign of the allergic reaction (25).

AIRWAY MANAGEMENT

When one needs to emergently secure an airway, there are certain principles to remember: oxygenation even without removal of carbon dioxide can save the patient's life, and the complete inability to oxygenate will cause brain damage within 3 minutes. Therefore, as long as a needle can be placed in the trachea and oxygen can be given, the patient can be kept alive until a surgical airway can be obtained.

Percutaneous kits are available to perform emergency cricothyroidotomies; the operator must be able to complete the procedure in < 3 minutes, and preferably the procedure should be completed within 1 minute.

If a patient is not actively vomiting or otherwise soiling the airway, then mask ventilation should be attempted. Successful mask ventilation can require 2 or more hands, and an oral and/or nasal airway. Mask ventilation is all that is required if aspiration is not a risk and the operator is not expert at tracheal intubation. The complications of mask ventilation include damage to the eyes, insufflation of the stomach, and possible regurgitation.

Intubation of the trachea can be done via conventional laryngoscopy; this procedure requires practice. A laryngeal mask can be placed at the patient's glottic opening by pushing it into the patient's mouth and down the pharynx; proper placement of the laryngeal mask may require less practice and training than conventional laryngoscopy. The laryngeal mask does not protect against aspiration, but has been utilized in patients whose tracheas cannot be intubated using conventional laryngoscopy. Operators with expertise in tracheal intubation may encounter patients where conventional laryngoscopy is unsuccessful. An algorithm is then to be followed; depending on the status of the patient, either the procedure is aborted or a surgical airway is obtained (Figure 1) (26).

Situations where conventional laryngoscopy may be difficult include restriction of the oral airway, reduced pharyngeal space, noncompliant submandibular tissue, limited atlanto-occipital extension, and partial airway obstruction. Small mouth openings are encountered in patients who have temporomandibular joint disease, scarring near the mouths, congenital and surgical deformities, large tongues, and diseased teeth. The pharyngeal space can be decreased by edema and by masses. The submandibular tissue can be altered by infection (Ludwig's angina), by scarring as from burns, by surgery, by radiation, and by cancer. Patients who cannot extend their necks include patients in a Halo-jacket, those with ankylosing spondylitis, cervical disc disease, or cervical spinal injuries. Airway obstruction occurs when there is epiglotitis, pedunculated tumors and cysts in the airways, large tonsils, mediastinal and subcutaneous emphysema, or edema is present.

SUGGESTED READINGS

1. Nelson BJ, Weinert CR, Bury CL, et al: Intensive care unit drug use and subsequent quality of life in acute lung injury patients. *Crit Care Med* 2000; 28:3626-3630
    An assessment of the correlation between posttraumatic stress disorders and the quantity of sedation received by 24 (out of 36) patients who were discharged from the hospital and filled out their postdischarge questionnaires.

2. Brook AD, Ahrens TS, Schaiff R, et al: Effect of a nursing-implemented sedation protocol on the duration of mechanical ventilation. *Crit Care Med* 1999; 27:2609-2615
    Documents that the use of a protocol for sedation reduced the duration of mechanical ventilation, the intensive care unit and hospital lengths of stay, and the need for tracheostomies in patients who had acute respiratory failure.

3. Kress JP, Pohlman AS, O'Connor MR, et al: Daily interruption of sedative infusions in critically ill patients undergoing mechanical ventilation. *N Engl J Med* 2000; 343:1471-1477
    The daily interruption of the infusions of sedatives and narcotics decreased the quantity of drugs administered and decreased the length of stay in the ICU as well as the duration of mechanical ventilation.

4. Cook DJ, Walter SD, Cook RJ, et al: Incidence of and risk factors for ventilator-associated pneumonia in critically ill patients. *Ann Intern Med* 1998; 129:433-440
    Described the variables associated with the development of ventilator-associated pneumonia. Notably the administration of sedation and paralytic drugs was found more frequently in patients who developed nosocomial pneumonia.

5. Rotondi AJ, Chelluri L, Sirio C, et al: Patient's recollections of stressful

experiences while receiving prolonged mechanical ventilation in an intensive care unit. *Crit Care Med* 2002; 30:746-752

A 32-item questionnaire was used to collect data on patients' stressful psychological and physical experiences. Out of 817 patients, 100 patients survived and could remember their ICU experiences, whereas 50 survived and could not remember their experiences.

6. Inouye SK, Bogardus ST, Charpentier PA, et al: A multicomponent intervention to prevent delirium in hospitalized older patients. *N Engl J Med* 1999; 340:669-676

Describes interventions that can be done in the hospital that decrease the incidence of delirium in elderly medical patients.

7. Silverstein JH, Bloom HG, Cassel CK: Geriatrics and anesthesia. *Clin Anesthesiol* 1999; 17:8-12

A review of the changes in the elderly, with emphasis on changes in the drugs in the elderly.

8. Volles DF, McGory R: Pharmacokinetic considerations. *Crit Care Clin* 1999; 15:55-75

Review of opioids and the effects of liver and kidney disease on the drugs metabolisms.

9. Cammarano WB, Wiener-Kronish JP: Analgesics, tranquilizers and sedatives. *In:* Cardiac Intensive Care. First Edition. Brown DL (Ed). Philadelphia, WB Saunders, 1998, pp 591-602

Chapter on narcotics and sedatives commonly utilized in coronary care unit.

10. Cammarano WB, Pittet J-F, Weitz S, et al: Acute withdrawal syndrome related to the administration of analgesic and sedative medications in adult intensive care unit patients. *Crit Care Med* 1998; 26:676-684

A retrospective study of patients in the intensive care unit who met the criteria of withdrawl and the quantities of drug they received.

11. Lowson SM, Sawh S: Adjuncts to analgesia; sedation and neuromuscular blockade. *Crit Care Clin* 1999; 15:119-137

Review of the use of sedation, neuromuscular blockade and antidepressants in the ICU.

12. Bailey PL, Stanley TH: Intravenous opioid anesthetics. *In:* Anesthesia. Fourth Edition. Miller RD (Ed). New York, Churchill Livingstone, 1994, pp 291-388

Chapter on narcotics utilized in both the operating room and in intensive care units.

13. Ornstein E, Matteo RS: Effects of opioids. *In:* Geriatric Anesthesiology. First Edition. McLeskey CH (Ed). Baltimore, Williams & Wilkins, 1997, pp 249-260

Chapter on the effect of aging on the metabolism of opioids.

14. Peng PWH, Sandler AN: A review of the use of fentanyl analgesia in the management of acute pain in adults. *Anesthesiology* 1999; 90:576-99

A review of the pharmacology and uses of fentanyl.

15. Egan TD, Lemmens HJM, Fiset P, et al: The pharmacokinetics of the new short-acting opioid remifentanil in healthy adult male volunteers. *Anesthesiology* 1993; 79:881-892

The description of the characteristics of remifentanil in healthy men.

16. Song D, Whitten CW, White PF: Use of remifentanil during anesthetic induction: A comparison with fentanyl in the ambulatory setting. *Anesth Analg* 1999; 88:734-736

Compares the effects of fentanyl to remifentanil.

17. Reves JG, Glass PSA, Lubarsky DA: Nonbarbiturate intravenous anesthetics. *In:* Anesthesia. Fourth Edition. Miller RD (Ed). New York, Churchill Livingstone, 1994, pp 291-388

Chapter on drugs utilized for intubations in both the operating room and in intensive care units.

18. Fragen RJ: Effects of barbiturates, benzodiazepines, and other intravenous agents. *In:* Geriatric Anesthesiology. First Edition. McLeskey CH (Ed). Baltimore, Williams & Wilkins, 1997, pp 249-260

Chapter on the effect of aging on the metabolism of these intravenous drugs.

19. Smith I, White PF, Nathanson M, et al: Propofol-an update on its clinical use. *Anesthesiology* 1994; 81:1005-1043

A review of the pharmacology and uses of propofol.

20. Brown RH, Wagner EM: Mechanisms of bronchoprotection by anesthetic induction

agents. Propofol versus ketamine. *Anesthesiology* 1999; 90:822-828
Investigation in sheep of the mechanisms of bronchoprotection of ketamine and propofol.

21. Eames WO, Rooke GA, Sai-Chuen Wu R, et al: Comparison of the effects of etomidate, propofol and thiopental on respiratory resistance after tracheal intubation. *Anesthesiology* 1996; 84:1307-1311
Seventy-five patients were induced with 1 of these drugs, and respiratory resistance was measured.

22. Kohrs R, Durieux ME: Ketamine: Teaching an old drug new tricks. *Anesth Analg* 1998; 87:1186-1193
Review of ketamine and its possible neuroprotective effects.

23. Flexner C: Drug therapy: HIV protease inhibitors. *N Engl J Med* 1998; 338:1281-1292
A review of the protease inhibitors utilized in HIV patients.

24. Caldwell JE, Miller RD: Muscle relaxants in the intensive care unit. *Hospital Physician* 1996; 32:11-24
A review of muscle relaxants and their use in the intensive care unit.

25. Toh KW, Deacock SJ, Fawcett WJ: Severe anaphylactic reaction to cisatracurium. *Anesth Analg* 1999; 88:462-464
A case report and discussion regarding allergic reactions to muscle relaxants.

26. Benumof JL: Laryngeal mask airway and the ASA difficult airway algorithm. *Anesthesiology* 1996; 84:686-699
A review of the use of the laryngeal mask when faced with patients who have difficult airways.

PAIN, DELIRIUM, AND ISCHEMIA IN THE PERIOPERATIVE PERIOD

Jeanine P. Wiener-Kronish, MD, FCCP

Objectives

- To review the JCAHO requirements regarding Pain Management Standards
- To review the scientific concepts regarding pain, and to learn indications and complications of epidural and intrathecal narcotics
- To review concepts regarding delirium and concepts regarding preventive interventions
- To review concepts regarding perioperative myocardial ischemia and postoperative infarction

Key Words: pain, delirium, postoperative care, ischemia, infarction

JCAHO PAIN MANAGEMENT STANDARDS

The Joint Commission on Accreditation of Healthcare Organizations (JCAHO) has issued 6 new standards. The deadline for implementation of these standards was January 2001. These standards are: a) recognition of the right of individuals to appropriate assessment and management of pain, b) assessment of pain as well as the nature and the intensity of pain in all patients, c) establishment of policies and procedures that support the appropriate prescribing or ordering of effective pain medications, d) education of patients and families about effective pain management, e) addressing the individual's needs for symptom management in the discharge planning process, and f) integration of pain management into the organization's performance measurement and improvement program.

The hospital will have to demonstrate its commitment to pain management. For example, signs should be posted stating that "as a patient in this hospital, you can expect: a) to receive information about pain and pain relief measures, b) treatment by concerned staff committed to pain prevention and management, c) a quick response to your reports of pain, d) your reports of pain will be believed, e) state-of-the-art pain management, and f) dedicated pain-relief specialists."

NEW CONCEPTS REGARDING PAIN

Physiological pain is initiated by specialized sensory nociceptor fibers that are in peripheral tissues; these fibers are only activated by noxious stimuli. The sensory inflow generated by these nociceptors activates neurons in the spinal cord, which get to the cortex via a relay in the thalamus. However, there is plasticity to the system in that repeated stimuli of the nociceptors can cause progressive increases in the response. Therefore, pain is not a passive consequence of the transfer of a defined peripheral input to a pain center in the cortex, but an active process generated partly in the periphery and partly within the CNS by multiple plastic changes that can affect the gain in the system (1).

Gender Differences in Opioid-Mediated Analgesia

Opioids appear to be more effective analgesics for female patients than men. Females have reported greater pain relief from kappa opioid agonists after dental surgery. Furthermore, a review of investigations of patient-controlled analgesia documents that males consumed more opioids, suggesting that opioids may be less effective in men than in women. There is also vast literature documenting sex differences in pain perception. Much more investigation is needed prior to making definitive statements about gender differences in analgesia.

Chronic Pain

Often, patients in the ICU have underlying malignancies or other conditions that are associated with chronic pain. The ICU healthcare practitioner must be aware that different strategies need to be utilized when treating chronic pain conditions in comparison to acute pain, and that a pain-free state may not be achievable in these patients. The assessment of chronic pain should include a psychosocial evaluation, and treatment usually requires multimodal therapy, including medications of several different types. Antidepressants, membrane-stabilizing agents, and nonsteroidal anti-inflammatory drugs have been to shown to be useful in the management of patients with chronic pain. Also, neuroblockade and neuroaugmentation techniques have been shown to be of use in these patients (2, 3). Recently, intrathecal methylprednisolone was documented as an effective therapy for postherpetic neuralgia (4). Furthermore, gabapentin has been documented as a successful treatment of diabetic neuropathy, postherpetic neuralgia, and reflex sympathetic dystrophy (5). Thus, the treatment and management for chronic pain syndromes are quite different from acute pain due to surgery or due to a procedure. Patients who have chronic pain and are critically ill will need different drugs and different treatment modalities.

Postoperative Pain and Pain Relief

Pain is the outcome of an extremely complex process involving neurotransmitters and neuromodulators at all levels of the neuraxis; pain is an integration of noxious stimuli, affective traits, and cognitive factors (6). Several investigations in experimental animals and in patients have documented that pre-emptive analgesia improves the quality of postoperative pain management (7). Pre-emptive analgesia can decrease the sensitization of the central nervous system that would ordinarily amplify subsequent nociceptive input; preemptive analgesia requires the administration of local anesthesia or other pain medication prior to the development of pain (8). Patients who have more severe pain preoperatively will require larger quantities of pain medication perioperatively than patients who deny pain or have infrequent pain preoperatively (9).

The choices for pharmacologic postoperative pain relief therapy for hospitalized patients include the administration of nonsteroidal anti-inflammatory medications, the administration of narcotic or narcotic-like medications parentally into the epidural space or into the cerebrospinal fluid. The administration of nonsteroidal anti-inflammatory drugs can decrease the total dose of narcotic medication required for postoperative pain control. However, nonsteroidal anti-inflammatory drugs should not be administered to patients with renal insufficiency, or with a history of ulcer disease or with bleeding tendencies. Patients who have undergone craniotomies or major vascular surgery are therefore not considered good candidates for these medications.

The intrathecal administration of narcotics is not as popular as the administration of these medications into the epidural space because of the duration of the analgesia and the respiratory depression and headaches that can be associated with this procedure (10). Usually, only 1 dose of intrathecal opioid is given; thus, the duration of pain relief is a problem for some patients. After the administration of 0.5 to 1.0 mg of intrathecal morphine, 15 to 22 hours of analgesia has been reported (10, 11). Nonetheless, intrathecal opioids are now utilized for perioperative analgesia for cardiac surgeries, vascular surgeries, and hip surgeries, and patients receive parenteral narcotics if the spinal narcotic is insufficient for pain relief. Another reason intrathecal opioids have been underutilized is the fear of respiratory depression. The incidence of this event in a recent report was 3% of 6,000 patients (180 patients) who had received intrathecal preservative-free morphine, 0.2 - 0.8 mg, plus 25 mcg of fentanyl; none of the patients required intubation, and all of the patients responded to naloxone infusions without reversal of their analgesia (11). Pruritus (37% incidence) and nausea and vomiting (25% incidence) occurred at the same frequency that is seen after the administration of parenteral or epidural opioids (10-13). (Pruritus should be treated with naloxone, rather than diphenhydramine, as it is not due to histamine release). Finally, there is a

When neuraxial anesthesia (epidural/spinal anesthesia) or spinal puncture is employed, patients anticoagulated or scheduled to be anticoagulated with low molecular weight heparins or heaparinoids for prevention of thromboembolic complications are at risk for developing an epidural or spinal hematoma, which can result in long-term or permanent paralysis.

The risk of these events is increased by the use of indwelling epidural catheters for administration of analgesia or the concomitant use of drugs affecting hemostasis, such as nonsteroidal anti-inflammatory drugs (NSAID's), platelet inhibitors, or other anticoagulants. The risk also appears to be increased by traumatic or repeated epidural or spinal puncture.

Patients should be frequently monitored for signs and symptoms of neurological impairment. If neurological compromise is noted, urgent treatment is necessary. The physician should consider the potential benefit versus risk before neuraxial intervention in patients anticoagulated or to be anticoagulated for thromboprophylaxis (see also **WARNINGS, Hemorrhage, and PRECAUTIONS, Drug Interactions)**.

Figure 1. Warning on box of low-molecular-weight heparin.

fear of severe postdural puncture headaches that can require an epidural blood patch for relief. This complication and therapy occurred in 0.37% of 6,000 patients who received intrathecal opioids (10-13). However, the investigators admitted that intrathecal opioids were not offered to patients who had a history of frequent headaches.

One benefit of intrathecal opioids is the cost; the cost of intrathecal morphine or fentanyl is about one-third of the cost of these agents administered as epidural opioids (13). The administration of epidural opioids is associated with similar complications to the intrathecal administration of opioids. The incidence of dural puncture with epidurals ranges between 0.16% to 1.3%, and the incidence of headache in the group of patients that had a puncture is between 16% and 86% (12, 13). A unique complication to the epidural approach is the formation of epidural hematomas. The incidence of epidural hematomas appears to be very rare unless the patient is anticoagulated or has a coagulation disorder (13). There have been epidural hematomas reported in patients who have received low-molecular-weight heparin and then underwent placement of epidural catheters (14). There have been 3 separate national advisory panels on this issue, and warnings are now included in all packages of low-molecular-weight heparins (Figure 1). Because of these reports, guidelines have been generated; our local practice is to not place epidural catheters

for 12 hours after the last dose of low-molecular-weight heparin (14).

Epidural catheters can be placed at either the lumbar or thoracic vertebral level. The complications of placing epidural catheters at the thoracic level are comparable to the complications of lumbar catheter placement (12, 13). Thoracic epidurals with local anesthetics are usually utilized in patients undergoing thoracic or high abdominal operations, as they can give selective pain relief to these areas without affecting bowel function or lower extremity function. The placement of the epidural catheter farther away from the lumbar spinal segments providing the motor innervation to the lower extremities decreases the risk of their motor blockade (12, 13).

Local anesthetics and narcotics are often administered in combination via epidural catheters. Investigations have documented improved perioperative outcomes with this technique, including improved pulmonary function, decreased pulmonary complications, and decreased sedation (12, 13). Similarly, the administration of local anesthetics via an epidural catheter appears to reduce postoperative ileus, reduce the requirements of systemic opioids, and decrease the duration of hospitalization after abdominal surgery (12, 13). The local anesthetic appears to be the important agent in achieving these outcome benefits (12, 13). However, as local anesthetics have significant hemodynamic side effects that depend on the extent of the neural blockade and

Pain, Delirium, and Ischemia in the Perioperative Period
Diagnostic Criteria for Delirium
(Based on *Diagnostic and Statistical Manual of Mental Disorders*, Fourth Edition)

---

1. Disturbance of consciousness (that is, reduced clarity of awareness of the environment) in conjunction with reduced ability to focus, sustain, or shift attention

2. A change in cognition (such as memory deficit, disorientation, or language disturbance) or the development of a perceptual disturbance that is not better accounted for by a preexisting, established, or evolving dementia

3. Development of the disturbance – during a brief period (usually hours to days) and a tendency for fluctuation during the course of the day

4. Evidence from the history, physical examination, or laboratory findings that the disturbance is caused by

    a. A general medical condition
    b. A substance intoxication or side effect
    c. A substance withdrawal
    d. Multiple factors

Modified from the American Psychiatric Association by permission.

Figure 2. Diagnostic criteria for delirium (based on Diagnostic and Statistical Manual of Mental Disorders, Fourth Edition). Reproduced from Rummans TA, Evans JM, Krahn LE, et al: Delirium in elderly patients: Evaluation and management. *Mayo Clin Proc* 1995; 70:990

can cause motor blockade, which precludes postoperative ambulation; small doses of local anesthetic are administered in combination with opioids via the epidural catheters to obtain pain relief, minor nerve blockade, and to produce minimal side effects from both agents (15). For example, when given a solution of 0.05% ropivacaine (a new local anesthetic that causes less motor blockade than bupivicaine) and 1 mcg/mL fentanyl administered at 8 mL/hr via an epidural catheter, postoperative patients obtained optimal pain relief without motor blockade (15). It is important to note that patients are only allowed to ambulate with assistance when they are receiving these agents, and specific orders are required regarding additional pain medication.

POSTOPERATIVE ASSESSMENT

Postoperative patients remain in the hospital when they: a) have undergone procedures that require substantial therapy for pain, b) have lost a lot of blood or are bleeding, or c) cannot eat, drink, breathe, or think after the operation. In fact, the criteria for discharge after ambulatory surgery include stable vital signs, a stable mental status, the absence of severe pain, the ability to ambulate (if that was present preoperatively), evidence that urination is normal, and the ability to drink fluids.

Initial assessment of postoperative patients should include an assessment of the respiratory and cardiovascular systems. All patients are given supplemental oxygen in the immediate postoperative period; supplemental

Evaluation of Delirium

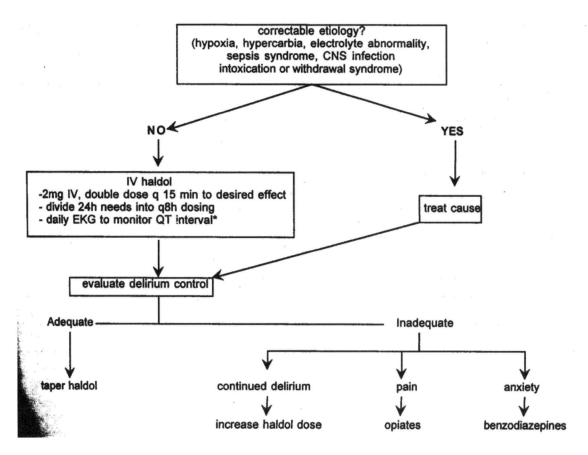

Figure 3. Diagram of the evaluation and treatment of delirium. Reproduced with permission from Gropper M, Wiener Kronish J: Postoperative care. *Dr. Wachter's Hospital Medicine,* In Press.

oxygen should be continued in all patients who have ongoing risks of hypoxemia. This risk exists in patients who have had surgeries of the thorax or upper abdomens, when receiving large doses of parenteral narcotics, or when lung disease or preexisting hypoxemia are present. Patients who have had central venous cannulation (or attempted cannulations) and patients who have had new tracheostomies, nephrectomies, or other operations in close proximity to the diaphragm should have a postoperative chest radiograph to exclude pneumothoraces.

Hypertension and hypotension are common in the immediate postoperative period. Hypotension is associated with blood or volume loss, and with perioperative myocardial ischemia or infarction. Serial hematocrits or hemoglobin

concentrations must be obtained and evidence of bleeding should be sought in all persistently hypotensive patients. An assessment of the patient's volume status may be required; comparisons of the volume of administered fluids to the volume of fluid lost or excreted must be done. The surgeons should be contacted early to discuss whether re-exploration may be required. Measurement of the patient's volume status may require the placement of either a central venous catheter or a pulmonary arterial catheter, depending on the underlying cardiac function or, in certain situations, by obtaining a cardiac echocardiogram. An electrocardiogram should be obtained when adult patients are hemodynamically unstable, and it should be compared to the preoperative cardiogram. Treatment should be initiated quickly;

RISK FACTORS FOR DELIRIUM AND INTERVENTION PROTOCOLS

TARGETED RISK FACTOR AND ELIGIBLE PATIENTS	STANDARDIZED INTERVENTION PROTOCOLS	TARGETED OUTCOME FOR REASSESSMENT
Cognitive impairment* All patients, protocol once daily; patients with base-line MMSE score of <20 or orientation score of <8, protocol three times daily	Orientation protocol: board with names of care-team members and day's schedule; communication to reorient to surroundings Therapeutic-activities protocol: cognitively stimulating activities three times daily (e.g., discussion of current events, structured reminiscence, or word games)	Change in orientation score
Sleep deprivation All patients; need for protocol assessed once daily	Nonpharmacologic sleep protocol: at bedtime, warm drink (milk or herbal tea), relaxation tapes or music, and back massage Sleep-enhancement protocol: unit-wide noise-reduction strategies (e.g., silent pill crushers, vibrating beepers, and quiet hallways) and schedule adjustments to allow sleep (e.g., rescheduling of medications and procedures)	Change in rate of use of sedative drug for sleep+
Immobility All patients; ambulation whenever possible, and range-of-motion exercises when patients chronically non-ambulatory, bed or wheelchair bound, immobilized (e.g., because of an extremity fracture or deep venous thrombosis), or when prescribed bed rest	Early-mobilization protocol: ambulation or active range-of-motion exercises three times daily; minimal use of immobilizing equipment (e.g., bladder catheters or physical restraints)	Change in Activities of Daily living score
Visual impairment Patients with <20/70 visual acuity on binocular near-vision testing	Vision protocol: visual aids (e.g., glasses or magnifying lenses) and adaptive equipment (e.g., large illuminated telephone keypads, large-print books, and fluorescent tape on call bell), with daily reinforcement of their use	Early correction of vision, ≤48 hr after admission
Hearing impairment Patients hearing ≤ 6 of 12 whispers on Whisper Test	Hearing protocol: portable amplifying devices, earwax disimpaction, and special communication techniques, with daily reinforcement of these adaptations	Change in Whisper Test score
Dehydration Patients with ratio of blood urea. nitrogen to creatinine>18, screened for protocol by geriatric nurse-specialist	Dehydration protocol: early recognition of dehydration and volume repletion (i.e., encouragement of oral intake of fluids)	Change in ratio of blood nitrogen to creatinine

*The orientation score consisted of results on the first 10 items on the Mini-Mental State Examination (MMSE). Sedative drugs included standard hypnotic agents, benzodiazepines, and antihistamines, used as needed for sleep.

Figure 4. Risk factors for delirium and intervention protocols.

crystalloid can be administered once several diagnoses have been excluded, including pulmonary edema, myocardial ischemia, and infarction (not including right-sided myocardial infarction).

Postoperative hypertension is associated with pain, volume overload, hypercarbia, acidosis, full bladder, preexisting hypertension, and agitation. Patients with essential hypertension have altered baroreflex control of heart rate and have circulatory instability perioperatively, with increased periods of hypertension and tachycardia (16). The mechanism for the increased perioperative circulatory lability in postoperative hypertensive patients may be due to sympathetic hyperactivity, reduced parasymapathetic responsiveness, or both (16). Hypertension should be treated perioperatively; severe hypertension should be treated with short-acting intravenous medications (i.e., esmolol or labetolol) that are utilized for hypertensive emergencies. More modest levels of hypertension can be treated with intravenous agents and/or by the administration of oral agents once the patient is stable.

Changes in mental status must be rapidly investigated. Confusion and agitation can reflect hypoxemia, myocardial ischemia, hypoglycemia, hyperglycemia, or other metabolic derangements, as well as cerebral insults (carotid occlusion, cerebral embolism, and subarachnoid or intracerebral hemorrhage). Mental status changes or agitation should *not* be attributed to the presence of an endotracheal tube or to pain without excluding these other diagnoses.

Perioperative Neurologic Complications

Postoperative delirium is commonly encountered; 14% to 56% of hospitalized patients develop delirium (17). The development of delirium is associated with increases in the length of hospitalization, increases in the requirements of institutionalization, and accounts for increased expenditures ($4 billion in 1994!) (17-22). Delirium, an acute confusional state (Figure 2), is usually caused by multiple factors; the patient often has 1 or more risk factors, and hospital-related insults lead to the development of delirium. Risk factors include age, cognitive impairment, poor functional status, abnormal preoperative electrolytes, noncardiac thoracic surgery, aortic aneurysm surgery, and alcohol ingestion (17-22). Conditions in the hospital that appear to be associated with the development of delirium include the use of physical restraints, use of bladder catheters, malnutrition, administration of > 3 medications, hypoxemia, electrolyte disturbances, renal failure, pain, infection, hypercarbia, patient restrictions, alcohol withdrawl, and the administration of benzodiazepines or meperidine (17-22). Elderly

patients are at extremely high risk for delirium given their illnesses and the routine care that occurs in critical care units. Many of the hospital activities associated with increased patient delirium are routinely practiced in ICUs, including the use of patient restraints, bladder catheterization, the administration of sedatives and psychoactive drugs, allowing naps and altering sleep patterns, loud noise levels day and night, and lack of physical exercise.

Benzodiazepines have pharmacokinetic and pharmacodynamic changes in the elderly that make their use problematic in this group. The half-life of diazepam increases to nearly 60 hours in patients age 70 years and older (19). Psychoactive drugs may have to be discontinued in delirious patients to determine the cause(s) of the state; haldol or short-acting opiates can be given to control the confusional state (Figure 3).

Recently, an intervention strategy was tested on elderly (> 70 years of age) hospitalized patients with risk factors for delirium to determine whether the interventions could decrease the episodes of delirium in these patients (17). The interventions included: board with names of care-team members, discussions of current events, word games, warm milk or herbal tea for sleep, decreasing noise on the ward, back massages and relaxation tapes, range-of-motion exercises, no physical restraints, magnifying lenses, portable amplifying devices, and encouragement of oral intake of fluid (Figure 4). There were 90 episodes of delirium in the control group and 62 episodes in the group of patients receiving the interventions; the control group had 161 days of delirium, whereas the experimental group had 105 days. Thus, the incidence of delirium was significantly lower in the intervention group than in the usual care group. There was also a significant reduction in the rate of use of sedative drugs for sleep in the intervention group compared to the usual care group. Finally, the cost of the intervention averaged $327/patient, and an estimated cost of intervention per case of delirium prevented was $6,341. This is similar to the estimated costs for prevention of a fall ($7,727-$11,834), or to the estimated costs to prevent a myocardial infarction ($19,800-$42,900) (17).

Perioperative strokes occur in 1% to 6% of patients undergoing cardiothoracic surgery. The risk factors for stroke include prior neurologic deficits, heart failure, carotid artery bruits, a diagnosis of chronic obstructive lung disease, and the development of atrial tachyarrhythmias (23). Another surgical procedure associated with perioperative strokes is carotid artery endarterectomy; the incidence of perioperative stroke depends on the frequency with which hospital staff performs this procedure (24). In hospitals where a benefit for endarterectomy has been found, the 5-year risk of stroke is 4.8% (compared to a 10.6 % risk in the medical group) (24). Evaluation for stroke should be considered when patients have a sudden change in mental status, there is a delay in awakening after anesthesia, or the patient has developed focal deficits. Urgent evaluation is mandatory to distinguish ischemic from hemorrhagic causes.

Perioperative Ischemia and Infarction

Cardiac morbidity is still the leading cause of death after surgery. Patients at major risk for perioperative ischemia and infarction include those who have unstable angina, decompensated congestive heart failure, significant arrhythmias, or who have severe valvular disease (25). Patients with an intermediate risk for cardiac events are those with stable angina, prior myocardial infarction, diabetes mellitus, or with compensated congestive heart failure (25). Other risk factors are considered "minor" and include advanced age, heart rhythm other than sinus, history of cerebrovascular event, uncontrolled hypertension, and low functional status (25). Drugs that decrease the risk for perioperative ischemia include atenolol and clonidine (26-28). Other drugs are under active investigation. Notably, beta-blockers have not been found to significantly increase airway resistance in patients with chronic obstructive lung disease, and should be given to such patients when they are at risk for ischemia or have had myocardial infarctions (29). Beta-blockers are contraindicated in patients with moderate or severe asthma.

Cardiac surgery and other surgeries release creatine kinase, thereby complicating the biochemical diagnosis of perioperative myocardial infarction. In cardiac surgery, not only is there release of skeletal muscle, there is some degree of myocardial injury from the procedures. Cardiac troponin I levels are routinely elevated after cardiac surgery to about 3 ng/mL without perioperative myocardial infarction. Therefore, higher levels (usually > 10 ng/mL) are necessary for the diagnosis of infarction after cardiac surgery.

SUGGESTED READINGS

1. Woolf CJ, Salter MW: Neuronal plasticity: Increasing the gain in pain. *Science* 2000; 288:1765-1768
   Reviews the new scientific discoveries regarding the plasticity of pain response.
2. Practice Guidelines for Chronic Pain Management. *Anesthesiology* 1997; 86:995-1004
   Practice guidelines for the practitioners involved with chronic pain management.
3. Levy MH: Pharmacologic treatment of cancer pain. *N Engl J Med* 1996; 335:1124-1132
   Review of choices for pain relief in cancer patients.
4. Kotani N, Kushikata T, Hashimoto H, et al: Intrathecal methylprednisolone for intractable postherpetic neuralgia. *N Engl J Med* 2000; 343:1514-1519
   A randomized controlled trial of intrathecal methylprednisolone compared to intrathecal lidocaine or no treatment for 4 weeks. The intrathecal treatment showed significant and long-lasting improvement in pain.
5. Mao J, Chen LL: Gabapentin in pain management. *Anesth Analg* 2000; 91:680-687
   A review of the efficacy of gabapentin treatment in the management of neuropathic pain.
6. Sidall PJ, Cousins MJ: Spinal pain mechanisms. *Spine* 1997; 22:98-104
   Review of spinal pain mechanisms.
7. Kundra P, Gurnani P, Bhattacharya A: Preemptive epidural morphine for postoperative pain relief after lumbar

laminectomy. *Anesth Analg* 1997; 85:135-138
Epidural morphine improves postoperative pain.

8. Gottschalk A, Smith DS, Jobes DR, et al: Preemptive epidural analgesia and recovery from radical prostatectomy. *JAMA* 1998; 279:1076-1082
Even in the presence of aggressive postoperative pain management, preemptive epidural analgesia significantly decreases postoperative pain during hospitalization and long after discharge.

9. Slappendel R, Weber EWG, Bugter MLT, et al: The intensity of preoperative pain is directly correlated with the amount of morphine needed for postoperative analgesia. *Anesth Analg* 1999; 88:146-148
Patients with severe preoperative pain require large quantities of pain medication perioperatively.

10. Gwirtz KH, Young JV, Byers RS, et al: The safety and efficacy of intrathecal opioid analgesia for acute postoperative pain. Seven years experience with 5,969 surgical patients at Indiana University Hospital. *Anesth Analg* 1999; 88:599-604
The report documents the safety and problems with giving intrathecal morphine and fentanyl for postoperative pain relief.

11. Chaney MA, Furry PA, Fluder EM, et al: Intrathecal morphine for coronary artery bypass grafting and early extubation. *Anesth Analg* 1997; 84:241-248
Describes the use of intrathecal morphine in cardiac surgery patients and how this technique does not delay extubation.

12. Ballantyne JC, Carr DB, deFerranti S, et al: The comparative effects of postoperative analgesic therapies on pulmonary outcome: Cumulative meta-analyses of randomized, controlled trials. *Anesth Analg* 1998: 86:598-612
A meta-analyses of randomized, control trials to assess the effects of analgesic therapies on postopreative pulmonary function.

13. Liu S, Carpenter RL, Neal JM: Epidural anesthesia and analgesia: Their role in postoperative outcome. *Anesthesiology* 1995; 82:1474-1498

Review of epidural anesthesia, and its influence on organ function and hospitalization.

14. Harlocker T, Wedel D: Spinal-epidural blockade and perioperative low molecular weight heparin; smooth sailing on the Titanic. *Anesth Analg* 1998; 86:1163-1166
Discusses the issue of epidural hematomas and low molecular weight heparin.

15. Liu SS, Moore JM, Luo AM, et al: Comparison of 3 solutions of ropivacaine/fentanyl for postoperative patient-controlled epidural analgesia. *Anesthesiology* 1999; 90:727-733
Discusses the new local anesthetic ropivacaine and the volume and concentration factors involved in epidural analgesia.

16. Parlow JL, Begou G, Sagnard P, et al: Cardiac baroreflex during the postoperative period in patients with hypertension. *Anesthesiology* 1999; 90:681-692
Investigation of perioperative heart rate control in hypertensive patients. Clonidine improves heart rate control, and therefore could prevent perioperative tachycardia and ischemia.

17. Inouye SK, Bogardus ST, Charpentier PA, et al: A multicomponent intervention to prevent delirium in hospitalized older patients. *N Engl J Med* 1999; 340:669-676
Describes interventions that can be done in the hospital that decrease the incidence of delirium in elderly medical patients.

18. Rummans TA, Evans JM, Krahn LE, et al: Delirium in elderly patients: Evaluation and management. *Mayo Clin Proc* 1995; 70:989-998
A review of the evaluation and management of delirium in the elderly.

19. Marcantonio ER, Juarez G, Goldman L, et al: The relationship of postoperative delirium with psychoactive medications *JAMA* 1994; 272:1518-1522
Nested case-control study of pscyhoactive medications and the development of delirium.

20. Marcantonio ER, Goldman L, Mangione CM, et al: A clinical prediction rule for delirium after elective noncardiac surgery. *JAMA* 1994; 271:134-139

A prospective cohort study to predict delirium after surgery.

21. Inouye SK, Charpentier PA: Precipitating factors for delirium in hospitalized elderly persons. *JAMA* 1996; 275:852-857
   Two prospective cohort studies in tandem to investigate the precipitating factors for delirium in medical patients.

22. Lynch EP, Lazor MA, Gellis J, et al: The impact of postoperative pain on the development of postoperative delirium. *Anesth Analg* 1998; 86:781-785
   Surgical patients were interviewed daily; higher levels of pain were associated with the development of delirium.

23. Roach GW, Kanchuger M, Mangano CM, et al: Adverse cerebral outcomes after coronary bypass surgery. *N Engl J Med* 1996; 335:1857-1863
   Prospective study of 2,108 patients undergoing cardiac surgery.

24. Caplan LR: Stroke treatment; promising but still struggling. *JAMA* 1998; 279:1304-1306
   Editorial regarding 3 reports of carotid endarterectomy trials.

25. Coley CM, Eagle KA: Preoperative assessment and perioperative management of cardiac ischemic risk in noncardiac surgery. *Curr Probl Cardiol* 1996; pp 294-382

A comprehensive review of preoperative cardiac risk assessment.

26. Mangano DT, Layug EL, Wallace A, et al: Effect of atenolol on mortality and cardiovascular morbidity after noncardiac surgery. *N Engl J Med* 1996; 335:1713-1720
   Prospective trial of atenolol documenting improvement in mortality.

27. Wallace A, Layug B, Tateo I, et al: Prophylactic atenolol reduces postoperative myocardial ischemia. *Anesthesiology* 1998; 88:7-17
   Further investigation into data on atenolol trial reveals decreased ischemia of the patients who lived longer.

28. Stuhmeier K-D, Mainzer B, Cierpka J, et al: Small, oral dose of clonidine reduces the incidence of intraoperative myocardial ischemia in patients having vascular surgery. *Anesthesiology* 1996; 85:706-712
   Two micrograms per kg of oral clonidine given 90 minutes prior to surgery was compared to placebo. Perioperative myocardial ischemic episodes were decreased.

29. Reynolds RJ, Burford JG, George RB: Using β-blockers safely in asthma and COPD patients. *J Respir Dis* 1982; 3:95-113
   Discusses the safe use of β-blockers in these patients.

POISONINGS AND OVERDOSE

Janice L. Zimmerman, MD, FCCP, FCCM

Objectives

- To describe physical examination and laboratory findings suggestive of specific poisons
- To outline general measures for the resuscitation and stabilization of the overdose patient
- To discuss indications and contraindications of interventions to decrease absorption of poisons from the gastrointestinal tract
- To describe indicated interventions and antidotes for poisons and substances of abuse that are likely to result in the need for ICU admission

Key Words: poisoning; substance abuse; toxicology; gastric lavage; charcoal; antidotes

TABLE OF ABBREVIATIONS

CNS   central nervous system
ECG   electrocardiogram
GHB   γ-hydroxybutyrate
GI   gastrointestinal
INH   isoniazid
NAC   N-acetylcysteine
SSRIs   selective serotonin reuptake inhibitors

Intentional and accidental poisonings and substance abuse frequently result in the need for critical care support. The critical care physician should possess the ability to predict and manage complications of known overdoses as well as to offer a differential diagnosis for patients in whom the toxic substance is unknown. In many cases, only supportive care is necessary until the effects of the toxin diminish. However, some poisonings require specific antidotes or interventions to decrease morbidity and mortality. The contribution of poisonings or substances of abuse to other critical illnesses must be recognized. General management principles of poisonings and substance abuse that are pertinent to intensive care management are presented, as well as interventions for specific overdoses that the intensivist is likely to encounter.

CLINICAL PRESENTATION

Patients with potential overdose may be asymptomatic or present with life-threatening toxicities. The absence of symptoms on initial examination does not preclude potential deterioration and development of more severe symptoms. Life-threatening toxicities that often require intensive management include coma, seizures, respiratory depression, hypoxemia, arrhythmias, hypotension, hypertension, and metabolic acidosis.

Diagnosis

The diagnosis of the exact substance involved in an overdose or poisoning should never take precedence over resuscitation and stabilization of the patient (see "Management"). However, the initial evaluation of the patient may identify characteristic signs and symptoms that will enable the physician to make a specific diagnosis quickly and assist in directing optimal therapy.

History

Information regarding the substance ingested, the quantity taken, and the time of ingestion should be accurately collected, if possible. Establishing the time of ingestion is important to assess the significance of presenting symptoms. It is important to discern what drugs the patient may be able to access, such as cardiac medications, antidepressants, etc.

Physical Examination

Vital signs and the neurologic examination are particularly helpful in the initial evaluation of a patient. Tables 1 and 2 list drugs associated with specific changes in vital signs and neurologic alterations. Of the vital signs, blood pressure is probably the least helpful in determining the specific poisoning agent. In many poisonings, hypotension may be the terminal manifestation of multisystem insufficiency. Tachypnea must also be regarded as fairly nonspecific and may result as a compensatory response to metabolic acidosis or hypoxemia due to pulmonary edema. Although the initial neurologic examination may be pertinent, it is also important to follow changes in neurologic function over time. Hypoactive bowel sounds may be associated with narcotic or anticholinergic agents and hyperactive bowel sounds may result from poisoning with organophosphates.

Table 1. Clues to diagnosis in poisoning: Vital signs

Vital Signs	Increased	Decreased
Blood pressure	Amphetamines/cocaine Anticholinergics Ephedrine Sympathomimetics	Antihypertensives Cyanide Cyclic antidepressants Ethanol Narcotics Organophosphates/carbamates Sedative/hypnotics
Heart rate	Amphetamines/cocaine Anticholinergics Carbon monoxide Cyanide Cyclic antidepressants Ethanol Sympathomimetics Theophylline	Barbiturates β-blockers Calcium channel blockers Cholinergics Digitalis glycosides Sedative/hypnotics Organophosphates/carbamates γ-hydroxybutyrate
Respiratory rate	Amphetamines Anticholinergics Hydrocarbons Carbon monoxide Organophosphates/carbamates Salicylates Theophylline	Alcohols Barbiturates Narcotics Sedative/hypnotics γ-hydroxybutyrate
Temperature	Amphetamines/cocaine Anticholinergics β-blockers Cyclic antidepressants Salicylates Sympathomimetics Theophylline	Barbiturates Carbon monoxide Ethanol Hypoglycemic agents Narcotics Sedative/hypnotics

Table 2. Clues to diagnosis in poisoning: Neurologic findings

Pupils	*Pinpoint (miotic)*	*Dilated (mydriatic)*
	Barbiturates (late)	Alcohol
	Cholinergics	Anticholinergics
	Narcotics (except meperidine)	Antihistamines
	Organophosphates	Barbiturates
	Phenothiazine	Ethanol
	Phencyclidine	Meperidine
		Phenytoin
		Sympathomimetics
Nystagmus	Alcohols	Phencyclidine
	Carbamazepine	Phenytoin
	Carbon monoxide	Sedative/hypnotics
Seizures	Amphetamines	Lithium
	Anticholinergics	Organophosphates
	Carbon monoxide	Phencyclidine
	Cocaine	Phenothiazines
	Cyanide	Salicylates
	Cyclic antidepressants	Strychnine
	γ-Hydroxybutyrate	Theophylline
	Isoniazid	

Table 3. Toxidromes

Poisoning Syndrome	Symptoms
Cholinergic (SLUDGE)	Salivation, lacrimation, urination, defecation, GI upset, emesis. Also, bradycardia, fasciculations, confusion, miosis
Anticholinergic	Dry skin, hyperthermia, mydriasis, tachycardia, delirium, thirst
Sympathomimetic	Hypertension, tachycardia, seizures, CNS excitation, mydriasis
Narcotic	Miosis, respiratory depression, depressed level of consciousness
Sedative/hypnotic	Depressed level of consciousness, respiratory depression, hyporeflexia

GI, gastrointestinal; CNS, central nervous system

Toxidromes

Findings on physical examination may enable the physician to characterize the poisoning into a classic "toxidrome." This categorization may allow the physician to direct diagnostic evaluation and define appropriate therapy (Table 3).

Laboratory Examination

Effective use of the laboratory may supplement the history and physical examination. An arterial blood gas measurement will detect hypoxemia, hypercarbia, and significant acid-base disorders in poisonings. In combination with electrolytes, a significant anion gap acidosis may be diagnosed. The detection of an osmolal gap (> 10) through comparison of the measured osmolality with calculated osmolality—[(2 x sodium + glucose/18) + (blood urea nitrogen/2.8)]—may indicate the presence of methanol, ethanol, ethylene glycol, acetone, or isopropyl alcohol.

An electrocardiogram (ECG) should be obtained in unstable patients and when cardiotoxic drug ingestion is suspected.

Qualitative toxicology screens are performed on urine samples. These tests report only the presence or absence of a substance and are limited by the testing available at an institution. Qualitative toxicology screens are helpful in evaluating coma of unknown cause, distinguishing between toxicosis and psychosis, and choosing a specific antidote (rarely). Qualitative test results seldom change the initial management of poisoned patients. Quantitative analyses provide serum levels and may direct specific therapies in selected cases. Quantitative levels that are particularly helpful in the patient with unknown poisoning are acetaminophen and salicylate levels. Other quantitative levels that may be useful include carbamazepine, carboxyhemoglobin, ethanol, methanol, ethylene glycol, theophylline, phenytoin, lithium, barbiturates, digoxin, and cyclic antidepressant levels. Although cyclic antidepressant levels are often the only measurements available to confirm antidepressant ingestion, the levels correlate poorly with toxicity.

MANAGEMENT
Resuscitation and Stabilization

The initial priorities are airway, breathing, and circulation ("ABCs"). Intubation may be necessary to support oxygenation and ventilation or to protect the airway. Hypotension from toxins is most commonly due to venous pooling, rather than myocardial depression, and should be initially treated with isotonic fluids, rather than vasopressor agents. High-flow oxygen should be routinely administered to the poisoning victim, pending assessment of oxygenation by arterial blood gas or pulse oximetry.

In the patient with depressed level of consciousness, the following additional interventions should be considered:

- 50% glucose (25 to 50 g)
- 100 mg of thiamine intravenously
- Naloxone (0.4 to 2 mg iv), especially with classic findings of miosis and respiratory depression

- Flumazenil—not routinely recommended; consider in patients who have a clinical course compatible with a sedative overdose. Flumazenil is contraindicated in known cyclic antidepressant overdoses and in chronic benzodiazepine users because of the risk of seizures.

Nonspecific Therapy

Following initial stabilization, nonspecific interventions are used to decrease absorption from the gastrointestinal (GI) tract or to enhance elimination. GI decontamination can be attempted with gastric emptying procedures (induced emesis, gastric lavage), adsorption of drugs (activated charcoal), and increasing transit through the GI tract (cathartics, whole bowel irrigation).

Induced Emesis. The use of induced emesis with ipecac is not recommended in adults. Ipecac is effective in inducing vomiting but is not necessarily effective in recovering toxins. Contraindications to the use of ipecac include hydrocarbon or corrosive ingestion, absent gag reflex, depressed mental status, a risk for central nervous system (CNS) depression or seizures, and pregnancy. At best, induced emesis eliminates ≤ 50% of the ingested toxin. Potential complications include aspiration pneumonitis, Mallory-Weiss tear, and protracted emesis, which delays the use of activated charcoal.

Gastric Lavage. Gastric lavage is performed in the adult with a 36- to 40-French Ewald tube inserted orally. Lavage is performed with aliquots of 100 to 200 mL of normal saline or water. Previous studies indicated that the greatest benefit of lavage in obtunded patients occurs within 1 hour of ingestion, but subsequent studies have failed to confirm any benefit. Current recommendations suggest that gastric lavage should not be employed routinely, and should be considered only in life-threatening ingestion when lavage can be instituted within 1 hour of ingestion. The airway must be protected in patients with depressed level of consciousness. Lavage is contraindicated in acid or alkali ingestions because of possible esophageal perforation and in the presence of a severe bleeding diathesis. Complications of lavage include aspiration pneumonitis, esophageal perforation, and cardiovascular instability.

Activated Charcoal. Activated charcoal is the single best intervention in poisonings and should be administered in most cases of orally ingested toxins. The greatest benefit is probably within the first hour after ingestion. The appropriate dose of charcoal (1 g/kg) may be administered by an orogastric or nasogastric tube if patient cooperation is limited. Substances not adsorbed by activated charcoal include iron, lithium, cyanide, strong acids or bases, alcohols, and hydrocarbons. The use of charcoal in acetaminophen poisoning has been questioned because of the potential absorption of the antidote N-acetylcysteine (NAC). In these cases, it is best to administer charcoal since many ingestions are multiple drug overdoses, and charcoal will adsorb acetaminophen. If a toxic ingestion of acetaminophen is confirmed, the charcoal slurry can be removed prior to the use of NAC. The only contraindication to the use of charcoal is known or suspected GI perforation.

Current recommendations for decreasing GI absorption of toxins emphasize the use of activated charcoal despite lack of proven benefit. In patients who are critically ill on hospital presentation or who have a potentially life-threatening ingestion, gastric lavage plus activated charcoal can be considered, although the benefit of lavage has not been established.

Cathartics. Cathartics are routinely administered with charcoal, based on the assumption that they decrease GI transit time, help limit drug absorption, and serve as a useful adjunct to charcoal therapy. However, there is no evidence of efficacy. Sorbitol is the most commonly used cathartic. Care must be taken with the very young and elderly patients because electrolyte abnormalities can ensue due to diarrhea.

Whole Bowel Irrigation. Whole bowel irrigation involves large volumes of polyethylene glycol electrolyte solution given over time (1 to 2 L/hr) to mechanically cleanse the bowel. This method has been recommended for ingested substances that are not well adsorbed by activated charcoal (i.e., iron and lithium), ingestions of sustained-release or enteric-coated products, and ingestions of illicit drug packets. In many cases, this method may not be practical; further study is required to identify any benefit in toxic ingestions. Contraindications to this intervention include ileus, GI obstruction or perforation, hemodynamic instability, and intractable vomiting; CNS or respiratory depression and inability to cooperate are relative contraindications.

Enhanced Elimination. Measures to increase elimination of toxic substances attempt to enhance the normal detoxification mechanisms performed by the liver and kidney. Multiple doses of charcoal for drugs with an enterohepatic circulation may have the greatest potential utility. This technique may be helpful in poisonings with barbiturates, carbamazepine, dapsone, and theophylline. Although multiple doses of charcoal have been used in poisonings with cyclic antidepressants, digoxin and phenytoin, proof of effectiveness is lacking. The dosing regimen has not been standardized, but currently not < 12.5 g/hr or an equivalent amount at other intervals is recommended. Smaller doses administered more frequently may decrease the occurrence of vomiting. Repeat doses of charcoal should not contain a cathartic. Care must be taken to ensure that adequate gastric emptying occurs before administration of a subsequent dose.

Forced diuresis to accelerate renal excretion of drugs has little clinical effect and may predispose the patient to volume overload. Alkaline diuresis is effective in promoting the elimination of barbiturates and salicylates. Two ampules of sodium bicarbonate can be added to 1 L of D5W solution, and the rate of administration should be determined by the patient's ability to handle the fluid load and the maintenance of urine pH > 7. Acidification of the urine has been proposed for ingestions involving phencyclidine, strychnine, amphetamines, and quinine. However, the metabolic consequences of acidification weigh against any clinical usefulness of this measure. Dialysis may be considered for ingestions involving water-soluble substances of low-molecular weight. Drug overdoses in which dialysis may be beneficial include alcohols, amphetamines, phenobarbital, lithium, salicylates, theophylline, and thiocyanate.

Table 4. Toxins and antidotes/antagonists

Toxin	Antidote
Acetaminophen	N-acetylcysteine
Arsenic/mercury/ gold/lead	BAL (dimercaprol)
Benzodiazepines	Flumazenil
β-blocker	Glucagon, calcium (?)
Calcium-channel blocker	Calcium, glucagon
Carbon monoxide	Oxygen, hyperbaric oxygen
Coumarin derivatives	Vitamin K_1
Cyanide	Nitrites, thiosulfate, hydroxocobalamin
Digoxin	Digoxin-specific Fab fragments
Ethylene glycol	Ethanol, fomepizole
Heparin	Protamine
Oral hypoglyemic agents/insulin	Glucose 50%, somatostatin
Iron	Deferoxamine
Isoniazid	Pyridoxine
Methanol	Ethanol, fomepizole
Narcotics	Naloxone
Nitrites	Methylene blue
Organophosphates/ carbamates	Atropine, pralidoxime

Hemoperfusion is useful with the same compounds that are dialyzable and involves the passing of blood through a filtering device that contains charcoal or a synthetic resin as an absorbent. Charcoal hemoperfusion may be helpful in elimination of carbamazepine, phenobarbital, phenytoin, and theophylline. Hemodialysis and hemoperfusion are efficient methods of removing poisons but are costly, require trained personnel, and may be associated with complications. Use of continuous arteriovenous or venovenous hemoperfusion in poisoning has been reported on a limited basis, but no data demonstrate an impact on outcome.

SPECIFIC THERAPY

Although management of many toxic ingestions involves only the nonspecific therapy outlined above, some toxins have specific interventions or antidotes. Table 4 lists toxins and their respective antidotes. Specific poisonings are discussed in detail below. Attention should be directed to managing those poisonings that most frequently result in death: analgesics; antidepressants; stimulants and street drugs; cardiovascular drugs; alcohols; and sedative and hypnotics.

SPECIFIC POISONINGS AND SUBSTANCES OF ABUSE
Acetaminophen

Although the intensivist is unlikely to care for a patient with a pure acute acetaminophen overdose, knowledge of appropriate management is important in multiple drug overdoses. Acetaminophen levels should be obtained in all multiple drug overdoses ≥ 4 hours after ingestion. Levels plotted on the Rumack-Matthew nomogram will suggest the need for NAC therapy (140 mg/kg oral loading dose; 70 mg/kg orally every 4 hours for 72 hours). NAC serves as a substitute for glutathione, which normally metabolizes toxic metabolites of acetaminophen. Lavage may be considered if appropriate to decrease absorption. Charcoal interferes only slightly with the effectiveness of NAC, and the dose of NAC does not require adjustment. NAC is most effective in the first 8 hours but is recommended up to 24 hours after a significant ingestion. It is also reasonable to administer NAC > 24 hours after ingestion if toxic levels of acetaminophen are present. Late administration of NAC may also be potentially beneficial in fulminant hepatic failure due to acetaminophen toxicity. There are no firm guidelines for administration of NAC in chronic ingestions or multiple ingestions over time. A course of NAC should be strongly considered if hepatic enzymes are elevated at presentation. Antiemetics are frequently needed to improve tolerance of oral NAC. The local Poison Control Center should be contacted for other NAC regimens such as intravenous administration for refractory vomiting or shorter courses of therapy.

Recommendations for management of extended-release forms include determination of acetaminophen levels 4 and 8 hours after ingestion and initiation of NAC if either level is potentially toxic.

Alcohols

Although infrequent, ethylene glycol and methanol ingestions can result in significant morbidity and mortality. Clinical manifestations, metabolic derangements, and management are similar for both alcohols.

Cardiopulmonary and neurologic symptoms may include pulmonary edema, hypotension, ataxia, seizures, and coma. Abdominal pain, nausea, and vomiting are frequent. Visual disturbances (blurred vision, photophobia, blindness, optic disc hyperemia) are clues to methanol toxicity, and the finding of calcium oxalate crystals in urine may indicate ethylene glycol ingestion. Significant symptoms may be delayed up to 24 hours after methanol ingestion. Both ingestions are classically characterized by an anion gap metabolic acidosis and an osmolal gap. An anion gap metabolic acidosis may not be present initially if sufficient time has not elapsed for metabolism to toxic acids or high levels of ethanol prevent metabolism of other alcohols. An osmolar gap may not be present in late presentations if the alcohol has already been metabolized to acid. Most institutions are unable to provide blood levels of methanol or ethylene glycol in a timely manner, and treatment is initiated based on the clinical history and acid-base status.

Treatment of ethylene glycol and methanol includes the following:

- Maintenance of a secure airway
- Gastric lavage—only if instituted within 1 hour of ingestion
- Activated charcoal if other substances are potentially ingested (does not adsorb alcohols)
- 50% glucose if indicated
- Thiamine, folate, multivitamin supplement
- Ethanol orally or intravenously to maintain blood level at 100 to 150 mg/dL—Ethanol is preferentially metabolized by alcohol dehydrogenase
- Fomepizole (4-methylpyrazole), which does not cause CNS depression, may substitute for ethanol
- Hemodialysis for visual impairment, renal failure, pulmonary edema,

significant or refractory acidosis, level of > 25 mg/dL
- Bicarbonate for acidosis is advocated by some clinicians.

Isopropyl alcohol is more potent than ethanol and results in similar manifestations at lower doses. Isopropyl alcohol ingestions are characterized by an osmolar gap but no metabolic acidosis. Treatment is supportive and may require intubation and mechanical ventilation for respiratory depression. Hemodialysis is reserved for evidence of hypoperfusion and failure to respond to supportive therapy.

Amphetamines/Methamphetamines

Amphetamines, methamphetamines, and related agents have enjoyed varying popularity as drugs of abuse. These drugs cause release of catecholamines, which results in a sympathomimetic toxidrome characterized by tachycardia, hyperthermia, agitation, hypertension, and mydriasis. Hallucinations (visual and tactile) and acute psychosis are frequently observed. Acute adverse consequences include myocardial ischemia and arrhythmias, seizures, intracranial hemorrhage, stroke, rhabdomyolysis, necrotizing vasculitis, and death.

An amphetamine-like drug, 3-4-methylenedioxymethamphetamine, is a designer drug associated with "rave" parties. It is commonly known as ecstasy, XTC, and MDMA, and acts as a stimulant and hallucinogen. Complications are usually a result of drug effects and nonstop physical activity.

Management of amphetamine intoxication is primarily supportive. Gastric lavage has little role, since absorption following oral ingestion is usually complete at the time of presentation. A careful assessment for complications should be made including measurement of core temperature, obtaining an ECG, and evaluating laboratory data for evidence of renal dysfunction and rhabdomyolysis. Intravenous hydration for possible rhabdomyolysis is warranted in individuals with known exertional activities pending CPK results. Benzodiazepines, often in high dosage, are useful for control of agitation.

Benzodiazepines

A benzodiazepine receptor antagonist, flumazenil, is available as a diagnostic tool and adjunctive treatment for benzodiazepine overdoses. Flumazenil should not be considered a substitute for intubation in patients with significant respiratory depression. Its use is contraindicated in suspected cyclic antidepressant overdoses and in patients physically dependent on benzodiazepines due to the risk of seizures. The initial dose of flumazenil is 0.2 mg over an interval of 30 seconds, followed by doses of 0.3 mg and 0.5 mg every minute up to a cumulative dose of 3 mg. Resedation is likely due to the short half-life of flumazenil (0.7 to 1.3 hours) compared with benzodiazepines.

β-Blockers

β-adrenergic blockers produce toxicity through bradycardia and hypotension. Hypotension often results from negative inotropic effects rather than bradycardia. Glucagon is considered the initial drug of choice since it produces chronotropic and inotropic effects and does not compete with the *β*-receptor. An initial dose of 2 to 3 mg of glucagon is given intravenously and an infusion of 2 to 5 mg/hr can be initiated, adjusted for desired clinical effects and then tapered over 12 hours as indicated. Transcutaneous pacing and transvenous pacing may be considered in cases refractory to glucagon. Additional drugs that have had variable efficacy in *β*-blocker overdoses include atropine, epinephrine, isoproterenol, and dopamine. Phosphodiesterase inhibitors such as amrinone and milrinone, intra-aortic balloon pump, or cardiopulmonary bypass may be considered if there is no response to these interventions. In a number of cases, calcium and insulin euglycemia have been reported to be beneficial.

Calcium-Channel Blockers

Calcium-channel blocker overdose should be considered in the hypotensive, bradycardic patient, particularly those with a history of hypertension. Ten milliliters of 10% calcium chloride should be administered intravenously in the presence of hemodynamic instability. Calcium is effective in reversing negative inotropic effects and conduction abnormalities in ~ 50% of overdoses. As in *β*-blocker overdose, glucagon may have beneficial effects. Transcutaneous and transvenous pacing are additional options in refractory cases. Successful treatment has also been reported with amrinone and insulin euglycemia (insulin 0.1-10 U/kg/hr and glucose 10-75 g/hr).

Carbon Monoxide

Carbon monoxide has 240 times the affinity for hemoglobin as oxygen. Carboxyhemoglobin reduces oxygen-carrying capacity and also shifts the oxyhemoglobin dissociation curve to the left. Carbon monoxide also exerts direct cellular toxic effects. Although the diagnosis of carbon monoxide poisoning is confirmed by an increased carboxyhemoglobin level, decisions for aggressive therapy with 100% oxygen should be based primarily on a clinical history suggestive of exposure. High-flow oxygen or intubation with administration of 100% oxygen should be initiated as soon as possible while confirmatory tests are obtained. An ECG, chest radiograph, and arterial blood gas measurement should be obtained to assess the level of toxicity. The finding of metabolic acidosis implies significant exposure with inadequate oxygen availability at the tissue level. The use of hyperbaric oxygen in the setting of carbon monoxide poisoning is controversial but should be considered for any patient with a depressed level of consciousness, focal neurologic abnormality, or cardiac instability.

Cocaine

Significant morbidity and mortality are associated with cocaine use by all routes, including nasal insufflation, intravenous, smoking, and oral. Toxicities include CNS hemorrhage (subarachnoid and intraparenchymal), cerebrovascular accidents, seizures, noncardiogenic pulmonary edema, arrhythmias, hypertension, myocardial ischemia, barotrauma, bowel ischemia, hyperthermia, and rhabdomyolysis. These potential morbidities should be considered in any critically ill cocaine abuser, and treatment should be initiated as indicated. Chest pain thought to be ischemic usually responds to nitroglycerin and/or benzodiazepines. Phentolamine is considered a second-line agent. Aspirin is recommended but thrombolysis should be considered only when other interventions have failed and immediate angiography and angioplasty are not available. In the case of severe hypertension, labetalol may be the drug of choice since it has both α- and β-adrenergic blocking properties. In most cases, intravenous fluid hydration should be instituted until rhabdomyolysis can be excluded. Rhabdomyolysis is enhanced by high environmental temperatures and increased physical activity. The agitation and combativeness frequently associated with cocaine use can usually be controlled with benzodiazepines. If frank psychosis is present, neuroleptics such as haloperidol are indicated, although there is a theoretical concern of lowering the seizure threshold.

Cyanide

Cyanide exposure is rare, but may occur in occupational settings involving metal extraction, electroplating, chemical synthesis, and firefighting. Cyanide inhibits cytochrome oxidase, which halts oxidative phosphorylation. Metabolic acidosis and decreased oxygen consumption result. Symptoms include nausea and vomiting, agitation, and tachycardia. Serious poisonings can result in seizures, coma, apnea, hypotension, and arrhythmias. Additional complications include rhabdomyolysis, hepatic necrosis, and acute respiratory distress syndrome. Diagnosis may be difficult in the absence of an exposure history. A cyanide antidote kit (Taylor Pharmaceuticals, San Clemente, CA) is used for management.

- Amyl nitrite pearls are an immediate source of nitrite to induce methemoglobinemia. Methemoglobin has a higher affinity for cyanide than cytochrome oxidase.
- 10% sodium nitrite iv to induce methemoglobinemia

- 25% sodium thiosulfate iv enhances conversion of cyanide to thiocyanate, which is excreted by the kidneys.

Hydroxocobalamin has been used in Europe for cyanide poisoning and relies on the formation of nontoxic cyanocobalamin (vitamin B_{12}). Mixed evidence exists for use of hyperbaric oxygen in cyanide poisoning.

Cyclic Antidepressants

Antidepressant overdoses account for the second largest number of deaths from poisoning in the United States. Toxicities include arrhythmias, seizures, depressed level of consciousness, and hypotension. Life-threatening events occur within the first 6 hours of hospitalization; most often, they occur within 2 hours of presentation. Serum levels may confirm ingestion, but these levels do not correlate with toxicity. Altered mental status is the best predictor of a significant ingestion and risk of complications. Cyclic antidepressants slow sodium influx into myocardial cells resulting in intraventricular conduction delays, wide complex arrhythmias, and negative inotropy. The ECG may be normal in significant ingestions or demonstrate a QRS > 0.10 seconds or amplitude of the terminal R wave in AVR ≥ 3 mm. Management should include the following:

- Maintain a secure airway
- Stabilize vital signs
- ECG monitoring
- Consider gastric lavage
- Activated charcoal
- Alkalinization of blood with sodium bicarbonate to pH of 7.45 to 7.55 for prolonged QRS or wide complex arrhythmias.
- $MgSO_4$ for torsades de pointes
- Benzodiazepines for seizures
- Norepinephrine or phenylephrine for refractory hypotension rather than dopamine
- Additional doses of activated charcoal for significant morbidity

Sodium bicarbonate uncouples the cyclic antidepressant from the myocardial sodium channels and alkalinization with bicarbonate may be superior to hyperventilation.

In an animal study, hypertonic saline was most effective in treatment of a wide QRS complex, but this therapy has not been evaluated in humans. Bicarbonate may also be beneficial for seizures and hypotension unresponsive to other interventions. Physostigmine is not indicated in cyclic antidepressant overdose.

Gamma-Hydroxybutyrate

Gamma-hydroxybutyrate (GHB) is a naturally occurring metabolite of γ-aminobutyric acid, which was banned in 1991 due to reported toxicities. Clinical effects of GHB ingestion may include hypothermia, loss of consciousness, coma, respiratory depression including arrest, seizure-like activity, bradycardia, hypotension, and death. Concomitant use of alcohol results in synergistic CNS and respiratory effects. More recently, γ-butyrolactone (GBL) and 1, 4-butanediol (BD), which are precursors of GHB, have been abused with resultant manifestations similar to GHB. The benefit of activated charcoal is unknown due to the rapid absorption of these substances. Although patients usually recover spontaneously in 2 to 96 hours, supportive therapy with airway protection and mechanical ventilation may be necessary. Use of physostigmine to reverse CNS effects is not recommended. A GHB withdrawal syndrome of agitation and delirium has been reported in high dose, frequent abusers.

Isoniazid (INH)

INH toxicity produces seizures (often intractable), an anion gap metabolic acidosis, coma, and hepatic toxicity. The treatment of choice is intensive supportive care and the use of pyridoxine (vitamin B_6 5 g iv or a dose equivalent to the amount of INH ingested). Hemoperfusion or hemodialysis may be considered, particularly in patients with renal insufficiency.

Lithium

Although arrhythmias are reported, neurologic abnormalities are the major manifestation of acute and chronic lithium toxicity. CNS manifestations include lethargy, dysarthria, delirium, seizures, and coma.

Symptoms of GI distress, polyuria, and polydipsia may be present. Patients who chronically ingest lithium are more prone to toxic effects. Serum lithium levels of > 2.5 to 4 mmol/L may be considered life threatening, depending on the clinical circumstances. Whole bowel irrigation may be considered in serious toxicity since lithium is not adsorbed by charcoal. Volume resuscitation should be aimed at restoring adequate urine output, but forced diuresis is not effective in enhancing lithium excretion. Diuretics can worsen toxicity and should be avoided. Hemodialysis is indicated in life-threatening toxicity, which may include renal dysfunction, severe neurologic dysfunction, volume overload or levels of $\geq$ 4 mmol/L in acute ingestion or $\geq$ 2.5 mmol/L in chronic ingestions. Due to redistribution between intracellular and extracellular compartments, a rebound increase in lithium level can occur 6 to 8 hours after dialysis. Continuous arteriovenous and venovenous hemodiafiltration have also been used to remove lithium and may be associated with less rebound. Sodium polystyrene sulfonate has been suggested to decrease lithium absorption, but evidence of clinical benefit is lacking and complications of hypokalemia, hypernatremia, and fluid overload may result.

Narcotics

Naloxone should be used to reverse the morbidity of respiratory depression and depressed level of consciousness associated with narcotic overdose. An initial dose of 2 mg should be administered intravenously unless the patient is known to be addicted, in which case lower initial doses should be used to prevent sudden withdrawal symptoms. Doses > 2 mg may be required to reverse the effects of propoxyphene, codeine, pentazocine, methadone, oxycodone, hydrocodone, and fentanyl. Naloxone can be administered at doses up to 10 mg and occasionally up to 20 mg. Naloxone can also be administered by the intramuscular, sublingual, and endotracheal routes if intravenous access is not established. Continuous infusion may be necessary since virtually all narcotics have a longer half-life than naloxone. The initial hourly infusion dose should be one-half to two-thirds of the amount in milligrams that was needed to initially reverse the respiratory depression. Noncardiogenic pulmonary edema may also occur with narcotics and can be managed with supportive care that may require intubation and mechanical ventilation.

Organophosphates and Carbamates

Organophosphate/carbamate poisoning exerts potential deleterious effects on 3 systems: a) muscarinic (parasympathetic) system, inducing bronchorrhea, bradycardia, and SLUDGE syndrome (Table 3); b) nicotinic autonomic system, resulting in muscle weakness; and c) CNS, including confusion, slurred speech, and central respiratory depression. Pulmonary toxicity from bronchorrhea, bronchospasm, and respiratory depression is the primary concern. Both intravenous atropine and pralidoxime (1 to 2 g initially) are indicated. Atropine does not reverse nicotinic manifestations; therefore, patients with significant respiratory muscle weakness require the use of pralidoxime. Large amounts of atropine may be required, and the initial dose is usually 2 to 4 mg, repeated every 5 minutes. The end point of atropinization is clearing of secretions from the tracheobronchial tree. An intermediate syndrome of respiratory paralysis, bulbar weakness, proximal limb weakness, and decreased reflexes may develop 24 to 96 hours after resolution of the cholinergic crisis. Poisoning with nerve gases such as sarin also results in a cholinergic syndrome requiring similar management.

Salicylates

Salicylates are found in many over-the-counter preparations. Patients with chronic rather than acute ingestions of salicylates are more likely to require intensive care. Symptoms of salicylate poisoning include tinnitus, nausea and vomiting, and depressed level of consciousness. In addition, fever, an anion gap metabolic acidosis, coagulopathy, prolonged prothrombin time, transient hepatotoxicity, and noncardiogenic pulmonary edema may be present. The clinical presentation of salicylate

toxicity may be mistaken for sepsis. The Done nomogram used to estimate the severity of an acute salicylate overdose may not reliably correlate with observed toxicity. Gastric lavage may be considered for significant ingestions, and activated charcoal should be administered. Alkalinization of the urine is indicated to enhance salicylate excretion if serum levels are > 35 mg/dL. Hemodialysis may be indicated with levels of > 100 mg/dL, refractory seizures, persistent alteration in mental status, or refractory acidosis.

Selective Serotonin Reuptake Inhibitors

Poisoning with selective serotonin reuptake inhibitors (SSRIs) is usually less severe than poisoning with cyclic antidepressants. Acute overdoses may result in nausea, vomiting, dizziness, and less commonly, CNS depression and arrhythmias. Therapeutic doses, or overdoses of SSRIs alone, or in combination with other agents, can cause serotonin syndrome, which may be life threatening. This syndrome may be precipitated by SSRIs, monoamine oxidase inhibitors, serotonin precursors (L-tryptophan), lithium, meperidine, and nonselective serotonin reuptake inhibitors (e.g., imipramine, meperidine, trazodone). Clinical manifestations include altered mental status (agitation, coma), autonomic dysfunction (blood pressure fluctuation, hyperthermia, tachycardia, diaphoresis, diarrhea), and neuromuscular abnormalities (tremor, rigidity, myoclonus, seizures). Management of an overdose should include activated charcoal, but the benefit of gastric lavage has not been determined. Intensive supportive care may be necessary, including cooling, sedatives, anticonvulsants, and mechanical ventilation. The role of other agents, such as serotonin antagonists (propranolol, cyproheptadine, methysergide), bromocriptine, or dantrolene in the treatment of serotonin syndrome is currently unclear. Most cases of serotonin syndrome resolve in 24 to 72 hours.

Theophylline

Theophylline toxicity is characterized by nausea, vomiting, and agitation. More serious complications include dysrhythmias and seizures. Toxicity is more likely to occur following chronic theophylline use compared with an acute overdose in an individual not taking theophylline. Gastric lavage and activated charcoal should be utilized to decrease GI absorption. An initial theophylline level should be obtained, as well as a subsequent level 1 hour later. Unfortunately, sustained-release preparations of theophylline may form conglomerates in the stomach and allow for continued absorption, despite aggressive interventions. Hypokalemia is commonly present in theophylline overdose and should be treated aggressively to prevent any contribution to the initiation of arrhythmias. Seizures are often poorly responsive to phenytoin but may respond to benzodiazepines. Any patient with a life-threatening complication and/or a level of > 60 mg/L with chronic ingestion or a level of > 80 to 90 mg/L with an acute ingestion should be considered for hemoperfusion or hemodialysis. Multiple doses of charcoal are indicated to enhance elimination of theophylline in patients with less severe manifestations.

Herbal Medicine/Dietary Supplements

Herbal medicines are the most common form of alternative therapy in the United States, and can be marketed without testing for safety or efficacy. Poisoning may result from product misuse, contamination of the product, or through interaction with other medications. Cardiac toxicity may result from aconitine and cardiac glycosides. Aconitine or related compounds are common ingredients in Asian herbal medications. Symptoms include paresthesias, hypersalivation, dizziness, nausea, vomiting, diarrhea, and muscle weakness. Sinus bradycardia and ventricular arrhythmias can occur. No antidote is available, but atropine may be considered for bradycardia or hypersalivation. Cardiac glycosides or digoxin-like factors can be found in many herbal preparations, particularly teas and laxatives. Toxicity is similar to digoxin toxicity with visual disturbances, nausea, vomiting, and arrhythmias. A digoxin level should be obtained but may not correlate with clinical findings since numerous cardiac glycosides will not crossreact in the digoxin immunoassay. With significant toxicity, digoxin-specific antibodies should be administered. CNS stimulation is characteristic of preparations containing ephedrine and pseudoephedrine, which are often found in products marketed as herbal ecstasy. A typical sympathomimetic syndrome can result with tachycardia, hypertension, mydriasis, and agitation. Seizures, stroke, myocardial infarction, arrhythmias, liver failure, and death have also been reported. Supportive care is indicated similar to management of other sympathomimetic syndromes. Ginkgo biloba has been reported to result in spontaneous bleeding including subdural hematomas, which may be due to antiplatelet activating factor effects. Treatment for bleeding includes supportive care and blood products as needed. Garlic may also result in bleeding due to inhibition of platelet aggregation, and ginseng has been associated with hypoglycemia. Contaminants found in some products such as mercury, arsenic, lead, antihistamines, etc. may contribute cause toxicities.

SUGGESTED READINGS

1. American Academy of Clinical Toxicology; European Association of Poisons Centres and Clinical Toxicologists. Position statement: Gastric lavage. *J Toxicol Clin Toxicol* 1997; 35:711-19

2. American Academy of Clinical Toxicology; European Association of Poisons Centres and Clinical Toxicologists. Position statement: Single-dose activated charcoal. *J Toxicol Clin Toxicol* 1997; 35:721-24

3. American Academy of Clinical Toxicology; European Association of Poisons Centres and Clinical Toxicologists. Position statement: Whole bowel irrigation. *J Toxicol Clin Toxicol* 1997; 35:753-62

4. American Academy of Clinical Toxicology; European Association of Poison Centres and Clinical Toxicologists. Position Statement and practice guidelines on the use of multi-dose activated charcoal in the treatment of acute poisoning. *J. Toxicol Clin Toxicol* 1999; 37: 731-751

5. Ang-Lee MK, Moss J, Yuan C-S: *JAMA* 2001; 286:208-16

6. Barceloux DG, Krenzelok EP, Olson R, et al: American Academy of Clinical Toxicology practice guidelines on the treatment of ethylene glycol poisoning. *J Toxicol Clin Toxicol* 1999; 37:37-560

7. Bardin PG, van Eden SF, Moolman JA, et al: Organophosphate and carbamate poisoning. *Arch Intern Med* 1994; 154:1433–1441

8. Brent J, McMartin K, Phillips S, et al: Fomepizole for the treatment of ethylene glycol poisoning. *N Engl J Med* 1999; 340:832-8

9. Brent J, McMartin K, Phillips S, et al: Fomepizole for the treatment of methanol poisoning. *N Engl J Med* 2001; 344:424-9

10. Bryan TM, Skop BT, Mareth ER: Pathophysiology and management of the serotonin syndrome. *Ann Pharmacother* 1996; 30:527–533

11. Cox J, Wang RY: Critical consequences of common drugs: Manifestations and management of calcium-channel blocker and β adrenergic antagonist overdose. *Emerg Med Rep* 1994; 15:83–90

12. Glauser J: Tricyclic antidepressant poisoning. *Cleveland Clin J Med* 2000; 67:704-19

13. Goldfrank LR, Flomenbaum NE, Lewin NA, et al (Eds): Goldfrank's Toxicologic Emergencies. Sixth Edition. Stamford, CT, Appleton and Lange, 1998

14. Hall AH, Rumack BH: The treatment of acute acetaminophen poisoning. *J Intensive Care Med* 1986; 1:29–32

15. Ko RJ: Adulterants in Asian patent medicines (letter). *N Engl J Med* 1998; 339:847

16. Lange RA, Hillis LD: Cardiovascular complications of cocaine use. *N Engl J Med* 2001; 345:351-58

17. Li J, Stokes SA, Woeckner A: A tale of novel intoxication. A review of the effects of gamma-hydroxybutyric acid with recommendations for management. *Ann Emerg Med* 1998; 31:729–736

18. Manoguerra AS: Gastrointestinal decontamination after poisoning—Where is the science? *Crit Care Clin* 1997; 4:709–725

19. Martin TG: Serotonin syndrome. *Ann Emerg Med* 1996; 28:520–526

20. Pimentl L, Trommer L: Cyclic antidepressant overdoses. *Emerg Med Clin North Am* 1994; 12:533–547

21. Pond SM, Lewis-Driver DJ, Williams GM, et al: Gastric emptying in acute overdose: A prospective randomized controlled trial. *Med J Aust* 1995; 163:345–349

22. Sessler CN: Theophylline toxicity: Clinical features of 116 consecutive cases. *Am J Med* 1990; 88:567–576

23. Spitalnic SJ, Wang RY: Updating salicylate toxicity. *Emerg Med Rep* 1993; 14:173–180

24. Trujillo MH, Guerrero J, Fragachan C, et al: Pharmacologic antidotes in critical care medicine: A practical guide for drug administration. *Crit Care Med* 1998; 26:377–391

25. Yuan TH, Kerns WP, Tomaszewski CA, et al: Insulin-glucose as adjunctive therapy for severe calcium channel antagonist poisoning. *J Toxicol Clin Toxicol* 1999; 37:463

26. Zimmerman JL, Rudis M: Poisonings. *In*: Critical Care Medicine. Parrillo JE, Dellinger RP (Eds), Mosby, Inc, St. Louis, 2001, pp 1501-24

SEVERE HYPERTENSION

Stuart L. Linas, MD

Objectives

- To diagnose and manage severe hypertension
- To characterize and compare pharamacologic agents to treat these disorders

Key Words: hypertension; pharmacologic treatment; diagnosis; cardiovascular disease

TABLE OF ABBREVIATIONS

ACE	angiotensin-converting enzyme
BP	blood pressure
CNS	central nervous system
dP/dt	maximal change in pressure over time; shearing force of cardiac impulse
MAO	monoamine oxidase
MAP	mean arterial pressure

Of the 40% of the adults with hypertension in the United States, one-fourth to one-third of this group have moderate-to-severe hypertension (diastolic pressure of > 104 mm Hg). While the majority of these adults remain asymptomatic for many years, a small percent of this group will experience rapid acceleration of blood pressure (BP) elevation which, if uncontrolled, may lead to death within months. Whether the hypertension is due to 1 of a number of secondary causes or progression of preexisting essential hypertension, this so-called "hypertensive crisis" is characterized by markedly elevated BP in association with end-organ dysfunction, such as central nervous system (CNS) disturbances or acute left ventricular dysfunction. There is no single, absolute pressure range at which hypertensive crisis can be said to occur. Rather, the immediate risk of morbidity depends on the patient's age, gender, previous BP, and rate of pressure increase. Patients with long-standing hypertension may tolerate diastolic pressures of 110 to 120 mm Hg without immediate morbidity, while previously normotensive persons, children, and gravid females may develop complications at much lower values (as low as a diastolic pressure of 100 mm Hg). The presence of end-organ dysfunction or vascular injury mandates emergent therapy, even in cases where the diastolic pressure is only modestly increased. This chapter focuses on the various clinical hypertensive settings that mandate specific therapies and characterizes and compares a number of the pharmacologic agents used in the treatment of these disorders.

CLASSIFICATION OF HYPERTENSION (1–3)

Although a number of terms have been used to classify severe hypertension, the most useful classification is based on the clinical requirement to reduce BP (1). Conditions entailing an immediate risk of serious morbidity within hours of presentation mandate the most aggressive treatment and are termed "hypertensive crises." This category (Table 1) includes the severely hypertensive patient with 1 of the following conditions: acute CNS disturbances; hypertensive encephalopathy; acute cardiovascular emergencies including aortic dissection, pulmonary edema, ischemic cardiac syndromes, malignant hypertensions; catecholamine excess states; and hypertensive obstetrical emergencies. Although management of each of these conditions is individualized, these hypertensive crises generally require hospitalization with intensive care and parenteral therapy.

A second group of disorders (Table 2), which have been labeled with various confusing terms such as "hypertensive urgencies," include severe hypertension in association with chronic conditions such as stable angina; chronic congestive heart failure; chronic renal failure; transient ischemic attacks; or previous

Table 1. Most frequent causes of hypertensive crisis'

Malignant hypertension
Hypertensive encephalopathy
Preeclampsia/eclampsia
Scleroderma renal crisis
Acute pulmonary edema
Acute myocardial infarction
Unstable angina
Acute aortic dissection
Intracranial hemorrhage,
   ischemic stroke, or
   subarachnoid hemorrhage
Catecholamine Excess States
   Pheochromocytoma
   MAO/tyramine interaction
   Antihypertensive withdrawal
   Cocaine intoxication

MAO, monoamine oxidase.

Table 2. Other causes of severe hypertension

Severe hypertension (diastolic pressure of > 115 mm Hg) in association with 1 or more of the following:
   Chronic renal failure
   Chronic congestive heart failure
   Stable angina
   Transient ischemic attacks
   Previous cerebrovascular accident
   Perioperative hypertension
   Renal transplant recipients
   Spinal cord injuries

cerebrovascular accident; perioperative hypertension; renal transplant recipients; and spinal cord injuries. Generally, these patients have diastolic pressures of > 115 mm Hg, but the absolute level of pressure leading to eventual complications is variable. In these conditions, the risk of complications from the BP elevation is not immediate, and the risk of morbidity due to overaggressive therapy mandates a more gradual BP reduction that extends over a period of hours to days. Most hypertensive urgencies require observation in an inpatient or emergency room setting; however, the majority of patients will respond well to oral therapy.

The third and probably most common treatment category, termed "severe uncomplicated hypertension," includes patients who present with severely elevated BP (diastolic pressures of ≥ 115 mm Hg) who are asymptomatic, with the exception of mild, nonspecific symptoms, such as headache or fatigue. Initial evaluation of these patients with severe uncomplicated hypertension indicates no immediate evidence of end-organ damage. Such patients are typically seen in emergency room settings where they present for medication refills, or in whom the severely elevated BP is incidentally discovered. Despite sometimes markedly elevated pressures (e.g., diastolic pressure of 140 mm Hg in the chronic hypertensive), these patients are at low risk for immediate complications. Hypertension-related morbidity tends to occur over a period of months to years. A gradual pressure reduction over a few days with oral therapy in the outpatient setting is most appropriate. Frequently, merely restarting a previously effective regimen and making follow-up arrangements is all that is necessary. Although medical-legal issues may pressure physicians into loading these patients with medication to observe on-the-spot BP control, this practice has been questioned as having no clear rational scientific basis.

Hypertension is also distinguished according to cause as primary (essential) or secondary. Although > 90% of patients with mild-to-moderate hypertension have primary hypertension, > 20% of the patients with severe hypertension have secondary causes including renal parenchymal diseases, renovascular hypertension, or drug use. In patients with malignant hypertension, the number with secondary hypertension is > 50%.

MALIGNANT/ACCELERATED HYPERTENSION (1–3)

Malignant/accelerated hypertension is a specific syndrome in which there is markedly elevated pressure in conjunction with hypertensive neuroretinopathy (2, 3). Fundoscopic examination demonstrates flame-shaped hemorrhages and cotton-wool spots (accelerated hypertension) or papilledema (malignant hypertension). As the prognosis for both conditions is identical, the term "malignant hypertension" is used for both. Untreated malignant hypertension is a rapidly fatal disorder, with > 90% mortality within 1 year. The causes of death are renal failure (19%), congestive heart failure (13%), renal failure plus congestive heart failure (48%), stroke (20%), myocardial infarction (1%), and aortic dissection (1%). Important predictors of longevity at the time of presentation include level of renal function and degree of retinopathy.

The secondary causes of malignant hypertension are listed in Table 3. One of the most common causes is renovascular hypertension related to fibromuscular dysplasia or atherosclerosis. The frequency of this condition varies among populations, with a racial predilection for Caucasians. Forty-three percent of Caucasians but only 7% of African Americans with malignant hypertension have renovascular disease. Up to 20% of cases of malignant hypertension occur in patients who have been diagnosed with underlying chronic glomerulonephritis.

Other common renal causes include reflux nephropathy (particularly in children), and analgesic nephropathy.

Clinical Features of Malignant Hypertension

The overall incidence of malignant hypertension has declined in recent decades. The mean age on presentation is 40 to 50 years, and the disease is rare in patients aged > 65 years. Males predominate over females by 2:1, and the incidence is higher in African Americans than Caucasians. Smoking has been found to increase the risk factor by 2.5 to 5-fold. Average diastolic pressure among malignant hypertensive patients is 120 to 130 mm Hg. In 85% of patients, headache is the most common presenting symptom, located in the occipital or anterior part of the head, with a steady quality, and often worst in the morning. The majority (60%) also complain of visual blurring and occasionally blindness. Thirty percent complain of generalized fatigue or malaise. Neurologic signs include focal deficits, stroke, or transient ischemic attacks, confusion, or somnolence. Ischemic chest pain or left ventricular

Table 3. Most frequent causes of secondary malignant hypertension

Primary Renal Disease
  Chronic glomerulonephritis
  Reflux nephropathy
  Analgesic nephropathy
  Acute glomerulonephritis
  Radiation nephritis
  Chronic lead intoxification
Renovascular Hypertension
Endocrine Hypertension
  Pheochromocytoma
Systemic vasculitis
Atheroembolic renal crisis
Scleroderma renal crisis
Drugs
  Oral contraceptives
  Nonsteroidal anti-inflammatory agents
  Atropine
  Corticosteroids
  Sympathomimetics
    Cocaine
    Nasal recongestants
Antihypertensive withdrawal
Severe burns

dysfunction may be present. Physical examination often indicates evidence of left ventricular hypertrophy due to long-standing antecedent hypertension. Another common complaint is weight loss in over half of these patients. It is caused by diuresis induced by high levels of circulating renin and angiotensin as the hypertension enters the malignant phase. Patients often present with intravascular volume depletion, which has strong implications for treatment.

Careful fundoscopic examination is the key to the diagnosis of malignant hypertension. While the presence of Keith and Wagener stage I or II lesions, with arteriolar sclerosis or arteriovenous compressions, indicates the presence of long-standing hypertension, the presence of flame-shaped hemorrhages or cotton-wool spots (Keith and Wagener stage III), or papilledema (stage IV), collectively termed hypertensive neuroretinopathy, implies the failure of CNS autoregulation, and confirms the diagnosis of malignant hypertension.

Laboratory features are relatively nonspecific. Evidence of intravascular hemolysis is common and can make it difficult to differentiate this disorder from primary vasculitis with secondary hypertension. Indicators of a highly stimulated renin-angiotensin-aldosterone axis include hypokalemia and metabolic alkalosis, and the abnormalities may persist for months after adequate BP control. Evidence of renal involvement includes elevated urea nitrogen and creatinine. The urinalysis often shows proteinuria and hematuria, with occasional erythrocyte casts.

Pathogenesis of Malignant Hypertension

At the point of transition from benign to malignant hypertension, diffuse microvascular lesions develop, leading to progressive increases in systemic vascular resistance and BP. Although the exact initiating event is unclear, considerable evidence suggests that mechanical stress in the arteriolar wall leads to disruption of endothelial integrity. Other vascular-toxic influences have been proposed, including immunologic factors, and hormones such as circulating angiotensin II, catecholamines, and vasopressin. Regardless of the exact inciting mechanism, the resulting diffuse endovascular damage leads to activation of the coagulation cascade, platelet microaggregation, and endovascular hemolysis. Myointimal proliferation of the arteriolar wall results in progressive luminal narrowing. Central to the transition to the malignant phase is the intense activation of the renin-angiotensin system seen in most patients, resulting from primary renovascular disease, or from progressive renal ischemia from arteriolar narrowing. A vicious cycle ensues, with renin-angiotensin activation increasing systemic pressures, further damaging the vasculature and inducing higher renin release due to ischemia. During this progressive malignant phase, the majority of patients experience progressive sodium and water loss believed to be due to a pressure-induced diuresis. This condition may exacerbate renin release, thereby leading to a paradoxical worsening of hypertension.

Pathology of Malignant Hypertension

Although diffuse arteriolar lesions are prominent in the kidneys, other organs are affected, including pancreas, liver, and gastrointestinal tract. The hallmark of this disease is fibrinoid necrosis of the renal afferent arteriole, with necrosis of the entire arteriolar wall and swelling presumably from leakage of fibrin and other plasma elements from the endovascular space. Alternating segments of wall necrosis with areas of intact vascular constriction may lead to a "sausage string" appearance. Proliferative endarteritis of the renal interlobular artery is the second characteristic lesion, with a concentric onion-skin appearance and marked luminal compromise. Ischemic glomerular obsolescence can be seen distal to occlusive lesions. Marked hyperplasia of the juxtaglomerular apparatus results in the high renin state.

Hypertensive Encephalopathy

Hypertensive encephalopathy is a distinct clinical entity resulting from rapid increases in perfusion pressures that exceed CNS blood flow autoregulation. Diastolic pressure is typically $\geq$ 140 mm Hg. Hypertensive neuroretinopathy is usually present, but may be absent when pressure increases are very abrupt, such as in acute glomerulonephritis or in catecholamine excess states. Within 12 to 48 hours, signs and symptoms of CNS dysfunction develop, including headache, nausea, vomiting, weakness, confusion, somnolence, seizures, and coma. Focal neurologic defects are not common. The onset of symptoms tends to be slower than ischemic stroke or cerebral bleed. Untreated, coma and death may follow in 24 to 48 hours. The hallmark of hypertensive encephalopathy is its reversibility within 1 to 12 hours of adequate BP reduction. Hypertensive encephalopathy needs to be distinguished from other causes of encephalopathy (Table 4).

The pathogenesis of hypertensive encephalopathy involves the breakthrough of CNS blood flow autoregulation leading to endovascular damage. Extravasation of plasma proteins and brain edema follow, causing the neurologic abnormalities. Brain edema, petechiae, and microinfarctions are found on pathologic examination.

GENERAL PRINCIPLES OF TREATMENT (1, 4)

In hypertensive crises, prompt, aggressive therapy is necessary to prevent progressive injury (1, 4). However, care must be taken to avoid overtreatment, as profound, precipitous decreases in BP can result in CNS hypoperfusion with catastrophic consequences. Watershed stroke, paraplegia, permanent blindness, and death have been reported due to overaggressive antihypertensive treatment. While cerebral blood flow is autoregulated in normal subjects between mean arterial pressures (MAPs) of 60 to 120 mm Hg, the autoregulatory range is shifted to higher values (typically 120 to 160 mm Hg) in chronic hypertensives. Although the autoregulatory range is reset in chronic hypertensives, the lower limit of the autoregulatory range is ~ 25% below the resting MAP. Mild symptoms of globally low CNS flow, such as nausea, yawning, hyperventilation, clamminess, and syncope, begin to develop well below the lower limit of autoregulation, when MAP drops by $\geq$ 50%.

Because of these considerations, it is recommended that the BP be acutely reduced by no more than 25% to 30% in hypertensive emergencies, to approximately the lower limit of CNS blood flow autoregulation. Thus, initial treatment goals are typically a BP of 160 to

Table 4. Differential diagnosis of hypertensive encephalopathy

Cerebral infarction
Subarachnoid or intracerebral hemorrhage
Subdural or epidural hematoma
Brain tumor
Seizure disorders
CNS vasculitis
Encephalitis
Meningitis

CNS, central nervous system.

170/100 to 110 mm Hg, or MAP of $\geq$ 120 mm Hg. Further reductions toward normotensive levels should be carried out only gradually over several days to weeks, allowing time for the cerebral vasculature to readjust autoregulatory range. Important exceptions to this general recommendation exist, however. Elderly patients with carotid stenosis are particularly susceptible to CNS hypoperfusion. BP management in patients with stroke or intracranial bleeding is controversial, as the loss of CNS blood flow autoregulation and the presence of brain edema necessitate maintaining high systemic pressures to provide adequate cerebral perfusion. In acute aortic dissection, the immediate goal of therapy is BP reduction to normotensive levels or below. Likewise, in previously normotensive subjects with abrupt increases in BP, normotension may be the goal.

The recommended rapidity of initial BP reduction varies with different conditions. When faced with a hypertensive crisis, therapy should begin immediately without waiting for test results that would delay treatment. In general, the most rapid reduction, e.g., 15 to 30 minutes, should be induced in patients with the cardiovascular emergencies of acute dissection, unstable angina, or congestive heart failure with pulmonary edema. In patients with malignant hypertension or hypertensive encephalopathy, a more controlled titration of BP reduction over 1 to 3 hours is satisfactory. In cases of intracranial events, such as stroke or bleeding, treatment must be still more gradual (6 to 12 hours) for careful control.

The decision to use oral or parenteral antihypertensive therapy largely follows from the classification of the situation. In general, crises are best treated parenterally, with intensive care monitoring by arterial cannulation or automated BP cuff measurement. Controversy exists as to the management of the relatively asymptomatic malignant hypertensive. Although oral medication under close observation has been used successfully, we prefer initial parenteral therapy. The progressive breakdown of CNS autoregulation in these patients enhances the sensitivity to ischemia with abrupt decreases in BP. Intravascular volume depletion occurs in many malignant hypertensive patients and enhances the sensitivity to precipitous increases in pressure. Overshoot hypotension is easily avoided with short-acting, titratable, parenteral agents (5).

Nitroprusside remains the most useful intravenous agent for hypertensive crises. It has a favorable hemodynamic profile of preload, as well as afterload reduction without direct cardiac effects, and also allows titration of the dose for minute-to-minute pressure control. Other agents, such as trimethaphan, diazoxide, labetalol, etc., have characteristics desirable in more limited clinical circumstances. A common mistake in the management of these patients is the premature discontinuation of parenteral therapy, leading to a rebound in BP. Oral therapy should begin only after the pressure has been stabilized, and the parenteral agent should only then be slowly weaned.

Most noncritical hypertensive situations and cases of uncomplicated severe hypertension can be managed with oral therapy. The decision for inpatient observation must be individualized. Patient reliability is a major consideration. One error commonly made with oral therapy is the failure to take orthostatic BP measurements. Smooth, controlled BP reduction in supine patients may turn to frank hypotension on standing, particularly in the volume-depleted patient.

Diuretics

The initial evaluation should include an estimate of the intravascular volume status. For those patients with clear intravascular volume overload, as in dilated congestive heart failure, initial diuretic therapy is appropriate. However, the majority of patients with malignant hypertension have some degree of intravascular volume depletion. In such patients, the initial use of diuretics is contraindicated, as is the restriction of sodium intake. Gentle volume expansion with crystalloid is sometimes useful in stabilizing the initial therapeutic response in very sensitive, hypovolemic patients. Many vasodilators, used effectively as initial therapy, stimulate reflex cardiovascular responses, which result in compensatory salt and water retention. Over the course of several days of therapy, this regimen may result in considerable volume overload and pseudotolerance to therapy. At this

point, initiation of diuretic therapy is a useful maneuver to restore the efficacy of the antihypertensive agent.

TREATMENT OF SPECIFIC DISORDERS

Uncomplicated Malignant Hypertension (1, 4)

Expeditious therapy begins with the goal of achieving 25% reductions in MAP or diastolic pressure of 100 to 110 mm Hg within 1 to 3 hours (Table 5). In patients with neuroretinopathy but no other signs or symptoms of end-organ failure, the need for parenteral therapy is debated. While there are reports of successful management with oral medication, even without hospitalization, we limit this approach to the exceptional patient. Since the arteriolopathy of malignant hypertension includes fixed anatomic lesions, the initiation of treatment often results in acute decrements in renal function, owing to the loss of perfusion pressure through fixed arteriolar lesions. In patients initially presenting with azotemia, renal function may worsen dramatically, necessitating the adjustment of medication doses and even precipitating the need for renal replacement therapy. Continued antihypertensive treatment is mandatory to halt the progression of arterial damage. Some patients with little or no renal function early in the course of treatment recover some renal function over the ensuing weeks or months. Among the parenteral agents, nitroprusside remains the standard. Because some patients are highly sensitive to treatment, low starting doses of $\geq$ 0.3 μg/kg/min are recommended, with titration every 3 to 5 minutes until the desired effects are reached. A number of parenteral agents have been used as successful alternatives. Labetalol, a combined α- and nonselective β-adrenergic antagonist, has rapid onset following intravenous administration and tends to result in consistent, smooth BP reductions when given either by drip or by a minibolus method. Diazoxide, a potent direct arteriolar dilator with a rapid onset, has a long history of successful use in hypertensive emergencies, including malignant hypertension. It is a preferred alternative to nitroprusside in cases where

Table 5. Recommendations for reducing blood pressure in hypertensive crisis

Clinical Situation	Recommended	Drugs To Avoid
Hypertensive encephalopathy	Nitroprusside, labetalol, diazoxide	Clonidine, β-blockers, hydralazine, diazoxide
Malignant hypertension	Nitroprusside, labetalol, diazoxide, dihydropyridine, calcium antagonists, enalaprilat	Diuretics, monotherapy with clonidine
Cerebral infarction	Nitroprusside, labetalol	Hydralazine, diazoxide, minoxidil
Intracerebral hemorrhage	Nitroprusside, labetalol	Hydralazine, diazoxide, minoxidil
Subarachnoid hemorrhage	Nimodipine, nitroprusside	Hydralizine, diazoxide, minoxidil
Aortic dissection	Nitroprusside plus β-blocker, trimethaphan, labetalol	Hydralizine, diazoxide, minoxidil
Adrenergic crisis	Phentolamine, nitroprusside plus β-blocker, labetalol	Monotherapy with β-blockers
Antihypertensive withdrawal	Phentolamine, nitroprusside, labetalol, resume initial drug	
Acute pulmonary edema	Nitroprusside, intravenous nitroglycerin	Systolic failure, β-blockers, verapamil, diltiazem, labetalol
Ischemic heart disease or myocardial infarction	Nitroglycerin plus β-blocker, nitroprusside, labetalol	Hydralazine, diazoxide, minoxidil
Eclampsia	Labetalol, methyldopa, hydralazine	ACE inhibitors, nitroprusside

ACE, angiotensin-converting enzyme.

intensive care monitoring is not feasible. As both labetalol and diazoxide have a duration of action of many hours, care must be taken to avoid overshoot hypotension.

Other new parenteral agents with a rapid onset deserve mention. Nicardipine, a parenteral calcium-channel antagonist of the dihydropyridine class, and enalaprilat, an angiotensin-converting enzyme (ACE) inhibitor, and Fenoldopam a Dopadrenergic receptor agonist. These agents have hemodynamic characteristics that suggest a potential role in the treatment of malignant hypertension. As only small numbers of patients have been studied with these agents, recommendations for their use await further trials. Drugs that are to be avoided as initial treatment for the malignant hypertension include diuretics and β-blockers as single agents. β-blockers decrease cardiac output while increasing peripheral vascular resistance, thus worsening the existing hemodynamic derangements already present.

Hypertensive Encephalopathy

Hypertensive encephalopathy, if left untreated, can progress to coma and death in 24 to 48 hours. It is a diagnosis of exclusion, however, and consideration must be given to other neurologic processes (Table 4). The diagnostic feature of hypertensive encephalopathy is its rapid resolution with BP control. Azotemic patients seem to have a higher risk of hypertensive encephalopathy.

Although management is similar to treatment for malignant hypertension, the presence of CNS ischemia and edema dictate that particular care be exercised in protecting cerebral perfusion. Hence, parenteral therapy with intensive care monitoring is clearly indicated. The MAP should be reduced by 25% over 2 to 3 hours initially; overshoot must be avoided, as neurologic complications have been reported from MAP reductions of ≥ 40%. In previously normotensive patients, including eclamptics, BP should be normalized. If the patient's mental status worsens with treatment, the pressure should be allowed to increase and then the pressure should be reduced more slowly. If the patient's mental status fails to improve, one should reconsider other CNS diseases and the diagnosis of hypertensive encephalopathy. Lumbar puncture should be avoided due to the risk of herniation. The pressure should be gradually lowered to normal ranges over several days to allow restoration of autoregulation. In choosing an antihypertensive agent, one should focus on its effect on global as well as regional cerebral flow, on its effect on intracranial pressure, and especially on neurologic or sedating side effects, which confuse the neurologic assessment.

Nitroprusside is the agent of first choice. At low doses, nitroprusside is known to increase cerebral blood flow, which can theoretically increase intracranial pressure; higher doses are without this effect. Labetalol is a reasonable alternative, with its rapid action and lack of sedating side effects. Diazoxide has the theoretical advantage of causing little or no change in cerebral blood flow. However, because of the long duration of action, these latter 2 agents must be titrated very carefully. Drugs to be avoided include centrally acting agonists, such as clonidine, because of sedation. β-blockers reduce cardiac output and may worsen CNS ischemia. The efficacy of hydralazine is unpredictable, and it can induce patchy cerebral perfusion with a steal of flow

from ischemic areas. Calcium-channel blockers must be used cautiously, as increased cerebral blood flow due to these agents may raise intracranial pressure.

Ischemic Stroke (6)

Hypertension is a common consequence of ischemic cerebral infarction (6). The hypertension tends to improve spontaneously within the first 24 hours. Systemic pressure is often labile, and failure of cerebral blood flow autoregulation in ischemic and infarcted areas increases the risk of worsened ischemia with even small reductions in pressure. For these reasons, pharmacologic BP control in this condition is controversial. Although there is no good evidence that overall prognosis is improved with treatment of mild-to-moderate hypertension, most authors agree that in extreme cases (diastolic pressures of > 120 mm Hg), acute treatment is warranted. Nitroprusside, beginning at low doses, is preferred because of the ability to control pressure on a minute-by-minute basis. The initial goal should be 160 to 170/100 to 110 mm Hg, achieved smoothly over the first 24 hours, with further gradual reduction toward normal levels over the next several days.

The cerebrovascular selective calcium-channel blocker, nimodipine, is currently under investigation for routine use in ischemic stroke, with mixed results at present. In a meta-analysis of 5 randomized trials, 2 subgroups were found to benefit: a) those patients ≥ 65 years old; and b) those patients who present with severe neurologic deficits. Agents which have sedating effects, which increase intracranial pressure, or which exacerbate cerebral perfusion inhomogeneity should be avoided (7).

Subarachnoid Hemorrhage (7)

Management of patients with subarachnoid hemorrhage is significantly different from management of patients with ischemic stroke, because the presence of extravasated blood induces intense vasospasm in neighboring vessels. This vasospasm, which typically develops between days 4 and 12, is the leading cause of postoperative morbidity. Hypovolemia is associated with increased vasospasm, and there is evidence that volume expansion may help some patients. The use of nimodipine is proven to reduce ischemic brain injury, even at doses which have little effect on the systemic BP. Markedly elevated pressures (> 200/120 mm Hg) increase the risk of rebleeding and should be treated with 20% to 25% reduction in MAP over 6 to 12 hours, but not < 160 to 180/100 mm Hg. Nitroprusside or labetalol is often required.

Intracerebral Hemorrhage

Unlike in ischemic stroke, patients with intracerebral hemorrhage uniformly present with hypertension, which is persistent beyond the first week. Recommendations for BP control are difficult, because the prominent cerebral edema and elevated intracranial pressure make cerebral perfusion critically dependent on systemic BP. Intracranial pressure should be monitored, and only extreme elevation of systemic pressure, e.g., diastolic presure of $\geq$ 130 mm Hg, should be treated. Acute pressure reduction should be limited to 20%, and nitroprusside is preferred. Because of the very high levels of circulating catecholamines, propranolol is often added when nitroprusside alone is ineffective. Alternatives include labetalol, but the long duration of action increases the risk of overshoot hypotension. While small hemorrhages may be managed like ischemic infarctions, the poor prognosis of large hemorrhage makes further treatment recommendations difficult. Barbiturates reduce MAP modestly, while they markedly reduced the intracranial pressure; they should be considered in severe cases.

Head Trauma

In severe head trauma, brain edema contributes directly to ischemic injury and mortality. The main goal of therapy is, therefore, to control intracranial pressure. With the failure of cerebral blood flow autoregulation that follows injury, systemic hypertension can worsen intracranial pressure elevation. Severe hypertension should be treated, but the cerebral perfusion pressure, the difference between MAP and intracranial pressure, should be maintained > 50 mm Hg to prevent CNS ischemia.

Nitroprusside is used, and propranolol may be added if necessary. Labetalol or nitroglycerin are alternatives.

Aortic Dissection

Patients with aortic dissection can present with a dramatic picture of severe, often tearing, pain in the chest, back, or abdomen, accompanied by diaphoresis, nausea, or vomiting. If this condition is untreated, 25% die in the first 24 hours and 60% to 70% die in the first 2 weeks. Patients at risk for dissection include those with advanced atherosclerosis, Marfan's syndrome, Ehler's Danlos syndrome, and coarctation of the aorta. Clues to the diagnosis include discrepancies in peripheral pulses and mediastinal widening on chest radiograph. Computed tomography scans of the thorax are widely available for emergency use and should be considered as a first diagnostic choice. Transthoracic echocardiography is not sensitive. Transesophageal echocardiography is sensitive in distinguishing between proximal and distal dissection. Magnetic resonance imaging is also useful but involves moving patients from the intensive care unit setting. Dissection begins as tears in the intima of the aorta are propagated by both elevated BP and by the shearing force of the cardiac impulse (dP/dt). The enlarging hematoma may lead to occlusion of branch vessels, resulting in myocardial infarction, stroke, spinal cord or bowel infarction, acute renal failure, and ischemic legs. Renal arterial involvement may trigger renin release from the ischemic kidney, leading to refractory hypertension. Dissection to the aortic root can precipitate acute aortic insufficiency; rupture of the ascending aorta leads to hemopericardium and tamponade.

Antihypertensive therapy should begin immediately when dissection is strongly suspected, before confirmation of the diagnosis. The BP should be lowered to normotensive levels or below, with the resolution of pain as the therapeutic goal. Equally important is reduction of dP/dt. The most widely used regimen is the combination of propranolol and nitroprusside. To prevent reflex cardiac stimulation, propranolol is given first, with a test dose of 0.5 mg iv, followed by 1 mg every 5 minutes until the heart rate approaches 60 beats/minute. Nitroprusside is then titrated to a systolic pressure of 100 to 120 mm Hg or to as low as 70 to 80 mm Hg, as needed to alleviate pain, a marker of continued propagation of the dissection.

An alternative regimen, preferred by some clinicians because of a more potent reduction in dP/dt, is the ganglionic blocking agent, trimethaphan. The rapid onset (1 to 2 minutes) and short duration (10 minutes) allows precise pressure control. Mild reflex increases in heart rate are treated with β-blockade. Disadvantages of this agent include parasympathetic blockade resulting in paralytic ileus and bladder atony, and the development of tachyphylaxis after 24 to 96 hours of use. Labetalol has also been used successfully, alone or in combination with nitroprusside. However, its long duration of action is a disadvantage in patients undergoing emergency surgery. Agents to be avoided include hydralazine and diazoxide, which cause reflex cardiac stimulation.

Following initial BP control and definitive diagnosis, further therapy depends on the site of dissection. In general, dissections involving the ascending aorta (proximal, type A) are surgically repaired. Distal dissections (type B), which involve only the descending aorta distal to the left subclavian artery, are managed medically if uncomplicated. Oral medication used for chronic treatment include β-blockers, labetalol, verapamil, diltiazem, methyldopa, reserpine, and guanethidine. Even normotensive individuals should continue medications to keep the heart rate and shear forces low.

Pulmonary Edema

Many patients who present with pulmonary edema have longstanding antecedent hypertension with concentric left ventricular hypertrophy and well-preserved systolic contraction. As has been shown in animal experiments, abrupt increases in cardiac afterload due to increased systemic resistence results in acute diastolic dysfunction. With poor diastolic relaxation, the left ventricle requires markedly elevated filling pressures, leading to pulmonary venous hypertension and edema. In contrast to the traditional therapy for dilated congestive heart failure, diuretic and inotropic agents are not indicated. Rather, acute reduction of afterload with vasodilators improves diastolic relaxation and lowers pulmonary venous pressure. Nitroprusside is often used in this situation. Modest decreases in pressure improves symptoms markedly. Nitrates can be added to enhance reductions in preload. Chronically, patients may be treated with angiotensin-converting enzyme (ACE) inhibitors, or calcium-channel antagonists, with or without β-blockers, as these agents have been shown to improve diastolic function and cause regression or concentric left ventricular hypertrophy.

For the uncommon patient who presents with hypertensive congestive heart failure with a dilated, poorly contractile left ventricle, negative inotropic agents should be avoided. Diuretics and nitroprusside plus morphine sulfate or nitroglycerin are effective. Enalaprilat, the intravenous form of the ACE inhibitor enalapril, may also be useful.

Coronary Artery Disease (8)

Hypertension in the setting of myocardial ischemia should be controlled (8). Increases in sympathetic tone and catecholamine release result in increases in afterload and left ventricular wall tension. Prompt afterload and modest preload reduction are necessary, and enhancement of coronary blood flow is desirable. In the setting of unstable angina, intravenous nitroglycerin is the agent of choice. By dilating intercoronary collaterals more than small resistance arterioles, perfusion is enhanced to ischemic myocardium. Calcium-channel antagonists and labetalol have also been successfully used. In contrast, other vasodilators, such as nitroprusside, dilate resistance arterioles predominantly, thereby resulting in a steal of blood flow away from ischemic areas. Thus, nitroprusside is reserved for cases refractory to initial nitrate therapy.

Hypertension in the setting of acute myocardial infarction often resolves over the course of a few hours with sedation and pain control alone. Considerable evidence demonstrates that the early use of β-blocking agents may reduce ultimate infarction size. When systemic pressures remain elevated above a diastolic pressure of 100 mm Hg, antihypertensive treatment is indicated. Nitroglycerin is preferred, but nitroprusside and labetalol have been used successfully. Pressure is reduced quickly to near normotensive levels, taking care to avoid overshoot hypotension, which can worsen coronary perfusion. Therapy can usually be weaned within 24 hours.

Perioperative Hypertension

Uncontrolled hypertension is an undisputed risk factor for mortality in the surgical patient. Induction of anesthesia may result in rapid and wide fluctuations in BP, leading to intraoperative hypotension, stroke, myocardial ischemia, or acute renal failure. Whenever possible, surgery should be deferred until diastolic pressure is controlled below 110 mm Hg. In chronic hypertensive patients who are administered adequate treatment, the immediate postoperative doses of medications should be reduced and only gradually increased to preoperative doses.

Postoperative hypertension is extremely common after coronary bypass, carotid endarterectomy, renal revascularization, and coarct repair. BP control is important to reduce the risk of bleeding from suture lines. Although nitroprusside is widely used, some prefer to use nitroglycerin for the postcoronary bypass patient. Trimethaphan, because of its inhibition of bowel function, is contraindicated postoperatively.

Catecholamine-Associated Hypertension

A number of conditions are associated with emergent hypertension due to a hyperadrenergic state (Table 1) in conjunction with monoamine oxidase (MAO) inhibitor therapy, and withdrawal from centrally acting α_2-agonists or β-blockers. Pheochromocytoma is a very rare cause of hypertension. Excess catecholamine secretion results in sustained BP elevation in the majority of cases, while peripheral catecholamine uptake and storage lead to paroxysmal symptoms. Symptoms include headache, palpitations, hypertension, anxiety, abdominal pain, and diaphoresis. Often, patients will present with orthostatic pressure

changes. For hypertensive emergency, the treatment of choice is the short-acting parenteral α-agonist phentolamine, given in 5 to 10 mg iv boluses every 5 minutes until pressure is controlled. Nitroprusside has also been effective as initial therapy. Following BP reduction, β-blockade is generally added to control tachycardia or arrhythmias. As in all catecholamine excess states, β-blockers should never be given first, as the loss of β-adrenergically-mediated vasodilation will leave β-adrenergically-mediated vasoconstriction unopposed and will result in increased pressure. Definitive therapy of pheochromocytoma includes surgical removal of the tumor. In preparation for surgery, an oral agent regimen of the nonselective α-agonist phenoxybenzamine, with β-blocker subsequently added, is used. Two weeks of this regimen is preoperatively recommended to allow the intravascular volume to normalize. Labetalol has been effective in treating pheochromocytoma-related hypotension, but only in selected patients. β-blockade by this agent exceeds its α-blocking effect, and actual precipitation of severe hypertension has been reported.

Excess catecholamine-related hypertension can result from ingestion of sympathomimetic agents such as cocaine, amphetamines, phencyclidine, phenylpropanolamine (diet pills), decongestants such as ephedrine and pseudoephedrine, and other agents including atropine, ergot alkaloids, and tricyclic antidepressants. Critically elevated pressures can result, and cases complicated by seizures, myocardial infarction, aortic dissection, and stroke have been reported. Treatment is similar to pheochromocytoma crisis, with nitroprusside or phentolamine and subsequent β-blocker therapy. The duration of the hypertension is self limited and resolves after a number of hours.

The abrupt discontinuation of chronic β-blocker therapy or centrally acting α-agonist antihypertensives such as clonidine, methyldopa, or guanabenz can lead to overshoot hypertension. This condition is due to rebound sympathetic outflow, occurring 12 to 72 hours after the last dose, and is accompanied by symptoms such as headache, diaphoresis, anxiety, nausea, tachycardia, and abdominal pain. In cases of moderate hypertension, simply restarting the antihypertensive may be all that is necessary. For those with critically elevated pressures, nitroprusside or phentolamine is effective, and the oral medication may be restarted once pressures have been controlled.

In patients on MAO-inhibitor therapy, ingestion of foods containing tyramine sympathomimetic amines, or tricyclic antidepressants precipitate hyperadrenergic hypertension. Tyramine is metabolized by an alternative pathway to octopamine, which releases catecholamines from peripheral sites by acting as a false neurotransmitter. Again, in severe cases, nitroprusside or phentolamine is used, with the addition of β-blockade as needed for tachycardia. The episodes are self limited and last $\leq$ 6 hours.

Eclampsia

During normal pregnancy, BP is decreased and then slowly increases toward the normal range during the third trimester. Preeclampsia, with proteinuria, edema, and relatively increased pressures (defined as $\geq$ 140 mm Hg), generally occurs in young primigravidas beyond the 20th week of gestation. In this condition, despite visible edema, intravascular volume is low and the renin-angiotensin system is activated. Progression to seizures constitutes eclampsia, and may occur with diastolic pressures of only 100 mm Hg. General therapy includes bed rest and parenteral magnesium. Diuretics are contraindicated, given the low intravascular volume. Antihypertensive treatment is begun in the case of eclampsia or when the diastolic pressure approaches 105 mm Hg. To avoid compromising placental blood flow, the goal of therapy should be diastolic pressure of 90 to 100 mm Hg. Because of its well-established record of safety in this setting, hydralazine is the preferred agent. The dose is 5 to 10 mg iv every 20 minutes until the pressure is controlled. Unlike many other antihypertensives, hydralazine increases placental blood flow. Intravenous methyldopa may be added when hydralazine alone is not effective. In cases where these agents are ineffective, alternatives are controversial. Diazoxide is recommended by

some, but its relaxant effect on uterine smooth muscle inhibits labor, and it crosses the placenta and can cause fetal hyperglycemia and hyperbilirubinemia. Nitroprusside is used only in refractory cases and then only briefly, in preparation for cesarean section. Trimethaphan causes meconium ileus and should not be used. ACE inhibitors can cause fetal acute renal failure and are contraindicated. Nifedipine appears useful.

Hypertension Associated With Renal Failure

In the setting of malignant hypertension, renal failure is common. Aggressive treatment can arrest and reverse renal damage. Initially, however, renal function may deteriorate with therapy and dialysis may be required. Dialysis is rarely needed in patients presenting with creatinine of $\leq$ 4.5 mg/dL ($\leq$ 300 μmol/L). In the majority of patients, renal function improves beginning after 2 weeks of therapy. Long-term experience demonstrates that in malignant hypertensive patients who require dialysis due to renal failure, up to 50% of these patients will regain function and discontinue the need for dialysis. When the combined length of both kidneys is $\geq$ 20.2 cm, recovery can be expected, whereas, if the length is $\leq$ 14.2 cm, recovery is unlikely.

Nitroprusside is effective initial parenteral therapy, but it carries a particular risk of thiocyanate toxicity when renal function is reduced. Thiocyanate levels should be monitored, and the duration of therapy should be kept to < 72 hours whenever possible. Of the oral agents, calcium antagonists and minoxidil are effective and safe. ACE inhibitors may cause hyperkalemia in undialyzed patients with significant renal insufficiency.

Other Hypertensive Situations

Scleroderma renal crisis is a particularly aggressive form of malignant hypertension in which proliferative endarteritis precedes hypertension. The incidence among patients with scleroderma is 8% to 13%, and it is more common among African Americans. Progression to end-stage renal disease occurs in 1 to 2 months without treatment. Aggressive pressure control with ACE inhibitors is the appropriate treatment, and it leads to a long-term survival rate of ~ 50%. Corticosteroid use should be avoided. One-fourth of patients with extensive second- and third-degree burns develop severe hypertension in the first few days; this condition is likely due to the high levels of circulating catecholamines and renin. Nitroprusside or phentolamine is a successful therapeutic agent. Patients with transverse spinal cord lesions at the T6 level or higher, including patients with Guillain-Barré syndrome, have autonomic dysreflexia in which a noxious stimulus in a dermatome below the level of the lesion can trigger a massive sympathetic discharge. This autonomic dysfunction leads to severe hypertension, bradycardia, diaphoresis, and headache. In > 90% of cases, distention of bladder or bowel is responsible, and prompt decompression leads to a resolution of the hypertension. Drugs that have been used successfully include nitroprusside, phentolamine, and labetalol.

Hypertension in renal transplant recipients may be due to a variety of causes, including acute rejection, vascular anastomotic stenosis, obstructive uropathy, corticosteroid use, cyclosporine, and native kidney renin release. Careful consideration should be given for each of these patients. Oral calcium-channel antagonists are effective and well tolerated in these patients. Severe or malignant hypertension due to excess aldosterone production is very rare, with a few case reports of aldosterone secreting adenomas and tumors of the ovary and kidney. The endocrine profile of malignant hypertension can mimic primary hyperaldosteronism for many months of successful antihypertensive treatment. Drugs associated with the development of severe or malignant hypertension include cyclosporine, erythropoietin, amphotericin B, lithium, and amitriptyline. Erythropoietin-associated hypertension is treated with phlebotomy and dose reduction in conjunction with antihypertensive drugs. Diabetics on β-blockers can experience severe hypertension with hypoglycemic episodes, presumably due to catecholamine release.

ANTIHYPERTENSIVE AGENTS (1)

The following section details the characteristics of each agent. Parenteral agents are summarized in Table 6, and oral agents are listed in Table 7.

Intravenous Agents

Nitroprusside

Nitroprusside, of the parenteral agents, is the most broadly used. It is a direct vasodilator of both arterioles and venous capacitance vessels and reduces both preload and afterload. Cardiac and uterine smooth muscle are not affected and there are no CNS side effects. Its rapid onset (1 to 2 minutes) and short half-life (3 to 4 minutes) allow rapid titration to BP. The initial infusion rate should be ≤ 0.3 µg/kg/min and can be titrated by 1 µg/kg/min every 3 to 4 minutes to a maximum dose of 10 µg/kg/min. The drug is metabolized to cyanide, which is rapidly converted in the liver to thiocyanate. Cyanide toxicity may rarely occur in patients with hepatic dysfunction and should be suspected in cases of refractory hypotension, unexplained metabolic acidosis, or venous hyperoxemia. It is treated with sodium nitrite followed by sodium thiosulfate infusion. Thiocyanate is excreted by the kidney with a half-life of 1 week. Toxicity may be seen in patients with renal dysfunction on significant doses for long periods, when plasma thiocyanate levels exceed 10 mg/dL. Signs include loss of antihypertensive effect, lactic acidosis, vomiting, mental status disturbances, and seizures. In patients with renal dysfunction, nitroprusside infusion should be limited to 72 hours when possible, and thiocyanate levels should be monitored. Toxicity is reversible when the drug is discontinued and can be treated with dialysis. Tachyphylaxis to nitroprusside does not develop in the absence of thiocyanate toxicity, but, like all potent vasodilators, resistance to therapy can emerge due to reflex cardiac stimulation, activation of the renin-angiotensin system, and sodium and water retention.

Table 6. Parenteral agents used in hypertensive crisis

Drug	Onset	Duration	Dose	Comments
Nitroprusside	Seconds	2–4 mins	0.3 µg/kg/min; maximum: 10 µg/kg/min	Risk of cyanide (liver failure) or thiocyanate (renal failure) toxicity; avoid use for 72 hrs in renal failure
Diazoxide	1–2 mins	4–12 mins	25- to 75-mg bolus over 30 secs every 5 to 10 mins; maximum dose: 600 mg	May exacerbate myocardial ischemia
Labetalol	2–5 mins	3–5 hrs	20-mg bolus over 2 mins followed in 10 mins by 40-mg boluses thereafter; 20-mg bolus over 2 mins	May precipitate heart block or asthma; avoid if β-blockers are contraindicated
Trimethaphan	1–2 mins	10 mins	0.5 mg/min; 0.5 to 2 mg/min infusion; maintenance: 2 to 5 mg/min	Causes paralytic ileus and bladder atony; tachyphylaxis within 96 hrs
Nitroglycerin	1–2 mins	3–5 mins	5 µg/min; maintenance: 5 to 100 µg/min	Dose required is highly variable
Hydralazine	5–10 mins	3–9 hrs	5-mg bolus; 1- to 5-mg bolus every 15 to 20 mins	Especially useful in preeclampsia/ eclampsia
Phentolamine	1–2 mins	15–30 mins	1-mg bolus; 1- to 5-mg bolus every 5 to 10 mins; maximum: 20 to 30 mg	Intermittent maintenance dose as needed; may exacerbate peptic ulcer disease
Propranolol	2–5 mins	6–8 hrs	1- to 3-mg bolus over 1 to 3 mins; repeat in 5 mins, if necessary	Use as adjunct only, not as single agent
Enalaprilat	10–15 mins	6 hrs	0.625 to 1.25 mg; repeat every 4 to 6 hrs	Caution use in patients with volume depletion

Table 7. Oral agents used in severe hypertension

Calcium-Channel Antagonists
    Dihydropyridines
Angiotensin-converting enzyme inhibitors
Direct-Acting Vasodilators
    Hydralazine 50 to 100 mg twice a day
    Minoxidil 5 to 20 mg twice a day
Adjunctive Therapy
    β-blockers
    Loop diuretics

Labetalol

Labetalol is a combined α- and β-adrenergic antagonist with relative selectivity for β-blockade by 7-fold on intravenous administration. BP reduction is by redution in systemic vascular resistance with little or no change in cardiac output, heart rate, or cerebral blood flow. Onset is rapid (5 minutes), and duration of action is 3 to 6 hours, with combined renal and hepatic drug clearance. Pressure reduction is smooth and predictable with minibolus or intravenous drip infusion. By minibolus, 20 mg is given slowly over 2 minutes, followed in 10 minutes by 40 mg and subsequently 40 to 80 mg every 10 minutes. The maximum intravenous loading dose is 300 mg. Alternatively, a 20-mg bolus can be followed by administration of 0.5- to 2.0-mg/min drip. The availability of labetalol for oral administration simplifies the transition to an oral regimen. The oral dose begins at 200 mg twice daily to a maximum of 1200 mg/day. The combined α- and β-blocking properties of this drug make it particularly useful in aortic dissection or catecholamine excess states, although paradoxical worsening of hypertension has occasionally been seen in cases of pheochromocytoma. Labetalol should not be used in patients with sinus bradycardia, atrioventricular block, congestive heart failure, or reactive airway disease.

Trimethaphan Camsylate

Trimethaphan blocks both cholinergic and adrenergic ganglionic transmission, resulting in both preload and afterload reduction. A marked reduction in dP/dt makes this agent primarily useful in the treatment of aortic dissection. Reflex chronotropic stimulation is mild and may be treated with a β-blocking agent. Rapid onset (102 minutes) and short duration (10 minutes) enable accurate titration of dose. Infusion is begun at a rate of 0.5 mg/min and increased in 3- to 5-minute increments to a maximum rate of 5 mg/min. Metabolism is believed to be by cholinesterase. When using this agent, the patient's head should be elevated to increase efficacy. Pseudotolerance due to salt and water retention occurs, and true tachyphylaxis within 96 hours limits its use. Adverse reactions include orthostatic hypotension, paralytic ileus, bladder atony, mydriasis, cycloplegia, dry mucous membranes, and respiratory depression at higher doses due to a curare-like effect. Use is contraindicated in patients with glaucoma.

Diazoxide

Diazoxide is a powerful arteriolar dilator without effects on venous capacitance. Significant reflex cardiac activation occurs, with increases in heart rate and cardiac output, stimulation of renin production, and renal sodium and water retention. Onset is rapid (1 to 2 minutes), and the duration is 4 to 12 hours, with combined renal and hepatic clearance. The drug is given in miniboluses of 25 to 75 mg every 5 to 10 minutes or infusion of 15 mg/min for 10 to 30 minutes to a total dose of 150 to 600 mg. Pretreatment with a β-blocking agent increases efficacy. It is highly protein bound. Protein binding is reduced in uremia, dictating lower doses in patients with renal failure. The use of diazoxide is primarily limited to those cases where nitroprusside is preferred but intensive care monitoring is not possible, and to obstetrical emergencies refractory to hydralazine. Adverse reactions include hyperglycemia, arrest of labor, and myocardial ischemia. High protein binding can displace other drugs, such as warfarin. Contraindications to use include aortic dissection, myocardial infarction, angina, and stroke.

Nitroglycerin

In low doses, nitroglycerin primarily decreases preload by venodilation; at higher doses, it is also a mild arterial dilator. Nitroglycerin also dilates large coronary arteries and intercoronary collateral vessels, and increases subendocardial perfusion. This beneficial effect on myocardial blood flow makes it the agent of choice in hypertensive patients with acute myocardial infarction, angina, ischemic congestive heart failure, and postcardiac bypass. The onset is rapid (1 to 2 minutes) with brief duration (3 to 5 minutes). Infusion is begun at a rate of ≤ 5 μg/min and maximum dose is 100 μg/min.

Hydralazine

Hydralazine is a pure arterial vasodilator with less potency and predictability of response than diazoxide. It is the vasodilator of choice in pregnant patients. Onset after intravenous bolus is 10 to 30 minutes, with a duration of action of 3 to 9 hours. The drug is excreted by the kidneys. Initial dose in the pregnant patient is 5 mg iv, with an additional 5 to 10 mg every 15 to 20 minutes. There is significant variability in the dose and frequency required. Reflex stimulation of heart rate, cardiac output, and volume retention often leads to pseudotolerance. Use of hydralizine should be avoided in patients with coronary artery disease, stroke, and aortic dissection.

Phentolamine Mesylate

This nonselective α-antagonist is useful in the treatment of catecholamine excess states. It is both an arterial and venous dilator. Onset is rapid (1 to 2 minutes) and duration is brief (15 to 30 minutes) allowing close titration. The initial intravenous dose of 1 mg is followed by 1 to 5 mg every 5 to 10 minutes to a maximum total of 20 to 30 mg. Subsequent intermittent dosing is continued as necessary. Adverse reactions include tachycardia arrhythmias (in the absence of β-blockade), abdominal pain, and diarrhea. Phentolamine stimulates gastric secretions and should not be used in patients with peptic ulcer disease.

β-Blockers

Given alone, β-blockers increase systemic vascular resistance and depress cardiac output and glomerular filtration rate, and are generally not appropriate monotherapy for severe or malignant hypertension. They are used as adjunct therapy for their negative inotropic and chronotropic effects. Propranolol is a nonselective β-antagonist with a half-life of 4 hours. Intravenous dose is 1 to 3 mg at a rate of 1 mg/min, followed by a second dose, if necessary. Oral doses vary from 80 to 230 mg/day divided 3 or 4 times daily. Metoprolol is β_1 selective and has a slightly longer half-life. The initial injection of 5 mg is followed in 2 to 5 minutes by a second and subsequently a third injection, if necessary. Oral therapy is 100 to 400 mg/day, divided twice a day. β-blocker therapy is contraindicated in patients with bradycardia, significant atrioventricular block, congestive cardiomyopathy, and reactive airway disease.

Enalaprilat

This rapidly acting (10 minutes) precursor of the ACE inhibitor, enalapril, has been shown in small studies to be effective in hypertensive emergencies. The dose is 0.625 to 1.25 mg iv over a 5-minute period, repeated every 6 hours. Volume-depleted patients and malignant hypertensive patients have increased sensitivity to ACE inhibitors because of the high renin-angiotensin state. The specific role of enalaprilat in hypertensive emergencies has not yet clearly been defined.

Other Agents

Intravenous verapamil has been used successfully for hypertensive emergencies, but, unfortunately, the doses necessary tend to cause an unacceptably high incidence of cardiac conduction abnormalities. The experience with diltiazem has been very limited. Fenoldopam, a novel dopamine-1 receptor antagonist with salutary effects on renal blood flow, has shown promise in the treatment of severe hypertension. Methyldopa, reserpine, and other rauwolfia alkaloids can no longer be recommended for use in severe hypertension.

Oral Agents

Calcium-Channel Antagonists

Among the many oral agents that are effective in the treatment of severe hypertension, calcium-channel blockers are the most frequently used. Calcium antagonists do not exacerbate bronchospasm, angina, or peripheral ischemia. They are free from CNS side effects. There is a theoretical cytoprotective effect to ischemic tissue with calcium- channel antagonists. The acute effects of calcium-channel blockers on renal function are likewise favorable, with afferent vasodilation opposing the effects of norepinephrine and angiotensin II. Renal vasodilation results in increased renal blood flow and glomerular filtration rate in most patients. Of the 3 classes of calcium antagonists, the derivatives of dihydropyridine are the most useful for hypertension. The other 2 classes, represented by diltiazem and verapamil, affect cardiac contractility and conduction to a greater extent.

Nifedipine is the most extensively used calcium-channel antagonist for severe hypertension and has a generally predictable response effective in a high percentage of patients. Onset after an oral dose of 10 to 20 mg is in the range of 20 and 30 minutes, with a 4- to 6-hour duration of action. Although "sublingual" administration is frequently discussed, actual absorption probably occurs in the stomach, and this route should not be used. Reduction in vascular resistance tends to be proportional to the initial state of vascular tone. Reflex tachycardia is mild, and cardiac output usually changes little due to the small negative inotropic effect. Cerebral vasodilation can contribute to increased intracranial pressure, a concern in patients with hypertensive encephalopathy.

Overshoot hypotension has been reported, usually in hypovolemic patients or in those patients who use diuretics. Use of the sustained release preparation prevents this problem and can be used in less urgent situations. It has been used successfully in malignant hypertension. Adverse reactions include headache, facial flushing, and a burning sensation in the legs. Mild ankle edema is common due to increased capillary perfusion pressure, but this is usually not associated with weight gain.

The number of dihydropyridine-related calcium antagonists is growing, but there is little evidence of individual drug advantages. Their role in the treatment of severe hypertension is still evolving. Isradipine and Amlodipine have somewhat less negative inotropic actions than Nifedipine. Nicardipine is available for both oral and intravenous administration. Following administration, cardiac output is increased because of an apparent complete lack of negative inotropic effect, but reflex chronotropic action appears to be less than with Nifedipine. Nicardipine crosses the blood-brain barrier and may be useful in the treatment of subarachnoid hemorrhage. Nimodipine is primarily a cerebral vasodilator with only weak antihypertensive effects. The drug is approved for use in subarachnoid hemorrhage. In addition, it may benefit some cases of ischemic stroke. Felodipine is a more potent peripheral vasodilator than Nifedipine, with little or no negative inotropic or cardiac conduction effects. In 1 study, its effectiveness was found to be comparable to minoxidil in severe chronic hypertensives.

Angiotensin-Converting Enzyme Inhibitors

ACE inhibitors are extremely valuable in the management of chronic hypertension because of the favorable effects on hemodynamics and freedom from adverse side effects. Inhibition of angiotensin II production reduces systemic vascular resistance with little tachycardia. Cardiac output is improved in patients with congestive heart failure but shows little change in others. Preferential dilation of the renal efferent arteriole is beneficial in patients with glomerular hyperfiltration. ACE inhibitors also have a favorable effect on cerebral blood flow autoregulation by shifting the range to lower values. Captopril, the first of these agents and the shortest acting, has been used successfully by the oral and sublingual routes in treating hypertensive emergencies and urgencies in small trials. It should be used with extreme caution in the hypovolemic or malignant hypertensive patients, however, because first-dose hypotension can occur. Scleroderma crisis is the single hypertensive emergency in which ACE inhibitors are the first-line agents. All of the currently available ACE inhibitors probably have comparable efficacy. Adverse effects include cough, taste disturbances, hyperkalemia, leukopenia, proteinuria, and allergic reactions. Patients with bilateral renal artery stenosis often experience reversible acute renal failure with ACE-inhibitor therapy. Use in pregnancy is contraindicated.

Direct-Acting Vasodilators

Minoxidil is the most powerful vasodilator available in oral form. Its action is purely arteriolar, without venous dilation or direct cardiac effects. Reflex increases in heart rate, cardiac output, and volume retention are marked with minoxidil and generally mandate addition of other agents to prevent pseudotolerance and unpleasant side effects. The starting dose is 2.5 mg twice daily and is increased every few days to a maximum dose of 40 mg/day. A β-blocker is added for tachycardia, with high doses often necessary. As fluid retention becomes evident, diuretics are added, typically furosemide 20 to 40 mg twice daily. Most patients who are refractory to other antihypertensive regimens can be controlled successfully on this so-called "triple therapy." The development of hypertrichosis with chronic therapy limits patient tolerance in females, however. Other adverse effects include pericardial effusions, and exacerbation of angina. Transient flattening or inversion of T waves on electrocardiogram are frequently noted, and are of unknown significance.

REFERENCES

1. Nolan CR, Linas SL: Accelerated/malignant hypertension. *In:* Diseases of the Kidney. Schrier RW, Gottshalk C (Eds). Boston, Little Brown, 1997, pp 1475–1554
2. Kitiyakara C, Guzman NJ: Malignant hypertension and hypertensive emergencies. *J Am Soc Nephrol* 1998; 9:133–142
3. Zampaglione B, Pascale C, Marchisio M, et al: Hypertensive urgencies and emergencies. Prevalence and clinical presentation. *Hypertension* 1996; 27:144–147
4. Gifford RWJ: Management of hypertensive crises. *JAMA* 1991; 266:829–835
5. Zell KR, Von Kuhnert L, Matthews C: Rapid reduction of severe asymptomatic hypertension. A prospective, controlled trial. *Arch Intern Med* 1989; 149:2186–2189
6. Phillips SJ: Pathophysiology and management of hypertension in acute ischemic stroke [clinical conference]. *Hypertension* 1994; 23:131–136
7. Feigin VL, Rinkel GJ, Algra A, et al: Calcium antagonists in patients with aneurysmal subarachnoid hemorrhage: A systematic review [see comments]. *Neurology* 1998; 50:876–883
8. Ryan TJ, Anderson JL, Antman EM, et al: ACC/AHA guidelines for the management of patients with acute myocardial infarction: Executive summary. A report of the American College of Cardiology/American Heart Association Task Force on Practice Guidelines (Committee on Management of Acute Myocardial Infarction). *Circulation* 1996; 94:2341–2350

MYOCARDIAL INFARCTION

Steven M. Hollenberg, MD

Objectives

- To review the diagnosis of myocardial infarction, with emphasis on diagnostic pitfalls
- To understand indications, contraindications, and use of thrombolytic therapy
- To understand the role of cardiac catheterization, angioplasty, and surgical revascularization
- To review medical therapy of acute myocardial infarction
- To review complications of acute myocardial infarction

ANATOMY OF ACUTE INFARCTION

Definitions

Ischemic heart disease results from an inadequate level of coronary blood flow to meet myocardial oxygen demand. The heart extracts oxygen nearly maximally at baseline, and so increases in demand must be met by commensurate increases in coronary blood flow. Myocardial infarction occurs when prolonged ischemia causes myocardial necrosis.

Myocardial ischemia is associated almost immediately with failure of contraction. Although this can result in part from myocardial necrosis, areas of nonfunctional but viable myocardium can also cause or contribute to the development of systolic dysfunction. This reversibly dysfunctional myocardium comes under 2 main categories: stunning and hibernation. Myocardium reperfused after ischemia may exhibit profound contractile dysfunction despite restoration of normal blood flow, but may recover eventually; this transient postischemic dysfunction is termed "stunning." Hibernating myocardium is a state of persistently impaired myocardial function at rest due to severely reduced coronary blood flow, and can be viewed as a response that reduces myocardial contractile function in an area of hypoperfusion so as to restore equilibrium between flow and function, thus minimizing the potential for ischemia or necrosis. Both stunned and hibernating myocardium have contractile reserve, and function of both may improve with time and/or revascularization.

Pathogenesis

Myocardial infarction is usually due to thrombus formation within a coronary artery, most often resulting from rupture of an atherosclerotic plaque. Classification of infarctions into those which are transmural and those which are nontransmural has been largely abandoned due to the recognition that electrocardiographic criteria are neither sensitive nor specific to make this distinction. Infarctions can be usually into Q-wave infarctions, which are usually transmural and most often result from total coronary occlusion, and non-Q-wave infarctions, which are usually subendocardial and result from subtotal coronary occlusion. More recently, myocardial infarction has been divided based on the presence of ST-segment elevation at presentation. This classification is useful clinically because patients with ST-elevation MI are eligible for thrombolytic therapy, and patients with non-ST elevation MI are not.

Distribution of the Major Coronary Arteries

The left anterior descending coronary artery (LAD) supplies the anterior left ventricle, anterior septum, and usually the left ventricular apex; the LAD has septal and diagonal branches. Anterior infarction is seen in electrocardiographic (EKG) leads V_1 to V_5. The right coronary artery (RCA) supplies the inferior left ventricular wall, usually the inferior septum, most of the right ventricle, and the sinus node. The RCA is dominant (that is, it gives rise to a posterior descending artery and so supplies left ventricular myocardium in the inferior septal region) in 80% of patients. Inferior infarction is seen in EKG leads II, III, and aVF. The circumflex coronary artery runs in the atrioventricular (A-V) groove; obtuse marginal (OM) branches supply the lateral and posterolateral left ventricle. Lateral infarction is seen in EKG leads I, aVL, V_5, and V_6.

DIAGNOSIS OF ACUTE INFARCTION

The diagnosis of acute myocardial infarction is made on the basis of a compatible clinical presentation, electrocardiographic changes, and a rise and fall in enzymes indicative of myocardial damage. The differential diagnosis of acute infarction includes dissecting aortic aneurysm, pericarditis, pulmonary processes such as pulmonary embolism, pneumonia, and pneumothorax, gastrointestinal processes such as esophageal or peptic ulcer disease and cholecystitis, and costochondritis.

The classic electrocardiographic feature of acute infarction is ST segment elevation, followed by T wave inversion and ultimate development of Q waves. The diagnosis can be limited in the presence of pre-existing left bundle-branch block (LBBB) or permanent pacemaker. Nonetheless, new LBBB with a compatible clinical presentation should be treated as acute myocardial infarction and treated accordingly. True posterior MI, which usually accompanies inferior infarction, can be subtle; hallmarks include prominent R waves, tall upright T waves, and depressed ST segments in leads V_1 and V_2. The clinician must also be careful not to be fooled by electrocardiographic "imposters" of acute infarction, which include pericarditis, J-point elevation, Wolff-Parkinson-White syndrome, and hypertrophic cardiomyopathy.

The classic biochemical marker of acute myocardial infarction is elevation of creatine phosphokinase (CPK) levels. The CPK MB isoenzyme is found primarily in cardiac muscle, and only small amounts are present in skeletal muscle and brain. CPK peaks during the first 24 hours and then decreases rapidly. Lactate dehydrogenase (LDH) levels peak at 72 to 96 hours and may be used to detect recent infarction, which is associated with an increase in the LDH_1 isoenzyme.

Elevations in troponin T and troponin I are more specific biochemical markers of cardiac muscle damage. Their use is becoming more widespread, and has superceded use of CPK MB in many settings. Troponins are more sensitive and specific for the detection of myocardial damage, and troponin elevation in patients without ST elevation (or in fact, without elevation of CPK-MB) identifies a subpopulation at increased risk for complications. Troponins may not be elevated until 6 hours after an acute event, and once elevated, remain high for days to weeks, limiting their utility to detect late reinfarction.

THROMBOLYTIC THERAPY FOR ACUTE MYOCARDIAL INFARCTION

Early reperfusion of an occluded coronary artery is indicated for all eligible candidates. Thrombolytic therapy has been proven to decrease mortality in patients with ST segment elevation; patients treated early derive the most benefit. Indications and contraindications for thrombolytic therapy are listed below. Contraindications can be regarded as absolute or relative.

Indications

- Symptoms consistent with acute myocardial infarction
- EKG showing 1-mm (0.1 mV) ST elevation in at least 2 contiguous leads, or new left bundle-branch block
- Presentation within 12 hours of symptom onset
- Absence of contraindications

Contraindications

Absolute

- Active internal bleeding
- Intracranial neoplasm, aneurysm, or A-V malformation
- Stroke or neurosurgery within 6 weeks
- Trauma or major surgery within 2 weeks which could be a potential source of serious rebleeding
- Aortic dissection

Relative

- Prolonged (> 10 minutes) or clearly traumatic cardiopulmonary resuscitation*

- Severe uncontrolled hypertension
  (> 200/110 mm Hg)*
- Trauma or major surgery within 6 weeks
  (but more than 2 weeks)
- Pre-existing coagulopathy
- Active peptic ulcer
- Infective endocarditis
- Pregnancy
- Chronic severe hypertension

* Could be an absolute contraindication in low-risk patients with myocardial infarction

THROMBOLYTIC AGENTS

Streptokinase (SK) is a single-chain protein produced by α-hemolytic streptococci, which produces a systemic lytic state for about 24 hours. SK is given as a 1.5-million-unit iv infusion over 1 hour. Hypotension with infusion usually responds to fluids and a decreased infusion rate, but allergic reactions are possible. Hemorrhagic complications are the most feared side effect, with a rate of intracranial hemorrhage of approximately 0.5%.

Tissue plasminogen activator (t-PA) is a recombinant protein that is more fibrin-selective than streptokinase and produces a higher early coronary patency rate. Based on the favorable results of the Global Utilization of Streptokinase and Tissue Plasminogen Activator for Occluded Coronary Arteries (GUSTO) trial, t-PA is usually given in an accelerated regimen consisting of a 15 mg bolus, 50 mg iv over the initial 30 minutes, and 35 mg over the next 60 minutes; adjustment for weight is preferred for patients < 67 kg. Allergic reactions do not occur because t-PA is not antigenic, but the rate of intracranial hemorrhage may be slightly higher than that with SK, around 0.7%.

Reteplase (r-PA), is a deletion mutant of t-PA with an extended half-life, and is given as 2 10 mg boluses 30 minutes apart. Reteplase was originally evaluated in angiographic trials, which demonstrated improved coronary flow at 90 minutes compared to t-PA, but subsequent trials showed similar 30-day mortality rates. Why enhanced patency with r-PA did not translate into lower mortality is uncertain.

Tenecteplase (TNK-tPA) is a genetically engineered t-PA mutant with amino acid substitutions that result in prolonged half-life, resistance to plaminogen-activator inhibitor-1, and increased fibrin specificity. TNK-tPA is given as a single bolus, adjusted for weight. A single bolus of TNK-tPA has been shown to produce coronary flow rates identical to those seen with accelerated t-PA, with equivalent 30-day mortality and bleeding rates. Based on these results, single-bolus TNK-tPA is an acceptable alternative to t-PA that can be given as a single bolus.

Other new thrombolytics include *lanoteplase* (n-PA), a deletion mutant of t-PA with prolonged half-life that is given as a single bolus (120,000 U/kg). Angiographic studies demonstrated increased TIMI 3 flow with n-PA compared to t-PA and an equivalent 30-day mortality rate, but a higher rate of bleeding. *Staphylokinase*, a plasminogen activator produced by certain strains of *Staphylococcus aureus*, is as potent as t-PA and significantly more fibrin-specific. Staphylokinase, however, has a short half-life, is antigenic, and induces antibody formation. Site-directed mutagenesis as well as conjugation with polyethylene glycol are being used in an attempt to reduce the immunogenicity of Staphylokinase and to increase its plasma half-life.

The ideal thrombolytic agent has not yet been developed. Newer recombinant agents with greater fibrin specificity, slower clearance from the circulation, and more resistance to plasma protease inhibitors are being studied.

COMBINATION FIBRINOLYTIC AND ANTI-PLATELET THERAPY IN ACUTE ST-SEGMENT ELEVATION MYOCARDIAL INFARCTION

Thrombolytic monotherapy for acute ST segment elevation myocardial infarction is successful in achieving normal (TIMI grade 3) flow in only approximately 50% - 60% of cases. Furthermore, fibrinolysis activates platelets, which causes further thrombus formation and subsequent reocclusion and reinfarction in a significant number of patients. Researchers have proposed that the combination of a glycoprotein IIb/IIIa inhibitor with a reduced dose of fibrinolytics would maximize inhibition of platelet aggregation without an increase in the most serious bleeding complications. Although early studies showed improved patency, (manifested by a larger percentage of patients with TIMI 3 flow), convincing data that this approach improves clinical outcomes is lacking.

"Facilitated" early percutaneous coronary intervention refers to planned percutaneous coronary intervention after reduced dose pharmacological reperfusion therapy. This strategy has been shown to be feasible with an acceptable safety profile. Studies are currently underway to determine whether this combined approach could provide the optimal reperfusion strategy.

PRIMARY ANGIOPLASTY IN ACUTE MYOCARDIAL INFARCTION

Rapid restoration of coronary blood flow is the initial goal of therapy for acute myocardial infarction. As many as one-half to two-thirds of patients presenting with acute myocardial infarction may be ineligible for thrombolytic therapy, and these patients should be considered for primary PTCA. Primary PTCA can achieve reperfusion of the infarct vessel without the risk of bleeding associated with thrombolytic therapy. In experienced hands, initial success rates exceed 90%. Complications include reinfarction in 2% to 4% (a rate lower than with thrombolytics), distal embolization of thrombus, ventricular arrhythmias, and transient but severe hypotension associated with the Bezold-Jarisch reflex, which is more common with reperfusion of the right coronary artery.

The major advantages of primary PTCA over thrombolytic therapy include a higher rate of Thrombolysis in Myocardial Infarction (TIMI) trial grade 3 (normal) flow and a lower risk of intracranial hemorrhage. Several randomized trials have suggested that PTCA is preferable to thrombolytic therapy for AMI patients at higher risk, including those over 75 years old, those with anterior infarctions, and those with hemodynamic instability. The largest of these trials is the GUSTO-IIb Angioplasty Substudy, which randomized 1,138 patients. At 30 days, there was a clinical benefit in the combined primary endpoints of death, nonfatal reinfarction, and nonfatal disabling stroke in the patients treated with PTCA compared to t-PA, but no difference in the "hard" endpoints of death and myocardial infarction at 30 days.

It should be noted that these trials were performed in institutions in which a team skilled in primary angioplasty for acute myocardial infarction was immediately available, and that this allowed for prompt reperfusion of the infarct-related artery. More important than the method of revascularization is the time to revascularization, and this should be achieved in the most efficient and expeditious manner possible. If primary PTCA can be performed in a timely manner (within 60 minutes) by highly experienced personnel, this may be the preferred method of revascularization, since it offers more complete revascularization with improved restoration of normal coronary blood flow and detailed information about coronary anatomy. When performing PTCA will require a substantial time delay, and in less experienced hands, thrombolytic therapy may be preferable. Retrospective studies have suggested that in the community setting (as opposed to PTCA performed as part of a controlled clinical trial), mortality rates after myocardial infarction with routine primary PTCA and thrombolytic therapy are currently equivalent.

There are certain subpopulations, however, in which primary PTCA is clearly preferred. Revascularization for patients with cardiogenic shock is discussed in the Heart Failure syllabus.

Situations in Which PTCA is Clearly Preferable to Thrombolytics in Acute Myocardial Infarction

- Contraindications to thrombolytic therapy
- Cardiogenic shock
- Patients in whom uncertain diagnosis prompted cardiac catheterization which revealed coronary occlusion

Situations in Which PTCA May be Preferable to Thrombolytics in Acute Myocardial Infarction

- Elderly patients (> 75 years)
- Hemodynamic instability
- Large anterior infarction

- Patients with a prior myocardial infarction or prior coronary artery bypass grafting

CORONARY STENTING FOR ACUTE MYOCARDIAL INFARCTION

Primary angioplasty for acute myocardial infarction results in a significant reduction in mortality but is limited by the possibility of abrupt vessel closure, recurrent in-hospital ischemia, reocclusion of the infarct-related artery, and restenosis. The PAMI Stent Trial was designed to test the hypothesis that routine implantation of an intracoronary stent would reduce angiographic restenosis and improve clinical outcomes compared to primary balloon angioplasty alone. This large, randomized, multicenter trial involving 900 patients did not show a difference in mortality at 6 months but did show improvement in ischemia-driven target vessel revascularization and less angina in the stented patients compared to PTCA alone.

Glycoprotein IIb/IIIa receptor antagonists inhibit the final common pathway of platelet aggregation, and their use in percutaneous intervention is becoming almost routine. The ReoPro and Primary PTCA Organization Randomized (RAPPORT) Trial compared the glycoprotein IIb/IIIa inhibitor abciximab to placebo in 483 patients with acute ST segment elevation MI undergoing primary PTCA. The trial showed no difference in the primary endpoint of death, nonfatal MI, or any repeat revascularization procedure at 6 months, but the incidence of death, reinfarction, or urgent revascularization was lower with abciximab versus placebo at 7 days; bleeding complications, which occurred mostly at arterial access sites, were more common with abciximab. The ADMIRAL Trial (Abciximab Before Direct Angioplasty and Stenting in MI Regarding Acute and Long Term Follow Up) was the first placebo-controlled study to evaluate abciximab as an adjunct to primary PTCA and stenting in acute myocardial infarction patients. Abciximab used in conjunction with stenting improved coronary patency before stenting and resulted in a nearly 50% relative risk reduction in the incidence of death, recurrent MI, and urgent revascularization at 30 days, although this was associated with an increased incidence of minor bleeding.

OTHER INDICATIONS FOR ANGIOPLASTY IN ACUTE MYOCARDIAL INFARCTION

In patients who fail thrombolytic therapy, salvage PTCA is indicated, although the initial success rate is lower than that of primary angioplasty, reocclusion is more common, and mortality is higher. The RESCUE trial focused on a subset of acute myocardial infarction patients with anterior infarction and showed a reduction in the combined endpoint of death or congestive heart failure at 30 days in the group receiving salvage PTCA.

There is no convincing evidence to support empirical delayed PTCA in patients without evidence of recurrent or provokable ischemia after thrombolytic therapy. The TIMI IIB trial and other studies suggest that a strategy of "watchful waiting" allows for identification of patients who will benefit from revascularization.

MEDICAL THERAPY FOR MYOCARDIAL INFARCTION

Aspirin

Unless contraindicated, all patients with suspected myocardial infarction should be given aspirin, 160 to 325 mg. This should be accomplished within the first 10 minutes of hospital evaluation, and the aspirin should be chewed to accelerate absorption. Aspirin has been shown to reduce mortality in acute infarction to the same degree as thrombolytic therapy, and its effects are additive to thrombolytics. In addition, aspirin reduces the risk of reinfarction.

Once begun, aspirin should probably be continued indefinitely. Aspirin irreversibly inactivates platelet cyclooxygenase, inhibiting platelet aggregation and reducing the release of platelet-derived vasoconstrictors such as serotonin and thromboxane A_2. Recent data suggest that the anti-inflammatory effects of aspirin may play a role in inhibiting plaque rupture as well. Toxicity with aspirin is mostly gastrointestinal; enteric-coated preparations may minimize these side effects.

Heparin

Administration of full-dose heparin after thrombolytic therapy with t-PA is essential to diminish reocclusion after successful reperfusion. Dosing should be adjusted to weight, with a bolus of 80 U/kg and an initial infusion rate of 18 U/kg/hr, with adjustment to keep the partial thromboplastin time (PTT) between 50 and 70 seconds. Heparin should be continued for 24 to 48 hours.

Low molecular weight heparins (LMWH) have several theoretical advantages over unfractionated heparin. Because of a higher resistance to inactivation by platelet factor 4 and a lower affinity for heparin-binding proteins, LMWHs have a more predictable pharmacokinetic profile, greater bioavailability and longer plasma half-life, all of which result in more predictable and reliable anticoagulant effects. LMWHs may be given once or twice daily as subcutaneous injections at fixed or weight-adjusted doses, thus simplifying administration and eliminating the need for laboratory monitoring and dose adjustment.

LMWHs have been studied in several large randomized trials in patients with unstable angina or non-Q wave MI. In both the Efficacy and Safety of Subcutaneous Enoxaparin in Non-Q-Wave Coronary Events (ESSENCE) study and the TIMI 11B trial, the combined endpoint of death, myocardial infarction, or recurrent ischemia at 14 days was significantly reduced (15% relative risk reduction) with enoxaparin therapy compared to unfractionated heparin. The data regarding other LMWHs have not been as positive as the enoxaparin data, with no significant benefit from dalteparin treatment in patients already on aspirin. Specific considerations with the use of LMWH include decreased clearance in renal insufficiency and the lack of a commercially available test to measure its anticoagulant effect.

Nitrates

Nitrates have a number of beneficial effects in acute myocardial infarction. They reduce myocardial oxygen demand by decreasing preload and afterload, and may also improve myocardial oxygen supply by increasing subendocardial perfusion and collateral blood flow to the ischemic region. Occasional patients with ST elevation due to occlusive coronary artery spasm may have dramatic resolution of ischemia with nitrates. In addition to their hemodynamic effects, nitrates also reduce platelet aggregation. Despite these benefits, the recently reported GISSI-3 and ISIS-4 trials failed to show a significant reduction in mortality from routine acute and chronic nitrate therapy. Nonetheless, nitrates are still first-line agents for the symptomatic relief of angina pectoris and when myocardial infarction is complicated by congestive heart failure.

Our practice is to administer sublingual nitroglycerin to all patients presenting with chest pain, unless the systolic blood pressure is < 100 mm Hg or evidence of right ventricular infarction is present. For patients with persistent chest pain, intravenous nitroglycerin is infused at 10 µg/min and increased in increments of 5 to 10 µg/min every 5 minutes until the pain resolves.

The major adverse effects of nitrates are hypotension and headache. Nitrates should be used with great caution in patients with right ventricular infarction, who may not tolerate decreases in filling pressure. Similarly, precipitous decreases in blood pressure in patients presenting with inferior myocardial infarction should raise the suspicion of right ventricular involvement. Nitrate-induced hypotension is usually caused by vasodilation and is treated with rapid bolus infusion of intravenous fluids.

B-Blockers

The β-blockers are beneficial both in the early management of myocardial infarction and as long-term therapy. In the pre-thrombolytic era, early intravenous atenolol was shown to significantly reduce reinfarction, cardiac arrest, cardiac rupture, and death. For patients receiving t-PA, immediate β-blockade with metoprolol resulted in a significant reduction in recurrent ischemia and reinfarction.

Administration of intravenous β-blockade should be strongly considered for patients presenting with acute myocardial infarction, especially those with continued ischemic discomfort and sympathetic hyperactivity manifested by hypertension or tachycardia. Therapy should be avoided in patients with moderate or severe heart failure, hypotension, severe bradycardia or heart block, and severe bronchospastic disease. Metoprolol can be given as a 5-mg iv bolus, repeated every 5 minutes for a total of 3 doses. Because of its brief half-life, esmolol may be advantageous in situations where precise control of the heart rate is necessary or rapid drug withdrawal may be needed if adverse effects occur.

Oral β-blockade should be initiated in all patients who can tolerate it, even if they have not been treated with intravenous β-blockers. The major side effects include exacerbation of heart failure, hypotension, conduction abnormalities, and bronchospasm.

Angiotensin-Converting Enzyme Inhibitors

Angiotensin-converting enzyme (ACE) inhibitors are known to reduce mortality and improve symptoms in patients with symptomatic left ventricular dysfunction from a variety of causes, and to prevent progression to symptomatic heart failure in patients with asymptomatic left ventricular dysfunction. Several large randomized trials, most recently the Heart Outcomes Prevention Evaluation (HOPE) study, have demonstrated that ACE inhibitors decrease mortality after myocardial infarction. This improved survival is additive to the benefits of aspirin and β-blockers. The mechanisms responsible probably include limitation in the progressive left ventricular dysfunction and enlargement (remodeling) that often occurs after infarction, but a reduction in ischemic events was seen as well. Recent studies have suggested that ACE inhibition can ameliorate endothelial dysfunction in atherosclerosis.

Although the trials have demonstrated a benefit with ACE inhibition for all patients postinfarction, patients with significant left ventricular dysfunction (ejection fraction < 40%) have the most to gain. ACE inhibition should be started early, preferably within the first 24 hours after infarction. Immediate intravenous ACE inhibition with enalaprilat has not been shown to be beneficial. Patients should be started on low doses of oral agents (captopril 6.25 mg 3 times daily) and rapidly increased to the range demonstrated beneficial in clinical trials (captopril 50 mg 3 times daily, enalapril 10 to 20 mg twice daily, lisinopril 10 to 20 mg once daily, or ramipril 10 mg once daily).

Calcium Antagonists

Randomized clinical trials have not demonstrated a mortality benefit for calcium-channel blockers for routine use after myocardial infarction. In fact, meta-analyses suggest that high doses of the short-acting dihydropyridine nifedipine increase mortality in myocardial infarction. Adverse effects of calcium-channel blockers include bradycardia, atrioventricular block, and exacerbation of heart failure. Patients with non-Q-wave myocardial infarction who are not in congestive heart failure, however, appear to have a significant reduction in reinfarction and recurrent ischemia when treated with diltiazem.

Although routine administration of calcium blockers in acute myocardial infarction is not indicated, these agents are useful for patients whose postinfarction course is complicated by recurrent angina, because these agents not only reduce myocardial oxygen demand but also inhibit coronary vasoconstriction. For hemodynamically stable patients, diltiazem can be given, starting at 60 to 90 mg orally every 6 to 8 hours. In patients with severe left ventricular dysfunction, long-acting dihydropyridines without prominent negative inotropic effects such as amlodipine, nicardipine, or the long-acting preparation of nifedipine may be preferable; increased mortality with these agents has **not** been demonstrated.

Antiarrhythmics

Routine prophylactic administration of lidocaine is no longer recommended. Even though lidocaine increases the frequency of premature ventricular contractions and of early ventricular fibrillation, overall mortality is not decreased. In fact, meta-analyses of pooled data have demonstrated *increased* mortality from the routine use of lidocaine.

Nonetheless, lidocaine infusion is clearly indicated after an episode of sustained ventricular tachycardia or ventricular fibrillation, and should be considered in patients with nonsustained ventricular tachycardia. Lidocaine is administered as a bolus of 1 mg/kg (not to exceed 100 mg), followed by a second bolus of 0.5 mg/kg 10 minutes later, along with an infusion at 1 to 3 mg/min. Lidocaine is metabolized by the liver, and so lower doses should be given in the presence of liver disease, in the elderly, and in patients who have congestive heart failure severe enough to compromise hepatic perfusion. Toxic manifestations primarily involve the central nervous system, and can include confusion, lethargy, slurred speech, and seizures. Because the risk of malignant ventricular arrhythmias decreases after 24 hours, lidocaine is usually discontinued after this point. For prolonged infusions, monitoring of lidocaine levels (therapeutic between 1.5 and 5 g/mL) is sometimes useful.

Intravenous amiodarone is an alternative to lidocaine for ventricular arrhythmias. Amiodarone is given as a 150 mg IV bolus over 10 minutes, followed by 1 mg/min for 6 hours, then 0.5 mg/min for 18 hours.

Perhaps the most important point in the prevention and management of arrhythmias after acute myocardial infarction is maintaining normal serum potassium and magnesium levels. Serum electrolytes should be followed closely, particularly after diuretic therapy. Routine administration of magnesium has not been shown to reduce mortality after acute myocardial infarction, but empiric administration of 2 grams of intravenous magnesium in patients with early ventricular ectopy is probably a good idea.

COMPLICATIONS OF ACUTE MYOCARDIAL INFARCTION

Postinfarction Angina and Infarct Extension

Causes of ischemia after infarction include decreased myocardial oxygen supply due to coronary reocclusion or spasm, mechanical problems which increase myocardial oxygen demand, and extracardiac factors such as hypertension, anemia, hypotension, or hypermetabolic states. Nonischemic causes of chest pain, such as postinfarction pericarditis and acute pulmonary embolism, should also be considered.

Immediate management includes aspirin, β-blockade, iv nitroglycerin, heparin, consideration of calcium-channel blockers, and diagnostic coronary angiography.

Postinfarction angina is an indication for revascularization. PTCA can be performed if the culprit lesion is suitable, recognizing that acute outcomes and long-term patency may not be as good as those with elective angioplasty. CABG should be considered for patients with left main disease, 3 vessel disease, and those unsuitable for PTCA. If the angina cannot be controlled medically or is accompanied by hemodynamic instability, an intra-aortic balloon pump should be inserted.

Ventricular Free Wall Rupture

Ventricular free wall rupture typically occurs during the first week after infarction. The classic patient is elderly, female, and hypertensive. Free wall rupture presents as a catastrophic event with shock and electromechanical dissociation. Salvage is possible with prompt recognition, pericardiocentesis, and thoracotomy. Emergent echocardiography or pulmonary artery catheterization can help make the diagnosis.

Ventricular Septal Rupture

Septal rupture presents as severe heart failure or cardiogenic shock, with a pansystolic murmur and parasternal thrill. The hallmark finding is a left-to-right intracardiac shunt ("step-up" in oxygen saturation from right atrium to right ventricle). It can be difficult to distinguish from mitral regurgitation on pulmonary artery catheter tracing. Both can produce dramatic "v" waves in the pulmonary artery occlusion pressure (PAOP) tracing. Echocardiography can help make the distinction. Surgical repair is required.

Acute Mitral Regurgitation

Papillary muscle *dysfunction* is common after inferior myocardial infarction but is rarely important hemodynamically; the characteristic holosystolic apical murmur of mitral regurgitation is typically present. Papillary muscle *rupture*, on the other hand, presents dramatically with marked hemodynamic compensation; consisting of pulmonary edema and shock; a murmur may or may not be present due to decreased cardiac output. Acute management includes afterload reduction with nitroprusside and intra-aortic balloon pumping as temporizing measures. Definitive therapy is surgical valve repair or replacement.

Right Ventricular Infarction

Right ventricular infarction occurs in as many as 30% of patients with inferior infarction and is clinically significant in 10%. Patients present with hypotension, elevated neck veins, and clear lung fields. Although these patients appear to be in cardiogenic shock, right ventricular infarction carries a better prognosis.

The diagnosis is made by identifying ST elevation in right precordial leads or by characteristic hemodynamic findings on right heart catheterization (elevated right atrial and right ventricular end-diastolic pressures with normal to low PAOP and low cardiac output). Echocardiography can demonstrate depressed right ventricular contractility and can help differentiate right ventricular infarction from tamponade, which may present with similar clinical and hemodynamic findings.

Treatment, in addition to rapid reperfusion of the occluded coronary artery if necessary, includes fluid resuscitation with normal saline boluses to increase left ventricular filling pressure and inotropic therapy with dobutamine or possibly amrinone to stimulate RV contractility. Patients who do not respond rapidly to fluids need hemodynamic monitoring to guide therapy. For continued hemodynamic instability, intra-aortic balloon pumping may be useful, particularly because elevated right ventricular pressures and volumes increase wall stress and oxygen consumption and decrease right coronary perfusion pressure, exacerbating right ventricular ischemia. Nitrates should be avoided because of their propensity to reduce right ventricular preload, resulting in decreased cardiac output.

Cardiogenic Shock

Cardiogenic shock as a complication of acute myocardial infarction carries a high mortality rate, approaching 60% to 90% in some series. It is considered in detail in the section on acute heart failure in the intensive care unit. Hemodynamically, cardiogenic shock is defined as a cardiac index < 1.8 L/min/m^2 with an elevated PAOP, generally > 18 mm Hg. Prompt reperfusion of the occluded coronary artery is the only way to reduce the mortality associated with cardiogenic shock. Because thrombolytic therapy alone does not appear to be very effective in cardiogenic shock, primary PTCA is recommended. An intra-aortic balloon pump should be placed before the PTCA to stabilize the patient and enhance coronary blood flow and reduce myocardial oxygen demand. Urgent coronary artery bypass surgery may be an alternative if prompt angioplasty is not feasible.

KEY POINTS

1. Myocardial infarction is diagnosed by a compatible clinical history, evolution of characteristic EKG changes, and an increase and decrease in cardiac enzymes.
2. All patients with suspected myocardial ischemia should be given aspirin upon presentation to the emergency department.
3. Acute reperfusion of the occluded coronary artery is the key to achieving a good outcome. The promptness of reperfusion is more important than the mode by which it is accomplished.
4. Thrombolytic therapy or mechanical reperfusion should be considered up to 12 hours after the onset of symptoms.
5. *All* patients should receive β-blockers after acute myocardial infarction, except those who cannot tolerate them.
6. Routine prophylactic administration of lidocaine is no longer recommended. Keep the serum potassium levels high. Consider administration of magnesium in patients with frequent ventricular ectopy.
7. Patients with cardiogenic shock should be stabilized with an intra-aortic balloon pump and revascularized if possible by angioplasty or bypass surgery.
8. Echocardiography is extremely useful for the diagnosis of complications after myocardial infarction. Invasive hemodynamic monitoring may be necessary in some cases as well.
9. Prognosis after myocardial infarction is most closely related to the degree of left ventricular impairment.
10. Not all akinetic myocardium is dead after myocardial infarction; consider the presence of myocardial stunning or hibernation.

SUGGESTED READING

1. β-Blocker Heart Attack Trial Research Group: A randomized trial of propranolol in patients with acute myocardial infarction. I. Mortality results. *JAMA* 1982; 247:1707-1714
   3,837 patients were randomized to oral propranolol or placebo started 5 to 21 days after myocardial infarction. β-Blockade reduced mortality from 7.2% versus 9.8%, a 26% reduction.

2. CAPTURE Investigators: Randomised placebo-controlled trial of abciximab before and during coronary intervention in refractory unstable angina: the CAPTURE Study. *Lancet* 1997; 349:1429-35
   1,265 patients with unstable angina randomized to glycoprotein IIb/IIIa inhibition with abciximab or placebo 24 hours prior to planned percutaneous coronary intervention. Abciximab reduced death, infarction, or revascularization from 15.9% to 11.3%, a 29% reduction.

3. Cohen M, Demers C, Gurfinkel EP, et al: A comparison of low-molecular-weight heparin with unfractionated heparin for unstable coronary artery disease. Efficacy and Safety of Subcutaneous Enoxaparin in Non-Q-Wave Coronary Events Study Group. *N Engl J Med* 1997; 337:447-52
   3,171 patients with angina at rest or NQMI randomized to LMWH (enoxaparin) or unfractionated heparin. At 14 and 30 days the risk of death, myocardial infarction, or recurrent angina was significantly lower with enoxaparin.

4. Fibrinolytic Therapy Trialists' (FTT) Collaborative Group: Indications for fibrinolytic therapy in suspected acute myocardial infarction: Collaborative overview of early mortality and major morbidity results from all randomised trials of more than 1000 patients. *Lancet* 1994; 343:311-322
   Excellent compilation of the randomized trials of thrombolytic therapy in MI, emphasizing the direct relationship between early treatment and improved outcomes.

5. Grines CL, Browne KF, Marco J, et al: A comparison of immediate angioplasty with thrombolytic therapy for acute myocardial infarction. *N Engl J Med* 1993; 328:673-679
   395 thrombolytic-eligible patients randomized to t-PA or primary angioplasty for myocardial infarction. Primary angioplasty was successfully accomplished in almost 90% of patients. For the group as a whole, mortality was not significantly decreased with angioplasty (2.6% versus 6.5%, p = 0.06), but the combined endpoint of death or reinfarction was decreased (5.1% versus 12%).

6. Gruppo Italiano per lo Studio della Sopravvinza nell'Infarto Miocardico (GISSI): Effectiveness of intravenous thrombolytic treatment in acute myocardial infarction. *Lancet* 1986; 2:397-402
   The landmark study of 11,712 patients, which demonstrated a 19% reduction in mortality with intravenous streptokinase

7. GUSTO Investigators: An international randomized trial comparing 4 thrombolytic strategies for acute myocardial infarction. *N Engl J Med* 1993; 329:673-682
   A mega-trial of 41,021 patients randomized to accelerated t-PA or streptokinase. Accelerated t-PA reduced mortality from 7.3% to 6.3% (reduction, 14%) compared to streptokinase, with a slight increase (0.2%) in the rate of disabling stroke.

8. GUSTO Angiographic Investigators: The effects of tissue plasminogen activator, streptokinase, or both on coronary-artery patency, ventricular function, and survival after acute myocardial infarction. *New Engl J Med* 1993; 329:1615-1622
   Angiographic substudy of the GUSTO trial in which patients underwent coronary angiography at 90 minutes. The degree of coronary flow (TIMI grade) was directly related to outcome, validating the open artery hypothesis. Improved flow was seen with t-PA compared to streptokinase, but normal (TIMI grade 3) flow was present in only 55% of patients at 90 minutes.

9. Gutstein DE, Fuster V: Pathophysiology and clinical significance of atherosclerotic plaque rupture. *Cardiovasc Res* 1999; 41:323-333
   Excellent review of current concepts of the causes of plaque rupture in acute coronary syndromes.

10. Hochman JS, Sleeper LA, Webb JG, et al: Early revascularization in acute myocardial infarction complicated by cardiogenic shock. *N Engl J Med* 1999; 341:625-634
    Landmark trial of 302 patients with MI and cardiogenic shock randomized to an early invasive strategy or aggressive medical management. The early invasive strategy reduced 30-day mortality from 556.0 to 46.7% (p = 0.11), and, as reported later, 1-year mortality was reduced from 66.4 to 53.3% (p = 0.03).

11. ISIS-2 Collaborative Group: Randomised trial of intravenous streptokinase, oral aspirin, both, or neither among 17,187 cases of suspected acute myocardial infarction: ISIS-2. *Lancet* 1988; 2:349-360
    Aspirin alone reduced mortality in patients with acute myocardial infarction by 23%, and streptokinase alone reduced mortality by 25%. The combination of the 2 decreased mortality by 42% without increasing stroke rates. It has become widespread practice since this study to administer aspirin acutely to almost every patient presenting with an acute myocardial infarction.

12. ISIS-4 (Fourth International Study of Infarct Survival) Study Group: ISIS-4: A randomised factorial trial assessing early oral captopril, oral mononitrate, and intravenous magnesium sulphate in 58,050 patients with suspected acute myocardial infarction. *Lancet* 1995; 345:669-685
    Oral captopril, started early upon admission, decreased mortality after acute myocardial infarction (from 7.7% to 7.2%, reduction of 7%). Oral nitrates or intravenous magnesium did not reduce mortality.

13. LATE Study Group: Late assessment of thrombolytic efficacy (LATE) study with alteplase 6 - 24 hours after onset of acute myocardial infarction. *Lancet* 1993; 342:759-766
    Thrombolytic therapy with t-PA reduced 35-day mortality when given 6 to 12 hours after the onset of symptoms, but not beyond that time.

14. Libby P: Current concepts of the pathogenesis of the acute coronary syndromes. *Circulation* 2001; 104:365-372
    An excellent review of the concepts of the pathogenesis of acute ischemic syndromes.

15. Montalescot G, Barragan P, Wittenberg O, et al: Platelet glycoprotein IIb/IIIa inhibition with coronary stenting for acute myocardial infarction. *N Engl J Med* 2001; 344:1895-1903
    300 patients with acute MI randomized to abciximab plus stenting or placebo plus stenting. Abciximab improved coronary patency before stenting, the success rate of the stenting procedure, the rate of coronary patency at 6 months, left ventricular function, and clinical outcomes.

16. Ohman EM, Armstrong PW, Christenson RH, et al: Cardiac troponin T levels for risk stratification in acute myocardial ischemia. *N Engl J Med* 1996; 335:133-1341
    Cardiac troponin T levels, CK-MB levels, and electrocardiograms were analyzed in 855 patients presenting with acute coronary syndromes. Mortality within 30 days was directly correlated with troponin T levels, and troponin T level was an independent risk marker. The study showed that troponin levels allow for further stratification of risk when combined with standard measures.

17. Pfeffer MA, Braunwald E, Moye LA, et al: Effect of captopril on mortality and morbidity in patients with left ventricular dysfunction after myocardial infarction. Results of the Survival and Ventricular Enlargement Trial. *N Engl J Med* 1992; 327:669-677
    Captopril reduced mortality 19% in asymptomatic patients with postinfarction ejection fractions < 40%.

18. Rogers WJ, Canto JG, Lambrew CT, et al: Temporal trends in the treatment of over 1.5 million patients with myocardial infarction in the United States from 1990 to 1999. *J Am Coll Cardiol* 2000; 36:2056-2063
    Results from this registry document the percentage of patients treated with different therapies after myocardial infarction. Care is improving, but some interventions proven to reduce mortality after myocardial infarction are still underutilized.

19. Ryan TJ, Anderson JL, Antman EM, et al: American College of Cardiology/American Heart Association guidelines for the management of patients with acute myocardial infarction. 1999 Update. A report of the American College of

Cardiology/American Heart Association Task Force on Practice Guidelines. *J Am Coll Cardiol* 1999; 34:890-911
A comprehensive consensus statement regarding the indications for various invasive diagnostic and therapeutic maneuvers, when to consider temporary pacemakers, and the appropriate roles of assorted pharmacologic interventions.

20. Scandinavian Simvastatin Survival Study Group. Randomised trial of cholesterol lowering in 4,444 patients with coronary heart disease: The Scandinavian Simvastatin Survival Study (4S). *Lancet* 1994; 344:1383-1389
The first trial to demonstrate a mortality benefit from lipid-lowering therapy. Long-term therapy with simvastatin improved survival and decreased coronary events in patients with coronary artery disease and elevated cholesterol.

21. Yusuf S, Sleight P, Pogue J, et al: Effects of an angiotensin-converting-enzyme inhibitor, ramipril, on cardiovascular events in high-risk patients. *N Engl J Med* 2000; 342:145-153
9,297 high-risk patients (55 or older, with vascular disease or diabetes plus one other cardiovascular risk factor) randomized to ramipril or placebo for a mean of 5 years. Ramipril significantly reduced the rates of death, myocardial infarction, and stroke.

HEART FAILURE AND CARDIAC PULMONARY EDEMA

Steven M. Hollenberg, MD

Objectives

- To review the definition, demographics, and etiology of congestive heart failure diagnosis
- To understand the pathophysiology of the heart failure syndrome
- To review general treatment goals and medical therapy for heart failure, with an emphasis on acute heart failure in the intensive care unit
- To understand the etiology and pathophysiology of cardiogenic shock
- To review initial and definitive management of cardiogenic shock

DEFINITION AND EPIDEMIOLOGY

Congestive heart failure (CHF) can be defined as the inability of the heart to provide an adequate cardiac output without invoking maladaptive compensatory mechanisms. Congestive heart failure affects more than 3 million patients in the U.S., nearly 1.5% of the adult population. Every year, 400,000 patients develop heart failure for the first time, and CHF results in 1,000,000 hospital admissions per year in the U.S. Congestive heart failure is a major cause of cardiovascular death (estimated at 200,000/year), and a major cause of morbidity and mortality as well. CHF is now the most common reason for hospitalization in the elderly, and an estimated $8 billion is spent on heart failure annually.

The causes of heart failure are numerous, and are listed in Table 1. The predominant causes, however, are ischemia, hypertension, alcoholic cardiomyopathy, myocarditis, and idiopathic cardiomyopathy. Coronary artery disease is increasing, both as a primary cause and as a complicating factor.

Heart failure can be broken down into several different classifications: acute versus chronic, left-sided versus right-sided, systolic versus diastolic dysfunction. Most patients in the

intensive care unit have acute left-sided heart failure and present with pulmonary edema, which is not usually difficult to diagnose. It is important for the clinician, however, to distinguish between systolic and diastolic dysfunction. Although CHF results most commonly from decreased systolic performance, diastolic dysfunction, defined clinically as cardiogenic pulmonary congestion in the presence of normal systolic performance, is becoming more common as a cause of CHF as the U.S. population ages.

PATHOPHYSIOLOGY

Heart failure is a syndrome caused not only by the low cardiac output resulting from compromised systolic performance, but also by overly active compensatory mechanisms. Myocardial damage from any cause can produce myocardial failure. To compensate for the reduced cardiac output of a failing heart, an elevation in ventricular filling pressure occurs in an attempt to maintain output via the Frank-Starling law. These elevated diastolic filling pressures can compromise subendocardial blood flow and cause or worsen ischemia. With continued low cardiac output, additional compensatory mechanisms come into play, including sympathetic nervous system stimulation, activation of the renin-angiotensin system, and vasopressin secretion. All of these mechanisms lead to sodium and water retention and venoconstriction, increasing both preload and afterload. These increases in preload and afterload, although initially compensatory, can exacerbate the heart failure, because elevated preload increases pulmonary congestion, and elevated afterload impedes cardiac output.

DIAGNOSIS OF PULMONARY EDEMA

The symptoms and signs of congestive heart failure relate both to low cardiac output and

Table 1. Etiologies of Congestive Heart Failure

Ischemic
Hypertensive
Idiopathic
Valvular
Peripartum
Familial
Toxic
    Alcoholic
    Radiation
    Drug-related (anthracyclines)
    Heavy metals (cobalt, lead, arsenic)
Metabolic/nutritional
Systemic diseases
    Hypothyroidism
    Connective tissue disease
    Diabetes
    Sarcoidosis
Infiltrative
    Amyloidosis
    Hemochromatosis
Tachycardia-induced
Autoimmune

elevated ventricular filling pressures. Low output produces the symptoms of weakness and fatigue and an ashen appearance, sometimes with mottling. Increased left-sided filling pressures result in symptoms of pulmonary congestion such as dyspnea, cough, orthopnea, and paroxysmal nocturnal dyspnea, as well as signs which may include tachycardia, pulmonary rales, a diffuse, enlarged, and laterally displaced point of maximal impulse, an S_3 and S_4 gallop, a murmur of mitral regurgitation. Elevated right-sided preload can lead to symptoms such as anorexia, nausea, and abdominal pain, along with signs of systemic congestion such as jugular venous distension, a right-sided S_3 gallop, a murmur of tricuspid regurgitation, hepatomegaly, ascites, and peripheral edema.

Patients in the intensive care unit often present with acute heart failure and pulmonary edema. Their presentation can be dramatic with sudden onset of shortness of breath and tachypnea with use of accessory muscles. Crackles and often wheezing can be heard throughout the lung fields, at times obscuring some of the cardiac auscultatory findings. Hypotension and evidence of peripheral vasoconstriction and hypoperfusion may be present if cardiac output is decreased. The differential diagnosis of cardiac pulmonary

edema includes other causes of acute dyspnea such as pulmonary embolism, pneumothorax, and bronchial asthma and causes of noncardiac pulmonary edema such as aspiration, infection, toxins, or trauma.

Initial evaluation of the patient with pulmonary edema should include an electrocardiogram and chest x-ray. The electrocardiogram may show evidence of myocardial ischemia, infarction, or arrhythmias. The chest x-ray can demonstrate cardiomegaly along with pulmonary infiltrates. Echocardiography can be extremely useful to evaluate systolic performance and the presence of regional wall motion abnormalities suggestive of ischemia. Valvular abnormalities can be diagnosed rapidly as well. Invasive hemodynamic monitoring may be useful, not so much to make the diagnosis as to guide pharmacologic therapy in the decompensated patient.

GENERAL TREATMENT GOALS

The goals of congestive heart failure therapy are to control symptoms, improve exercise tolerance, prolong life, and where possible, to correct the underlying cause. In the critical care setting, control of symptoms and correction of underlying causes are emphasized. It is important to realize that different therapies can have different effects on these goals.

The therapeutic agents can be viewed in the light of the pathophysiologic mechanisms of CHF development. Fluid restriction, diuretics, and venodilators decrease cardiac preload. Angiotensin converting enzyme (ACE) inhibitors counteract activation of the renin-angiotensin system and reduce afterload as well. Arterial dilators can also reduce afterload. Inotropic agents can improve cardiac pump function and increase output. Beta-blockers can counteract sympathetic activation and are being used more commonly in chronic heart failure management, but have little role in acute CHF.

HEART FAILURE THERAPY

Diuretics

Diuretics cause renal sodium and water loss, resulting in decreased preload and pulmonary and systemic congestion. In the intensive care unit, loop diuretics such as furosemide are usually chosen initially because of their rapid onset and are given as intravenous boluses. Part of the rapid effect of furosemide may relate to venodilation.

If intermittent bolus doses of loop diuretics are ineffective or poorly tolerated due to large fluid shifts and consequent hypotension, continuous infusion may be preferable. The dosage is titrated to the desired effect. Alternatively, another diuretic with a different mechanism of action, such as metolazone or chlorthiazide, may be added.

Use of diuretics can lead to significant hypokalemia or hypomagnesemia, which can predispose the patient to arrhythmias. Careful addition of a potassium-sparing diuretic can be considered in some settings. A recent trial showed decreased mortality in chronic heart failure when spironolactone at low doses was added to maximal therapy.

NITRATES

Nitrates are still first-line agents for the symptomatic relief of angina pectoris and when myocardial infarction is complicated by congestive heart failure. Given the high incidence of coronary artery disease in patients with congestive heart failure, use of nitrates to reduce preload is often desirable. In severely decompensated CHF, intravenous nitroglycerin is preferred because of questionable absorption of oral and transdermal preparations and for ease of titration. Intravenous nitroglycerin should be started at 5 µg/min and increased in increments of 5 µg/min every 3 to 5 minutes as needed for symptomatic relief. The major adverse effects of nitrates are hypotension and headache.

ANGIOTENSIN-CONVERTING ENZYME INHIBITORS

Angiotensin-converting enzyme (ACE) inhibitors have been shown to reduce mortality and improve symptoms in patients with symptomatic left ventricular dysfunction from a variety of causes, and to prevent progression to symptomatic heart failure in patients with asymptomatic left ventricular dysfunction. Several large randomized trials have recently demonstrated that ACE inhibitors decrease mortality after myocardial infarction. The benefits result in part from limitation in progressive left ventricular dysfunction and enlargement (remodeling).

ACE inhibitors can be given intravenously in the acute setting if necessary, or started orally once the patient is more stable. Patients should be started on low doses and titrated upward to the range demonstrated beneficial in clinical trials (captopril 50 mg 3 times daily, enalapril 10 to 20 mg twice daily, or lisinopril 10 to 40 mg once daily).

ANGIOTENSIN RECEPTOR BLOCKERS

An alternative approach to inhibiting the effects of angiotensin II is use of agents that block the angiotensin II receptor (ARBs). Since these agents do not increase bradykinin, the incidence of some side effects, such as cough and angioedema, is greatly reduced. The hemodynamic effects of ARBs have been shown in a number of trials to be similar to those of ACE inhibitors. Although some trials, most recently the Valsartan in Heart Failure (Val-Heft) Trial, have suggested equivalent mortality reductions with ARBs and ACE inhibitors, the number of heart failure patients treated with ARBs and followed for mortality is still relatively small. The most recent guidelines do not support initiation of ARBs instead of ACE inhibitors to decrease mortality in patients with heart failure, and addition of beta-blockers rather than ARBs to ACE inhibitors is preferable. In patients who cannot tolerate ACE inhibitors, however, ARBs are a good alternative.

VASODILATORS

Nitroprusside is a balanced arterial and venous vasodilator which causes direct relaxation of smooth muscle by activating guanylate cyclase. The rapid onset and reversibility of action of nitroprusside make it an especially useful drug in the critical care setting. Nitroprusside reduces arteriolar resistance and venous tone to an equivalent extent, lowering both systemic vascular resistance and left and right ventricular filling pressures. Nitroprusside can increase stroke volume in heart failure by means of cardiac unloading. Venodilation decreases filling pressures and can decrease left ventricular wall stress in addition to relieving pulmonary congestion. Nitroprusside is used in acute cardiogenic pulmonary edema, decompensated congestive heart failure, mitral insufficiency, aortic insufficiency, and is a drug of choice for malignant hypertension. Nitroprusside may also be useful in low cardiac output syndromes in conjunction with inotropic therapy.

Nitroprusside is given by continuous intravenous infusion. In heart failure, nitroprusside is started at 10 µg/min and increased by 10 µg/min every 5 to 15 minutes; a decrease of 20 to 50% in wedge pressure and an increase of 20 to 40% in cardiac output is considered a positive response. Individual responses are highly variable, but most patients show a beneficial effect at 1-2 µg/kg/min. In pulmonary edema with hypertension, the starting dose is the same but is increased more rapidly, in increments of 20 µg/kg every 3 to 5 minutes. Doses required to treat hypertension are generally considerably higher than those used in heart failure.

The major complication of nitroprusside therapy is hypotension. A hypotensive response should always prompt consideration of whether the filling pressures are lower than expected. If the hypotension does not respond promptly to discontinuation of the infusion and fluid administration, dopamine may be necessary. The other major toxicity of nitroprusside therapy results from accumulation of cyanide or thiocyanate. This usually occurs only in patients who have been receiving high doses of nitroprusside for 72 hours or more, commonly in patients with renal insufficiency or failure. Cyanide inhibits oxidative phosphorylation and leads to metabolic acidosis. Treatment of cyanide toxicity involves facilitation of its metabolism to thiocyanate with thiosulfate and sodium nitrite. Thiocyanate toxicity may present with confusion, hyperreflexia, and convulsions.

Hydralazine reduces afterload by directly relaxing smooth muscle. Its effects are almost exclusively confined to the arterial bed. In normal subjects, the hypotensive actions of hydralazine provoke a marked reflex tachycardia, but this response is often blunted in with heart failure. Hydralazine is effective in

increasing cardiac output in heart failure, and improves mortality in chronic congestive heart failure when given in conjunction with oral nitrates.

In the critical care unit, intravenous hydralazine is often preferable to oral dosing, infused slowly over 20 minutes to minimize hypotension. Doses start at 5 to 10 mg, and can be increased to 20 mg given every 6 to 8 hours. Oral doses range from 25 to 100 mg every 6 hours, but some patients may need much higher doses due to malabsorption. Tachycardia develops with hydralazine therapy in some patients. This mandates caution in administering the drug to patients with known or suspected ischemic heart disease. Prolonged administration of hydralazine is attended by the development of a lupus-like syndrome in up to 20% of patients.

DIGOXIN

Digitalis, which has been used to treat heart failure for more than 200 years, works by inhibiting Na-K-dependent ATPase activity, causing intracellular sodium accumulation and increasing intracellular calcium via the sodium-calcium exchange system. Digoxin improves myocardial contractility and increases cardiac output, but is a mild inotrope when compared to catecholamines. When used chronically for CHF in conjunction with diuretics and ACE inhibitors, digoxin has been shown to reduce symptoms and decrease hospital admissions, but it has no effect on mortality. Digoxin has a slow onset and long half-life (for digoxin, 36 hours) compared to the catecholamines. It has a narrow toxic/therapeutic ratio, and individual hemodynamic responses to acute digitalis administration are highly variable. For these reasons, digoxin has a role for the control of supraventricular tachycardias but is not often useful as an inotrope in the critical care unit.

INOTROPIC AGENTS

In severe decompensated heart failure, inotropic support may be initiated. Dobutamine is a selective β_1-adrenergic receptor agonist which can improve myocardial contractility and increase cardiac output without inducing marked changes in heart rate or systemic vascular resistance. Dobutamine is the initial inotropic agent of choice in patients with decompensated acute heart failure and adequate systolic blood pressure. Dobutamine has a rapid onset of action, and a plasma half-life is 2 to 3 minutes; infusion is usually initiated at 5µg/kg/min and then titrated. Tolerance to the effect of dobutamine may develop after 48-72 hours, possibly due to down-regulation of adrenergic receptors. Some studies have suggested continued improvement in functional status and hemodynamics for several weeks after a 3-day infusion of dobutamine. The mechanism of this prolonged benefit is unclear; some improvements in metabolic function and mitochondrial ultrastructure have been seen. Dobutamine has the potential to exacerbate hypotension in some patients, and can precipitate tachyarrhythmias.

Milrinone is a phosphodiesterase inhibitor milrinone with both positive inotropic and vasodilatory actions. Because milrinone does not stimulate adrenergic receptors directly, it may be effective when added to catecholamines or when β-adrenergic receptors have been down-regulated. Compared to catecholamines, phosphodiesterase inhibitors have minimal chronotropic and arrhythmogenic effects.

Although clearly useful to improve hemodynamics in the acute setting, controversy has arisen regarding use of inotropic agents (other than digoxin) as outpatient maintenance therapy for chronic heart failure. Concerns have included exacerbation of arrhythmic complications, either by induction of myocardial ischemia or by independent pathways, and perpetuation of neurohumoral activation, which might accelerate the progression of myocardial damage. Milrinone was recently examined in a prospective manner in order to determine whether its use could reduce hospitalization time following an acute heart failure exacerbation. Although these observations did not demonstrate any advantage for patients treated with milrinone, patients whom the investigators felt "needed" acute inotropic support were not included in the trial, thereby biasing the enrollment toward a less severely afflicted cohort. Therefore, the utilization of such agents today remains at the discretion of the clinician. The proof that these agents have beneficial

effects on hard clinical endpoints remains elusive, but their hemodynamic effects render them tempting alternatives in decompensated patients.

Inotropic infusions need to be titrated carefully in patients with ischemic heart disease to maximize coronary perfusion pressure with the least possible increase in myocardial oxygen demand. Invasive hemodynamic monitoring can be extremely useful to allow for optimization of therapy in these unstable patients, because clinical estimates of filling pressure can be unreliable, and because changes in myocardial performance and compliance and therapeutic interventions can change cardiac output and filling pressures precipitously. Optimization of filling pressures and serial measurements of cardiac output (and other parameters, such as mixed venous oxygen saturation) allow for titration of inotropes and vasopressors to the minimum dosage required to achieve the chosen therapeutic goals, thus minimizing the increases in myocardial oxygen demand and arrhythmogenic potential.

BETA BLOCKERS

Although perhaps counterintuitive on hemodynamic grounds, there is now compelling evidence that beta blockers are beneficial not only for patients with acute myocardial infarction complicated by heart failure, but also with chronic heart failure from all causes. These agents can, however, be problematic during the acute phase of heart failure, as they can depress contractility. When given for heart failure indications per se, beta blockers should be introduced when the patient is in a well compensated and euvolemic state, typically in the ambulatory setting and at minimal doses.

Patients who experience an exacerbation of heart failure while on maintenance beta-blocker therapy, particularly at a higher dose, present a previously rare dilemma that is becoming more common. No controlled observations are available to guide therapy, so current practice remains largely at the discretion of individual clinicians. Since a decrease in or discontinuation of the dose of maintenance beta-blocker therapy should result in an abrupt increase in exposure of myocardial beta receptors to endogenous catecholamines, the effect could be comparable to administration of exogenous catecholamines in a non-beta-blocked patient. Therefore, it seems rational to apply the same standards to modification of beta-blocker dosage as one does to institution of catecholamine therapy in the management of decompensated heart failure. An innovative alternative which may lessen the risk of acute increase in catecholamine exposure while allowing temporary increase in inotropic state would be to maintain the beta-blocker regimen at or near baseline while administering a non-catecholamine inotropic agent such as milrinone. This approach may reduce the risk of deleterious side effects in patients deemed to require inotropic therapy, although there is little supporting data in this regard.

CARDIOGENIC SHOCK

Cardiogenic shock can be defined as a state of inadequate tissue and cellular perfusion resulting from cardiac dysfunction. Defined clinically, this includes decreased cardiac output and evidence of tissue hypoxia in the presence of adequate intravascular volume. Hemodynamic criteria include sustained hypotension (systolic blood pressure less than 90 mm Hg or 30 mm Hg below basal levels for at least 30 minutes) and a reduced cardiac index (less than 2.2 L/min/m^2) in the presence of elevated pulmonary capillary wedge pressure (greater than 15 mm Hg).

Etiology

The most common cause of cardiogenic shock is an extensive acute myocardial infarction, although a smaller infarction in a patient with previously compromised left ventricular function may also precipitate shock. Shock presenting with a delayed onset may result from infarct extension, reocclusion of a previously patent infarct artery, or decompensation of function in the non-infarct zone due to metabolic abnormalities. Cardiogenic shock can also be caused by mechanical complications such as acute mitral regurgitation, rupture of the interventricular septum, or free wall rupture, or by large right ventricular infarctions. Other

causes of cardiogenic shock include myocarditis, end-stage cardiomyopathy, valvular heart disease, and myocardial dysfunction after prolonged cardiopulmonary bypass shock. In the most recent report of the SHOCK (SHould we emergently revascularize Occluded Coronaries for shocK) trial registry of 1,160 patients with cardiogenic shock, 74.5% had predominant left ventricular failure, 8.3% acute mitral regurgitation, 4.6% ventricular septal rupture, 3.4% isolated right ventricular shock, 1.7% tamponade or cardiac rupture, and 8% had other causes.

Pathophysiology

Cardiac dysfunction in cardiogenic shock is usually initiated by myocardial infarction or ischemia. The myocardial dysfunction resulting from ischemia worsens that ischemia, setting up a vicious cycle. Systolic myocardial dysfunction decreases stroke volume and cardiac output, leading to hypotension, which decreases coronary perfusion pressure, which can exacerbate ischemia. The increased ventricular diastolic pressures that result from heart failure reduce the pressure gradient for coronary blood flow, and the additional wall stress elevates myocardial oxygen requirements, also worsening ischemia. Tachycardia reduces the time available for diastolic filling, further compromising coronary blood flow. Decreased cardiac output compromises systemic perfusion, which can lead to lactic acidosis. Compensatory vasoconstriction in response to decreased perfusion can increase afterload, producing further strain on an already compromised left ventricle.

Cardiogenic shock also leads to diastolic myocardial dysfunction. Infarction and ischemia decrease diastolic compliance, increasing left ventricular diastolic pressures and leading to pulmonary edema. Pulmonary congestion can cause hypoxemia, which can also contribute to ischemia.

Diagnosis and Initial Management

Cardiogenic shock is an emergency. After recognizing the presence of shock, the clinician must perform the clinical assessment required to understand its cause while initiating supportive therapy before shock causes irreversible damage to vital organs. The challenge is that since speed is important to achieve a good outcome, evaluation and therapy must begin simultaneously. While the evaluation must be thorough, neither overzealous pursuit of a diagnosis before stabilization has been achieved nor overzealous empiric treatment without establishing the underlying pathophysiology is desirable. A practical approach is to make a rapid evaluation initially, based on a limited history, physical examination, and specific diagnostic procedures. The diagnosis of circulatory shock at the bedside is made by the presence hypotension along with a combination of clinical signs indicative of poor tissue perfusion, including oliguria, a clouded sensorium, and cool, mottled extremities indicative of reduced blood flow to the skin. Cardiogenic shock is diagnosed after documentation of myocardial dysfunction and exclusion of nonmyocardial factors such as hypovolemia, hypoxia, and acidosis. Patients with cardiogenic shock usually have symptoms and signs of heart disease, including elevated filling pressures, gallop rhythms, and other evidence of heart failure. A murmur of mitral regurgitation, aortic stenosis, or ventricular septal defect may be heard. An electrocardiogram should be performed immediately; other initial diagnostic tests ordinarily include a chest x-ray, arterial blood gas, electrolytes, complete blood count, and cardiac enzymes.

Echocardiography is an excellent initial tool for confirming the diagnosis of cardiogenic shock and for sorting through the differential diagnosis, and should be routinely done early. Echocardiography provides information on overall and regional systolic function, and can rapidly diagnose mechanical causes of shock such as papillary muscle rupture and acute mitral regurgitation, acute ventricular septal defect, and free wall rupture and tamponade. Unsuspected severe mitral regurgitation is fairly common. In some cases, echocardiography may reveal findings compatible with right ventricular infarction.

Invasive hemodynamic monitoring is critical for confirming the diagnosis and for guiding pharmacologic therapy. The hemodynamic profile of cardiogenic shock includes a pulmonary capillary wedge pressure greater than 15 mm Hg and a cardiac index less than 2.2 L/min/m^2. It should be recognized that optimal filling pressures may be higher than this in individual patients due to left ventricular diastolic dysfunction. Right heart catheterization may reveal an oxygen step-up diagnostic of ventricular septal rupture or a large "v" wave suggestive of severe mitral regurgitation. The hemodynamic profile of right ventricular infarction includes high right-sided filling pressures in the presence of normal of low wedge pressures.

Initial Management

General Considerations

Maintenance of adequate oxygenation and ventilation are critical. Many patients require intubation and mechanical ventilation early in their course, if only to reduce the work of breathing and facilitate sedation and stabilization before cardiac catheterization. Some recent studies have suggested that use of continuous positive airway pressure in patients with cardiogenic pulmonary edema can decrease the need for intubation, but the studies are small and need to be evaluated with some caution; failure of noninvasive ventilation occurred at least half of the time.

Electrolyte abnormalities should be corrected, because hypokalemia and hypomagnesemia predispose to ventricular arrhythmias. Relief of pain and anxiety with morphine sulfate (or fentanyl if systolic pressure is compromised) can reduce excessive sympathetic activity and decrease oxygen demand, preload, and afterload. Arrhythmias and heart block may have major effects on cardiac output, and should be corrected promptly with antiarrhythmic drugs, cardioversion, or pacing. Measures that have been proven to improve outcome after myocardial infarction and are routinely employed, such as nitrates, beta blockers, and angiotensin-converting enzyme inhibitors, have the potential to exacerbate hypotension in cardiogenic shock, and should be withheld until the patient stabilizes.

Following initial stabilization and restoration of adequate blood pressure, tissue perfusion should be assessed. If tissue perfusion remains inadequate, inotropic support or intra-aortic balloon pumping should be initiated. If tissue perfusion is adequate but significant pulmonary congestion remains, diuretics may be employed. Vasodilators can be considered as well, depending on the blood pressure.

Fluids

The initial approach to the hypotensive patient should include fluid resuscitation unless frank pulmonary edema is present. Patients are commonly diaphoretic and relative hypovolemia may be present in as many as 20% of patients with cardiogenic shock. Fluid infusion is best initiated with predetermined boluses titrated to clinical endpoints of heart rate, urine output, and blood pressure. Ischemia produces diastolic as well as systolic dysfunction, and thus elevated filling pressures may be necessary to maintain stroke volume in patients with cardiogenic shock. Patients who do not respond rapidly to initial fluid boluses or those with poor physiologic reserve should be considered for invasive hemodynamic monitoring.

Optimal filling pressures vary from patient to patient; hemodynamic monitoring can be used to construct a Starling curve at the bedside, identifying the filling pressure at which cardiac output is maximized. Maintenance of adequate preload is particularly important in patients with right ventricular infarction.

Vasopressor Agents

When arterial pressure remains inadequate, therapy with vasopressor agents may be required to maintain coronary perfusion pressure. Maintenance of adequate blood pressure is essential to break the vicious cycle of progressive hypotension with further myocardial ischemia. Dopamine increases both blood pressure and cardiac output, and is usually the initial choice in patients in the presence of systolic pressures less than 80 mm Hg. When hypotension remains refractory, norepinephrine may be necessary to maintain organ perfusion pressure. Phenylephrine, a selective alpha-1 adrenergic agonist, may be a good choice when tachyarrhythmias limit therapy with other vasopressors. Vasopressor infusions need to be

titrated carefully in patients with cardiogenic shock to maximize coronary perfusion pressure with the least possible increase in myocardial oxygen demand. It is also mandatory to ensure that filling pressures are optimal. Hemodynamic monitoring is useful in this regard.

Inotropic Agents

In patients with inadequate tissue perfusion and adequate intravascular volume, cardiovascular support with inotropic agents should be initiated. Dobutamine, a selective β1-adrenergic receptor agonist, can improve myocardial contractility and increase cardiac output, and is the initial agent of choice in patients with systolic pressures greater than 80 mm Hg. Dobutamine may exacerbate hypotension in some patients, and can precipitate tachyarrhythmias. Use of dopamine may be preferable if systolic pressure is less than 80 mm Hg, although tachycardia and increased peripheral resistance may worsen myocardial ischemia. In some situations, a combination of dopamine and dobutamine can be more effective than either agent alone.

Milrinone is a phosphodiesterase inhibitor that increases intracellular cyclic AMP by mechanisms not involving adrenergic receptors, producing both positive inotropic and vasodilatory actions. This effect may be important in patients with chronic heart failure, in whom chronic elevation of circulating catecholamine levels can produce down-regulation of beta-adrenergic receptors. Milrinone has minimal chronotropic and arrhythmogenic effects compared to catecholamines. In addition, because milrinone does not stimulate adrenergic receptors directly, its effects may be additive to those of the catecholamines. Milrinone, however, has the potential to cause hypotension and has a long half-life; in patients with tenuous clinical status, its use is often reserved for situations in which other agents have proven ineffective. Standard administration of milrinone calls for a bolus loading dose of 50 μg/kg followed by an infusion of 0.5 μg/kg/min, but many clinicians eschew the loading dose (or halve it) in patients with marginal blood pressure.

PATIENTS WITH ADEQUATE TISSUE PERFUSION AND PULMONARY CONGESTION

In patients whose primary abnormality after initial resuscitation from cardiogenic shock is pulmonary congestion but who appear to have adequate tissue perfusion, diuretics may be employed. Bolus doses of loop diuretics are usually employed, but continuous infusion may be more effective in patients with tenuous hemodynamics. Vasodilators should be used with extreme caution in the acute setting due to the risk of precipitating further hypotension and decreasing coronary blood flow.

After blood pressure has been stabilized, however, vasodilator therapy can decrease both preload and afterload. Sodium nitroprusside is a balanced arterial and venous vasodilator that decreases filling pressures and can increase stroke volume in patients with heart failure by reducing afterload. Nitroglycerin is an effective venodilator that reduces the pulmonary capillary occlusion pressure and can decrease ischemia by reducing left ventricular filling pressure and redistributing coronary blood flow to the ischemic zone. Both agents may cause acute and rapid decreases in blood pressure, and dosages must be titrated carefully; invasive hemodynamic monitoring can be useful in optimizing filling pressures when these agents are used.

FURTHER MANAGEMENT

Although it has been demonstrated convincingly that thrombolytic therapy reduces mortality in acute myocardial infarction, the benefits of thrombolytic agents in patients with cardiogenic shock are less certain. No trials have demonstrated that thrombolytic therapy reduces mortality in patients with established cardiogenic shock, although the patient numbers are small since most thrombolytic trials have excluded patients with cardiogenic shock at presentation.

The failure of thrombolytic therapy to improve survival in patients with cardiogenic shock probably results from lower rates of reperfusion in these patients. Reasons for decreased thrombolytic efficacy in cardiogenic shock probably include hemodynamic, mechanical, and metabolic factors. Some small studies support the notion that vasopressor therapy to increase aortic pressure improves thrombolytic efficacy.

Intra-aortic balloon counterpulsation (IABP) reduces systolic afterload and augments diastolic perfusion pressure, increasing cardiac output and improving coronary blood flow. These beneficial effects, in contrast to those of inotropic or vasopressor agents, occur without an increase in oxygen demand. IABP is efficacious for initial stabilization of patients with cardiogenic shock. Small randomized trials in the prethrombolytic era, however, failed to show that IABP alone increases survival. IABP alone does not produce a significant improvement in blood flow distal to a critical coronary stenosis. IABP is probably not best used as an independent modality for the treatment of cardiogenic shock, but may be an essential support mechanism to allow definitive therapeutic measures to be undertaken. In hospitals without direct angioplasty capability, stabilization with IABP and thrombolysis followed by transfer to a tertiary care facility may be the best management option. IABP may be useful as an adjunct to thrombolysis in this setting by increasing drug delivery to the thrombus, by improving coronary flow to other regions, by preventing hypotensive events, or by supporting ventricular function until areas of stunned myocardium can recover. Retrospective studies have shown that patients with cardiogenic shock in the community hospital treated with IABP placement followed by thrombolysis had improved in-hospital survival and improved outcomes after subsequent transfer for revascularization, although selection bias is clearly a confounder.

Pathophysiologic considerations favor aggressive mechanical revascularization for patients with cardiogenic shock due to myocardial infarction. Patients with cardiogenic shock are candidates for direct angioplasty, which can achieve brisk flow in the infarct artery in most patients. Retrospective trials examining the effect of angioplasty on mortality in patients with cardiogenic shock found consistently that patients with successful reperfusion have much better outcomes than those without.

The recently reported SHOCK trial is a landmark study because it contains the only randomized, controlled, prospective data addressing revascularization in patients with cardiogenic shock. The SHOCK trial randomly assigned patients with cardiogenic shock to receive optimal medical management—including IABP and thrombolytic therapy—or to cardiac catheterization with revascularization using PTCA or CABG. The trial enrolled 302 patients and was powered to detect a 20% absolute decrease in 30-day all-cause mortality rates. Mortality at 30 days was 46.7% in patients treated with early intervention and 56% in patients treated with initial medical stabilization, but this difference did not reach statistical significance (p = 0.11). At 6 months, the absolute risk reduction was 13% (50.3% compared with 63.1%, p = 0.027). Subgroup analysis showed a substantial improvement in mortality rates in patients younger than 75 years of age at both 30 days (41.4% versus 56.8%, p=0.01) and 6 months (44.9% versus 65.0%, p=0.003).

It is important to note that the control group (patients who received medical management) had a lower mortality rate than that reported in previous studies; this may reflect the aggressive use of thrombolytic therapy (64%) and balloon pumping (86%) in these controls. These data provide indirect evidence that the combination of thrombolysis and IABP may produce the best outcomes when cardiac catheterization is not immediately available. The trial was underpowered to detect the primary end point, but the improved survival with revascularization at 6 months and in patients younger than 75 years of age strongly supports the superiority of a strategy of early revascularization in most patients with cardiogenic shock.

The role of newer developments in PTCA for acute myocardial infarction in patients with cardiogenic shock remains to be defined. Recent reports have suggested that placement of coronary stents may improve outcome, either after failed or suboptimal PTCA or as a primary approach. A recent study of direct PTCA in patients with shock reported a success rate of 94%, with placement of stents

in 47%; in-hospital mortality was 26%. The role of adjunctive antiplatelet therapy is also evolving. Glycoprotein IIb/IIIa inhibitors have been shown to improve short-term clinical outcomes after angioplasty, especially in patients at high risk for complications. Published experience with platelet glycoprotein IIb/IIIa receptor inhibition in cardiogenic shock is limited, but extrapolation from other settings suggests that they may play an important adjunctive role in shock patients who undergo angioplasty.

In centers where angiography is not available, support with intraaortic balloon pumping and administration of thrombolytic agents is another alternative, with prompt transfer to a facility with the capability to provide revascularization; retrospective analyses have suggested that this strategy improves outcome.

KEY POINTS

1. Congestive heart failure is becoming more prevalent as the United States population ages.

2. Coronary artery disease is increasing as a cause of and contributing factor to congestive heart failure.

3. Heart failure is a syndrome caused not only by compromised systolic performance but also by compensatory mechanisms, which are initially beneficial but ultimately exacerbate the heart failure.

4. The goals of congestive heart failure therapy are to control symptoms, improve exercise tolerance, prolong life, and where possible, to correct the underlying cause with an emphasis on symptom control and correction of underlying causes in the critical care setting. Different therapies can have different effects on these goals.

5. Fluid restriction, diuretics, and venodilators decrease cardiac preload and reduce systemic and pulmonary congestion.

6. Angiotensin converting enzyme (ACE) inhibitors counteract activation of the renin-angiotensin system and reduce afterload as well. Arterial dilators can also reduce afterload. These agents should be started at low doses but titrated aggressively to maximal tolerated dosages.

7. Inotropic agents can improve cardiac pump function and increase output, but need to be titrated carefully in critically ill patients. Invasive hemodynamic monitoring can be extremely useful to allow for optimization of therapy with inotropes in unstable patients. This will allow the minimum dosage required to achieve the chosen therapeutic goals to be used, minimizing the increases in myocardial oxygen demand and arrhythmogenic potential.

8. Cardiogenic shock usually results from a myocardial infarction and is a medical emergency. The key to achieving a good outcome is an organized approach with rapid diagnosis and prompt initiation of therapy to maintain blood pressure and cardiac output.

9. Expeditious coronary revascularization is crucial in patients with cardiogenic shock. When available, emergent cardiac catheterization and revascularization with angioplasty or coronary surgery appears to improve survival and represents standard therapy at this time.

10. In hospitals without direct angioplasty capability, stabilization of patients with cardiogenic shock with IABP and thrombolysis followed by transfer to a tertiary care facility may be the best option.

SUGGESTED READING

1. Hollenberg SM, Parrillo JE: Reversible causes of severe myocardial dysfunction. *J Heart Lung Transplant* 1997; 16:S7-12
   Review of causes and mechanisms of reversible myocardial dysfunction.

2. Martin SJ, Danziger LH: Continuous infusion of loop diuretic in the critically ill: A review of the literature. *Crit Care Med* 1994; 22:1323-1329
   Review of continuous furosemide infusion in the critical care setting.

3. Stevenson LW, Dracup KA, Tillisch JH: Efficacy of medical therapy tailored for severe congestive heart failure in patients transferred for urgent cardiac transplantation. *Am J Cardiol* 1989; 63:461-4

Hemodynamic-guided therapy in patients referred for transplantation led to clinical improvement in a substantial fraction, obviating the need for transplantation.

4. Digitalis Investigation Group: The effect of digoxin on mortality and morbidity in patients with heart failure. *N Engl J Med* 1997; 336:525-33
   A large multicenter randomized, controlled trial of digoxin or placebo added to diuretics and ACE inhibitors in patients with congestive heart failure. Digoxin reduced hospital admissions for CHF, but had no effect on mortality.

5. CONSENSUS Trial Study Group: Effects of enalapril on mortality in severe congestive heart failure. Results of the Cooperative North Scandinavian Enalapril Survival Study (CONSENSUS). *N Engl J Med* 1987; 316:1429-1435
   ACE inhibition reduced mortality in patients with class IV heart failure.

6. Cohn JN, Johnson G, Ziesche S, et al: A comparison of enalapril with hydralazine-isosorbide dinitrate in the treatment of chronic congestive heart failure. *N Engl J Med* 1991; 325:303-310
   ACE inhibitors were superior to the combination of nitrates and hydralazine in patients with class II and III heart failure.

7. Hollenberg SM, Parrillo JE: Shock. *In*: *Harrison's Principles of Internal Medicine.* Fauci AS, Braunwald E, Isselbacher KJ, et al (Eds). New York, McGraw-Hill, 1997, pp 214-222
   One approach to the diagnosis, pathophysiologic mechanisms, and management of shock.

8. Goldberg RJ, Yarbebske J, Lessard D, Gore JM: A two-decades (1975 to 1995) long experience in the incidence, in-hospital and long-term case-fatality rates of acute myocardial infarction: A community-wide perspective. *J Am Coll Cardiol* 1999; 33:1533-1539
   Results of the Worcester Heart Attack Study showing a consistent incidence of cardiogenic shock; (7.5%), with

consistent mortality up to the last 4 years studied, when a decrease was noted.

9. Hochman JS, Buller CE, Sleeper LA, et al: Cardiogenic shock complicating acute myocardial infarction - etiologies, management and outcome: A report from the SHOCK Trial Registry. SHould we emergently revascularize Occluded Coronaries for cardiogenic shocK? *J Am Coll Cardiol* 2000; 36:3 Suppl A:1063-1070
   Final results of a registry for the SHOCK trial randomizing patients with cardiogenic shock to immediate catheterization and revascularization or thrombolysis and delayed catheterization.

10. Hochman JS, Sleeper LA, Webb JG, et al: Early revascularization in acute myocardial infarction complicated by cardiogenic shock. *N Engl J Med* 1999; 341:625-634
    Landmark study randomizing 302 patients with cardiogenic shock on the basis of left ventricular failure to emergency revascularization or initial medical stabilization. Overall mortality at 30 days was 9.3% lower in the revascularization group (46.7% versus 56.0%), but this did not reach statistical significance. (p = 0.11) The difference was significant, however, at 6 months, and in patients less than 75.

11. Hollenberg SM, Kavinsky CJ, Parrillo JE: Cardiogenic shock. *Ann Intern Med* 1999; 131:47-59
    A brief review of cardiogenic shock.

12. Anderson RD, Ohman EM, Holmes DR, Jr., et al: Use of intraaortic balloon counterpulsation in patients presenting with cardiogenic shock: Observations from the GUSTO-I Study. Global Utilization of Streptokinase and TPA for Occluded Coronary Arteries. *J Am Coll Cardiol* 1997; 30:708-715
    72% of the patients in the GUSTO trial had cardiogenic shock; IABP appears to be underutilized in these patients in this analysis.

13. Berger PB, Holmes DR, Jr., Stebbins AL, Bates ER, Califf RM, Topol EJ: Impact of an aggressive invasive catheterization and revascularization strategy on mortality in patients with cardiogenic shock in the Global Utilization of Streptokinase and Tissue Plasminogen Activator for Occluded Coronary Arteries (GUSTO-I) trial. An observational study. *Circulation* 1997; 96:122-127
    In the GUSTO trial, a strategy of early angiography and revascularization was associated with decreased mortality in cardiogenic shock.

14. Antoniucci D, Valenti R, Santoro GM, et al: Systematic direct angioplasty and stent-supported direct angioplasty therapy for cardiogenic shock complicating acute myocardial infarction: In-hospital and long-term survival. *J Am Coll Cardiol* 1998; 31:294-300
    Observational study of direct PTCA for cardiogenic shock. 47% of patients received stents, and open arteries with normal (TIMI grade 3 flow) were achieved in 85% of all patients. In-hospital mortality was 26%, and 6-month mortality was 29%.

15. Barron HV, Every NR, Parsons LS: Use of intra-aortic balloon counterpulsation in patients with cardiogenic shock complicating acute myocardial infarction: data from the National Registry of Myocardial Infarction 2. *Am Heart J* 2001; 141:933-939
    Registry data suggesting improved outcomes with IABP use in patients with cardiogenic shock.

16. Kovack PJ, Rasak MA, Bates ER, Ohman EM, Stomel RJ: Thrombolysis plus aortic counterpulsation: Improved survival in patients who present to community hospitals with cardiogenic shock. *J Am Coll Cardiol* 1997; 29:1454-1458
    Retrospective analysis; mortality with thrombolytics plus IABP was 33%, significantly better than thrombolytics alone (68%).

ENDOCRINE CRISES

James A. Kruse, MD, FCCM

Objectives

- Recognize the causes, signs, and symptoms of life-threatening hormonal imbalances involving the thyroid, pancreatic, adrenal, and pituitary glands
- Identify the optimal laboratory tests for rapidly confirming these disorders
- Review strategies for initiating treatment of specific endocrine emergencies
- Understand important pearls and caveats regarding their management

Key Words: Adrenal insufficiency; diabetes insipidus; diabetic ketoacidosis; hyperosmolar-nonketotic dehydration syndrome; hypoglycemia; myxedema coma; pheochromocytoma; thyroid storm

INTRODUCTION

Endocrine emergencies other than glycemic disturbances are uncommon, even in the ICU setting. Nevertheless, every intensivist must be able to identify these disorders, select appropriate initial laboratory tests for their confirmation, and provide emergency pharmacologic and supportive treatment.

THYROID STORM

Thyroid storm is a state of life-threatening thyrotoxicosis caused by abnormally high levels of circulating free thyroxin (FT_4) or tri-iodothyronine (T_3). It is usually due to hyperthyroidism, but can also be caused by overdose of exogenous thyroid hormone preparations. The most common etiology of both compensated hyperthyroidism and thyroid storm is Graves' disease, an autoimmune disorder caused by circulating thyroid-stimulating

immunoglobulins. Toxic nodular goiters are the next most common cause. Other etiologies include thyroiditis, thyroid adenomas, metastatic thyroid cancer, pituitary tumors, and struma ovarii, but thyroid storm from these etiologies is rare. Besides thyroid replacement preparations, a variety of other drugs can induce hyperthyroidism, including iodine, amiodarone and lithium. Transition from compensated thyrotoxicosis to thyroid storm is frequently precipitated by an intercurrent illness, trauma, surgery, or some other physiologic stress.

The signs and symptoms of thyrotoxicosis are given in Table 1. Proptosis and pretibial myxedema occur only in patients with Graves' disease. Sinus tachycardia and other supraventricular tachydysrhythmias, particularly atrial fibrillation and atrial flutter, are common in all forms of thyrotoxicosis. In contrast to ordinary thyrotoxicosis, thyroid storm is characterized by severity of these manifestations, particularly the cardiovascular and central nervous system features.

In most cases of thyrotoxicosis, the thyroid-stimulating hormone (TSH) level is abnormally low and the FT_4 is abnormally high. The total thyroxin level can be misleading due to various factors that can affect thyroxin binding to plasma proteins. An older method to obviate this detraction is performance of the T_3 resin uptake test along with the total thyroxin concentration. The product of these 2 assay results yields the free thyroxin index (FTI). This value has increased diagnostic accuracy over total thyroxin, but it is still inferior to the FT_4 assay. Older TSH assay methods were unable to quantify low levels of the hormone and therefore could only detect hypothyroidism, not hyperthyroidism.

Table 1. Signs and symptoms of thyrotoxicosis

Symptoms	*Signs*
Heat intolerance	Tachycardia, atrial fibrillation
Nervousness	Tremors, hyperreflexia
Fatigue	Systolic hypertension
Generalized weakness	Widened pulse pressure
Anorexia	Goiter
Weight loss	Signs of high-output congestive heart failure
Diarrhea	Proptosis
Dyspnea (due to congestive heart failure)	Pretibial myxedema
Angina pectoris (if underlying coronary disease)	Hyperthermia
	Changes in cognition

However, the newer (so-called *sensitive*) TSH assays are now widely available and can quantify levels within the thyrotoxic range. TSH can be elevated in the face of hyperthyroidism, due to excessive TSH secretion by the pituitary, but this is a rare cause of hyperthyroidism and even rarer as a cause of thyroid storm. Another rare form of hyperthyroidism is T3-thyrotoxicosis, in which T3 rather than T4 is responsible for the thyrotoxicosis. The FT4 concentration can be normal in this variant.

Thyroid function test results tend to be more severely abnormal in patients with thyroid storm than in patients with more compensated forms of thyrotoxicosis. However, there are no specific cut-off test levels that clearly separate these 2 entities. Thus, although the diagnosis of thyrotoxicosis can be made on the basis of laboratory testing, thyroid storm remains a clinical diagnosis. Nonspecific laboratory findings that may be seen in hyperthyroidism include hyperglycemia, hypercalcemia, and hyperbilirubinemia.

There are 3 alternatives for definitively treating hyperthyroidism: surgical removal of the thyroid, radioactive iodine ablation, and long-term pharmacologic therapy that blocks thyroid hormone synthesis. Only the latter treatment is used in the treatment of thyroid storm. Propylthiouracil (PTU) is the treatment of choice for inhibiting thyroid hormone synthesis in thyroid storm. The drug is typically given as a loading dose of 1,000 mg followed by 250 mg every 6 hours. An alternative drug having the same mechanism of action is methimazole. Both drugs can cause agranulocytosis, so patients must be monitored for this complication.

Several adjunctive pharmacologic measures are commonly employed in the treatment of thyroid storm to inhibit peripheral conversion of T4 to T3 and to blunt the effects of excess circulating thyroid hormones. The most important of these is the use of a ß-adrenergic blocking drug to blunt the cardiovascular effects of thyrotoxicosis, such as tachycardia and hypertension. Unless contraindicated, propranolol should be employed routinely. If necessary, it can be administered by slow IV injection in increments of 1 to 2 mg, up to a total of 10 mg initially. Typical oral doses are 20 to 120 mg every 6 hours, titrated to effect.

An oral iodine preparation such as Lugol's solution (e.g., 1 mL every 8 hours), iodine-containing radiocontrast material (e.g., 0.5 to 1.0 g of sodium ipodate daily), or potassium iodide (e.g., as 5 drops of saturated solution of potassium iodide every 6 hours), or parenteral sodium iodide (e.g., up to 1 g of sodium iodide IV every 8 hours initially) is often used to block release of thyroid hormone stored within the gland. However, iodine-containing agents must not be administered until 1 hour after PTU has been started, lest they stimulate further synthesis of thyroid hormones. Lithium has also been used to block hormone release, but it is generally not recommended due to its low therapeutic index.

Corticosteroids, sodium ipodate, and propranolol inhibit peripheral conversion of T4 to T3. Propranolol has the advantage of also ameliorating the hyperadrenergic manifestations of thyrotoxicosis. Routine treatment with corticosteroids is recommended for patients with thyroid storm to cover for the possibility of relative adrenal insufficiency. Hydrocortisone can be used in doses of 100 to 300 mg/day for this purpose, and also to inhibit peripheral T4 to T3 conversion.

Most cases of thyroid storm should be managed in an ICU setting for close monitoring and provision of supportive measures. This includes monitoring and treatment of potentially life-threatening cardiovascular complications (e.g., dehydration, cardiac dysrhythmias, heart failure) and therapy aimed at the intercurrent illness or injury that provoked decompensation. Acetaminophen and cooling devices are employed for managing hyperthermia. Aspirin is commonly proscribed for this purpose because it theoretically could worsen thyrotoxicosis by displacing thyroxine from circulating proteins; however, it can be given if there is a compelling indication such as treatment of concomitant acute coronary syndrome.

MYXEDEMA COMA

Myxedema coma represents an extreme state of hypothyroidism. The hypothyroidism may be caused by prior treatment of hyperthyroidism (e.g., by thyroidectomy, radioactive iodine treatment, or propylthiouracil), or due to iodine deficiency, autoimmune thyroiditis, or therapeutic use of lithium or amiodarone. It usually occurs in elderly patients. As with thyroid storm, a provocative event, such as infection, operation, or trauma, frequently precipitates progression from compensated thyroidal illness to a life-threatening state. Signs and symptoms of hypothyroidism are shown in Table 2.

Deep tendon reflexes may be absent or hypoactive, often with an abnormally prolonged relaxation phase. Pleural and pericardial effusions can also occur. Since myxedema coma represents an advanced form of hypothyroidism, any of these manifestations can be present or severe. Alterations in consciousness are present by definition and can range from slowed mentation or confusional states to frank psychosis, or more classically, unresponsiveness. Hypoventilation and frank respiratory failure are common complications of myxedema coma. Bradycardia, conduction disturbances, and low-QRS voltage are common electrocardiographic abnormalities.

Nonspecific laboratory findings can include hyponatremia, hyperlipidemia, hypoglycemia, and elevated serum creatine phosphokinase activity. Arterial blood gas analysis typically reveals hypercapnia and hypoxemia. The key diagnostic laboratory findings are elevation of circulating TSH and depression of circulating FT4. A rare exception occurs when the hypothyroidism is caused by pituitary or hypothalamic failure (i.e., secondary or tertiary hypothyroidism, respectively), in which both TSH and FT4 levels are low.

Table 2. Signs and symptoms of hypothyroidism

Symptoms	*Signs*
Cold intolerance	Apathy, dulled sensorium
Lethargy	Bradycardia
Fatigue	Hypothermia
Daytime somnolence	Goiter, macroglossia
Constipation	Alopecia, puffy facies, dry skin,
Weakness	Hoarseness
Myalgias	Distant heart tones
Impaired cognition	Hypoactive reflexes

Acutely ill patients without thyroid disease frequently have abnormal circulating thyroid hormone levels, especially if they are severely ill. Differentiating this so-called *sick euthyroid syndrome* from true hypothyroidism becomes problematic when considering the possibility of hypothyroidism in critically ill patients. The most common laboratory findings in sick euthyroid patients are low levels of FT_4 and T_3. Both can be low if the severity of illness is marked, but T_3 is usually low even with more modest degrees of illness severity. In some cases, FT_4 levels can be elevated in this syndrome. TSH can be normal or abnormal in either direction, but it is less often affected by this syndrome than FT_4 and T_3. A frequent clue to the presence of euthyroid sick syndrome is the finding of high circulating levels of reverse tri-iodothyronine (rT_3), the inactive stereoisomer of the physiologically active form of T_3. Thyroid hormone supplementation is not necessary in patients with euthyroid sick syndrome.

Myxedema coma must be promptly identified so that specific hormone replacement therapy can be instituted. Typically recommended is a single IV loading dose of 300 to 500 µg of thyroxine, followed by daily maintenance doses of either 50 to 100 µg IV or 100 to 200 µg orally or enterally. Hydrocortisone (e.g., 100

mg IV every 8 hours) is recommended to treat any concomitant adrenal insufficiency, or avert adrenal crisis which may be precipitated by thyroid supplementation. To avoid inducing vasodilation-mediated hypotension, passive rewarming measures are generally preferred over vigorous active rewarming. The most common life-threatening manifestation of myxedema coma is respiratory failure. Patients often either present with overt respiratory failure or with an alteration of consciousness that otherwise necessitates endotracheal intubation and mechanical ventilation. Others do not require mechanical ventilation initially but develop respiratory failure shortly after hospital admission. Thus, close vigilance over respiratory status is essential, including blood gas monitoring to detect hypoventilation and hypoxemia.

ADRENAL FAILURE

The most common cause of this syndrome is autoimmune-mediated destruction of the adrenal glands. Other causes of primary adrenal insufficiency include infiltration of the glands by amyloidosis, sarcoidosis, infection, or neoplasm. Among infectious causes are meningococcal, pseudomonal, tuberculous, fungal, and viral infections involving the glands. The acquired immunodeficiency syndrome is associated with adrenal

Table 3. Signs and symptoms of adrenal insufficiency

Symptoms	*Signs*
Fatigue, myalgia, arthralgia	Fever
Generalized weakness	Abdominal tenderness
Orthostatic lightheadedness	Tachycardia
Anorexia, weight loss	Orthostatic or frank hypotension
Nausea, vomiting	Confusion
Abdominal pain	Vitiligo
Diarrhea	Hyperpigmented skin
Salt craving	Amenorrhea, galactorrhea

Table 4. Nonspecific laboratory findings in adrenal insufficiency

Serum biochemical tests	*Peripheral blood counts*
Hyponatremia and hyperkalemia	Anemia
Hypoglycemia	Neutropenia
Prerenal azotemia	Lymphocytosis
Hypercalcemia	Eosinophilia
Metabolic acidosis (normal anion gap)	

insufficiency, usually caused by adrenal involvement with cytomegalovirus or Kaposi's sarcoma. Other causes of adrenal failure are glandular hemorrhage or infarction, and use of the drugs ketoconazole and etomidate.

Secondary adrenal insufficiency is caused by lack of pituitary production of adrenocorticotropic hormone (ACTH), due to brain tumors, head trauma, stroke, pituitary surgery, radiation therapy to the brain, anoxic encephalopathy, or infiltrative brain diseases. The most common cause, however, is withdrawal of chronic corticosteroid therapy that has led to suppression of the pituitary-adrenal axis.

Signs and symptoms are given in Table 3. In patients with compensated adrenal insufficiency, acute adrenal crisis is frequently precipitated by an intercurrent illnesses (e.g., sepsis) or an operation. Volume depletion is less likely to occur in secondary causes because mineralocorticoid secretion is largely under the control of the renin-angiotensin system.

Hyperpigmentation is caused by high circulating levels of ACTH; thus, it is observed in primary but not secondary adrenal insufficiency.

Nonspecific laboratory findings are shown in Table 4. A random cortisol level < 15 μg/dL is abnormal in a severely stressed patient. However, definitive confirmation of the diagnosis is best accomplished using the synthetic ACTH stimulation test. The rapid stimulation test is conventionally performed by drawing a blood sample for baseline plasma cortisol measurement, then administering 250 μg of cosyntropin IV, and then repeating the plasma cortisol measurements on blood samples obtained 30 and 60 minutes following the cosyntropin injection. Presumptive treatment can be initiated after these 2 post-stimulation blood samples are drawn, while awaiting assay results. If the patient is unstable to the degree that delaying hormone replacement for an hour or so could be dangerous, 1 dose of dexamethasone can be administered at the same time stimulation testing is begun.

Table 5. Signs and symptoms (usually paroxysmal) of pheochromocytoma

Symptoms	*Signs*
Anxiety	Hypertension
Cutaneous flushing	Orthostatic blood pressure changes
Palpitations	Diaphoresis
Chest pain, dyspnea	Premature heart beats
Nausea, vomiting	Tachydysrhythmias
Abdominal pain	Tremors

(Dexamethasone does not cross-react with laboratory cortisol assays, whereas hydrocortisone does.) Adrenal failure is most likely present if the highest post-stimulation cortisol level is < 15 µg/dL. Levels > 18 µg/dL exclude most cases of adrenal insufficiency, but levels up to 25 mg/dL may represent an inadequate response patients that are profoundly stressed.

Definitive treatment for adrenal crisis is IV hydrocortisone (200 mg initially; followed by 300 mg per day, either as 100 mg every 8 hours or as a continuous infusion). Because it does not provide adequate mineralocorticoid activity, dexamethasone is not employed except when used as the initial dose to avoid interference with cortisol assays. Emergency treatment should also include vigorous fluid replacement using IV infusions of 5% dextrose in isotonic saline to treat associated hypoglycemia and volume depletion. Intensive care unit monitoring is necessary to ensure adequate fluid resuscitation and glycemic control, and to provide supportive measures.

PHEOCHROMOCYTOMA

This uncommon disorder is caused by a tumor, usually benign, consisting of catecholamine-producing chromaffin cells. The tumor typically arises in the adrenal medulla, but occasionally occurs at extra-adrenal sites. The most common extramedullary location is the organ of Zuckerkandl adjacent to the aortic bifurcation. Some cases are associated with multiple endocrine neoplasia syndrome types IIa or IIb, or with von Recklinghausen's disease.

Pheochromocytoma results in hypertension and other signs and symptoms of catecholamine excess (Table 5). The hypertension can be sustained or paroxysmal, and hypertensive crisis can occur. A typical paroxysm lasts for about 30 minutes and consists of marked hypertension associated with headache, diaphoresis, and palpitations. Orthostatic hypotension or exacerbation of hypertension with postural changes sometimes occurs. Any of the signs and symptoms of congestive heart failure and acute or chronic complications of hypertension can also occur.

The diagnosis of pheochromocytoma is conventionally made by demonstrating increased 24-hour urinary excretion of catecholamines (epinephrine and norepinephrine) and their byproducts (vanillylmandelic acid and metanephrines). Measurement of plasma catecholamine concentrations also has diagnostic utility. Normal urinary metanephrines or normal plasma catecholamines, however, do not reliably exclude pheochromocytoma. The single best biochemical screening test is the plasma metanephrine assay. Normal plasma concentrations of these metabolites essentially exclude the possibility of

Table 6. Signs and symptoms of hypoglycemia

Neuroglycopenic manifestations	*Adrenergically mediated manifestations*
Confusion	Anxiety
Headache	Diaphoresis
Visual disturbances	Tremulousness
Behavorial changes	Tachycardia
Delirium	Palpitations
Stupor or coma	Nausea, vomiting
Seizures	Weakness

pheochromocytoma. Several provocative tests have been described, but have little if any role in ICU patients.

In critically ill patients that are suspected of having pheochromocytoma, definitive diagnostic testing is best accomplished after the patient has stabilized and is no longer in need of intensive care. This is because many acute physiologic disturbances that are common in ICU patients (e.g., myocardial infarction, congestive heart failure, renal failure, sepsis, respiratory failure, anemia, hypoglycemia, hypothyroidism, peptic ulcer, dehydration, and coma) interfere with interpretation of biochemical assays for pheochromocytoma. A variety of drugs used in the acute care setting similarly interfere with diagnostic testing; e.g., catecholamines, other sympathomimetics, vasodilators, adrenergic blocking agents, and diuretics.

Once the diagnosis of pheochromocytoma is confirmed by biochemical testing, the next step is localization of the tumor. Although angiography and inferior vena cava blood sampling were commonly used in the past, these techniques have been supplanted by noninvasive methods, such as computed tomography, magnetic resonance imaging, and radiolabeled *m*-iodobenzylguanidine scintigraphy.

Definitive treatment is surgical removal. Although curative in most cases, surgery entails considerable risk of provoking hypertensive crisis. Therefore, it is delayed until the patient has been stabilized. This entails achieving adequate adrenergic blockade, controlling blood pressure, optimizing volume status, and treating any concomitant acute conditions. The conventional pharmacologic agent of choice for acute hypertensive emergencies in patients with pheochromocytoma is phentolamine mesylate, a short-acting a-adrenergic receptor blocker. The starting dose is 2 to 5 mg, given as an IV bolus, and repeated at intervals of 5 minutes or more until blood pressure is controlled. Sodium nitroprusside can also be used. For more chronic treatment, phenoxybenzamine (a long-acting a-adrenergic blocker) has been the conventional oral agent of choice. Typical dosing starts at 10 mg every 12 hours and is titrated to blood pressure control. ß-adrenergic blocking drugs are often unnecessary, but can be used adjunctively to control tachydysrhythmias. Use of ß-blocking drugs is contraindicated in patients that are not already receiving an a-adrenergic blocking drug, because the resulting unopposed a-adrenergic stimulation can precipitate hypertensive crisis. Other drugs that have been advocated include prazosin, metyrosine, and labetalol.

HYPOGLYCEMIA

Hypoglycemia can be due to excessive exogenous insulin (e.g., iatrogenic and intentional overdose), certain heritable inborn errors of carbohydrate metabolism (e.g., hereditary fructose intolerance and glycogen storage diseases), and various acquired disorders (e.g., sepsis; various malignancies; and hepatic, renal, or adrenal failure). Excessive insulin can be secreted by pancreatic tumors (i.e., insulinoma), and insulin-like factors can be secreted by certain nonpancreatic neoplasms (e.g., hepatoma, lymphoma, leukemia, sarcomas, and carcinoid tumors). Drug-induced hypoglycemia can occur with sulfonylurea agents, ethanol, pentamidine, ß-adrenergic blockers, quinine, quinidine, and disopyramide. Abruptly stopping dextrose containing parenteral nutrition infusions can also induce hypoglycemia.

Whipple's triad describes the classic diagnostic criteria for hypoglycemia — namely, symptoms of hypoglycemia, associated low blood glucose concentration (< 50 mg/dL), and symptom resolution after dextrose administration. Clinical signs and symptoms can be divided into neuroglycopenic manifestations and adrenergically mediated manifestations (Table 6). Signs and symptoms may be absent or blunted in patients concomitantly receiving a ß-adrenergic receptor blocking agent. In some cases, assays for insulin levels and C-peptide levels, drug testing, and provocative tests are required to pinpoint the specific cause of hypoglycemia.

Hypoglycemia has the potential to cause devastating and permanent neurologic injury if it is severe and prolonged; therefore, it must be considered a medical emergency. Acute treatment of hypoglycemia consists of 3 components. The first is to provide dextrose without delay. The initial treatment of choice is IV injection of 50 mL of a 50% dextrose solution. Blood can be sampled for glucose analysis if it does not delay dextrose administration. However, waiting for glucose assay results before administering dextrose is not advised. There is little harm in administering 1 dose of dextrose, even to patients that actually have hyperglycemia. The second measure is to institute a continuous IV infusion of dextrose. This is needed to prevent recurrence of hypoglycemia following metabolism of the bolus dose. In patients developing hypoglycemia while already receiving a dextrose infusion, the dextrose bolus should be followed by increasing the dextrose infusion rate, concentration, or both. The third measure is serial glucose testing to detect possible recurrences that may occur despite the above measures, and to allow titration of maintenance dextrose administration. Maintenance dextrose administration and serial glucose monitoring are particularly important for patients with an altered sensorium, since it will interfere with clinical detection of hypoglycemic symptoms.

Specific treatment may be indicated depending on the etiology (e.g., hydrocortisone for adrenal insufficiency, or activated charcoal administration for acute overdoses of oral hypoglycemic drugs). If the hypoglycemia is refractory to multiple IV boluses of dextrose, glucagon can be given along with additional dextrose. Glucagon is also useful for the initial treatment of hypoglycemia in unconscious patients lacking ready IV access, since the drug can be given intramuscularly. Diazoxide (e.g., as a continuous IV infusion at 300 mg/hour) has also been used in refractory cases; however, its vasodilator properties restrict its use to hemodynamically stable patients.

DIABETIC KETOACIDOSIS

Whereas insulin deficiency or resistance can lead to simple hyperglycemia, diabetic ketoacidosis (DKA) occurs when there is a complete or near-complete lack of insulin. It occurs commonly in children and young adults with new onset or established type I diabetes mellitus, due to noncompliance with insulin therapy or some intercurrent medical illness such as an infection. Signs and symptoms of DKA are shown in Table 7.

Key laboratory findings include hyperglycemia (typically 400 to 800 mg/dL), metabolic acidosis (due to excess production of acetoacetic and ß-

Table 7. Signs and symptoms of diabetic ketoacidosis

Symptoms	*Signs*
Malaise	Kussmaul breathing
Fatigue	Acetone breath odor
Polyuria	Altered level of consciousness
Thirst, polydipsia	Abdominal tenderness
Nausea, vomiting	Tachycardia
Abdominal pain	Orthostatic or frank hypotension

hydroxybutyric acid), and ketosis (due to accumulation of acetone and acetoacetic acid). The anionic dissociation products of ß-hydroxybutyric and acetoacetic acids result in elevation of the serum anion gap, present in most cases of DKA. Unlike acetone and acetoacetate, ß-hydroxybutyrate is not a true ketone and does not react to the standard nitroprusside test for serum or urine "ketone bodies." Serum potassium levels are usually high in DKA initially, despite a deficit of total body potassium caused by hyperglycemia-induced diuresis. The hyperkalemia, ascribable to the effects of insulin deficiency, usually abates shortly after insulin treatment is initiated. As a result, hypokalemia can be expected to develop early in the course of therapy, and potassium administration is nearly always required.

Treatment for DKA centers on the use of insulin and fluids, both given as IV infusions. Normal saline is administered initially until adequate intravascular volume replacement is achieved, and then hypotonic fluids are substituted to avoid or minimize development of hyperchloremia. After initiating IV fluids, regular insulin is administered as an IV bolus (0.1 to 0.2 u/kg), followed by a continuous IV infusion (0.1 u/kg per hour). The insulin infusion must be titrated against serial blood glucose measurements obtained at 1- to 2-hour intervals. Once the blood glucose concentration drops below about 250 mg/dL, the IV fluid composition is changed to include 5% dextrose in water or hypotonic saline. The IV insulin infusion is continued until ketoacidosis abates, as evidenced by near-normalization of serum total CO_2 content (e.g., $\geq$ 18 mmol/L) and normalization of the serum anion gap.

Frequent blood glucose monitoring is essential during continuous IV insulin infusions to minimize the chance of hypoglycemia, and to allow its detection should it occur. Serial blood testing is also necessary to monitor electrolyte levels and to assess the response of the ketoacidosis to therapy. Both hypokalemia and hypophosphatemia commonly develop during therapy. Potassium supplementation is generally started as soon as hyperkalemia is excluded or resolves. Although it has been conventionally given to patients with severe metabolic acidemia, no clear role for administration of sodium bicarbonate has been demonstrated. Specific diagnostic studies are utilized to exclude suspected precipitating factors, such as sepsis or myocardial infarction.

After the patient's blood glucose is below 250 mg/dL and ketoacidosis has abated, IV insulin can be stopped and intermittent (every 4 or 6 hours) subcutaneous insulin dosing substituted using a sliding scale of regular insulin coverage titrated to blood glucose levels. Half of the patient's usual dose of subcutaneously administered intermediate acting insulin can be given in 2 divided doses. Parenteral dextrose administration is stopped and an appropriate oral diet begun.

HYPEROSMOLAR-NONKETOTIC DEHYDRATION SYNDROME

Whereas DKA commonly occurs when there is an absolute lack of insulin, hyperosmolar-nonketotic dehydration syndrome (HONK) occurs in patients that can secrete sufficient insulin to ward off ketoacidosis but insufficient to prevent hyperglycemia. As with DKA and other endocrine crises, an intercurrent illness frequently precipitates this disorder. HONK most often occurs in older adults and common precipitating disorders include myocardial infarction, stroke, and sepsis.

Symptoms are similar to DKA, chiefly polyuria and polydipsia, but changes in mentation are more common and more severe in HONK. Severe volume depletion and severe hyperosmolar-induced alterations in central nervous system function are frequent enough occurrences in this syndrome to explain the alternative sobriquets *hyperosmolar nonketotic coma* and *hyperosmolar nonketotic dehydration*. The hyperglycemia of HONK is more severe than is generally seen in DKA, exceeding 800 mg/dL by definition, and occasionally exceeding 2,000 mg/dL. In addition, ketoacidosis is absent in classic HONK. As syndromes, HONK and DKA overlap such that some cases of DKA are associated with higher blood glucose levels than is typical, and some cases of HONK have a degree of ketoacidosis. Thus, it is not uncommon for patients with HONK to have mild ketosis or ketoacidosis.

The associated intracellular dehydration common in HONK tends to result in hypernatremia. On the other hand, hyperglycemia-induced elevation in plasma osmolality results in an osmotic shift of water from the intracellular compartment to the extracellular compartment, thereby tending to lower plasma sodium by dilution. Although this effect by itself would tend to increase intravascular volume, the associated osmotic diuresis more than countervails and leads to volume depletion. The net effect of these forces determines actual plasma sodium concentration.

Although the degree of hypernatremia is commonly used by clinicians as a means of estimating free water deficits in acutely ill patients, its use for this purpose can be misleading in patients with HONK. Free water deficits are proportional to effective plasma osmolality, which in the absence of hyperglycemia is normally proportional to changes in plasma sodium concentration. However, in HONK the sodium concentration may be normal or decreased (as described above) even though the plasma is hyperosmolar due to hyperglycemia. Even if the patient is hypernatremic, the degree of hypernatremia will underrepresent the free water deficit in so far as hyperglycemia has tempered plasma sodium concentration. One way to estimate free water deficits in this situation is to consider the adjusted serum concentration, after taking into account the expected effect of hyperglycemia on serum sodium concentration. The conventional formula for accomplishing this is to adjust the serum sodium concentration downward by 1.6 mmol/L for every 100 mg/dL elevation in glucose concentration. Applying this factor to the patient's reported serum sodium concentration allows the clinician to abstractly consider what the patient's sodium level would be if the same free water deficit were present but in the absence of hyperglycemia.

Management of the patient with HONK is similar to that of DKA. Since the degree of dehydration is often much worse than DKA, more vigorous fluid replacement is usually necessary. Fluid resuscitation should be initiated prior to giving insulin lest circulatory shock be precipitated or worsened. This can occur because administered insulin will drive glucose intracellularly, decreasing plasma osmolality and causing an osmotic shift of water from the intravascular compartment to the intracellular compartment, leading to worsening of hypovolemia. The choice of IV fluid composition initially is always normal saline. Even though hypotonic IV fluids would alleviate the hyperosmolar state more rapidly, they are less effective at

Table 8. Etiologies of diabetes insipidus

Central causes	*Nephrogenic causes*
Congenital forms	Congenital forms
Idiopathic, autoimmune	Polycystic kidney disease
Cerebrovascular aneurysm	Medullary sponge disease
Cerebral thromboembolism	Sickle-cell disease
Intracranial hemorrhage	Hypercalcemia
Brain tumor (e.g., craniopharyngioma)	Prolonged hypokalemia
Anoxic encephalopathy	Sarcoidosis
Meningitis, encephalitis	Lithium
Granuloma of the brain	Demeclocycline
Brain surgery (e.g., hypophysectomy)	Amphotericin B
Head trauma	Vinblastine

expanding intravascular volume. Treatment priority is given to correcting hypovolemia because the secondary hypoperfusion represents a greater immediate threat to life than does hyperosmolality.

DIABETES INSIPIDUS

Antidiuretic hormone (ADH) is secreted by the posterior pituitary and acts on the distal renal tubules and collecting ducts to increase their permeability to water. As a result, the presence of ADH allows reabsorption of water in the distal nephron and elaboration of concentrated urine. Diabetes insipidus (DI) occurs when water reabsorption by the distal nephron is curtailed. In central DI, this is due to lack of ADH secretion, whereas in nephrogenic DI, it is due to unresponsiveness of the distal nephron to the action of ADH (Table 8). In either case, the resulting obligatory urinary dilution leads to polyuria, signs and symptoms of volume depletion, and secondary polydipsia. Other manifestations are a reflection of the underlying cause.

The key laboratory finding in critically patients with DI is hypernatremia, although it is not specific for DI. Hypernatremia is usually absent in patients with DI that are not acutely ill. This is because subjects with an intact thirst mechanism, a normal level of consciousness, and free access to water will drink enough to prevent hypernatremia. Seriously ill patients frequently have an abnormal sensorium, lack independent access to water, and may have blunted thirst perception—factors that can lead to dehydration and hypernatremia in the absence of DI, and much more rapid development of severe dehydration and severe hypernatremia in those with DI.

Polyuria is not specific for DI. Other causes include water diuresis secondary to excess fluid intake or administration, diuretic administration, hyperglycemia, alterations in the renal medullary concentration gradient (so called "medullary washout"), and the polyuria that can occur after acute renal failure or relief of obstructive uropathy. Classically, the diagnosis of DI is made by a water deprivation test in which all fluid intake is proscribed, thereby provoking mild dehydration and hypernatremia, and then assessing the effect on urine output and concentrating ability. This test can be dangerous in acutely ill and unstable patients because provoking hypovolemia could lead to compromised organ perfusion or circulatory failure. It should not be utilized in the ICU setting. Furthermore, it is unnecessary in most critically ill patients with DI because they are usually already hypernatremic. The diagnosis can be made in these patients simply by demonstrating an inappropriately low urine osmolality (and a low ADH level) in the face of hypernatremia.

Water deprivation normally leads to hypernatremia and the production of hyperosmolar urine (> 800 mosm/kg H_2O). In complete central DI urine osmolality is < 300 mosm/kg H_2O, whereas in partial central DI it ranges between 300 and 800 mosm/kg H_2O. Plasma ADH concentration is normally > 2 pg/mL during water deprivation, up to 1.5 pg/mL in partial central DI, but undetectable in complete central DI. In nephrogenic DI, plasma ADH levels can exceed 5 pg/mL. Central and nephrogenic DI can be distinguished by measuring urine osmolality before and after challenge using the desmopressin (1 mg subcutaneously), an ADH analog. In healthy subjects this results in a < 5% increase in urine osmolality, whereas an increase of ≥ 50% is expected in complete central DI. An intermediate rise (10 to 50%) is consistent with partial central DI. No change is expected in nephrogenic DI since the nephron is refractory to ADH and its analogs.

The degree of polyuria observed in DI can sometimes be prodigious, in some cases exceeding 20 L/day. To obviate the development of severe volume depletion, frequent assays of serum sodium level, careful monitoring of fluid intake and output, and appropriate titration of IV fluid administration are imperative. IV normal saline should be administered to patients that have or develop hypovolemia or signs of circulatory embarrassment. Normal saline is used in this case—even though the patient is hypernatremic—because it expands intravascular volume more effectively than hypotonic fluids, and because correction of hypovolemia should take priority over correction of hyperosmolality. Once intravascular volume is replenished, hypotonic fluids can be substituted, targeting correction of half of the free water deficit

during the first 24 hours of therapy, and the remaining deficit over the next 48 hours or so. Ongoing fluid loss must be taken into account. Overhydration should be avoided. It can induce a water diuresis that, if marked, can lead to washout of the normal medullary concentration gradient and thereby sustain the polyuria even if the DI is corrected or an ADH analog is administered. Electrolyte deficiency states (i.e., hypokalemia, hypomagnesemia, and hypophosphatemia) can develop rapidly in some polyuric patients. Frequent monitoring of serum electrolytes is therefore in order to allow titrated replacement and avoid severe deficiencies.

For mild cases of DI in the ICU, adequate IV fluid replacement and vigilant monitoring will often suffice as supportive treatment. In patients with marked degrees of polyuria due to central DI, administration of an ADH analog is used to limit the polyuria and decrease the risk of dehydration. Several alternatives are available for hormonal replacement. Aqueous vasopressin (typically dosed as 1 to 10 u subcutaneously or intramuscularly) has a short duration of action that allows close titration, but its potent vasoconstricting effect can precipitate coronary ischemia in susceptible patients. Desmopressin (typically dosed as 2 to 4 μg/day subcutaneously or IV in 2 divided doses) is safer because it lacks the vasoconstrictive effect of vasopressin. It is also available in an intranasal formulation (typically dosed as 10 to 40 μg/day in 2 to 3 divided doses). Vasopressin tannate in oil is given intramuscularly, but is not commonly used in the ICU due to its long duration of action (up to 72 hours).

Treatment of nephrogenic DI requires the same attention to fluid and electrolyte balance; however, ADH analogs are generally of no benefit. Any drugs implicated as causative are stopped. Other etiologies are usually controllable by chronic treatment with thiazide diuretics, which induce mild volume contraction. This stimulates sodium and water reabsorption in the proximal renal tubules and thereby diminishes water delivery to the distal nephron, serving to limit the polyuria.

ANNOTATED BIBLIOGRAPHY

1. Smallridge RC: Metabolic and anatomic thyroid emergencies: A review. *Crit Care Med* 1992; 20:276
   Provides a detailed review of the pathophysiology, diagnosis, and management of thyroid storm and myxedema coma. Contains 154 references.

2. Oelkers W: Adrenal insufficiency. *N Engl J Med* 1996; 335:1206
   This report includes a good overview of various hormonal functional assessments, including provocative evaluations that are more complex than the rapid cosyntropin test.

3. Lamberts SWJ, Bruining HA, de Jong FH: Corticosteroid therapy in severe illness. *N Engl J Med* 1997; 337:1285
   An excellent review of hypoadrenalism, focusing on the problems of diagnosis and management in the setting of critical illness. Discusses the concept of occult relative adrenal insufficiency.

4. Lenders JWM, Keiser HR, Goldstein DS, et al: Plasma metanephrines in the diagnosis of pheochromocytoma. *Ann Intern Med* 1995; 123:101
   Compares the diagnostic sensitivity of plasma metanephrine measurement to measurement of plasma catecholamines and urinary metanephrines.

5. Service FJ (Ed): Hypoglycemic disorders. *Endocrinol Metab Clin North Am* 1999; 28(3):467
   This entire issue is devoted to hypoglycemia. Contains articles on physiology of glucose counterregulation to hypoglycemia, classification of hypoglycemic disorders, drug-induced causes, diagnostic approaches, and others.

6. Roberge RJ, Martin TG, Delbridge TR: Intentional massive insulin overdose: Recognition and management. *Ann Emerg Med* 1993; 22:228
   Diagnostic and treatment considerations for managing hypoglycemia due to insulin overdose. Presentation includes a case report followed by a question and answer discussion.

7. Kruse JA, Geheb MA: Diabetic ketoacidosis and hyperosmolar syndrome. *In:* Companion to Principles & Practice of Medical Intensive Care. Kruse JA, Parker MM, Carlson RW, et al (Eds). Philadelphia, W.B. Saunders, 1996, pp 386-391
   Succinct, practical information for management of these 2 related disorders.

8. Umpierrez GE, Khajavi M, Kitabchi AE: Review: Diabetic ketoacidosis and hyperglycemic hyperosmolar nonketotic syndrome. *Am J Med Sci* 1996; 311:225
   A detailed review of hyperglycemic emergencies.

9. Blevins LS, Wand GS: Diabetes insipidus. *Crit Care Med* 1992; 20:69
   A good general overview of the disorder.

10. Bichet DG: Nephrogenic diabetes insipidus. *Am J Med* 1998; 105:431
    Covers the pathophysiology of this disorder in detail. Contains excellent illustrations.

11. Zaloga GP, Carlson RW, Geheb MA (Eds): Endocrine crises. *Crit Care Clin* 1991; 7:1
    This entire bound issue is devoted to endocrine emergencies. Contains individual articles on thyroid, adrenal, pituitary, and glycemic crises.

12. Pacak K, Linehan WM, Eisenhofer G, et al: Recent advances in genetics, diagnosis, localization, and treatment of pheochromocytoma. *Ann Intern Med* 2001; 134:315
    An update on neurochemical diagnostics, localization imaging, and surgical management.

13. Viallon A, Zeni F, Lafond P, et al: Does bicarbonate therapy improve the management of severe diabetic ketoacidosis? *Crit Care Med* 1999; 27:2690

A descriptive study and review of literature on the treatment of DKA with sodium bicarbonate.

14. Kannan CR, Seshadri KG: Thyrotoxicosis. *Disease-A-Month* 1997; 43:601
    An extensive review of the topic, with 144 references.

15. Yamamoto T, Fukuyama J, Fujiyoshi A: Factors associated with mortality of myxedema coma: Report of 8 cases and literature survey. *Thyroid* 1999; 9:1167
    Examines the issue of high-dose versus low-dose thyroid replacement therapy for myxedema coma.

16. Singer I, Oster JR, Fishman LM: The management of diabetes insipidus in adults. *Arch Intern Med* 1997; 157:1293
    A comprehensive, practical review of short- and long-term management of patients with central and nephrogenic DI.

17. Genuth SM. Diabetic ketoacidosis and hyperglycemic hyperosmolar coma. *Cur Ther Endocrinol Metab* 1997; 6:438
    Tutorial review.

NUTRITIONAL SUPPORT OF THE STRESSED INTENSIVE CARE UNIT PATIENT

Frederick A. Moore, MD, FCCM; Margaret McQuiggan, MS, RD, CSM

Objectives

- Discuss the rationale for nutritional support and nutrient requirements of ICU patients
- Discuss the use of total parenteral nutrition in the ICU
- Discuss the use of enteral nutrition in the ICU

Key Words: injury stress response, nutritional assessment, metabolic cart, nitrogen balance, total parenteral nutrition, enteral nutrition, immune-enhancing nutrition, catheter-related sepsis

TABLE OF ABBREVIATIONS

AA	amino acid
ALI	acute lung injury
BEE	basal energy expenditure
CARS	compensatory anti-inflammatory response syndrome
CNS	central nervous system
CRS	catheter-related sepsis
FFA	free fatty acid
GALT	gut-associated lymphoid tissue
MOF	multiple organ failure
PNI	Prognostic Nutritional Index
PUFA	polyunsaturated fatty acid
REE	resting energy expenditure
RES	reticuloendothelial system
SIRS	systemic inflammatory response syndrome
TEN	total enteral nutrition
TPN	total parenteral nutrition
UUN	urine urea nitrogen

METABOLIC RESPONSE TO STRESS VERSUS STARVATION

A variety of conditions that require ICU care lead to a stereotyped metabolic response which is called the "injury stress response." Traditionally, this has been viewed to be a central nervous system (CNS) mediated endocrine response that increases circulating levels of the counter-regulatory hormones (catecholamines, corticosteroids, and glucagon). More recently, the systemic inflammatory response syndrome (SIRS) has been described, and it is recognized that a variety of its mediators (e.g., TNFα, IL-1, IL-2, IL-6) also play an important role in the injury stress response. Favorable modulation of the injury stress response is not currently feasible because the driving mechanisms are not understood. The best management options are to control the initiating insult and to provide high-risk patients exogenous substrates that support the metabolic environment.

The injury stress response increases resting energy expenditure (REE). The increase in REE is dependent both upon the type and severity of the insult (REE can increase as much as 100% after burns, 50% after sepsis, 40% after trauma, and 30% after major surgery). To meet this increased metabolic demand, endogenous substrates are mobilized. Glucose stores (i.e., 2000 - 3000 kcal glycogen) are quickly depleted, and gluconeogenesis (principally in liver, but also in kidney) produces glucose that is shunted to glucose-dependent tissues (brain, erythrocytes, inflammatory cells, wound tissue). Adipose tissue is stimulated to release free fatty acids (FFA) and glycerol. The rate of lypolysis, however, exceeds lipid oxidation. As a result, plasma triglyceride levels increase and considerable reesterification occurs in the liver. This process requires energy and creates futile cycles. The increase in protein catabolism is the most dramatic effect. Skeletal muscle protein (later constitutive protein stores) is broken down, and the released amino acids become the substrate for acute-phase protein synthesis, gluconeogenesis, and energy production. The injury stress response differs from chronic starvation in several important ways (Table 1).

With brief starvation (up to 72 hours) glucose stores are rapidly depleted and the body depends heavily on the breakdown of protein to provide amino acids as a primary energy source and as a source of new glucose for glucose-dependent tissues. These pathways provide about 85% of energy needs in this setting. In the absence of "stress," this process may be easily interrupted by providing exogenous substrate. After 72 hours of starvation, adaptive changes favor the mobilization of fat and reduce the breakdown of protein to a low level (30% of energy requirements). Fat becomes the principal source of energy (70%). With longer starvation, protein is further protected by a decrease in total energy requirements. As with brief starvation, the process is quickly and easily reversed by providing exogenous glucose alone (which returns the patient to the brief starvation pattern) or exogenous glucose and amino acids.

Nutritional support should be tailored to metabolic environment (Table 2). The stressed ICU patient compared to the starved patient requires more nonprotein calories (25 kcal/kg/day versus 20 kcal/kg/day) and more protein (1.3 g/kg/day versus 1.0 g/kg/day). As patients become more stressed, they become more catabolic and less tolerant to glucose (see "Hyperglycemia" section). As a result, the amount of protein administered is increased (from 1.3 to 2.0 gm/kg/day) and the percent of nonprotein calories as glucose is decreased (from 80% to 70%). Thus, the nonprotein calories to gram of nitrogen ratio is decreased from 120:1 to 80:1.

Persistent hypercatabolism dominates the metabolic response to critical illness (Figure 1). At first, the amino acid demands are met by skeletal muscle proteolysis. However, in a short period of time this "autocannibalism" progressively erodes crucial constitutive structure elements as well as circulating proteins. The resulting acute protein malnutrition is associated with cardiac, pulmonary, hepatic, gastrointestinal, and immunologic dysfunction. In essence, subclinical multiple organ dysfunction (MOF) evolves as the patient becomes progressively more immunosuppressed. Delayed infections then extend hypercatabolism with the progression to full-blown MOF. Based on this paradigm, a number of clinical studies were performed in the 1980s to determine whether early nutritional support could improve the outcome of high-risk patients. Unfortunately, many of these studies failed to generate

Table 1. Metabolic response of starved versus stressed patients

Metabolic Consequences	Starved	Stressed
Resting energy	↑	↑↑
Respiratory quotient	Low (0.7)	High (0.85)
Primary fuel	Fat	Mixed
Proteolysis	↑	↑↑↑
Urinary nitrogen loss	↑	↑↑↑
Constitutive proteins	↓	↓↓↓
Acute-phase proteins	–	↑↑↑
Gluconeogenesis	↑	↑↑↑
Ketone production	↑↑↑	↑

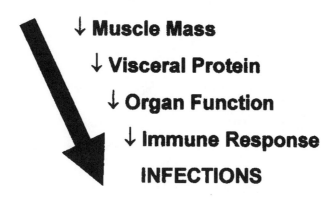

PERSISTENT HYPERCATABOLISM

↓ **Muscle Mass**

↓ **Visceral Protein**

↓ **Organ Function**

↓ **Immune Response**

INFECTIONS

MULTIPLE ORGAN FAILURE

Figure 1. Role of persistent hypercatabolism

Table 2. Nutritional support of starved versus stressed patients

Nutritional Support	Starved	Moderate Stress	Severe Stress
Nonprotein calories (kcal/kg/day)	20	25	25
- Glucose	100%	80%	70%
- Fat	EFA requirements	≤ 1 g/kg	≤ 1 g/kg
Protein (g/kg/day)	1.0	1.3	2.0
Nonprotein calories/ grams nitrogen	150:1	120:1	80:1

EFA, essential fatty acid; grams nitrogen = grams protein/6.25.

interpretable results, in large part due to the heterogeneous nature of the patients included in the studies. Most of the positive trials have been generated from burn and trauma patients. These patients tend to be young and free of confounding comorbid disease. Additionally, the severity of the burn/trauma injury can be quantitated so that a high-risk cohort of patients with persistent hypercatabolism can be identified for study enrollment. These studies have demonstrated that early nutrition improves outcome (improved nitrogen balance and

constitutive protein levels, improved immune function and decreased infections, decreased length of stay) and that the enteral route is preferred to the parenteral route. Whether these observations can be generalized to other ICU patient populations is not clear.

Modulate Immune Response

Despite tremendous advances in ICU care, nosocomial infections continue to be an unsolved problem. In large part, these late

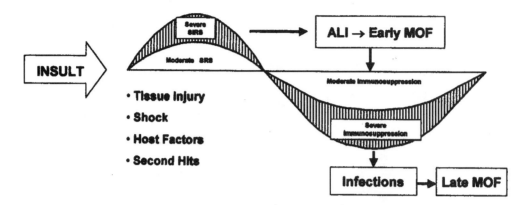

Figure 2. Dysfunctional regulation of inflammation. SIRS, systemic inflammatory response syndrome; ALI acute lung injury; MOF, multiple organ failure.

infections occur due to failure of local and systemic host defenses. While exact causes of late immunosuppression are not clear, it is now believed to occur in part as a result of dysfunctional regulation of inflammation (Figure 2). An initial insult (e.g., sepsis, trauma/burns, or major operation) precipitates early systemic hyperinflammation (i.e., SIRS), the amplitude and duration (generally 3 - 5 days) depends on the magnitude of the insult as well as some host factors. Severe SIRS can precipitate early MOF, which typically presents as acute lung injury (ALI). As time proceeds, certain components of this early SIRS are endogenously down-regulated to prevent unnecessary, potentially autodestructive inflammation. This is now referred to as the compensatory anti-inflammatory response syndrome (i.e., CARS). The resulting delayed immunosuppression, however, sets the stage for secondary infection which can either worsen early MOF, or trigger late MOF.

While various strategies have been proposed and tested to modulate this dysfunctional inflammatory response, the most promising approach to date has been the delivery of specific nutrients (generally via the gut) that exert pharmacologic immune-enhancing effects above and beyond the prevention of acute protein malnutrition (see previous section and later "Immune-Enhancing Formula" section). Glutamine is acknowledged to be the preferred

fuel of the enterocyte and is thought to stimulate lymphocyte and monocyte functions. Arginine promotes collagen synthesis required in wound healing and increases the number of total lymphocytes as well as the proportion of helper T cells. Additionally, arginine is the chief precursor of nitric oxide synthesis and has been shown to enhance delayed cutaneous hypersensitivity and lymphocyte blastogenesis. Traditional nutritional support includes a high proportion of plant-derived ω - 6 polyunsaturated fatty acid (PUFA). However, diets with a low ω - 6 PUFA and high fish-oil derived ω - 3 PUFA content are known to suppress the synthesis of cytokines that exhibit potent inflammatory activities, e.g., TNFα and Il-1β. Finally, exogenous nucleotides may be necessary in stressed states to maintain rapid cell proliferation and responsiveness.

Promote Gut Function

The dysfunctional gut is now believed to be the "reservoir for pathogens" that causes late MOF-associated infections (Figure 3). The initial insult (via ischemia/reperfusion, sepsis, inhibitory neuroendocrine reflexes) and emergency laparotomy (via anesthesia and bowel manipulation) cause an early ileus. Disuse (parenteral instead of enteral nutrition) and common ICU therapies (e.g., H$_2$-antagonists, narcotics, broad-spectrum antibiotics) promote

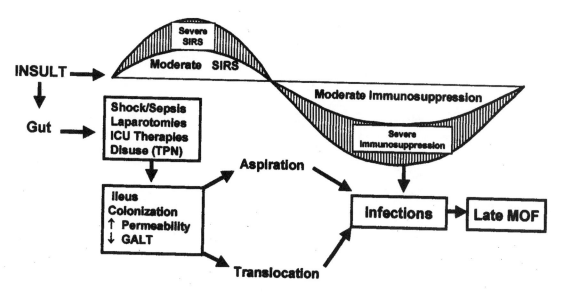

Figure 3. Role of gut in late infections. SIRS, systemic inflammatory response syndrome. MOF, multiple organ failure; GALT, gut-associated lymphoid tissue.

further gut dysfunction characterized by progressive ileus, colonization of the upper gut, increased permeability, and decreased gut-associated lymphoid tissue (GALT) function. Consequently, the upper gut becomes a reservoir for pathogens, and local and systemic defense mechanisms that prevent the spread of these organisms become impaired; the primary route of dissemination (i.e., aspiration versus translocation) is not clear. Although there is good epidemiologic evidence for this sequence of events, prospective randomized controlled trials of gut-specific therapies (e.g., selective gut decontamination, early enteral nutrition, and most recently immune-enhancing enteral formulas) that have consistently demonstrated a reduction in nosocomial infections (principally pneumonia) are the most convincing evidence. Thus, the provision of early enteral nutrition to promote more normal gut function is believed to prevent this cascade of events from occurring.

NUTRITIONAL ASSESSMENT

Medical history should be reviewed to determine the presence of factors that may predispose the patient to malnutrition, such as

weight loss, anorexia, vomiting, diarrhea, and decreased or unusual intake.

Physical examination focuses on an assessment of lean body mass (presence of muscle wasting), loss of subcutaneous fat, and the physical findings of micronutrition deficiencies (e.g. dermatitis, glossitis, poor wound healing).

Laboratory data should include constitutive protein concentrations and micronutrient concentrations (if clinical evaluation suggests possible deficiencies). Constitutive protein status is assessed by measuring serum concentrations of selected hepatically synthesized transport proteins that have been shown to correlate with nutritional status. These include albumin, transferrin, prealbumin, and retinol-binding protein. Depletion of visceral proteins may be categorized as mild, moderate, or severe (Table 3).

Anthropometric measurements include height, weight, and limb circumference. They are relatively insensitive to acute changes in nutritional status and are difficult to measure in patients with edema; therefore, they are mostly useful in monitoring patients requiring long-term nutritional support, such as home TPN. Body weight is the most commonly used of these

Table 3. Depletion of constitutive proteins

Protein	Normal Value	Mild	Moderate	Severe
Albumin (g/dL)	3.5-5.0	2.8-3.5	2.1-2.7	< 2.1
Transferrin (mg/dL)	200-400	150-200	100-150	< 100
Prealbumin (mg/dL)	10-40	10-15	5-10	< 5
Retinol-binding protein (mg/dL)	2.7-7.6	n/a	n/a	n/a

Data may also include measures of immune function (e.g., total lymphocyte count, delayed cutaneous hypersensitivity).

measures. Actual body weight should be interpreted in view of fluid status and relative to ideal weight for height or usual (e.g. pre-illness or pre-weight-loss) weight. Mid-arm muscle circumference correlates with somatic protein reserves, and triceps skin-fold thickness estimates the subcutaneous fat as compared to individuals of the same gender and age.

The Prognostic Nutritional Index (PNI) was developed using multivariate analysis to determine the relative value of various nutritional markers in predicting operative morbidity and mortality, and to develop a clinically applicable model to identify patients at risk for nutrition-based complications:

$$PNI = 158\% - 16.6(Alb) - 0.78(TSF) - 0.2(TFN) - 5.8(DH)$$

where Alb signifies albumin, TSF refers to triceps skinfold thickness, TFN signifies transferrin, and DH refers to delayed cutaneous hypersensitivity (number of responses). This predictive model has been used to enroll patients into clinical trials. Please note that the serum albumin is a very heavily weighted variable in this predictive model.

NUTRIENT REQUIREMENTS

The Harris-Benedict equation is a common method to estimate energy expenditure and thus to determine caloric requirements. The Harris-Benedict equation was derived from a population-based analysis in 1919, and is currently used to estimate basal energy expenditure (BEE) based on age, sex, height, and weight. The Harris-Benedict equations are as follows:

Men: BEE = 66 + (13.7 x weight) + (5 x height) - (6.8 x age)

Women: BEE = 665 + (9.6 x weight) + (1.9 x height) - (4.7 x age)

where weight is actual or in adjusted kg, height in cm, and age in years. The BEE represents energy requirements in the fasted, resting, nonstressed state. In the presence of metabolic stress, the BEE must be multiplied by an empirically derived stress factor to obtain an estimate of the caloric requirement. The numerical value for this empirically derived stress multiplication factor continues to be a source of controversy. In the not-too-distant past, the BEE was multiplied by stress factors as high as 3 in major stress settings such as in burn patients, resulting in estimated energy requirements and caloric intake as high as 5000 kcal/day. Complications of overfeeding, such as hypercapnia, hyperglycemia, and hepatic steatosis, have resulted in revisions of these stress multiplication factors. Currently, the usual stress multiplication factors range from 1.2 to 1.6 times the BEE. Needless to say, hypermetabolic injured and septic patients do not require 40 kcal/kg/day of nonprotein calories as was recommended in the past. Current recommendations for caloric support are in the range of 25 to 30 kcal/kg/day.

Metabolic gas analysis (also called metabolic cart or indirect calorimetry) measures inspired and expired concentrations of oxygen (O_2), carbon dioxide (CO_2), and nitrogen (N_2) as well as expired minute ventilation (V. E). Table 4 depicts typical values.

As expected, inspired O_2 (FIO_2) is greater than expired O_2 (FEO_2) because O_2 is being absorbed, and inspired CO_2 (FICO_2) is lower than expired CO_2 (FECO_2) because CO_2 is excreted. N_2 is neither absorbed nor excreted; therefore, the difference in FIN_2 and FEN_2 can be used to calculate inspired minute ventilation (V. I).

$$VI = \frac{FEN_2}{FIN_2} - VE$$

O_2 consumption (VO_2) can then be calculated as VO_2 = (VI x FIO_2) − (VE x FEO_2) and CO_2 production can be calculated as VCO_2 = (VE x FECO_2) − (VI x FICO_2).

From this information and a 24-hour urine urea nitrogen (UUN) determination, REE can be calculated using the Weir equation:

$$REE = 3.9 \times VO_2 + 1.1 \times VCO_2 - 2.8 \times UUN$$

The second commonly derived variable is the respiratory quotient (RQ). This is an indicator of net substrate oxidation and, hence, provides insight into substrate utilization. The RQ is calculated as follows:

$$RQ = VCO_2 / VO_2$$

The RQ for fat oxidation = 0.7, protein oxidation = 0.85, glucose oxidation = 1.0, and lipogenesis = 8.7 (see the following case example).

Case Example. A 68-year-old male with COPD has been on the ventilator for 7 days after an emergency laparotomy for perforated sigmoid diverticulitis. He is being considered for extubation and has spontaneous ventilatory parameters measured which include a minute ventilation of 13 L/min, tidal volume of 300 mL, vital capacity of 750 mL, and a negative inspiratory force of −30 cm H_2O. He is receiving TPN; it is questioned how TPN might contribute to his high minute ventilation. There are 2 ways that TPN might increase CO_2 production and thus increase minute ventilation. The first is by providing a high proportion of the nonprotein calories as glucose. Glucose oxidation has a higher RQ (1.0) than does fat oxidation (0.7). Therefore, a diet high in glucose will result in higher CO_2 production. This is most simply understood by reviewing the equations for glucose and fat oxidation.

Glucose Oxidation:

$$C_6H_2O_2 + 6\,O_2 \rightarrow 6\,CO_2 + 6\,H_2O$$

$$RQ = \frac{CO_2\ produced}{O_2\ consumed} = \frac{6\,CO_2}{6\,O_2} = 1.0$$

Lipid Oxidation:
$$2\,C_{54}H_{101}O_6 + 153\,O_2 \rightarrow 108\,CO_2 + 101\,H_2O$$

$$RQ = \frac{CO_2\ Produced}{O_2\ Consumed} = \frac{108\,CO_2}{153\,O_2} + 0.7$$

Thus, by providing a higher proportion of nonprotein calories as fat, CO_2 production may be decreased.

The *second* way that nutrition can contribute to excessive CO_2 production is by giving too many nonprotein calories. Excessive glucose is converted to fat.

Lipogenesis:
$$27\,C_6H_{12}O_2 + 6\,O_2 \rightarrow 2\,C_{55}H_{104}O_6 + 52\,CO_2 + 58\,H_2O$$

$$RQ = \frac{CO_2\ Produced}{O_2\ Consumed} = \frac{52\,CO_2}{6\,O_2} = 8.7$$

Of the 2 mechanisms proposed, the second is much more common. Please note, however, that this problem with TPN has been overemphasized. In most critically ill patients,

Table 4. Typical metabolic cart measurements

FIO_2	39.29%
FEO_2	35.7%
$FICO_2$	0.03%
$FECO_2$	3.32%
FIN_2	60.67%
FEN_2	60.98%

Table 5. Clinical condition and concomitant protein catabolism as indicated by levels of urinary nitrogen loss

Clinical Condition	Urinary Nitrogen Loss (g/day)
Nonstressed, starvation	< 8
Low stress (e.g., elective surgery)	8 – 12
Moderate stress (e.g., major trauma)	13 – 18
High stress (e.g., sepsis)	> 18

failure to wean is due to inadequate ventilatory endurance or unrecognized hypermetabolism. What these patients need is time to resolve their inflammatory response. Additionally, during this waiting period adequate nutrition and partial ventilatory support should be given to these patients to strengthen their skeletal muscles and diaphragms. Unfortunately, some clinicians, when faced with a difficult weaning situation, reflexively cut nutrition and allow their patients to starve. Additionally, clinicians try to assess whether this is occurring by obtaining a metabolic cart study. However, when using the metabolic cart in critically ill ventilated patients, it is frequently necessary to place the patient in full ventilatory support to get accurate numbers. Then, the patient is put back on a mode of partial ventilatory support. Unfortunately, things have changed because the patient is now expending energy to breathe. This is particularly worrisome in the difficult-to-wean patient in whom the work of breathing can consume 10% to 15% of their oxygen. Consequently, metabolic cart studies offer confounding information. Pragmatically, when a patient has sufficient ventilatory strength but is requiring marginally high minute ventilation (13 L/min), it is advised to cut nutrition in half the night before weaning ventilation. The next morning, place the patient on a T-piece and if this fails, the failure is not due to overfeeding.

UUN is measured as an indicator of the protein catabolic rate (i.e., stress) and is used to determine nitrogen balance. UUN represents 60% to 90% of the nitrogen excreted in the urine, and therefore, is a rough approximation of total urinary nitrogen (TUN). As the stress level increases, the concomitant increase in protein catabolism results in an increase in urinary nitrogen. Quantitatively, this can be interpreted as shown in Table 5.

Nitrogen balance is the difference between nitrogen intake and nitrogen output. Nitrogen intake is determined from dietary intake per day (grams of nitrogen = grams of protein / 6.25). Nitrogen output per day is determined by measuring UUN (gm) in a 24-hour urine collection and adding 4 g/day to approximate nonurea nitrogen loss in the urine plus other insensible N_2 losses (i.e., grams of UUN + 4 g/day). Nitrogen balance is calculated as follows:

Nitrogen balance = (g/day protein intake/6.25) - (g/day UUN) - 4 g/day

Traditionally, a prime goal in nutritional support has been to place the patient in +3 to +5 nitrogen balance. Traditional nitrogen balance studies are useful in patients with creatinine clearances > 50 mL/min. Once renal function is further compromised, calculations of protein catabolic rate are necessary. These require serial BUN ng/dL, serial weights, calculations of interdialytic time period, and urinary losses of nitrogen.

TOTAL PARENTERAL NUTRITION

Components of total pareneteral nutrition (TPN) include a) dextrose, b) fatty acids, c) amino acids, d) electrolytes, e) vitamins, f) trace minerals, and g) fluids. Nonprotein calories are provided as a balance of carbohydrate and fat. Dextrose monohydrate (caloric density 3.4 kcal/g) is the carbohydrate. Fat emulsions (caloric density 9 kcal/g) made from either soybean oil or a mixture of soybean oil and safflower oil provide fat calories and are the source of essential fatty acids (linoleic, linolenic, and arachidonic acids). Protein (caloric density 4 kcal/g) is provided as crystalline amino acids. Standard amino acid solutions contain a balance of essential and nonessential amino acids. The electrolyte cations, which include sodium, potassium, magnesium, phosphorus, and calcium, are admixed into the TPN solution using one of several anions. Acid-base status may be affected by the amount of chloride or acetate used in providing sodium and potassium. The concentrations of calcium and phosphorus are limited to avoid precipitation of a calcium phosphate salt. Multivitamin products that meet American Medical Association recommendations contain vitamins A, C, D, E, and the B vitamins, including folate, but not vitamin K, which must be added separately. A multitrace mineral product is added to provide copper, chromium, manganese, zinc, and selenium. Central TPN solutions are hyperosmolar and must be delivered through a large-lumen vein. When central access is unavailable or undesirable, parenteral nutrition with a dilute solution (< 800 mOsm/L) may be delivered through a peripheral vein for 7 to 10 days. Indications for its use in the ICU include:

1. Massive bowel resection
2. High output fistula refractory to elemental diet
3. Unable to meet > 60% of nutritional needs via enteral route by ICU day 8
4. Malabsorption
5. Persistent ileus or bowel obstruction
6. Perceived high risk for nonocclusive bowel necrosis (shock resuscitation, α-agonists, persistent severe distention or cramping)

Preoperative TPN

It is well documented that malnourished patients are at an increased risk for septic complications, problems with wound healing, longer hospital stays, and increased mortality. The unproved contention is that preoperative TPN can improve nutritional status and thereby reduce postoperative morbidity and mortality. Results of studies evaluating preoperative TPN and outcome are variable. Recent trials suggest that TPN may in fact promote postoperative septic complications. For the mild to moderately malnourished patients, the risks of preoperative TPN appear to outweigh the potential benefits. However, the small subgroup of patients who are severely malnourished appear to benefit from receiving 7 to 10 days of preoperative TPN. One of the confounding variables in the preoperative TPN trials is that many of the enrolled patients had cancer. Animal data show enhanced tumor growth with selected types of cancer when the animals are parenterally fed. Therefore, concern exists that preoperative TPN will simply promote tumor growth (i.e., you are feeding the tumor rather than the patient). This concern is supported by the clinical observation that TPN does not improve the nutritional status of patients with large tumors. Additionally, immunocompromised patients with cancer are at increased risk for infectious complications due to TPN.

Stress Formula TPN

These formulas have been modified to match the altered substrate utilization observed in stressed patients. Critical illness induces a hypercatabolic state (Figure 1). To blunt "autocannibalism" of endogenous protein stores, stress formula TPN provides increased amounts of exogenous amino acids. Specialty amino acid formulas which are designed to meet organ failure specific requirements include high branched-chain (HBC AA), hepatic failure (low aromatic AA), and renal failure (high essential AA). The use of these specialty formulas remains controversial because of the extra expense. Additionally, studies comparing HBC AA solutions with standard AA formulas in stressed patients have shown improvements in nitrogen retention, constitutive protein levels, and immune function, but have failed to demonstrate reduced morbidity or mortality. The use of specific organ failure formulas (hepatic and renal) has not been shown to improve nutritional status or outcome compared with standard AA solutions.

Glucose intolerance is common in critically ill patients. Consequently, meeting caloric needs with carbohydrate calories is difficult and may further exacerbate the complications associated with poor blood glucose control. Providing a proportion of the nonprotein calories as lipid facilitates attaining the desired caloric intake without "stressing" carbohydrate metabolism and meets essential fatty acid requirements. On the other hand, lipid particles are taken up by the reticuloendothelial system (RES) in a dose-dependent fashion. When lipid is given in high doses (> 2.5 g/kg/day) or infused over a short period (< 10 hours), the RES may become saturated with lipid and, hence, unable to scavenge microbes and other particulate matter. This may result in an increased susceptibility to sepsis. Furthermore, the currently available lipid emulsions are composed of long-chain fatty acids. Of these, linoleic acid (representing 50% - 65% by weight of the fatty acids) is the precursor for prostaglandin synthesis as well as other mediators of the inflammatory response, and may be immunosuppressive. It has been proposed that an excessive intake of linoleic acid may inhibit the immune system, facilitate the inflammatory response, and compromise the patient's ability to fight infection. Currently, patients should not receive > 1 g/ kg/day of lipid.

Monitoring TPN

TPN monitoring is done to a) determine the efficacy of the TPN therapy; b) determine changes in metabolic status (stress level); and c) detect complications associated with TPN. Measurements of efficacy in the acute care setting include weight, constitutive protein status (e.g., albumin, transferrin, prealbumin, and retinol-binding protein), nitrogen balance, and wound healing. However, it is important to remember that these levels are acutely decreased

by the stress insult alone. Following a stress insult, the liver "reprioritizes" its protein synthesis (i.e., decreases normal constitutive protein synthesis so that it can increase acute-phase protein synthesis), and this persists until the SIRS resolves. Metabolic status should be viewed first from the clinical perspective. Are there signs of SIRS with or without active infection? Is the patient hyperdynamic? What is the minute ventilation requirement? Metabolic status can be further assessed by laboratory variables that evaluate substrate tolerance (e.g., blood glucose and serum triglyceride concentrations) as well as protein catabolic rate (24-hour urine urea nitrogen). A metabolic gas study can document energy expenditure and respiratory quotient.

There are 4 categories of TPN-associated complications: a) nutritional (e.g., overfeeding, underfeeding, specific nutrient deficiencies or toxicities); b) metabolic (e.g., hyperglycemia, electrolyte, fluid, and acid-base imbalances, liver function abnormalities); c) infectious (i.e., catheter related sepsis); and d) mechanical (e.g., hemothorax, pneumothorax, subclavian vein thrombosis).

Refeeding Syndrome

Refeeding syndrome can occur with rapid and excessive feeding of patients with severe malnutrition due to starvation, alcoholism, delayed support, anorexia nervosa, and insufficient intracellular ions. As a result of ion fluxes into the cell with refeeding, serum phosphate, magnesium, potassium, and calcium levels can drop precipitously. In the case of blunted basal insulin secretion, severe hyperglycemia may arise. Symptoms include cardiac arrhythmias, confusion, respiratory failure, and even death. This can be prevented by initiating TPN at ~ 2/3 of the required goal predominantly by decreased dextrose kcal; then, gradually increased CHO kcal over 5 days while anticipating and correcting electrolyte abnormalities. Exogenous insulin may be required.

Table 6. Counterregulatory effects of hormones on glucose homeostasis

Hormone	Perturbs	Effect
Catecholamines	Glycogenlysis	↑
	Gluconeogenesis	↑
	Lipolysis	↑
	Insulin release	↓
Glucagon	Glycogenolysis	↑
	Gluconeogenesis	↑
	Ketogenesis	↑
Glucocorticoids	Gluconeogenesis	↑
	Catecholamine response	↑
	Insulin resistance	↑

Hyperglycemia

Critical illness is accompanied by increased plasma counterregulatory hormone levels, which have multiple effects on glucose homeostasis (Table 6). The end result is hyperglycemia with resistance to insulin.

Other factors that contribute to this "stress diabetes" include obesity, SIRS (TNFα, IL-1, IL-2, and IL-6), advanced age, exogenous steroid or catecholamines, increased free fatty acids, and nutritional support (parenteral route greater than enteral route).

The resulting hyperglycemia can adversely affect outcome through several mechanisms including a) glycosuria and inappropriate diuresis, b) increased risk of infection (by impairing neutrophil and immunoglobulin function), and c) exacerbation of cerebral edema.

Catheter-Related Sepsis

The pathogenesis of catherte-related sepsis (CRS) is straightforward. The indwelling catheter becomes contaminated and, over time, the bacteria or yeast proliferate, resulting in heavy local colonization, which then seeds the blood, resulting in bacteremia and signs of systemic sepsis. The catheter may have been contaminated a) at the time of insertion, b) later due to local skin colonization with bacteria or yeast which then tracked down the external surface of the catheter, and c) by hub contamination during manipulation which then tracked down the inside of the catheter. Other less-frequent sources of contamination include infusion of contaminated solutions or hematogenous seeding from a distal site of infection.

Preventative measures can be broken down into 3 categories a) catheter insertion, b) catheter care, and c) catheter removal. Important components of catheter insertion include skin preparation (chlorhexidine is more efficacious than alcohol or povidone iodine) and the use of maximal sterile barriers. Although it is commonly believed that multiple-lumen catheters have a higher rate of CRS compared to single-lumen catheters, randomized studies (which use rigorous central venous catheter protocols) show equal rates of CRS. Recent randomized trials indicate that CRS can be reduced by use of antibiotic or antiseptic bonded catheters. However, these catheters are considerably more expensive and should be used in select patients whose catheters are going to be in place for a prolonged period (e.g., 5 - 7 days). In regards to catheter care: a) dressing/tubing should be changed every 48 to 72 hours; b) antibiotic ointment is of questionable benefit (but is commonly used); and c) gauze dressing is superior to transparent dressing. Finally, removing the catheter at set intervals effectively reduces CRS, but must be weighed against the increased risk of mechanical complications associated with a new stick. Guidewire changes at set intervals are of debatable benefit in

Table 7. Indications for early enteral nutrition

Major Head Injuries: Glasgow Coma Scale score with an identifiable lesion on CT scan

Major Torso Trauma:
1. Major abdominal trauma defined by an Abdominal Trauma Index > 18
2. Anticipated prolonged LOS or mechanical ventilation with at least 2 of the following conditions:
    a. Injury to spleen, kidney, small bowel, or mesentery
    b. > 6 units transfusion requirement

Major Orthopedic Trauma: Two or more of the following:
1. > 6 units transfusion requirement
2. Major pelvic fracture (e.g., acetabular fx, vertical shear, open fx)
3. Two or more long-bone fractures

Major Chest Trauma: Combined multiple rib fractures and pulmonary contusions anticipated to require prolonged mechanical ventilation

Major Upper Gastrointestinal Surgery that precludes oral intake for > 5 days (e.g. esophagectomy, combined pancreatic-duodenal injury)

2nd *or* 3rd *Degree Burns* > 20%

Chronically Malnourished Patients anticipated to be NPO > 5 days:
1. Admission albumin < 2.5 g/dL
2. Recent weight loss > 10%
3. < 80% ideal body weight

Limited Physiologic Reserve anticipated to be NPO > 5 days:
1. Significant comorbid disease
    a. Lung disease: Chronic obstructive pulmonary disease requiring bronchodilators or steroids
    b. Liver disease: Admission bilirubin > 2.5 mg%, history of hepatic encephalopathy, or established cirrhosis
    c. Kidney disease: Chronic renal disease requiring dialysis or renal transplant
    d. Active malignancy
    e. Immune dysfunction: AIDS or current chemotherapy, or prednisone
2. Age > 70 years

---

reducing CRS, but may be an effective method of early diagnosis of local catheter colonization or local catheter infection.

ENTERAL NUTRITION

Enteral Route is Preferred to the Parenteral Route

The optimal route of substrate delivery is an ongoing debate and, like most good debates, it continues to evolve. TPN became widely available by the late 1970s. However, the enteral route was favored because it was safer and cheaper. By the mid-1980s, as a result of nutritional support teams, TPN had become reasonably safe and convenient because central venous catheters were being widely utilized in ICUs. An inappropriate fear of gastrointestinal intolerance discouraged the use of enteral nutrition, and by default TPN became the preferred route in the ICUs. By the late 1980s, however, clinical trials had convincingly demonstrated that enteral nutrition is well tolerated when delivered into the small bowel (see next section). Moreover, basic research observations offered compelling physiologic benefits for enteral feeding. Substrates (i.e.,

Table 8. Hermann Shock/Trauma ICU enteral formulary

Classification: *Product*	Immune-Enhancing: *Impact®*	Polymeric High-Protein: *Promote®*	Elemental: *Vivonex Plus®*	Renal: *Nepro®*
Kcal/mL	1.0	1.0	1.0	2.0
Protein (g/mL)	0.06	0.06	0.05	0.07
CHO (g/mL)	0.14	0.13	0.19	0.22
Fat (g/mL)	0.07	0.03	0.01	0.10
Na/K (mEq/L)	48/36	44/51	27/23	37/27
Phos/Mg (mEq/L)	800/270	1200/400	560/220	685/215
% H_2O	85	84	85	70
mOsm/kg H_2O	375	340	650	665
mL to meet RDA vitamin requirements	1500	1000	1800	947

Data may also include measures of immune function (e.g., total lymphocyte count, delayed cutaneous hypersensitivity).

nitrogen and glucose) delivered by the enteral route are better utilized than those administered parenterally. In addition, total enteral nutrition (TEN), compared with current TPN, prevents gastrointestinal mucosal atrophy, may attenuate the stress response to injury, maintains immunocompetence, and preserves normal gut flora. Finally, prospective, randomized, controlled trials have consistently shown that early TEN, when compared to TPN, is associated with reduced septic morbidity. Thus, today the enteral route is preferred. Considerable research efforts are being directed toward elucidating the mechanisms responsible for the improved outcomes (principally septic morbidity) associated with enteral nutrition and toward modifying TPN so that it can achieve the same outcomes in patients who cannot tolerate enteral diets.

How enteral feeding reduces septic morbidity is somewhat of an enigma. Multiple factors are likely involved. First, lack of enteral nutrition or lack of specific nutrients (e.g., glutamine, SCFA, fiber) may promote bacterial translocation. While bacterial translocation has been a popular endpoint in laboratory models, clinical studies have had a difficult time demonstrating that bacterial translocation is a common pathogenic event in critically ill patients. Second, excessive administration of glucose or lipids with TPN may worsen immunosuppression. This has been demonstrated in laboratory models, and 3 recent prospective randomized controlled trials of perioperative TPN have demonstrated that the TPN-fed patients, compared to control subjects who received no nutritional supplementation, have higher postoperative septic morbidity. Third, specific nutrients (e.g., glutamine, arginine, ω-3 fatty acids, and nucleotides) enhance immune effector cell function independent of preventing SIRS-induced acute protein malnutrition (see "Immune-Enhancing Formulas"). Fourth, stimulation of the enteric nervous system by enteral feeding enhances both local GALT and systemic mucosal-associated lymphoid tissue (MALT) function, which decreases the risk of nosocomial pneumonia.

Indications for Early Enteral Nutrition

Based on studies done in trauma patients, we believe early enteral nutrition is beneficial. Our indications are as shown in Table 7.

Prepyloric versus Postpyloric Feeding

This is another area of ongoing debate, but in this case considerable confusion exists because definitive data do not exist. Laboratory studies demonstrate that the stomach responds to stressful insults by decreasing its emptying and increasing its secretions. High nasogastric output in the acute phases of illness suggest that the same is true for humans. Additionally, manometry studies have documented that early antral atony is common in critically ill patients. Finally, recent studies have identified high gastric residuals to be the major cause for failure of gastric feedings in the ICU setting. On the other hand, small bowel motility and absorptive capacity appear to be relatively normal in the early phases of critical illness and clinical trials have convincingly demonstrated that early jejunal feeding is feasible in the vast majority of patients (roughly 85%). Additionally, it is preferred to no feeding or TPN because it promotes vital gut functions. As time proceeds, however, gastric emptying improves and gastric feeding then becomes feasible. Therefore, if you strive to feed sick patients early, the postpyloric route is preferred. If you feed not very sick patients or feed late, gastric feeding works and is preferred because it is more physiologic.

Formula Selection

Many of the early clinical trials were done with elemental formulas that were low in fat. It was assumed these would be better tolerated. However, in more recent studies, other types of formulas appear to be equally well tolerated. The numerous available formulas may be categorized into *polymeric formulas* (which contain nutrients in high molecular weight forms and require normal digestive and absorptive ability), *predigested formulas* (which contain 1 or more partially digested macronutrients or combinations of nutrients and can be absorbed in patients with compromised GI tracts), and *modular formulas* (which are composed of individual nutrients or combinations of nutrients but are nutritionally incomplete and intended for use as supplements or in combination with other products). Unfortunately, with exception of the immune-enhancing formulas (see next section), very little comparative data exists to guide clinicians in selecting the most appropriate formula for their ICU patients.

Table 8 depicts our ICU enteral formulary. We have developed a limited selection to meet the specific needs of our patient population. Our indications to use the formulas described in Table 8 are as follows:

Immune Enhancing Diet: These formulas should be used in patients who are at known risk for major septic complications and MOF:

1. Combined flail chest/pulmonary contusion anticipated to require prolonged mechanical ventilation.
2. Major abdominal trauma defined by an Abdominal Trauma Index > 18
3. Two or more of the following:
    a. > 6 units transfusion requirement
    b. Major pelvic fracture (e.g., acetabular fx, vertical shear, open fx)
    c. Two or more long-bone fractures
4. Nontrauma patients (e.g., major cancer operations) that the attending surgeon believes to be at risk for major septic morbidity.

Polymeric High Protein Formula: These formulas should be used in patients who do not meet the criteria for immune-enhancing diets, but who have normal digestive and absorptive capacity of the GI tract and are believed to have increased nitrogen requirements due to the presence of:

1. Major torso trauma
2. Major head injuries
3. Major upper GI surgery
4. Obese patients with moderate calorie need, but high protein needs.

Elemental Formulas: These formulas should be used in patients who have:

1.   Proven intolerance to the first formula used
2.   Not been fed enterally for > 8 days
3.   Pancreatitis
4.   Short gut
5.   High-output distal colonic or ileal fistula
6.   Persistent, severe diarrhea for > 48 hours while on polymeric formula
7.   Gastric regional CO_2 ($PrCO_2$) > 70, but < 90 for more than 8 hours (measured by gastric tonometry)
8.   Moderate distention > 24 hours.
Maintain elemental feeding for a minimum of 72 hours. Reinstate polymeric once all parameters are improved.

Renal Failure Formula:
1.   Renal failure requiring intermittent dialysis.

Degree of injury may merit formula dilution to ¾ strength to reduce viscosity and the addition of Promod (protein powder) to meet protein needs. Patients on continuous venous-venous hemo-dialysis (CVVHD) do not require renal formula.

Immune-Enhancing Enteral Formulas

Recent basic and clinical research suggests that the beneficial effects of enteral nutrition can be amplified by supplementing specific nutrients that exert pharmacologic immune-enhancing effects beyond the prevention of acute protein malnutrition. Such nutrients include glutamine, arginine, 4-3 PUFA, and nucleotides. At present, at least 3 immune-enhancing enteral formulas (i.e., enriched with various combinations of the above nutrients) are commercially available and have been tested in PRCTs. In this era of "evidence-based" medicine, these data are becoming increasingly difficult to dismiss. To date, there are at least 18 published, prospective, randomized, controlled trials (PRCT) where an immune-enhancing diet (IED) is compared with a standard enteral diet (SED) or no diet, and where the patient outcome was a predetermined end point (Table 9). Of the 18 PRCTs, 11 trials demonstrated improved outcome, 4 trials were highly suggestive of improved outcome, and 3 trials did not demonstrate any clinical outcome advantage.

Nonocclusive Bowel Necrosis

With wider application of enteral nutrition in ICU patients, this entity has emerged as a devastating complication. The incidence among patient populations described is < 0.3%; however, the mortality exceeds 50%. The pathogenesis is not understood. While gut hypoperfusion due to incomplete resuscitation is commonly stated to be the prelude, most cases of nonocclusive bowel necrosis occur in a delayed fashion in ICU patients with a complicated course (pneumonia, sepsis, renal failure) that requires progressively higher acuity care (e.g., nonconventional modes of ventilation, vasopressors, dialysis). Gastrointestinal signs and symptoms tend to occur late and as a result, clinical monitoring fails to detect this entity early in its course. The clinical presentation resembles bacterial sepsis.

CONTROVERSIES
Anabolic Compounds

The 4 major classes of anabolic compounds include recombinant human growth hormone (rhGH), insulin-like growth factor (IGF-1), anabolic steroids, and high-dose insulin. These drugs have been tested most extensively in burn patients where it has been observed that despite aggressive nutritional support, persistent metabolic stress and immobilization leads to major muscle wasting, which is a major obstacle in rehabilitation. RhGH is the most tested compound and has powerful anabolic effects on most body cells, either directly or by stimulating IGF-1 secretion. Relatively small trials have demonstrated accelerated donor site healing, improved muscle protein synthesis, decreased length of hospital stay, and improved mortality. A recent large multicenter trial, however, observed an increased mortality in critically ill patients who received rhGH. While there is no explanation for this increased mortality, this report has tempered enthusiasm for rhGH use in nonburned ICU patients.

Table 9. Assessment of patient outcome in 18 PRCTs comparing immune-enhancing diets (IED) versus standard enteral diets (SED) or no diet

First Author / Year (Journal)	Patient Type (Number)	IED	SED	Results with IED	Improved Outcome
Gottschlich 1990 *JPEN*	Burns (n=50)	Noncommercial Study Formula	Osmolite + Promote or Traumacal	↓ WI ↓ LOS	Yes
Daly 1992 *Surgery*	Cancer (n=77)	Impact	Non-Commercial Control Diet	↓ WC ↓ Infection	Yes
Brown 1994 *Pharmacotherapy*	Trauma (n=37)	Noncommercial Study Formula	Osmolite HN + Promod	— Infection	Yes
Moore 1994 *J Trauma*	Trauma (n=98)	Immun-Aid	Vivonex TEN	↓ IAA ↓ MOF	Yes
Bower 1995 *Crit Care Med*	Mixed ICU (n=296)	Impact	Osmolite HN	↓ Infection ↓ LOS	? Yes Subsets
Daly 1995 *Ann Surg*	Cancer (n=60)	Impact	Traumacal	↓ WC ↓ Infection ↓ LOS	Yes
Kudsk 1996 *Ann Surg*	Trauma (n=35)	Immun-Aid	Promote + Casec	↓ ABT ↓ Infection ↓ LOS	Yes
Senkel 1997 *Crit Care Med*	Cancer (n=154)	Impact	Non-Commercial Control Diet	↓ Late Infections	Yes
Mendez 1997 *J Trauma*	Trauma (n=43)	Noncommercial Study Formula	Osmolite HN + Promod	↑ ARDS	No
Saffle 1997 *J Trauma*	Burns (n=50)	Impact	Replete	------	No
Heslin 1997 *Ann Surg*	Cancer (n=154)	Impact	No Diet	------	No
Braga 1998 *Crit Care Med*	Cancer (n=154)	Impact	Non-Commercial Control Diet	↓ Infection ↓ LOS	? Yes Subsets
Atkinson 1998 *Crit Care Med*	Mixed ICU (n=369)	Impact	Non-Commercial Control Diet	↓ VentDays ↓ LOS	? Yes Subsets
Weimann 1998 *Nutrition*	Trauma (n=32)	Impact	Non-Commercial Control Diet	↓ SIRS ↓ MOF	? Yes Definitions
Senkel 1999 *Arch Surg*	Cancer (n=154)	Impact	Non-Commercial Control Diet	↓ Late Infections	Yes
Braga 1999 *Arch Surg*	Cancer (n=206)	Impact	Non-Commercial Control Diet	↓ Infection	Yes
Snyderman 1999 *Laryngoscope*	Cancer (n=129)	Impact	Replete	↓ Infection	Yes
Galban 2000 *JPEN*	Septic ICU (n=181)	Impact	Precitene Hiperproteico	↓ Late Infections	Yes

WI, wound infection; WC, wound complication; LOS, length of stay; Inf, infections; IAA intra-abdominal abscess; MOF, multiple organ failure; ABT, antibiotics; SIRS, systemic inflammatory response syndrome.

Osmolite®, Ross Laboratories, Columbus, OH; Promote®, Ross Laboratories, Columbus, OH; Traumacal®, Mead Johnson, Evansville, IN; Impact®, Novartis, Minneapolis, MN; ProMod®, Ross Laboratories, Columbus, OH; Immun-Aid®, McGaw, Irvine. CA; Vivonex® TEN, Novartis, Minneapolis, MN; Casec®, Mead Johnson, Evansville, IN; Replete®, Nestle, Deerfield, IL.

Pancreatitis

Acute pancreatitis induces severe hypercatabolism; without exogenous nutritional support, acute protein malnutrition can occur. TPN has been a standard of care to provide nutrients while "resting" the pancreas. However, recent studies have indicated that However, recent studies have indicated that enteral feeding into the jejunum in patients with acute pancreatitis is feasible. Compared with TPN, jejunal feeding does not cause increased pancreatic stimulation and is associated with reduced septic complications.

Obese Patients

Obesity affects one-third of Americans and is associated with a number of comorbid conditions that place patients at increased risk for ICU admission. Controversies concerning nutritional support of the obese patient include a) the definition of obesity, b) what body weight (ideal, actual, or adjusted) to use when estimating energy needs, and c) the amount of nonprotein calories and protein to administer. Obesity begins when an individual exceeds 120% of ideal body weight, which can be obtained with height/weight tables. Energy needs should be calculated using adjusted body weight, which is calculated by determining the obese patient's actual weight (ABW) and the ideal body weight (IBW). Then, 25% of the difference between these numbers is added to the IBW.

0.25 (ABW – IBW) + IBW = Adjusted Body Weight

This takes into account the increased lean body mass seen in obese patients. The adjusted body weight is then used in the Harris-Benedict equation (or other equations) to predict energy needs. Obese patients experience a similar metabolic response to critical illness. However, they tend to have more resistance to insulin and hyperlipidemia. "Letting them live off their excess fat" is an inappropriate strategy and if pursued will result in unnecessary and potentially harmful loss of lean body mass.

Obese patients should be started on nutritional support as early as their nonobese counterparts. While controversial, data are emerging that support the concept of "hypocaloric" feeding, where the obese patient is provided high protein (2 g/kg IBW/day), but low nonprotein calories (15 kcal/kg/day).

Specialized Formulas for Critically Ill Patients with Diabetes Mellitus

Formulas with reduced carbohydrate and increased fat loads are available for use in patients with diabetes mellitus. These formulas are more costly than standard formulas, and are marketed as being superior in maintaining glycemic control. However, individual responses may be variable. The use of standard high-protein formulas in an isocaloric or hypocaloric load, combined with appropriate insulin therapy, may be the most effective treatment for insulin resistance in the stressed, type-2 diabetic patient. Furthermore, gastric feedings with high-fat formulas in the diabetic patient with gastroparesis may be associated with delayed gastric emptying and increased risk of aspiration.

SUGGESTED READINGS

1. Rombeau JL, Rolandelli RG, Wilmore DW: Nutritional support. *In*: Scientific American Surgery. Wilmore DW, Brennan MF, Harken AH (Eds). New York, 1995
   This provides an algorithm and extensive explanation of nutritional management of ICU patients. This provides the information that is likely to be seen on the Surgical Critical Care exam.
2. Update In Intensive Care and Emergency Medicine 34: From Nutritional Support to Pharmacologic Nutrition in the ICU. Pichard C, Kudsk KA (Eds). Berlin, Springer-Verlag, 2000
   Provides "state of the art" discussion of traditional issues such as nutritional assessment and the metabolic response to critical illness, as well as new aspects of nutritional support such as modulation of the inflammatory response and host defense

barriers through specific macro- and micronutrients.

3. American Society of Parenteral and Enteral Nutrition: Guidelines for the use of parenteral and enteral nutrition in adult patients. *J Parent Ent Nutr* 1993; 17:1SA-26SA
Evidence-based consensus statement from the American Society of Enteral and Parenteral Nutrition (ASPEN) on indications for parenteral and enteral nutrition.

4. McClave SA, Snider HL: Understanding the metabolic response to critical illness: Factors that cause patients to deviate from the expected pattern of hypermetabolism. *New Horiz* 1994; 2:139-146
Nice overview of metabolic response to critical illness and factors that affect it.

5. McQuiggan MM, Marvin RG, McKinley BA, et al: Enteral feeding following major torso trauma: From theory to practice. *New Horiz* 1999; 7:131-140
Provide the rationale for early enteral nutrition in critically ill patients and outlines a protocol that insures implementation of enteral nutrition in the ICU.

6. Moore FA, Feliciano DV, Andrassy, et al: Enteral feeding reduces postoperative septic complications: A meta-analysis. *Ann Surg* 1992; 216:172-183
Meta-analysis of 8 prospective randomized trials that demonstrated that early enteral nutrition, compared to TPN, reduces postoperative septic morbidity.

7. Veterans Affair Total Parenteral Cooperative Study Group: Perioperative total parenteral nutrition in surgical patients. *N Engl J Med* 1991; 325:525-532
Large multicenter prospective randomized trial that demonstrated the preoperative TPN, compared to no nutritional supplementation, was associated with increased infectious morbidity. This has been confirmed by 2 more recent PRCTs. The only patients who appear to benefit from preoperative TPN were severely malnourished. Severe malnutrition represented only a small subset of the enrolled patients.

8. Talpers S, Romberger D, Bunce S, et al: Nutritionally associated increased carbon dioxide production: Excess total calories versus high proportion of carbohydrate calories. *Chest* 1992; 102:551-555
Demonstrates that CO_2 production did not significantly change when the carbohydrate to lipid ratio was changed during isocaloric feeding, but rose markedly as total caloric intake was increased above resting energy expenditure as a result of lipogenesis.

9. Takala J, Ruokonen E, Webster NR, et al: Increased mortality associated with growth hormone treatment in critically ill adults. *N Engl J Med* 1999; 341:785-792
Multicenter trial that demonstrated an increased mortality in critically ill patients requiring mechanical ventilation who were randomized to receive growth hormone.

10. Moore FA, Moore EE, Kudsk KA, et al: Clinical benefits of an immune-enhancing diet for early postinjury enteral feeding. *J Trauma* 1994; 37:607-615
Multicenter trial that demonstrated a reduction in intra-abdominal abscesses and MOF in patients randomized to an immune-enhancing formula compared to a standard enteral formula that had been used in previous nutritional trials.

11. DeWitt RC, Wu Y, Reneger KB, et al: Bombesin recovers gut-associated lymphoid tissue (GALT) and preserves immunity to bacterial pneumonia in mice receiving total parenteral nutrition. *Ann Surg* 2000; 231:1-7
Demonstrated that 5 days of TPN, compared to chow feeding, results in decreased GALT mass, decreased IgA levels in the gut and lung, and increased mortality to a clinically relevant septic challenge. Of note, these differences can be reversed by treating the TPN-fed animals with 3 days of the neuropeptide bombesin.

12. Marvin RG, McKinley BA, McQuiggan M, et al: Nonocclusive bowel necrosis occurring in critically ill trauma patients receiving enteral nutrition manifests no reliable clinical signs for early detection. *Am J Surg* 2000; 179:7-12
Thirteen cases of nonocclusive bowel necrosis were identified among 4,300 ICU patients (0.3%). The onset typically occurs

in the second week in high-acuity patients who have been tolerating enteral nutrition. Gastrointestinal signs of this entity occur late. Clinical presentation resembles bacterial sepsis with tachycardia, fever, and leukocytosis. Abdominal CT scanning is usual method of diagnosis.

ACUTE ABDOMEN / PANCREATITIS /BILIARY INFECTION

Frederick A. Moore, MD, FCCM

Objectives

- To discuss the diagnosis of intra-abdominal infection in ICU patients
- To discuss acute pancreatitis encountered in ICU patients
- To discuss biliary tract disease encountered in ICU patients
- To discuss common hollow viscus entities that cause an acute abdomen in ICU patients

Key Words*:* perforated duodenal ulcer; small bowel obstruction; bowel ischemia; pancreatitis; ascending cholangitis; acalculous cholecystitis; volvulus; diverticulitis

TABLE OF ABBREVIATIONS

BAT	blunt abdominal trauma
CHF	congestive heart failure
CT	computed tomography
DU	duodenal ulcer
ERCP	endoscopic retrograde cholangiopancreatography
GI	gastrointestinal
MRI	magnetic resonance imaging
NOBI	nonocclusive bowel ischemia
OF	organ failure
PRCT	prospective, randomized, controlled trial
PTC	percutaneous transhepatic cholangiography
SGD	selective gut decontamination
SIRS	systemic inflammatory response syndrome
TPN	total parenteral nutrition
VAP	ventilator-associated pneumonia

DIAGNOSIS OF INTRA-ABDOMINAL INFECTION IN ICU PATIENTS

In the late 1970s, nondirected exploratory laparotomy was recommended for ICU patients with unexplained progressive sepsis and organ failure (1). By the mid-1980s, it was recognized that many ICU patients were subjected to unnecessary laparotomies and that a variety of noninfectious insults (e.g., pancreatitis) could precipitate systemic hyperinflammation similar to bacterial sepsis (now referred to as systemic inflammatory response syndrome [SIRS]). Additionally, computed tomography scanning became widely available and has been documented to diagnose accurately a variety of intra-abdominal infections. Moreover, with the availability and success of percutaneous drainage, nondirected exploratory laparotomy has become a distinctly unusual diagnostic option. The possibility that an occult intra-abdominal infection is driving ongoing OF is still a frequent question pondered by intensivists. This diagnostic quandary can be approached by addressing the following questions.

Does the patient have concerning signs of progressive sepsis-induced organ failure?

Insight can be obtained by trending the clinical signs of SIRS (e.g., fever, tachycardia, and leukocytosis) and organ dysfunction (neurologic—metabolic encephalopathy; pulmonary—minute ventilation, oxygenation; cardiovascular—volume and ionotropic/vasopressor requirement, cardiac index/systemic vascular resistance; renal—creatinine and urine output; hepatic— bilirubin; gastrointestinal—ileus, intolerance to enteral nutrition; metabolic—glucose intolerance; lactate, oxygen consumption; hematologic—platelets, coagulopathy).

Is the source of sepsis-induced organ failure the chest versus the abdomen?

While other sources of infection (e.g., catheter-related sepsis, urinary tract infection, sinusitis) may cause an acute septic response, they rarely cause progressive OF. Ventilator-associated pneumonia (VAP) is the major confounder. It occurs frequently and can cause or worsen OF. Unfortunately, VAP is difficult to diagnose. Often, patients with intra-abdominal infections have 1 or more of the clinical criteria for pneumonia and the clinicians can be lolled into a false sense of security that they are treating a VAP. To avoid this confusion, it is helpful to categorize VAP as definite, probable, or possible. The use of bronchoalveolar lavage or protected specimen brush may be helpful in confirming the diagnosis when the clinical diagnosis is not definite.

What are the risks and the most likely cause of intra-abdominal infection?

While it is easy to order a battery of tests to be done over a couple of days that address all potential diagnoses, a critically ill patient may not tolerate this shotgun approach. The clinician needs to determine the relative urgency (e.g., CT scan tonight or tomorrow) and focus the work-up to minimize diagnostic delays and low-yield testing. Specific diagnoses have characteristic presentations (2–4). A review of recent abdominal operations can also provide important clues. Specific scenarios are associated with increased abdominal septic complications (e.g., hollow viscus perforation plus splenectomy, delayed treatment of perforated hollow viscus, resection of unprepped colon). It is also important to question the surgeons who performed the operation. They can provide the best risk assessment. A good abdominal examination can also be helpful. Important signs include localized tenderness and poor wound healing or infection. Recent intolerance to enteral nutrition is another valuable sign of an occult infection. Abdominal distention is a fairly nonspecific finding.

What are the most appropriate diagnostic tests (5, 6)?

Plain Radiographic Films. These films are universally available, inexpensive, safe, and they can be done at the patient's bedside. Obtain anteroposterior and left lateral decubitus views (ICU patients are not stable enough to be in the upright position). Check bowel gas pattern (i.e., obstruction or volvulus), presence of extra-luminal air (i.e., pneumoperitoneum or pneumo-retroperitoneum, pneumatosis intestinalis or portal vein air and unusual air/fluid levels), and abnormal calcifications (appendicalith, renal calculi, gallstones, chronic pancreatitis, and aortic aneurysm). This is a low-yield screening test.

Ultrasound. Ultrasound is usually available, relatively inexpensive, safe, and this procedure can be done at the patient's bedside. It is operator dependent (i.e., an ultrasound done in the middle of the night by an inexperienced practitioner may provide more misinformation than information), and it is less reliable with abdominal distention, obesity, recent surgery, and the presence of drains. It is ideal for gallbladder and biliary tree. Ultrasound is less accurate than CT scan for abscesses, but it should be used as a screening tool for patients who cannot be transported safely.

Computed Tomography. CT is usually available, but it is done outside the ICU (newer bedside technology lacks resolution). This procedure is operator independent, but reader dependent. Because of the risk of transport and costs of the test, the diagnostic yield needs to be considered (e.g., are the results going to change management?). CT can examine the entire abdomen and pelvis. It can detect accurately a variety of problems (abscesses, cholecystitis, biliary obstruction, pancreatic inflammation/plegmans/necrosis/cysts, appendicitis, diverticulitis, intestinal perforation/infarction).

Scintigraphy. Indium-labeled leukocyte scanning is preferred over Gallium scans. Gallium scans take longer and Gallium uptake by the bowel can be confused with localized infection. Indium-labeled leukocyte scans have similar accuracy as ultrasound and CT, but it takes at least 24 hours to get the results and it cannot be used to guide percutaneous drainage.

Magnetic Resonance Imaging (MRI). MRI has limited use in ICU patients due to constraints of a high magnetic field. It has a supplementary role if there is suspicion of extension into skeletal muscle, or if other imaging findings are ambiguous. It can be useful in differentiating abscess versus hematoma versus tumor.

Paracentesis/Peritoneal Lavage. Paracentesis and peritoneal lavage are universally available, relatively inexpensive, low risk, and these procedures can be done at the patient's bedside. Paracentesis should be performed on all septic patients with ascites to exclude peritonitis (both primary and secondary). Diagnostic peritoneal lavage is a well-documented test in the evaluation of abdominal trauma, but its role in nontraumatic disease is less well defined (7). It is an alternative to consider in the critically ill patient who cannot be transported easily for CT scanning and who have an equivocal physical examination, other medical problems that could account for symptoms (e.g., lower-lobe pneumonia with Gram-negative bacteremia) or septic shock of unknown etiology. Relative contraindications include obesity, portal hypertension, and previous abdominal operations.

ACUTE PANCREATITIS ENCOUNTERED IN ICU PATIENTS

Acute pancreatitis is believed to originate from inappropriate intracellular activation of digestive enzymes with autodigestion of the pancreas. This enzyme cascade activation establishes a noninfectious inflammatory response with activation of a variety of inflammatory cascades including complement bradykinin, histamine, and cytokines as well as recruitment of neutrophils and macrophages. In severe cases, the inflammation becomes systemic and causes remote organ dysfunction. The common histologic finding is microvascular endothelial injury. Acute pancreatitis is caused by alcohol or biliary tract disease in 90% of cases. The diagnosis of pancreatitis is suspected with a combination of clinical findings (e.g., fever, tachycardia, epigastric pain radiating into the back, abdominal tenderness) and laboratory studies (elevated white count, high amylase, high lipase). A number of possibilities exist in the differential diagnosis, and a CT scan is the most sensitive, noninvasive, diagnostic imaging test to confirm the diagnosis.

About a quarter of patients with acute pancreatitis will develop complications; most deaths occur in this group. Pancreatitis can be graded as mild or severe based on a variety of methods. The best method for grading the severity of pancreatitis is the "Ranson Criteria," which have been modified to create 2 similar systems: 1 for alcoholic pancreatitis; and the other for gallstone pancreatitis. Both systems incorporate 5 features measured at admission (e.g., for alcoholic pancreatitis: age > 55 years; white blood cell count of > 16,000 cells/mm^3, glucose > 200 mg/dL, LDH > 350 U/L, AST > 250 U/L), and 6 additional criteria determined during the initial 48 hours of hospitalization (e.g., for alcoholic pancreatitis: HCT decrease > 10 points, increase BUN > 5 mg/dL, serum Ca^{++} < 8 mg/dL, PaO$_2$ < 60 torr (< 8 kPa), base deficit > 4 mmol/L, fluid requirements > 6 L). When more than 3 criteria are met, the need for prolonged hospitalization and laparotomy increases. Most deaths occur in patients who meet more than 4 criteria. Mortality increases sharply with more than 6 criteria. The appearance of the pancreas on CT scan also adds to the prediction of adverse outcomes. High-resolution dynamic studies are used to identify pancreatic necrosis (i.e., lack of enhancement), which is at high risk to become infected.

Early in the disease process, patients with severe pancreatitis may experience fluid sequestration, acid-base abnormalities, electrolyte abnormalities, and renal failure. Acute severe pancreatitis can also cause early acute respiratory distress syndrome. Initial management is directed at correcting and monitoring for these problems. Nasogastric suction should be used to provide symptomatic relief. While a variety of agents (e.g., H$_2$-antagonists, glucagon, and octreotide) have been used to reduce pancreatic secretions, none have been shown to improve patient outcome. Acute pancreatitis induces severe hypermetabolism; without exogenous nutritional support, an acute protein malnutrition can occur. Total parenteral nutrition (TPN) has been a standard of care to provide nutrients while "resting" the pancreas. However, recent studies have indicated that enteral feeding into the jejunum in patients with acute pancreatitis is feasible. When compared with TPN, jejunal feeding does not cause increased pancreatic stimulation and is associated with reduced septic complications (8).

Secondary pancreatic infections (abscess or infected necrosis) are the most serious complications. Clinical studies (9, 10) have not demonstrated that the routine use of prophylactic antibiotics is beneficial. These studies are confounded by the entry of patients with mild-to-moderate pancreatitis and the use of antibiotics that do not achieve high concentrations within the pancreas or do not provide an adequate spectrum of antibacterial coverage (i.e., enterococci, streptococci, enteric Gram-negative rods, and Bacteroides). One recent prospective, randomized, controlled trial (PRCT) demonstrated that imipenem (which achieves high concentrations in the pancreas and has broad spectrum of coverage) is beneficial in severe pancreatitis. Thus, many physicians are using "prophylactic" antibiotics (e.g., imipenem or quinolones plus flagyl) in this setting. Similarly, recent PRCTs indicate that selective gut decontamination (SGD) reduced the incidence of pancreatic infections in severe pancreatitis, but SGD is not widely practiced in the United States (11). Pancreatic infections account for > 80% of the late deaths and early débridement is presumed to be beneficial. CT scanning remains the best method to identify suspected pancreatic infections. The classic findings of air bubbles in a peripancreatic fluid collection are diagnostic. Percutaneous aspiration of fluid collection for Gram staining culture is a sensitive method for confirming peripancreatic infections. Another late complication of acute pancreatitis is a development of pancreatic pseudocyst. This is a localized collection of pancreatic juice enclosed within a wall of fibrous or granulation tissue. Infected pseudocysts that cause sepsis in the ICU require external drainage. Percutaneous drainage may be appropriate for simple cysts containing thin fluid; laparotomy should be performed for septated collections which contain necrotic matter.

BILIARY TRACT DISEASE ENCOUNTERED IN ICU PATIENTS

Acute Cholecystitis. The vast majority of cases of acute cholecystitis are caused by gallstones. Cystic duct occlusion by an impacted stone initiates a chemical inflammatory process. As time progresses, secondary bacterial invasion of the inflamed obstructed gallbladder occurs in 50% of the cases (aerobic enteric organisms in 90%). If obstruction persists, severe disease (patchy gangrene, pericholecystic abscess, and empyema) develops. Acalculous cholecystitis is a condition that is classically encountered in critically ill ICU patients. Risk factors include elderly males with atheromatous vascular disease, diabetes, prolonged ileus, opiate administration, intravenous hyperalimentation (lack of enteral stimulation), multiple blood transfusions, and sepsis. The exact pathophysiology remains unknown, but the available data indicate that inflammation develops as a consequence of prolonged distention of the gallbladder, bile stasis, inspissation with sludge which results in mucosal injury, and thrombosis of blood vessels in the submuscular layer of the gallbladder. The inflammation is predominantly chemical (culture of aspirated gallbladder bile from these patients is positive in only 40% of the cases). When fully developed, the gallbladder shows marked edema of the seromuscular layer, mucosal ulceration, and focal necrosis. Gangrene is encountered in 25% of the cases. Acute emphysematous cholecystitis is another rare entity seen in ICU patients. This fulminant disease is caused by a mixed polymicrobial infection that includes gas-forming bacteria. The gallbladder may or may not contain any stones. The disease occurs predominantly in males and has a predilection for diabetic individuals. The presence of air within the gallbladder lumen, its wall, or the biliary tract on plain radiograph of the abdomen is characteristic.

The clinical picture of acute cholecystitis in most patients is readily recognizable (i.e., right upper quadrant pain and tenderness, fever, leukocytosis) and can be reliably confirmed by ultrasonography or scintigraphy examination. The number of false-positive results with scintigraphy (i.e., HIDA scan) can be reduced by administering intravenous morphine before the procedure. This opiate causes spasm of the sphincter of Oddi and thereby induces reflux of bile into the gallbladder if the cystic duct is patent. On the other hand, acute cholecystitis (especially acalculous) can be difficult to diagnose in the seriously ill ICU patient who is receiving narcotics and artificial ventilation. Awareness of this potential diagnosis is needed so that appropriate diagnostic investigations can be obtained to avoid missing this life-threatening complication. The diagnostic methods used include CT, ultrasonography, and scintigraphy. Ultrasonographic and CT findings indicative of acute acalculous cholecystitis include gallbladder wall thickness > 4 mm, pericholecystic fluid or subserosal edema with ascites, intramural gas, and sloughing of the mucosal membrane.

Initial treatment of acute cholecystitis includes nasogastric suction, intravenous fluid resuscitation, and broad-spectrum antibiotics. For patients who have either severe disease or significant comorbid disease (typical ICU patient), emergency surgical intervention is indicated for patients with established peritonitis (12). Urgent intervention is recommended for the following reasons: a) progression of the disease despite conservative management; b) failure to improve within 24 hours; c) presence of an inflammatory mass in the right hypochondrium; and d) detection of gas in the gallbladder or the biliary tree. Percutaneous cholecystostomy is a reasonable alternative for patients who are too ill to undergo an operation (13).

Acute Cholangitis. Cholangitis is caused by obstruction of the bile ducts. The resulting stasis promotes the development of infection. The most common cause is common bile duct stones. However, in patients who have undergone previous biliary operations, bile duct strictures are an equally frequent cause. Charcot triad (fever, jaundice, and right quadrant pain) should prompt the diagnosis of cholangitis. The additional findings of shock and mental confusion when added to the triad (the Reynold's pentad) suggests the presence of suppurative cholangitis, which may require more aggressive interventions. Laboratory values will reflect the existence of biliary obstruction (elevated bilirubin and alkaline phosphatase) and infection (increased leukocyte count and positive blood cultures).

Ultrasonography is a noninvasive modality that can be helpful in confirming the diagnosis of cholangitis (dilated bile ducts and stones). When the biliary tree is not dilated, ultrasonography may not detect common bile duct stones. Obstruction may be present without dilation in 60% to 70% of patients, especially in the early phases of disease. In diagnosing obstruction, scintigraphy has greater sensitivity than ultrasonography. MRI is sensitive in identifying small stones in the distal bile duct. Endoscopic retrograde cholangiopancreatography (ERCP) is another diagnostic modality that offers the possibility of therapeutic intervention.

Patients with clinical signs and laboratory findings consistent with cholangitis should undergo immediate fluid resuscitation and receive broad-spectrum antibiotics (to cover enterococcus, Gram-negative rods, and anaerobes). Most patients (up to 85%) respond to this treatment. However, for patients whose condition does not improve (i.e., "refractory cholangitis"), urgent biliary decompression is required. The 3 options include: a) surgical decompression; b) percutaneous transhepatic cholangiography (PTC); and c) ERCP. With increasing experience, endoscopists have shown that they are successful in decompressing the duct in 90% to 100% of patients with the use of biliary stents or limited sphincterotomy (14, 15). This method has become the preferred initial approach. For the patients in whom ERCP is not feasible or in whom the clinical condition continues to worsen, PTC or surgical decompression should be done. Both approaches are associated with complications. PTC may cause bleeding, bile leak, or exacerbation of sepsis, while surgical decompression is associated with a high mortality rate.

Gallstone Pancreatitis. The pathogenesis of gallstone pancreatitis is still debated. There are 2 conflicting theories. One theory is that the passage of a stone causes reflux of bile and the duodenal contents into the pancreatic duct. The other theory is that the migrating stone obstructs the pancreatic duct.

Regardless of whether reflux versus obstruction is the initiating event of pancreatic inflammation, in most patients, gallstone pancreatitis is a self-limiting disease that resolves after the stone passes into the duodenum. These patients deserve a definitive procedure, which in most cases would be a semielective cholecystectomy (high-surgical risk patients can be treated by ERCP sphincterotomy) (13). For patients whose stone does not pass, pancreatitis can become a severe life-threatening process. Surgical intervention of severe pancreatitis should be considered dangerous. ERCP management has emerged as a superior method (16, 17). The optimal time to intervene is controversial. Patients who fail conservative management and have hyperbilirubinemia should be considered candidates for urgent ERCP.

HOLLOW VISCUS ENTITIES THAT CAN CAUSE AN ACUTE ABDOMEN IN ICU PATIENTS

Perforated Duodenal Ulcer (DU). Perforated DU presents clinically as sudden onset of epigastric pain which radiates to the right scapula. Lower abdominal pain may also be present. Pain intensity peaks rapidly and does not typically diminish. This pain is caused by spillage of noxious gastric contents. The initial chemical peritonitis converts over 12 to 24 hours into bacterial peritonitis. Physical examination typically shows a rigid abdomen with peritoneal signs. Pneumoperitoneum is found commonly on upright abdominal radiographs, but may be absent in 20%.

Treatment of perforated DU begins with fluid resuscitation and correction of electrolyte abnormalities. Nasogastric suction is instituted routinely and broad-spectrum antibiotic therapy is begun. Nonoperative management is controversial. While morbidity and mortality may not be significantly worse, hospitalization time is longer with conservative therapy. Additionally, elderly patients are more likely to fail conservative management. Consequently, most surgeons would recommend early operation. With the improvement in medical therapy for peptic ulcer disease, the standard operation includes debridement and omental

patch closure. Definitive antiulcer operations should be reserved for patients who are stable and have a previous history of peptic ulcer disease.

Small Bowel Obstruction. History (crampy abdominal pain, emesis, distention, and opstipation) and physical examination (distention, hyperactive or hypoactive bowel sounds, tenderness) would prompt this diagnosis. Plain abdominal radiographs should be performed to further aid with the diagnosis. The classic findings are distended small bowel with air-fluid levels and absent air distal to the obstruction. Upper gastrointestinal (GI) study with thin barium may be diagnostic. A barium enema may be very useful in identifying a distal small bowel site of obstruction or in differentiating small bowel from proximal colon obstruction. The role of CT is still evolving. CT can locate the level of obstruction with a high degree of accuracy. CT scans can also help determine the causes of obstruction, including an abscess (that could be drained percutaneously), malignancy, or inflammatory bowel disease. Additional findings, such as free air or pneumatosis intestinalis, may prompt an earlier operation.

Patients who present with intestinal obstruction can have multiple electrolyte abnormalities. The more proximal the obstruction, the more nausea and vomiting the patient will have. A hypochloremic hypokalemic alkalosis is the most common derangement. Other laboratory abnormalities include contraction alkalosis, hemoconcentration, and prerenal azotemia. Electrolyte abnormalities should be corrected quickly with judicious use of isotonic fluids in anticipation of possible surgery. All patients who have a bowel obstruction should have a nasogastric tube placed. These tubes can decompress the stomach and remove gastric contents. This procedure will usually make the patient feel better and it decreases the risk of aspiration. The use of long intestinal tubes do not offer any benefit over conventional nasogastric tubes. Prompt operation is indicated in patients who present with the following conditions: a) closed loop obstruction (persistent pain, localized tenderness, and a single loop of small bowel on radiographs); b) incarcerated hernia; and c) complete bowel obstruction. Differentiating complete from partial bowel obstruction may be difficult, and an upper GI series is helpful. A trial of nonoperative therapy can be considered for patients with a partial bowel obstruction. A delay in surgical intervention in patients with complete bowel obstruction can lead to an increased incidence of bowel necrosis and mortality. There are no accurate preoperative signs to diagnose bowel necrosis. The 4 concerning signs include fever, tachycardia, localized abdominal tenderness, and leukocytosis.

Mesenteric Ischemia. Mesenteric ischemia is difficult to diagnose early because signs and symptoms are nonspecific until the condition is far advanced, at which point therapeutic intervention is frequently not successful. Mesenteric ischemia can occur as a result of: a) arterial occlusion (secondary either to an embolism or thrombosis); b) nonocclusive bowel ischemia (NOBI); or c) mesenteric venous thrombosis. Arterial embolism occurs in patients with underlying cause for embolism (75% originate in the heart), while arterial thrombosis in patients with preexisting mesenteric vascular lesions (prodromal syndromes of chronic ischemia are present in 50% of the patients) and a precipitating event, such as hypovolemia or hypoperfusion, are common. Successful management requires a high degree of suspicion. Nearly all patients will require fluid resuscitation. While fluid resuscitation is being accomplished, diagnostic studies should be conducted. All patients with peritonitis require early laparotomy. For patients without peritonitis, angiography is a first good study. If arterial occlusion is demonstrated, the patient can be taken to the operating room for attempted correction with an accurate road map and knowledge of the collateral circulation. If incomplete arterial occlusion is demonstrated, then consideration should be given to thrombolytic therapy.

NOBI generally occurs in patients who are ill for other reasons (such as myocardial infarction, major trauma, pancreatitis), are receiving drugs that decrease mesenteric perfusion (such as digitalis, vasopressors, and cocaine), and/or are receiving enteral nutrition (18). The onset of signs and symptoms of NOBI

is often more gradual than with arterial occlusion. The typical patient presents with systemic signs of bacterial sepsis associated with abdominal distention/tenderness and intolerance to enteral nutrition. Enteral nutrition and vasoconstrictors should be stopped. Resuscitation should be started to ensure good mesenteric perfusion. Abdominal plain films should be obtained. If these films cause concern but are not diagnostic, an abdominal CT scan should be obtained. NOBI is characterized by thickened distended bowel with pneumatosis intestinalis. These patients should be given broad-spectrum antibiotics. Urgent laparotomy is indicated for peritonitis and unremitting systemic sepsis. In patients with systemic causes for low mesenteric perfusion (e.g., congestive heart failure [CHF], vasoconstrictor therapy, recent cardiopulmonary bypass), angiography can be both diagnostic and therapeutic. The mesenteric vasoconstriction can be treated with selective intra-arterial infusion of a splanchnic vasodilator, such as papaverine.

Mesenteric venous thrombosis is even of more gradual onset and is very difficult to diagnose. Symptoms may develop over a period of days. The diagnosis is suspected on the basis of massive fluid losses and the presence of an underlying condition, such as CHF, polycythemia, sickle cell disease, carcinomatosis, and a variety of hypercoagulable conditions (e.g., deficiencies in antithrombin III, protein C, and protein S). If venous thrombosis is initially suspected, CT scan can often make the diagnosis. The diagnosis can also be confirmed by observing the venous phase of a mesenteric angiogram. Initial treatment is anticoagulation. Surgery is reserved for resection of dead bowel (venous thrombectomy is rarely successful).

A specific cause of colon ischemia is ligation of the inferior mesenteric artery during aortic surgery. In general, the initial management is as described above, with the exception that early protosigmoidoscopy should be done. Patients with disease limited to the mucosa (i.e., edematous mucosa with petechial hemorrhage and punctate ulcers) sometimes recover without surgery, but late strictures may occur. Laparotomy is indicated when there is evidence of sepsis or peritonitis.

Missed Hollow Viscus Injury Following Blunt Abdominal Trauma. As the traditional indications for nonoperative management of liver and spleen injuries have been liberalized, the issue of delayed diagnosis of hollow viscus injuries (HVIs) has emerged as an important topic for ICU practitioners (17). Blunt HVI is uncommon, occurring in ~ 1% of admitted patients. Early diagnosis can be difficult. Initial physical examination is often unreliable and findings, such as a "seat belt" sign (i.e., abdominal wall ecchymosis) or lumbar vertebral fractures, are not very sensitive. In most institutions, contrast enhanced CT scanning has replaced diagnostic peritoneal lavage, as in the initial modality to evaluate blunt abdominal trauma (BAT). Unfortunately, extravasation of contrast material from the perforated bowel during CT scanning is rarely seen, and other diagnostic signs of HVI (e.g., unexplained fluid, mesenteric streaking, abnormal small bowel morphology, and pneumoperitoneum) have uncertain sensitivities and specificities (18). Ultrasound is being used with increasing frequency in the initial evaluation of BAT, but even the most enthusiastic ultrasonographer acknowledges that this diagnostic modality will miss HVI. The clinical consequences of delayed diagnosis of HVI is another area of contention. Recent series in children have reported that diagnostic delay does not affect outcome. This has not been the experience in adults. Delayed diagnosis is associated with increased abdominal septic complications (especially duodenal perforations). Diagnostic delays can be minimized by diligent review of the initial CT scan, careful serial physical examinations, and liberal use of follow-up studies (e.g., c-loop contrast studies or repeat CT scans) in high-risk patients.

Large Bowel Obstruction. The 3 primary causes of large bowel obstruction are: a) carcinoma; b) diverticulitis; and c) volvulus. About 20% of colorectal cancer patients present with partial or complete obstruction. Presenting complaints include crampy abdominal pain, distention, and obstipation. Plain abdominal films are used to confirm the diagnosis and to possibly delineate the site of obstruction. Half of the patients have a competent ileocecal valve and are at risk to develop severe cecal distention

(i.e., > 12 cm) and perforation. Contrast enemas (use water soluble contrast if perforation is suspected) are useful to confirm the diagnosis as well as to determine the level and degree of obstruction. Sigmoidoscopy should be part of the early assessment of patients with suspected large bowel obstruction to exclude rectal cancer, stricture, or an inflammatory process, and it may be therapeutic in the case of sigmoid volvulus. Patients with perforation or complete obstruction should be resuscitated, given broad-spectrum antibiotics, and taken urgently to the operating room. Patients with partial obstruction may benefit by having gentle bowel prep and a colonoscopy prior to laparotomy.

Volvulus of the colon is a rare form of bowel obstruction where the patient typically presents with subacute symptoms and a history of previous "attacks." Volvulus is caused by an axial twist or folding of the bowel upon its mesentery. Successful management depends on early recognition and correct identification of the site (sigmoid in 50% to 70%; cecal in 20% to 30%; transverse and splenic flexure portions are rare). Plain abdominal films may provide useful information concerning the site in 50% of cases.

The classic radiographic finding of sigmoid volvulus includes a greatly dilated loop of colon lying in the right upper quadrant, with convergence of the loop directed toward the left lower quadrant. In equivocal cases, barium enema may be useful. Patients with clinical signs of colon necrosis or perforation should undergo urgent laparotomy. The remaining patients should undergo therapeutic endoscopy (rigid or flexible) to decompress the colon, which has a success rate of 80% to 90%. Nonoperative detorsion of sigmoid volvulus spares the patient an emergency operation, but recurrent volvulus is common; therefore, elective sigmoid resection is indicated.

Radiologic evidence of cecal volvulus is less characteristic (i.e., large featureless air collection in the left upper quadrant along with signs of small bowel obstruction), and up to 50% of the cases may initially be missed by the radiologist. In most cases, barium enema can reliably confirm the diagnosis. Endoscopic decompression is less successful than with sigmoid volvulus, and its use depends on the availability of an experienced endoscopist. As a result, management of cecal volvulus has remained largely surgical. The appropriate operative management when the detorsed cecum is viable is controversial. The argument is centered around the question balancing the risk of infectious morbidity with resection versus the risk of recurrence with cecopexy.

Ogilvie's syndrome (i.e., pseudo-obstruction of the colon) is an important entity to consider when entertaining the diagnosis of large bowel obstruction. It is associated with a variety of medical conditions, some of which are common in ICU patients (e.g., major nonabdominal operations or infections, hip fractures, electrolyte abnormalities, narcotics). The clinical presentation is abdominal distention with minimal tenderness. SIRS is unusual unless it is present from a secondary source (e.g., urinary tract infection or pneumonia). The pathogenesis is not clearly understood and is believed to be multifactorial. Plain radiographic films are generally diagnostic showing massive dilation of the colon. Other etiologies of mechanical large bowel obstruction may need to be excluded by contrast enema and/or endoscopy. Patients should be treated with nasogastric suction, correction of fluid and electrolytes, possible pharmacologic causes should be addressed, underlying infections should be diagnosed and treated. Serial examinations and daily abdominal films should be performed. If the cecum remains > 12 cm, colonoscopy should be performed (success rate 80% to 90%; recurrence rate 10% to 40%). Surgery should be reserved for clinical suspicion of impending perforation. If perforation is found, ileocecal resection with ileostomy and mucous fistula should be performed. If no perforation is found, tube cecostomy is preferred to formal cecostomy.

Diverticulitis. The clinical presentation can vary from a picture that looks like left-sided appendicitis to free perforation with diffuse peritonitis. Medical management should be started based on clinical diagnosis. Therapy consists of complete bowel rest, nasogastric decompression to relieve symptoms of obstruction, administration of broad-spectrum antibiotics, and volume resuscitation. Abdominal CT scan is the preferred method to confirm the diagnosis in critically ill patients.

CT reliably detects the location of the inflammation and provides valuable accessory information, such as the presence of an abscess, ureteral obstruction, or a fistula between the colon and the urinary bladder. The CT scan can also diagnose other causes of abdominal symptoms (e.g., ovarian abscess, a leaking abdominal aortic aneurysm). If a localized abscess exists, percutaneous drainage should be considered. This draining often allows the acute inflammatory process to resolve with antibiotics. The patient can then have a definitive, 1-stage resection with primary anastomosis done in a delayed fashion. If the abscess is low in the pelvis and cannot be approached safely through the abdominal wall, the transanal approach can be done, using ultrasound guidance. For acute free perforation, the patient requires urgent laparotomy. The goal is to remove the perforated segment and not attempt an anastomosis. The presence of a fistula to the bladder or vagina (usually in a woman who has had a hysterectomy) is seldom a cause for urgent surgical intervention. Bowel rest, intensive antibiotics, and TPN should be utilized until the acute inflammation resolves.

SUGGESTED READINGS

1. Polk HC, Shields CL: Remote organ failure: A valid sign of occult intra-abdominal infection. *Surgery* 1977; 81:310–313
   Early report of 6 patients who developed progressive organ failure; all had an intra-abdominal infection. Concluded that support of organ function without definitive drainage of intra-abdominal infections is only palliative.
2. Fisher RL: Gastrointestinal emergencies. *Crit Care Clin* 1995; 11:255–567
   Seven of the 14 chapters in this issue discuss topics pertinent to this lecture (i.e., abdomen as source of sepsis, biliary tract emergencies, medical management of pancreatitis, surgical management of pancreatitis, acute mesenteric ischemia, emergencies of inflammatory bowel disease, gastrointestinal emergencies in patients with acquired immunodeficiency syndrome).

3. Rege RV: Unusual aspects of gastrointestinal perforations. *Probl Gen Surg* 1985; 2:377–394
Reviews common and uncommon causes of gastrointestinal perforations.

4. Wittman DH, Syrrakos B, Wittman MM: Advances in the diagnosis and treatment of intra-abdominal infection. *Probl Gen Surg* 1993; 10:604–627
Comprehensive review of intra-abdominal infections.

5. McCarroll KA: Imaging in the intensive care unit. *Crit Care Clin* 1994; 10:247–459
Six of the 11 chapters in this issue discuss topics pertinent to this lecture (i.e., plain abdominal films, abdominal ultrasound, abdominal computed tomography scans, 2 chapters on nuclear medicine studies).

6. Norwood SH, Civetta JM: Abdominal CT scanning in critically ill surgical patients. *Ann Surg* 1985; 202:166–175
In this often-cited study, computed tomography scan was not positive for abscess prior to postoperative day 8, and only 55% of the examinations aided in or altered the diagnosis and < 30% altered management.

7. Richardson JD, Flint LM, Polk HC: Peritoneal lavage: A useful diagnostic adjunct for peritonitis. *Surgery* 1983; 94:826–829
Often-cited reference for the use of diagnostic peritoneal lavage in nontrauma patients. A total of 138 DPLs were performed, 77 had abnormal results of which 73 underwent laparotomy (65 necessary, 8 unnecessary). Of the 61 negative DPLs, 10 patients ultimately underwent laparotomy (4 necessary, 10 unnecessary).

8. Kalfarentzos F, Kehagias J, Mead N, et al: Enteral nutrition is superior to parenteral nutrition in severe acute pancreatitis: Results of a randomized, prospective trial. *Br J Surg* 1997; 84:1665–1669
Thirty-eight patients with acute severe pancreatitis were randomized to enteral nutrition (n = 18) or total parenteral nutrition (n = 20). Enteral nutrition was well tolerated. Patients receiving enteral nutrition had significantly fewer total complications and septic complications. Total parenteral nutrition was 3 times more expensive than enteral nutrition.

9. Golub R, Siddiqi F, Pohl D, et al: Role of antibiotics in acute pancreatitis: A meta-analysis. *J Gastrointest Surg* 1998; 2:496–503
A MEDLINE SEARCH identified 8 prospective, randomized, controlled trials. These trials were scored on a 10-point scale for quality, and the average study score was 7.5. Only 1 study showed a significant decrease in the mortality rate with the use of antibiotics. Three early trials using ampicillin showed no change in outcomes. Four later studies enrolled sicker patients and used antibiotics with a broader spectrum. A significant benefit in favor of antibiotics was found in these studies. These studies favored imipenem or a fluoroquinolone, which achieves excellent pancreatic tissue penetration. Conclusions: Patients with severe pancreatitis should receive prophylactic antibiotics.

10. Barie PS: A critical review of antibiotic prophylaxis in severe acute pancreatitis. *Am J Surg* 1996; 170:38S–43S
This is a nice review of a controversial topic. It outlines the clinical problem, basic laboratory studies, human pharmacology, the human prophylaxis trials using intravenous antibiotics and selective gut decontamination. It concludes that justification exists for the use of antibiotic prophylaxis in severe acute pancreatitis, but the data are insufficiently strong to mandate prophylaxis or to elevate it to the standard of care. Although its importance is unproven, it would make sense to choose an antibiotic regimen that achieves bactericidal concentrations in pancreatic tissue against most likely pathogens. Available data suggest that the combination of a fluoroquinolone plus metronidazole, or monotherapy with a carbapenem antibiotic, would be appropriate choices.

11. Luiten EJ, Hop C, Lange JF, et al: Differential diagnosis of Gram-negative versus Gram-positive infected and sterile pancreatic necrosis: Results of a randomized trial in patients with severe acute

pancreatitis treated with adjuvant selective decontamination. *Clin Infect Dis* 1997; 25:811–816

Patients who had severe acute pancreatitis without evidence for infected necrosis were randomly assigned to receive either selective gut decontamination (SGD) (n = 50) or standard therapy (n = 52). SGD consisted of: a) colistin sulfate, amphotericin, and norfloxacin as a sticky paste administered to the gums and as a rectal enema; and b) a short course of cefotaxime sodium until Gram-negative bacteria were eliminated from the oral cavity and rectum. Results: Infected necrosis occurred in 9 SGD patients (18%) and 20 control patients (37%, p = .03); the differences were related to a decrease in Gram-negative infections (SGD, 4; controls, 17). Compared with patients with sterile necrosis, the mortality rate was 1.6 times higher in patients with Gram-positive necrosis, 14.4 times higher in patients with Gram-negative necrosis, and 15.8 times higher in patients with mixed infection.

12. Lo C-M, Liu C-L, Fan S-T, et al: Prospective randomized study of early versus delayed laparoscopic cholecystectomy for acute cholecystitis. *Ann Surg* 1998; 227:461–467

Patients with a clinical diagnosis of acute cholecystitis were randomly assigned to early laparoscopic cholecystectomy within 72 hours of admission (early group, n = 45) or delayed interval surgery after initial medical treatment (delayed group, n = 41). Results: Eight of 41 patients in the delayed group underwent urgent operation (median 63 hours) because of spreading peritonitis (n = 3) and persistent fever (n = 5). Although the delayed group required less frequent modifications in operative technique and a short operative time, there was a tendency toward a higher conversion rate (23% versus 11%; p = .174) and complication rate (29% versus 13%, p = .07). For 38 patients with symptoms > 72 hours before admission, the conversion rate remained high after delayed surgery (30% versus 17%; p = .454). In addition, delayed laparoscopic cholecystectomy prolonged the total hospital stay (11 versus 6 days; p < .001) and recuperation period (19 versus 12 days; p < .001).

13. Sugiyama M, Tokuhara M, Atemi Y, et al: Is percutaneous cholecystectomy the optimal treatment for acute cholecystitis in the very elderly? *World J Surg* 1998; 22:459–463

Thirty-eight consecutive elderly patients (age > 80 years) with acute cholecystitis underwent urgent transhepatic percutaneous cholecystostomy (performed within 24 hours of admission in 31 patients and within 48 hours in 7 patients). Results: Percutaneous cholecystostomy was performed successfully in all patients, and there were no procedural-related complications. Prompt clinical improvement was achieved in 95% of patients. One patient required emergent cholecystectomy for persistent peritonitis, and 1 patient died from multiple organ dysfunction with terminal gastric carcinoma. Ten patients with cholelithiasis underwent successful elective cholecystectomy. Two patients underwent successful percutaneous cholecystolithotomy and have had no recurrent symptoms. Of 24 patients with calculous disease, 12 had the catheter removed without gallbladder or stone removal. Eight of these patients remained asymptomatic, but recurrent cholecystitis developed in 4 patients.

14. Suc B, Escat J, Cherqui D, et al: Surgery versus endoscopy as primary treatment in symptomatic patients with suspected common bile duct stones: A multicenter randomized trial. *Arch Surg* 1988; 133:702–708

In this prospective multicenter trial, patients with at least 1 of the following symptoms: jaundice, mild pancreatitis, mild cholangitis, increased alkaline phosphatase levels, or common duct stones or dilations on ultrasound were randomized to surgical treatment (ST) (n = 105), which consisted of cholecystectomy with cholangiogram and/or choledochotomy or endoscopic management (EM) (n = 97) consisted of ERCP with sphincterotomy and stone extraction (early cholecystectomy was mandatory if cholangitis or cholecystitis developed; otherwise, the necessity and timing of cholecystectomy were determined by the surgeon). All ST patients underwent operation, while EM was technically impossible in 6 cases. There were 3 deaths after EM (3%) and 1 after ST (1%). The difference was not statistically significant. The morbidity rate was 11% for both groups. Major complications were significantly more common after EM (13%) than after ST (4%). Minor complications were significantly more common after ST (7%) than after EM (0%). Retained stones were significantly more frequent after EM (20%) than after ST (6%). Additional procedures (after initial ST or EM) were required in 8% of ST patients and 29% of EM patients (p < .001).

15. Lai ECS, Mok FPT, Tan ESY, et al: Endoscopic biliary drainage for severe acute cholangitis. *N Eng J Med* 1992; 326:1582–1586
Eighty-two patients with severe acute cholangitis due to choledocholithiasis were assigned randomly to undergo surgical decompression of the biliary tract (41 patients) or endoscopic biliary drainage (41 patients), followed by definitive treatment. Results: Complications related to biliary tract decompression and subsequent definitive treatment developed in 14 patients treated with endoscopic biliary drainage and 27 treated with surgery (34% versus 66%, p > .05). The hospital mortality rate was significantly lower for the patients who underwent endoscopy (4 deaths) than for those treated surgically (13 deaths) (10% versus 32%, p < .03).

16. Fan S-TF, Lai ECS, Mok, FPT, et al: Early treatment of acute biliary pancreatitis by endoscopic papillotomy. *N Engl J Med* 1993; 328:228–232
Patients with acute biliary pancreatitis who were assigned randomly to 1 of 2 groups: 97 patients underwent within 24 hours after admission emergency endoscopic retrograde cholangiopancreatography (ERCP) followed by endoscopic papillotomy for ampullary and common bile duct stones, and 98 patients received initial conservative treatment and selective ERCP with or without endoscopic papillotomy only if their

condition deteriorated. Results: Emergency ERCP with or without endoscopic papillotomy resulted in a reduction in biliary sepsis as compared with conservative treatment (0 of 97 patients versus 12 of 98 patients, p = .001). There were no major differences in the incidence of local complications (10 patients in the group who received emergency ERCP versus 12 patients in the conservative-treatment group) or systemic complications (10 patients versus 14 patients) of acute pancreatitis between the 2 groups.

17. Siegel JH, Veerappan A, Cohen SA, et al: Endoscopic sphincterotomy for biliary pancreatitis: An alternative to cholecystectomy in high risk patients. *Gastrointest Endosc* 1994; 40:573–575
Prophylactic sphincterotomy was performed in 49 patients who presented with biliary pancreatitis more than once. The majority (39 patients) were treated electively after resolution of pancreatitis, while the remainder (10 patients) were treated urgently during their index admission because of continuing symptoms. No patient experienced recurrent pancreatitis over a mean follow-up period of 48 months. No mortality occurred and no significant morbidity was experienced.

18. Marvin RG, McKinley VA, McQuiggan M, et al: Nonocclusive bowel necrosis which occurs in critically ill trauma patients receiving enteral nutrition manifests no reliable clinical signs for early detection. *Am J Surg*, In Press
Review of 13 cases of nonocclusive bowel ischemia that occurred over a 5-year period. The typical presentation is delayed sepsis in a patient who requires high-acuity ICU care. Includes a review of the literature.

19. Allen GS, Moore FA, Cox CS, et al: Hollow visceral injury and blunt trauma. *J Trauma* 1998; 45:69–75
This large retrospective study confirms that an occult hollow viscus injury is a rare entity in both adults and children, but in contrast to smaller published series, delayed diagnosis (especially duodenal ruptures) is associated with increased abdominal septic complications).

20. Sherck J, Shatney C, Sensaki K, et al: The accuracy of computed tomography in the diagnosis of blunt small-bowel perforation. *Am J Surg* 1994; 168:670–675

This study provides the sensitivity and specificity of various computed tomography findings in predicting the presence of a hollow viscus injury (e.g., pneumoperitoneum: 45% sensitivity, 99% specificity; unexplained fluid 73% sensitivity; 98% specificity). Of note, contrast extravasation occurred in only 5 of 26 patients with hollow viscus injuries (sensitivities = 19%, specificity = 100%).

TRAUMA AND THERMAL INJURY

David J. Dries, MSE, MD, FCCP, FCCM

Objectives

- To identify the multisystem manifestations of trauma
- To recognize common patterns of presentation for cardiopulmonary injury
- To recognize evolving management of secondary brain injury
- To identify patients at high risk for venous thromboembolism following injury
- To recognize burn injury of various degrees and associated treatment options
- To assess and manage inhalation injury
- To review the latest available data regarding the outcome of burn injury

Key Words: Hemothorax; pneumothorax; secondary brain injury; venous thromboembolism; blunt cardiac injury; inhalation injury; duplex ultrasonography; low-molecular-weight heparin

TABLE OF ABBREVIATIONS

ATP   adenosine triphosphate
CPP   cerebral perfusion pressure
CSF   cerebrospinal fluid
CT   computed tomography
EAST Eastern Association for the Surgery of Trauma
ECG   electrocardiogram
GCS   Glasgow Coma Scale
ICP   intracranial pressure
MRI   magnetic resonance imaging
TBSA total body surface area

TRAUMA

Principal decision-making in the management of multiple organ injury rests with the trauma surgeon. The intensivist, however, is a critical component of the management team, particularly in the setting of blunt injury with multiple system dysfunction and less need for acute operative intervention. Certain types of injury have implications for all members of the trauma care team, both emergency department management and critical care support. All team members should, therefore, be able to identify and act immediately upon identification of injury and complications of initial treatment. The international process for injury identification and treatment is discussed in the *Advanced Trauma Life Support Course* published by the American College of Surgeons Committee on Trauma.

This chapter reviews recent developments and discusses common patterns of injury or complications of injury according to organ system.

Airway and Cervical Spine

The initial priority in the management of any injured patient is assessment and management of the airway. At the same time, care is taken to prevent movement of the cervical spine. All patients with blunt trauma are at risk for cervical spine injury. Patients with unknown cervical spine status and need of emergency airway control may be intubated safely by temporary removal of the immobilizing cervical collar, while in-line stabilization is maintained during intubation. After securing the airway, the collar is reapplied and the patient remains on log roll precautions until the complete spine status has been assessed. The choice of nasotracheal versus orotracheal intubation technique is based on provider preference and experience. Nasotracheal intubation, however, requires spontaneous respiration. In addition, no tubes should be passed through the nose of a patient who has midfacial trauma with a risk of cribriform plate fracture. When other means of airway control have failed, a surgical airway may be required.

Neurologic examination alone does not exclude a cervical spine injury. The integrity of the bony components of the cervical spine may be assessed in various ways. A variety of plain radiographs, computed tomography (CT) scans, or magnetic resonance imaging (MRI) scans may be obtained. The following patients are excluded from examination: a) those who cannot relate neurologic examination changes; b) those who are unresponsive due to either primary injury or the effects of pain medication; and c) those who receive muscle relaxants. Thus, recommendations were developed to determine the presence or absence of cervical spine instability.

The following recommendations were made for patients at risk for cervical spine injury:

- Patients who are alert, awake, and without mental status changes and neck pain and who have no distracting injuries or neurologic deficits may be considered to have a stable cervical spine and need no radiologic studies.

- All other patients should have at least a lateral view of the cervical spine, including the base of the occiput to the upper border of the first thoracic vertebra; and anteroposterior view showing the spinous processes of the second cervical through the first thoracic vertebra; and an open mouth odontoid view indicating lateral masses of the first cervical vertebra and the entire odontoid process. Axial CT scans with sagittal reconstruction may be obtained for any questionable level of injury or any area which cannot be adequately visualized on plain radiographs.

- Flexion and extension views of the cervical spine may be appropriate in patients complaining of significant neck pain with normal, plain radiograph results.

- Patients with neurologic deficits which may refer to a cervical spine injury require subspecialty consultation and MRI evaluation.

- Patients with an altered level of consciousness secondary to traumatic brain injury or other causes may be considered to

have a stable cervical spine if adequate 3-view plain radiographs and thin-cut axial CT images through C1 and C2 are normal.

- Most recent work suggests that CT scans may facilitate evaluation of C_1 to the top of C_3 in any head-injured or intubated patient. More and more centers are adding CT scans of the upper cervical spine when scans of the head are obtained after injury.

Cervical spine injury following blunt trauma reportedly occurs at a frequency of 4 to 6%. In the literature of cervical spine injury, there is little supporting evidence that defines the criteria for determining who gets cervical spine radiographs and who does not. Long-term follow-up to identify all cases of cervical spine injury missed in the acute setting is frequently unavailable. The true incidence of cervical spine injury is thus not known. The 3-view plain spine series (anteroposterior, lateral, and open-mouth odontoid view), supplemented by thin-cut axial CT imaging with sagittal reconstruction through suspicious areas or in adequately visualized areas, provides a false-negative rate of < 0.1%, if the studies are technically adequate and properly interpreted.

Tracheobronchial Injury

Tracheal or laryngeal disruption or fracture most commonly occurs at the junction of the larynx and the trachea. Signs and symptoms may include hoarseness, subcutaneous air, edema, or crepitus at the neck, but the patient may have minimal evidence of injury. The patient should be allowed to assume the position of comfort; this position may include sitting, if spinal injury is unlikely during the patient's initial assessment. Airway management by an experienced physician may include an awake tracheostomy. Cricothyroidotomy should be avoided.

Injury to the proximal trachea may be caused by blunt or penetrating trauma. Blunt injury to the cervical trachea occurs in < 1% inall patients with blunt trauma to the trunk. Injury to the larynx is the most common blunt injury. A direct blow to the trachea may cause compression or fracture of the cartilaginous ring, hematoma formation, bleeding, or airway obstruction. Injury to the trachea may also occur from the shoulder restraint harness of a seat belt. Proximal tracheal injuries may be caused by gunshot wounds or stab wounds to the neck. Hemoptysis and airway obstruction are signs that indicate the need for urgent access to the airway. Patients with subcutaneous air or dissecting air within the cervical fascia should be suspected for tracheal and/or esophageal injury.

Patients presenting with massive subcutaneous or mediastinal emphysema are suspected to have a distal tracheal or bronchus injury. Hemoptysis, hemopneumothorax, or a collapsed lung on plain chest radiograph confirms injury in the major intrathoracic airways. When chest tubes are placed and there is constant air loss, major airway disruption must be suspected. In this situation, bronchoscopy should be done as soon as possible to exclude a tracheal or large bronchial tear or proximal bronchial obstruction by a foreign body or secretions. Over 80% of traumatic tracheobronchial tears occur within 2.5 cm of the carina; lobar or segmental bronchi are seldom injured. Injury to the distal trachea is associated with severe compression trauma to the chest, particularly when the glottis is closed.

Airway control and ventilation may be difficult in these patients. A double lumen endotracheal tube may be required. Placement of these tubes requires skill and secretion management may be difficult. Surgical repair must be prioritized. If an airway can be established and maintained, other life-threatening problems, such as intra-abdominal hemorrhage, may be addressed. Repair of distal tracheal or bronchial injuries typically requires a thoracotomy. Postoperative management of these patients has several components. Repeat bronchoscopy may be required for secretion control. Mechanical ventilation should be provided to minimize the pressure within the airways. Use of pressure control modes of ventilation may be optimal.

Intrabronchial bleeding, manifest as hemoptysis and air hunger, is poorly tolerated and may lead rapidly to death due to alveolar flooding. Bleeding is typically caused by injury to bronchial arteries or fistulas between pulmonary veins, pulmonary arterial branches, and the bronchus. These patients may rapidly become hypoxic before other evidence of respiratory failure is apparent. In general, these patients should be positioned to facilitate drainage of blood out of the trachea. The uninvolved lung must be free of blood, if possible. Nasotracheal suctioning or bronchoscopy may be necessary to keep the bronchial tree clear and the contralateral lung expanded. For severe bleeding, a double lumen endotracheal tube may be inserted to confine the bleeding and protect the uninvolved lung. Where severe bleeding continues, thoracotomy should be performed with clamping of the involved bronchus at the hilum.

Rib and Pulmonary Parenchymal Injury

Rib fractures are frequently not detected on chest radiographs; the fracture may be documented by tenderness on physical examination. Pain control is essential for assuring adequate spontaneous ventilation. Where multiple adjacent rib segments are fractured, a flail chest may occur. The clinical manifestation of flail chest is paradoxical movement of the involved portion of the chest wall, i.e., inward movement of the segments during inhalation. Frequently, flail chest is associated with contusion of the underlying lung, pain, and hypoxemia. Less common is pneumothorax associated with an open thoracic wound. Open pneumothorax is generally associated with soft tissue deficit requiring dressings or closure and chest tube placement to reexpand the involved lung. Another complication of rib injury is hemothorax. Massive hemothorax is suggested by physical examination and the chest radiograph. Rapid loss of 1000 to 2000 mL of blood or ongoing blood loss of > 200 mL/hr through a chest tube is an indication for thoracotomy. In general, pneumothorax is associated with rib fractures and requires chest tube placement. Suction is applied routinely at approximately 20 cm H_2O. Any patient with a pneumothorax who requires a general anesthetic should have a chest tube in place. Perhaps the most feared complication of rib fracture is tension pneumothorax. Air is under pressure in the pleural space resulting in hemodynamic embarrassment and pulmonary dysfunction. This emergency should not be diagnosed by a chest radiograph. This clinical diagnosis is based on absent breath sounds, respiratory distress, jugular venous distention, and cardiovascular compromise. The trachea may deviate away from the side, requiring tube thoracostomy. Needle catheter placement into the pleural space at the second intercostal level in the midclavicular line may be necessary for urgent decompression of the involved hemithorax.

A common result of rib and chest wall injury is pulmonary contusion. Patients with penetrating trauma may have areas of hemorrhage surrounding a missile tract. The patient sustaining pulmonary contusion from blunt trauma may have a more globular or diffuse pattern of injury. Pulmonary contusion is usually diagnosed on the basis of the history of blunt chest trauma and findings of localized opacification on chest radiographs. The extent of pulmonary contusion is usually underestimated on plain film radiographs. CT scans evaluate and quantify pulmonary contusions. A scan demonstrating a large contusion (> 20%) increases the likelihood of prolonged ventilatory support for acute respiratory failure.

CT may also be useful in confirming the diagnosis of pulmonary contusion. One-third of pulmonary contusions do not manifest on plain radiographs until 12 to 24 hours after injury. More frequently than previously noted, CT scans have also demonstrated traumatic pneumatocele and parenchymal lacerations to the lung. Hypoxia may be the first evidence of severe pulmonary contusion. If the contusion is large enough or is bilateral, a significant decrease in lung compliance may also occur with associated increase in shunt fraction. The overall mortality rate of patients with pulmonary contusion is 15 to 16%. When chest wall injury is associated with this problem, particularly flail chest, the mortality rate approaches 45%.

Treatment is directed primarily at maintaining ventilation and preventing pneumonia. Progressive respiratory therapy to promote deep breathing, coughing, and mobilization is critical. Pain relief is essential for chest wall injuries. To this end, epidural analgesia is superior to intrapleural medication administration or rib blocks. The patient should be euvolemic, not dehydrated. Mechanical ventilation may be required in the hypoxic patient. This therapy may also be necessary in the patient with shock, increased work of breathing, coma, or significant preexisting lung disease.

Injury to Thoracic Aorta

Injury to the thoracic aorta is common among victims of high-speed motor vehicle crashes with an acute deceleration mechanism. Many victims of this injury are dead at the scene. An estimated 20% of the persons who sustain deceleration injury to the thoracic aorta live to reach the hospital due to containment of aortic rupture by connective tissue covering the aorta. Without recognition and treatment of this injury, 30% of these individuals will die within 12 hours, and 50% within 1 week. The mechanism of injury is a combination of differential deceleration of the mediastinal contents and force provided by the steering wheel or dashboard impacting the chest. Falls may also produce this injury. Most often, disruption occurs at the aortic isthmus, just distal to the origin of the left subclavian artery at the ligamentum arteriosum.

The initial anteroposterior chest radiograph is the single most important screening tool for injury to the thoracic aorta. Arteriography is the gold standard diagnostic study because of its ability to demonstrate the specific injury and reveal unsuspected vascular anomalies. Unfortunately, intimal flaps are being reported in up to 10% of studies. Most of these lesions resolve spontaneously and may be managed nonoperatively. In the emergency setting, newer spiral CT scans have become useful at rapidly diagnosing thoracic aortic injuries (particularly to the descending aorta) because of their greater speed and resolution. With a suspicious mechanism of injury, a clear chest radiograph is inadequate to rule out aortic injury. While mediastinal widening warrants aortography, 80% of the time the angiogram does not show injury to the thoracic aorta as the cause of mediastinal widening. Thus, latest generation CT imaging is becoming an acceptable method for evaluation of the widened mediastinum with aortography in cases requiring further definition.

Patients who are unstable at the scene of a crash or during the first 4 hours of hospitalization have a mortality rate of > 90%. Hemodynamically stable patients whose systolic blood pressure does not exceed 120 mm Hg during the first to 6 to 8 hours after injury have a survival rate of > 90%. Of the operative procedures for repairing injuries to the descending aorta, the most dreaded complication is paraplegia. Unfortunately, no one causative or preventative factor has been identified.

Various reports have suggested that operative management of injury to the descending aorta may be delayed in stable patients for a period that can range from hours to months. These individuals should receive an afterload-reducing agent or a drug to alter dP/dT (change in pressure over time), have their blood pressure maintained at or < 120/80 mm Hg, and have a stable mediastinal hematoma. Delayed reconstruction of chronic posttraumatic aneurysm of the descending aorta, using endovascular stented grafts, is also being reported. At this time, expeditious repair of injury to the descending aorta remains the most cost-effective approach with no additional risk of complications in adequately resuscitated patients.

Blunt Cardiac Injury

Cardiac injuries from blunt chest trauma are usually the result of high-speed motor vehicle crashes. Falls from heights, crushing injuries from motor vehicle crashes and falling objects, blast injuries, and direct violent trauma from assault are less common causes of blunt cardiac injury. Blunt trauma to the heart ranges from minor injuries to frank cardiac rupture. Minor injury is a nonspecific condition frequently termed cardiac contusion or myocardial contusion. Moderately severe lesions may include injury to the pericardium, valves, papillary muscles, and coronary vessels. The most severe of blunt cardiac injuries is the dramatic and often fatal condition of cardiac rupture.

The reported incidence of blunt cardiac injury depends on the modality and criteria used for diagnosis. The occurrence rate ranges from 8 to 71% in patients sustaining blunt chest trauma. The true occurrence rate remains unknown, as there is no diagnostic gold standard. The lack of such a standard leads to confusion with respect to making the diagnosis, thereby making the available literature difficult to interpret. Key issues involve identification of a patient population at risk for adverse events from blunt cardiac injury and then appropriately monitoring and treating these individuals. Conversely, patients who are not at risk for complications could be discharged from the hospital with appropriate follow-up.

The Eastern Association for the Surgery of Trauma (EAST) has recently reviewed studies that focused on the identification of blunt cardiac injury. Based on randomized, prospective data, they recommended that an admission electrocardiogram (ECG) should be performed in all patients in whom blunt cardiac injury was suspected. Additional recommendations included continuous ECG monitoring for 24 to 48 hours in patients where the initial ECG was abnormal. Similarly, if patients are hemodynamically unstable, evaluation should proceed with transthoracic echocardiography followed by transesophageal echocardiography, if an optimal study cannot be obtained. Finally, patients with coexisting cardiac disease and those with an abnormal admission ECG may undergo surgery if they are appropriately monitored. These individuals may require placement of a pulmonary artery catheter. The presence of sternal fracture does not predict the presence of blunt cardiac injury. To date, enzyme analysis is inadequate to identify patients with blunt cardiac injury.

Traumatic Brain Injury

Traumatic brain injury accounts for 40% of all deaths from acute injuries. It is the single most important factor in determining the outcome of various forms of trauma. Two hundred thousand victims with such injuries require hospitalization each year and often are permanently disabled. Many more persons suffer mild traumatic brain injury resulting in a physician visit or temporary disability. Individuals at greatest risk for traumatic brain injury are typically young and at the beginning of a potentially productive life. Thus, loss of potential income, cost of acute care, and continued expenses of rehabilitation and medical care are enormous. These realities mandate aggressive attention to the management of brain injury. Clinical factors associated with poorer outcome with head injury include:

- Midline shift on CT scan
- Systolic blood pressure < 90 mm Hg
- Intracranial pressure (ICP) > 15 mm Hg
- Age > 55 years
- Glasgow Coma Score < 8

Notably, head injury outcomes are determined by the number of secondary insults, not the injuries to other organ systems or body regions.

Given these realities, the most important concept in the recent treatment of brain-injured patients is the distinction between primary and secondary brain injury. Primary injury is that injury which occurs at the time of the traumatic incident and includes brain lacerations or other mechanical injuries to the brain at the moment of impact. After impact, the brain continues to be injured by various mechanisms, including the mechanical injury from cerebral edema or intracranial hematomas, ischemia from hypotension, cerebral edema or cerebral vascular dysregulation, hypoxia from inadequate ventilation, and secondary damage from a wide array of inflammation mediators. While prevention is the only strategy to avert primary brain injury, secondary injury can be prevented or at least blunted. Thus, the management of traumatic brain injury now includes increasing emphasis on the prevention of secondary insults.

The most important feature of the initial neurologic examination, the Glasgow Coma Scale (GCS), is designed to rapidly identify the severity of patient injury. Patients with GCS scores of 13 to 15 are considered to have mild head injuries. These individuals have an excellent prognosis and may not require hospitalization. They have a 3% chance of deteriorating into coma, and serial neurologic exams make this deterioration easy to detect. Individuals with GCS scores of 8 to 12 have moderate head injury. These patients do not

have normal neurologic examinations, but the severity of their injuries usually is not appreciated until the full GCS score is obtained. This group of patients has a 20% chance of declining into coma (GCS score of ≤ 8). Patients with severe head injury have the worst prognosis and require the most immediate care. All of these individuals require head CT scanning; except for select subpopulations, all of them require intracranial pressure (ICP) monitoring. As a group, there is a > 50% chance of an increased ICP; their depressed clinical examinations often preclude detection of changing neurologic status until their condition reaches catastrophic deterioration.

Evacuation of mass lesions has been the traditional focus of brain injury management throughout this century. The goal of removing space-occupying lesions is to prevent cerebral herniation. In previous studies among patients who talk and die, undetected hematomas were the principal cause of death. These are examples of patients who survive primary brain injury with the ability to talk and interact at some level, but who later succumb to preventable secondary brain injury. Cerebral herniation, representing the compression of critical neurologic centers against the retaining structures of the skull, is the common final pathway in these patients. Once herniation (regardless of the type) has occurred, patient outcome is dramatically affected. Studies over the last 50 years have demonstrated that once a patient herniates and slips into coma, the mortality rate reaches 33 to 41%, compared with mortality rates of 0 to 21% in patients who present with herniation before coma. Once a patient herniates and progresses to coma, hematomas must be evaluated within hours to avoid a significant risk of mortality.

After evacuation of mass lesions, emphasis is given to monitoring and control of ICP. ICP monitoring was introduced over 40 years ago as a means to quantify the study of brain swelling and cerebral edema. While the study of ICP initially focused on prevention of herniation by preventing swelling, it was soon apparent that keeping ICP from rising was a desirable end. As ICP rises, cerebral perfusion decreases and the threat of brain ischemia increases. Data are now emerging, however, that even in patients with adequate cerebral perfusion pressure (CPP), high ICP is associated with poor outcome. In the past, a variety of guidelines have been proposed for the optimal ICP level for treatment. Most current data place 25 mm Hg as the highest acceptable level for ICP at which treatment must begin. Modern methods of ICP monitoring include the ventriculostomy and intraparenchymal fiberoptic or strain-gauge devices. Subarachnoid bolts and epidural monitoring are used rarely or in select patient populations. Ventriculostomy carries an increased risk of infection and a slightly increased risk of bleeding. It is, however, the gold standard for ICP measurement.

Experimental work beginning in the mid-1980s demonstrated that ischemia is a significant threat to the head-injured patient. Ischemia had long been recognized as a factor in the outcome of head injury, but recent work has changed the paradigm through which head injury was viewed. Up to this time, the treatment priority has been control of cerebral edema and prevention of cerebral herniation. Any technique reducing ICP was thought to be good for the head-injured patient. By giving equal attention to ischemia, the current approach to the head-injured patient has evolved.

Ischemia is common following head injury. Autopsy findings have indicated that 60% of head-injured patients had ischemia. Cerebral blood flow on the first day after injury is less than half that of healthy individuals and may approach the ischemic threshold. In normal gray matter, cerebral blood flow is 50 mL/100 g/min of tissue, and in white matter, cerebral blood flow is 18 mL/100 g/min of tissue. Typical blood flow to gray matter within the first 8 hours after head injury is 30 mL/100 g/min of tissue, and in individuals with more severe injuries, cerebral blood flow as low as < 20 mL/100 g/min of tissue has been noted.

Improved recent understanding of cerebral blood flow coincides with multiple studies demonstrating disastrous consequences of hypotension in the setting of head injury. An increased death rate in head-injured patients with hypotension was documented in the National Traumatic Coma Data Bank, where the 2 most important factors related to outcome from head injuries were time spent with ICP of > 20 mm Hg and time spent with systolic pressure of < 90 mm Hg. These data suggest that patients with only a single episode of systolic blood pressure of < 90 mm Hg have a significantly worse outcome than those individuals who never experience this degree of hypotension.

Recent head injury management, therefore, places maintenance of adequate CPP as a goal equivalent to prevention of high ICP. The autoregulatory mechanisms in the brain are designed to maintain cerebral blood flow constant over a range of CPP between 50 and 150 mm Hg. This highly adaptive capacity allows the brain to see constant blood supply, despite changes in position and activity. In the severely injured brain, cerebral blood flow passively follows CPP. In the extreme case, with cerebral autoregulation disabled, cerebral ischemia results, as patients are maintained in a hypovolemic state with low mean arterial pressure to reduce cerebral blood volume and thereby ICP. In this practice, CPP was maintained below the autoregulatory threshold. Seemingly paradoxically, the best way to reduce ICP is to increase CPP into the autoregulatory range. This practice avoids hypotension and the ischemic damage that almost certainly attended the old practice of keeping patients with severe head injury "dry" and their arterial pressure low. At present, it is unclear what an adequate CPP is. Based on available data, including stepwise regression analysis, a CPP of 70 mm Hg has been suggested as a desirable level. Most head injury research protocols maintain this level.

Cerebral edema was thought to be aggravated by overzealous fluid administration, leading to increased intracranial pressure, brain ischemia and, ultimately, a poor outcome. However, in the patient with multiple injuries without head injury, aggressive volume resuscitation is a widely accepted method to maintain end-organ perfusion and adequate oxygen delivery. Traditional management strategies of the patient with severe head injury have changed with the knowledge of adverse effects of secondary brain insults. Much like the treatment of myocardial infarction for which the original zone of injury cannot be restored to normal, emphasis in the management of brain injury must be placed on avoidance of secondary insults to prevent extension of injury resulting from ischemia. An analysis of the Traumatic Coma Data Bank demonstrated that hypoxia and hypotension in the immediate period after head injury resulted in mortality rates of 28 and 50%, respectively. When the combined effect of hypoxia and hypotension during resuscitation was analyzed, the mortality rate increased to 57%. Later studies by other workers, using an algorithm guided by optimization of cerebral perfusion pressure, demonstrated a lower mortality in a cohort of patients thought to be similar to those enrolled in the Traumatic Coma Data Bank.

The second important consideration after avoidance of hypotension during resuscitation of the head-injured patient is the prevention of hypoxia. Hypoxia is 1 of the 5 top predictors of poor outcome in the National Traumatic Coma Data Bank, with 30 to 60% of severely head-injured patients presenting with hypoxia. While the optimal PaO_2 level in the head-injured patient has not been determined, available data suggest that a level of < 60 torr (< 8.0 kPa) is associated with poor outcome.

ICP is controlled with a variety of modalities. Our views on the use of these modalities and the management of head injury continue to evolve. Hyperventilation reduces ICP by reducing cerebral blood volume with increased cerebral vascular tone and induction of hypocapnia. Reduction in cerebral blood volume leads to intracranial blood volume loss and lower ICP. For many years, hyperventilation has been a primary means of reducing ICP. Hyperventilation can cause vasoconstriction independent of the metabolic demands of the brain. Hyperventilation may, therefore, reduce blood flow to the brain even if that reduction results in an ischemic injury. Recent studies, using jugular venous oximetry, have indicated that hyperventilation may produce cerebral ischemia. Other studies demonstrated that desaturation found in jugular venous blood is more common with hyperventilation than with other means employed for reduction in ICP. One prospective, randomized trial evaluated severely head-injured patients managed with hypocapnia versus normocapnia. The normocapnic group had better outcome at 3- and 6-month follow-up. Increasing evidence indicates that hyperventilation is an ICP treatment with high

cost, the threat of ischemia. Current management, therefore, includes use of less toxic means of reducing ICP, if available, rather than the use of hyperventilation. For example, drainage of cerebrospinal fluid (CSF) through ventricular drains should be started early with aggressive use of sedation, muscle relaxants, and administration of mannitol before resorting to hyperventilation.

Drainage of CSF and use of mannitol may be employed to control ICP and to optimize CPP. Some medical centers are facilitating drainage of CSF by placing ventriculotomy catheters when possible, as opposed to subarachnoid monitors, which do not allow for CSF removal. Drainage of CSF may be the first choice for the treatment of increased ICP. Mannitol is an osmotic diuretic given as a bolus, which develops an osmotic gradient between the blood and the brain. Mannitol may also act by improving cerebral blood flow through reduction in hematocrit and viscosity. Mannitol, however, cannot be given to hypotensive patients, as it will magnify shock states. In large doses, mannitol may lead to acute renal failure. If given as a constant infusion, mannitol may also open the blood-brain barrier and result in rebound cerebral edema. Mannitol drips, therefore, are not recommended. Serum osmolarity must be monitored in individuals who receive mannitol for control of ICP and optimization of CPP.

Recent developments in the care of the head-injured patient focus on the recognition of the importance of secondary brain injury as a determinant of prognosis. In studies of long-term outcome, the key elements of secondary brain injury, hypoxia and hypotension with secondary ischemia, are recognized to occur with increasing frequency. Optimal modalities to control secondary brain injury focus on maintenance of optimal CPP with the lowest possible ICP consistent with avoidance of cerebral ischemia. To control ICP, hyperventilation is now employed as an emergency tool rather than as a primary therapy.

Abdominal Organ Injury

The focus on management for intra-abdominal organ injury remains nonoperative.

The practitioner must be aware, however, of patients at greater risk for failure of that approach. Nonoperative management should be entertained only in hemodynamically stable patients. Identifying hemodynamically stable patients may be challenging in the setting of multiple injuries. A recent multicenter study of blunt splenic injury from the EAST included over 1,400 patients (age < 15 years) from 26 centers. Nonoperative management was attempted in 61% of these patients, with a resulting failure rate of 10.4%. Failure was associated with increasing age, Injury Severity Score (ISS), GCS, grade of splenic injury, and quantity of hemoperitoneum. Interestingly, other studies of nonoperative management of splenic injury suggest that many patients in high-risk categories can be managed nonoperatively, and that there is no increased mortality with failure of this approach.

Advances in nonoperative management have indicated differences between the spleen and liver. A high percentage of liver injuries appear to be manageable nonoperatively, and a somewhat lower proportion of liver injuries fail nonoperative management in comparison with blunt injury to the spleen. It has been speculated that liver injuries are more commonly associated with low-pressure venous injuries, and a greater proportion of spleen injuries are associated with arterial or arteriolar injury. Planned nonoperative management of the liver may be attempted in as many as 85% of patients with liver injuries; a failure rate of only 7% was found. In addition, significant improvement in outcome with nonoperative management was identified compared to operative management with respect to abdominal infection rates, transfusions, and length of hospital stay. Patients requiring operation due to hemodynamic instability may be successfully treated with packing. Evolution to nonoperative management in stable patients with high-grade injury results in lower mortality. In another major report from the University of Louisville, death secondary to blunt liver injury dropped from 8 to 2%; this improvement was attributed to improved methods of managing hepatic venous injuries. Proposed improvements in the management of hepatic venous injury include nonoperative

management in stable patients and willingness to employ gauze packing in unstable individuals.

As nonoperative management of abdominal solid organ injury continues to advance, missed blunt bowel injury has received increased attention. The sensitivity of CT scanning in defining bowel injury has been assessed by a variety of investigators. Recent reports suggest that sensitivity with latest-generation CT scans is as high as 94% for bowel injury, particularly if unexplained free fluid is considered a critical finding. A number of patients explored after CT scanning, however, have nontherapeutic laparotomies for bowel hematomas or contusions.

Abdominal Compartment Syndrome

A compartment syndrome is a condition in which increased pressure within a confined anatomic space adversely affects the function and viability of tissues contained within. Other confined anatomic spaces associated with compartment syndromes are the fascial spaces of the extremities, the globe as in glaucoma, and the cranial cavity as in epidural or subdural hematoma. Abdominal compartment syndrome is a condition in which sustained pressure within the abdominal wall, pelvis, diaphragm, and retroperitoneum adversely affect the function of the gastrointestinal tract and related extraperitoneal organs. Abdominal compartment syndrome is receiving widespread recognition as a complication of massive resuscitation following trauma, burns, or other surgical procedures (Table 1). Operative decompression is frequently required. Pressures below 10 mm of mercury within the abdominal cavity are normal. Short duration pressure increases frequently occur with coughing, valsalva maneuvers, defecation, and weight lifting. Surgical writers have graded abdominal hypertension into 3 intensity classes. First is mild abdominal hypertension where intraabdominal pressure ranges from 10-20 mm of mercury. In general, physiologic effects are minor and well tolerated. Moderate abdominal hypertension occurs with sustained elevation of intraabdominal pressure to 21-35 mm of mercury. Again, nonoperative therapy is frequently adequate, though operative decompression may be considered. Sustained elevation of intraabdominal pressure greater than 35 mm of mercury is an indication for operative abdominal decompression.

While a variety of measurement techniques for intraabdominal pressure exist, measurement of a fluid column related to intravesical pressure is probably most widely used. Some investigators actually transduce intravesical pressure to a signal on bedside monitors. Other methods to measure intraabdominal pressure include transduction of intragastric pressure or direct catheter methods within the abdominal cavity. A small number of investigators have reported measurement of inferior vena cava pressure utilizing transfemorally-placed catheters.

Intraabdominal hypertension has a variety of physiologic effects. In experimental preparations, animals die from congestive heart failure as abdominal pressure passes a critical threshold. Increased intraabdominal pressure significantly decreases cardiac output and left and right ventricular stroke work and increases central venous pressure, pulmonary artery wedge pressure, and systemic and pulmonary vascular resistance. Abdominal decompression reverses these changes. As both hemidiaphragms are displaced upward with increased intraabdominal pressure, decreased thoracic volume and compliance are seen. Decreased volume within the pleural cavities predisposes to atelectasis and deceases alveolar clearance. Pulmonary infections may also result. Ventilated

patients with abdominal hypertension require increased airway pressure to deliver a fixed tidal volume. As the diaphragm protrudes into the pleural cavity, intrathoracic pressure increases with reduction of cardiac output and increased pulmonary vascular resistance. Ventilation and perfusion abnormalities result, and blood gas measurements demonstrate hypoxemia, hypercarbia, and acidosis. Elevation of intraabdominal pressure also causes renal dysfunction. Control of intraabdominal pressure leads to reversal of renal impairment. Intraabdominal pressure as low as 15 to 20 mm of mercury may produce oliguria. Anuria is seen with higher intraabdominal pressures. Clearly, deterioration in cardiac output plays a role in diminished renal perfusion, but even when cardiac output is maintained at normal or supranormal values by blood volume expansion, impairment of renal function persists in the setting of intraabdominal hypertension. Renal dysfunction is also caused by compression of the renal vein, which creates partial renal blood outflow obstruction. Compression of the abdominal aorta and renal arteries may contribute to increased renal vascular resistance. Direct pressure on the kidneys may also elevate cortical pressures.

Other organs affected by increased intraabdominal pressure include the liver, where hepatic blood flow has been demonstrated to decrease with abdominal hypertension. It may be assumed that hepatic synthesis of acute phase proteins, immunoglobulins, and other factors of host defense may be impaired by reduced hepatic flow. Other gastrointestinal functions may be compromised by increased intraabdominal pressure. Splanchnic hypoperfusion may begin with intraabdominal pressure as low as 15 mm of mercury. Reduced perfusion of intraabdominal arteries, veins, and lymphatics may create changes in mucosal pH, translocation, bowel motility, and production of gastrointestinal hormones. Finally, intracranial hypertension is seen with chronic increase in intraabdominal pressure. Intracranial hypertension has been demonstrated to decrease when intraabdominal pressure is reduced in morbidly obese patients. Abdominal hypertension significantly increases intracranial

Table 1. Causes of Abdominal Hypertension

Peritoneal tissue edema diffuse peritonitis severe abdominal trauma
Fluid overload secondary to hemorrhagic or septic shock
Retroperitoneal hematoma
Reperfusion injury after bowel ischemia
Inflammatory edema secondary to acute pancreatitis
Ileus and bowel obstruction
Intraabdominal masses
Abdominal packing for hemorrhage
Closure of the abdomen under tension
Intraabdominal fluid accumulations

Modified from Wittman D: Compartment syndrome of the abdominal cavity. **In:** *Intensive Care Medicine. Irwin RS, Cerra FB, Rippe JM (Eds). Philadelphia, Lippincott-Raven, 1999, p 1890*

pressures at intraabdominal pressures routinely used during laparoscopy.

Operative decompression is the method of choice in the patient with severe abdominal hypertension and evidence of intraabdominal organ dysfunction. After decompression improvement in hemodynamics, pulmonary function, tissue perfusion, and renal function have been demonstrated in a variety of clinical settings. To prevent hemodynamic decompensation during decompression, intravascular volume should be restored, oxygen delivery maximized, and hypothermia and coagulation defects corrected. The abdomen should be opened under optimal conditions in the operating room, including hemodynamic monitoring with adequate venous access and controlled ventilation. Adjunctive measures to combat expected reperfusion wash out from byproducts of anaerobic metabolism include prophylactic volume loading and use of vasoconstrictor agents to prevent sudden changes in blood pressure. After decompression, the abdomen and the fascial gap is left open using one of a variety of temporary abdominal closure methods.

Pelvic Fracture

Substantial blunt force is required to disrupt the pelvic ring. The extent of injury is related to the direction and magnitude of the force. Associated abdominal, thoracic, and head injuries are common. Forces applied to the pelvis can cause rotational displacement with opening or compression of the pelvic ring. The other type of displacement seen with pelvic fractures is vertical, with complete disruption of the pelvic ring and the posterior sacroiliac complex.

Patients with pelvic ring injuries are easily subdivided into 2 groups on the basis of clinical presentation: a) those who are hemodynamically stable, and b) those who are hemodynamically unstable. There is a dramatic difference in the mortality rates between pelvic fracture patients who are hypotensive (38%) and those who are hemodynamically stable (3%). Hemodynamic instability and biomechanical pelvic instability are separate though related issues which tend to confuse the clinical picture.

The source of bleeding may be multifactorial and not directly related to the pelvic fracture itself. However, pelvic fracture blood loss that contributes to hemodynamic instability is a significant risk factor. Early fracture diagnosis and stabilization, using external skeletal fixation, are extremely important in the acute phase of patient management. Treatment of the patient is also directed by response to initial fluid resuscitation. It is essential to examine for other sources of hemorrhage (intrathoracic, intraperitoneal, external) in patients with evidence of ongoing bleeding. Retroperitoneal bleeding in a pelvic fracture patient usually arises from a low-pressure source, the cancellous bone at the fracture site or adjacent venous injury. Significant retroperitoneal arterial bleeding occurs in only ~10% of patients. Clinical evidence has suggested that provisional fracture stabilization, using a simple anterior external fixator or even "wrapping" in a bed sheet can control low pressure bleeding. Continued unexplained bleeding after provisional fracture stabilization suggests an arterial source. Angiography with embolization of the involved vessel is then indicated. Therapeutic angiography may also be required after abdominal exploration if a rapidly expanding or pulsatile retroperitoneal hematoma is encountered. In general, definitive operative stabilization of pelvic fractures is delayed 3 to 5 days to allow the patient to recover from acute injury.

Deep Venous Thrombosis and Thromboembolism

That deep venous thrombosis and thromboembolism occur after trauma is incontrovertible. The optimal mode of prophylaxis has yet to be determined. Low-dose heparin (5000 units subcutaneously 2 or 3 times daily) represents 1 pharmacologic treatment modality used for prophylaxis against deep venous thrombosis and pulmonary embolism. A meta-analysis of 29 trials and > 8,000 surgical patients demonstrated that low-dose heparin significantly decreased the frequency of deep venous thrombosis from 25.2% in patients with no prophylaxis to 8.7% in treated individuals. Similarly, pulmonary embolism was halved by low-dose heparin treatment (0.5% with treatment compared with 1.2% in controls). In double-blind trials, the occurrence rate of major hemorrhage was higher in patients treated with anticoagulation than in controls, but the difference in incidence was not significant. Minor bleeding complications, such as wound hematomas, were more frequent in low-dose heparin treatment patients (6.3%) than in controls (4.1%).

Unfractionated low-dose heparin has not been shown to be particularly effective in preventing venous thromboembolism in trauma patients. Two recent prospective trials demonstrated that low-dose heparin was not better in preventing deep venous thrombosis than no prophylaxis in patients with an Injury Severity Score of > 9. Sample sizes in these studies were small and statistical error could not be excluded. The results of low-dose heparin administration after injury with regard to pulmonary embolism were even more vague.

Defining the trauma patient at risk for venous thromboembolism is subjective and variable in the literature. The following injury patterns appear to differentiate high-risk patients for venous thromboembolism: closed-head injury (Glasgow Coma Scale Score of < 8), pelvis plus long-bone fractures (multiple long-bone fractures), and spinal cord injury. Greenfield and associates have developed a risk factor assessment tool for venous thromboembolism; preliminary evidence supported this risk factor assessment tool as a valid indicator of the development of venous thromboembolism. In this scale, risk factors are weighted; scores of < 3 represent low risk, scores of 3 to 5 represent moderate risk, and scores of > 5 represent high risk (Table 2).

When EAST reviewed the literature regarding the effectiveness of low-dose heparin for trauma patients, a clear recommendation could not be produced. Most studies showed no effect of low-dose heparin on venous thromboembolism. However, many of the studies examined suffered from methodologic errors or poor study design. Similarly, the use of sequential compression devices on the lower extremities in patients at risk for deep venous thrombosis is widely accepted; however, clinical studies demonstrating efficacy in trauma patients

Table 2. Risk-factor assessment tool for venous thromboembolism (VTE) in trauma

Risk Factor	Weight
Underlying Condition	
Obesity	2
Malignancy	2
Abnormal coagulation factors on hospital admission	2
History of VTE	3
Iatrogenic Factors	
Central femoral line > 24 hrs	2
≥ 4 Transfusions in first 24 hrs	2
Surgical procedure ≥ 2 hrs	2
Repair or ligation of major vascular injury	3
Injury-Related Factors	
AIS score of > 2 for chest	2
AIS score of > 2 for abdomen	2
AIS score of > 2 for head	3
Coma (GCS score of < 8 for > 4 hrs)	3
Complex lower-extremity fracture	4
Pelvic fracture	4
Spinal cord injury with paraplegia or quadriplegia	4
Age	
≥ 40 but < 60 yrs	2
≥ 70 but < 75 yrs	3
≥ 75 yrs	4
Total	

AIS, Abbreviated Injury Scales; GCS, Glasgow Coma Scale. Reproduced with permission from Greenfield LJ, Proctor ML, Rodriguez JL, et al: Posttrauma thromboembolism prophylaxis. *J Trauma* 1997; 42:100–103 are few. The mechanism of these devices is believed to be based on a combination of factors addressing venous stasis and hypercoagulability. These mechanisms are poorly understood at this time. The role of multimodality therapy to provide additional protection from venous thromboembolism in the setting of injury needs to be ascertained.

There is a wealth of randomized, prospective data supporting the use of low-molecular weight heparin as venous thromboembolism prophylaxis in orthopedic surgery. This literature is derived primarily from total hip replacement and knee replacement patients. We now have data suggesting that low-molecular weight heparin is superior to unfractionated heparin for prophylaxis in moderate- to high-risk trauma patients. Most data in many different types of patients confirm improved efficacy of low-molecular-weight heparin with the same or even less bleeding risk compared with prophylaxis with unfractionated heparin. Low-molecular heparin should be the standard form of venous thromboembolism prophylaxis in trauma patients with complex pelvic and lower extremity injuries as well as in those patients with spinal cord injuries. This agent is also safe for patients receiving craniotomy or nonoperative management of solid organ injury if started 24 or 72 hours after injury, respectively. Finally, literature is beginning to support the use of inferior vena cava filters in high-risk trauma patients without a documented occurrence of deep venous thrombosis or pulmonary embolism and who cannot be anticoagulated.

For established deep venous thrombosis or pulmonary embolism, anticoagulation is a well-established treatment. Current evidence suggests that a 3- to 6-month period provides adequate treatment for the first episode of deep venous thrombosis or pulmonary embolism in a patient without clotting abnormality. Patients in whom the risk of recurrent venous thromboembolism extends > 6 months may have anticoagulation extended indefinitely. In addition, patients whose injuries preclude the use of anticoagulants because bleeding would exacerbate their injuries should have consideration given to placement of a vena cava filter. Recent evidence also supported initial

treatment of venous thromboembolism with low-molecular-weight heparin.

Evaluation for deep venous thrombosis in the setting of injury receives continued study. Early identification of this complication would allow treatment to be initiated, thus decreasing the frequency and severity of complications. Studies in the nontrauma literature support the accuracy of both Doppler and duplex ultrasonography in the detection of deep venous thrombosis in the symptomatic patient. The overall accuracy of screening ultrasonography in the asymptomatic patient is less clear. Similarly, impedance plethysmography has high sensitivity and specificity in the detection of proximal deep venous thrombosis in symptomatic patients. Its low sensitivity in detecting deep venous thrombosis in asymptomatic patients precludes use as a surveillance technique in trauma patients at high risk for deep venous thrombosis. Logistical problems and complications associated with venography make the procedure less appealing than other noninvasive diagnostic measures. Venography still has a role in confirming deep venous thrombosis in trauma patients if diagnostic studies are equivocal. At present, it appears that future investigational efforts are best directed at developing the role of duplex ultrasonography in screening for deep venous thrombosis in the setting of injury.

Antibiotic Management

Much of the data surrounding antibiotic utilization in patients following injury comes from studies of patients with penetrating abdominal trauma. There are a wide variety of randomized prospective data available that support clear recommendations regarding the use of antibiotics in this patient group. While antibiotic therapy must be initiated prior to operation or in the emergency department, the intensivist should be aware of available recommendations regarding appropriate agents, duration of therapy, and the impact of shock and resuscitation.

In a clinical management update produced by the Practice Management Guidelines Workgroup of EAST, evidence regarding antibiotic utilization in penetrating abdominal trauma was reviewed. These writers suggest that there is sufficient randomized prospective data to recommend the use of only a single preoperative dose of prophylactic antibiotics with broad-spectrum aerobic and anaerobic coverage as a standard of care for trauma patients sustaining penetrating abdominal wounds. If no hollow viscus injury is noted subsequently, no further antibiotic administration is warranted. The second issue addressed is the duration of therapy in the presence of injury to any hollow viscus. Based on available prospective randomized data, there is sufficient evidence to recommend continuation of prophylactic antibiotics for only 24 hours even in the presence of injury to any hollow viscus. Unfortunately, there is insufficient data to provide meaningful guidelines for reducing infection risks in trauma patients with hemorrhagic shock. Vasoconstriction alters the normal distribution of antibiotics, resulting in reduced tissue penetration. To alleviate this problem, administered antibiotic doses may be increased 2- to 3-fold and repeated after every tenth unit of blood transfusion until there is no further blood loss. As the patient is resuscitated, antibiotics with activity against obligate and facultative anaerobic bacteria should be continued for periods dependent on the degree of identified wound contamination. Notably, aminoglycosides have been demonstrated to exhibit suboptimal activity in patients with serious injury, probably due to altered pharmacokinetics of drug distribution. Finally, a meta-analysis has examined studies assessing effectiveness of a single agent versus combination therapy containing aminoglycosides for penetrating wounds. This report concludes that single β-lactam agents were as effective as combination therapy in the setting of penetrating abdominal trauma.

Fewer data are available regarding the utilization of antibiotics in the patient following blunt injury. In the absence of monitoring device placement or the use of tube thoracostomy, antibiotics are not warranted. Many practitioners, however, believe Gram-positive antibiotic coverage is appropriate in the patient with tube thoracostomy or with invasive monitors of intracranial pressure. There are no randomized prospective data or multidisciplinary guidelines available to address this issue.

THERMAL INJURY

Thermal injury is a major public health problem for 2 to 2.5 million people who seek medical treatment in the United States each year. Thermal injury results in 100 - 150,000 hospitalizations and - 12,000 fatalities. Death rates are highest in the very young and the very old. Thirty-eight percent of the victims are < 15 years of age. An equal number of thermal injury victims are 15 to 44 years of age. Only 7% of thermal injury patients are > 65 years old, but the mortality in this age group is significant. Scalds are the most common form of childhood thermal trauma, while electrical and chemical injuries affect adults in the workplace. Factors shown to relate to mortality in thermal injury include the size of cutaneous involvement, age, and the presence or absence of inhalation injury. A discussion, based on available evidence, of optimal burn care, "Practice Guidelines for Burn Care," is slated for publication in the next several months. When available, appropriate care options will be available to all practitioners treating the burn patient.

Wound

Characteristics of skin affect patterns of cutaneous injury. Skin is very thin in infants and increases in thickness until 30 to 40 years of age. After this, skin progressively thins. Males have thicker skin than females. Average skin thickness is 1 to 2 mm. In general, dermis is 10 times thicker than associated epidermis. Cell types in the epidermis are predominately keratinocytes and melanocytes. The latter cells provide pigment generation against ultraviolet radiation. The predominant cell type in the underlying dermis, which is derived from the mesoderm, is the fibroblast, which produces collagen, elastin, ground substance of glycosaminoglycans, and proteoglycans. The dermis itself consists of a superficial papillary dermis and a thicker reticular dermis.

Table 3. Classification of burn depth

Degree of Burn	Depth of Tissue	Penetration Characteristics
First-degree	Partial thickness	Injury to the superficial epidermis, usually caused by overexposure to sunlight or brief heat flashes; classically, described as sunburn.
Second-degree	Superficial partial thickness	Injury is to the epidermis and upper layers of the dermis. Wounds characteristically appear red, wet, or blistered, blanchable, and extremely painful. Will heal within 3 weeks form epidermal regeneration from remaining remnants found in the tracts of hair follicles.
	Deep partial thickness	Injury is through the epidermis and may affect isolated areas of the deep thermal strata from which cells arise. This wound may appear red and wet or white and dry, depending on the extent of deep dermal damage. It heals without grafting but requires > 3 weeks with suboptimal cosmesis. Excision and split-thickness skin grafting are recommended.
Third-degree	Full thickness	Injury has destroyed both the epidermis and the dermis. The wound appears white, will not blanch, and is anesthetic. Tough, nonelastic, and tenacious coagulated protein (eschar) tissue may be present on the surface. This wound will not heal without surgical intervention.

Reproduced with permission from the Society of Critical Care Medicine.

The skin serves a number of critical functions. Unfortunately, all of these functions may be lost with thermal injury. Most importantly, the skin is a principal barrier against infection. Sebum (discussed in reference 8) has noted antibacterial properties. Skin also helps to maintain antigen presentation to immune cells and protects our fluid, protein, and electrolyte homeostasis. Skin has various sensory functions, affects heat preservation, and is associated with vitamin production.

In thermal injury, damage to the skin results from temperature of the thermal source and the duration of exposure. At 40 to 44° C, enzymatic failure occurs within the cell with rising intracellular sodium concentration and swelling due to failure of the membrane sodium pump. At exposure to 60° C, necrosis occurs in 1 hour with release of oxygen free radicals.

Three cutaneous zones of injury have been described:
- The *zone of coagulation* is the site of irreversible cell death with new eschar formation from local degradation of protein.
- The *zone of stasis* is the site of local circulatory impairment with initial cell viability. If ischemia follows in this zone, cell death will occur. Impaired circulation is thought to be secondary to platelet and neutrophil aggregates, fibrin deposition, endothelial cell swelling, and loss of erythrocyte deformability. These tissues are susceptible to secondary insults such as dehydration, pressure, overresuscitation, and infection. Measures implemented to minimize further tissue loss include

Table 4. Topical antimicrobial agents

Agent	Advantages	Disadvantages
Silver sulfadiazine	Painless application Broad spectrum Easy application Rare sensitivities	May produce transient leukopenia Minimal penetration of eschar Some Gram-negative species resistant
Mafenide acetate	Broad spectrum Easy application Penetrates eschar	Painful application Promotes acid-base imbalance Frequent sensitivity
Bacitracin, Polysporin	Painless application Nonirritating Transparent May be used on nonburn wounds	No eschar penetration
Silver nitrate (0.5% solution)	Painless application Broad spectrum Rare sensitivity Must be kept moist	No eschar penetration Electrolyte imbalances Discolors the wound and environment
Povidone-iodine	Broad spectrum	Painful application Systemically absorbed Requires frequent reapplication Discolors wounds
Gentamicin	Painless application Broad spectrum	Oto/nephrotoxic Encourages development of resistant organisms

Reproduced with permission from the Society of Critical Care Medicine.

nondesiccating dressings, careful fluid resuscitation, and topical antimicrobials.

- The *zone of hyperemia* is characterized by minimal cellular injury but prominent vasodilation and increased blood flow. Cell recovery generally occurs in this zone.

Vasoactive mediators, including thromboxane A_2 with platelet adherence and vasoconstriction, are seen in the burn wound. Beyond the vasoconstricting effects seen in the zone of stasis, the predominant effect and resuscitation issue are significant vasodilation and increased vascular permeability. The initial increase in vascular permeability may be related to short-term histamine release occurring soon after injury. The second longer period of vasodilation and increased vascular permeability is related to the release of a variety of vasoactive and oxidative products.

Wound Care

The degree of injury is assessed by the well-known rule of nines (Fig. 1). Anatomical criteria can also be employed to recognize the depth of injury and coincident likelihood of healing (Table 3). Partial-thickness injuries should heal within 3 weeks and leave the

Trauma and Thermal Injury

AREA	0 to 1	1 to 4	5 to 9	10 to 15	ADULT	% TOTAL
Head	19	17	13	10	7	
Neck	2	2	2	2	2	
Anterior Trunk	13	17	13	13	13	
Posterior Trunk	13	13	13	13	13	
Right Buttock	2.5	2.5	2.5	2.5	2.5	
Left Buttock	2.5	2.5	2.5	2.5	2.5	
Genitalia	1	1	1	1	1	
Right Upper Arm	4	4	4	4	4	
Left Upper Arm	4	4	4	4	4	
Right Lower Arm	3	3	3	3	3	
Left Lower Arm	3	3	3	3	3	
Right Hand	2.5	2.5	2.5	2.5	2.5	
Left Hand	2.5	2.5	2.5	2.5	2.5	
Right Thigh	5.5	5.5	8.5	8.5	9.5	
Left Thigh	5.5	5.5	8.5	8.5	9.5	
Right Leg	5	5	5.5	6	7	
Left Leg	5	5	5.5	6	7	
Right Foot	3.5	3.5	3.5	3.5	3.5	
Left Foot	3.5	3.5	3.5	3.5	3.5	
LUND & BROWDER CHART					**TOTAL**	

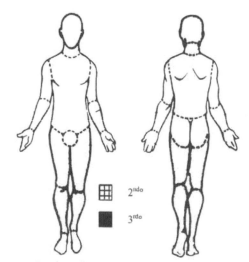

2^{ndo}

3^{rdo}

Figure 1. Patient skin assessment – percentage of body surface area at each age

stratum germinosum intact. Third-degree or full-thickness injuries involve all layers of epidermis and dermis. Some authors speak also of fourth-degree injuries, which involve deep structures such as tendon, muscle, and bone.

Local care begins with serial debridement of nonviable tissue and blisters. Topical antimicrobials, one of the major advances in burn wound care, are applied once or twice daily after washes with antiseptic solutions (Table 4). These topical antimicrobials are applied in occlusive dressings, which also help maintain fluid balance. The burn wound affords a warm, moist, protein-laden growth medium to Gram-positive and later Gram-negative bacteria. In general, systemic antibiotics are not employed in the initial days after injury.

Biologic dressings (cadaver allograft, porcine xenograft) are used for relatively clean wounds to reduce pain, bacterial colony counts, and fluid and protein loss. Rate of epithelialization is also increased, more so than with topical antimicrobials, which tend to cause relative inhibition of wound epithelialization.

- Biologic dressings may be placed on newly debrided partial-thickness wounds in anticipation of healing without surgery.
- Biologic dressings cover granulating excised wounds awaiting autografts.
- Biologic dressings gauge readiness of a wound for autografting (via early "take").
- Biologic dressings may facilitate removal of necrotic tissue from granulating wounds.

Where circumferential injury with second- or third-degree depth exists, the wound may need to be divided at the lateral aspects of extremities or on the torso to facilitate extremity perfusion or chest wall movement respectively. Division of wound eschar for this purpose is termed *escharotomy*. Usually, the need for escharotomy is clear within 48 hours of injury. Progressive tissue edema during resuscitation creates the need for escharotomy even if initial perfusion of circumferential torso burns is adequate. Abdominal wall escharotomy or laparotomy for abdominal compartment syndrome with respiratory embarrassment is sometimes required.

Wound Excision

Excision of burned tissue that will clearly not heal (determined by clinical assessment) is generally performed within 3 to 5 days of injury. Generally, we do not excise > 20% total body surface area (TBSA) at a time. If possible, wounds are covered with sheet or meshed autograft, harvested 3/ to 10/1000-inch thickness with a power dermatome from unburned sites. Good harvest sites are the thighs, back, and scalp. Grafts can be meshed onto the burn area in a ratio from 1:1 to 1:9 to increase coverage, with the assumption that the wound will reepithelialize within the mesh network. We generally do not use meshing > 1:3 due to increased incidence of contractures and graft shear. Cadaveric allograft can be used to cover excised areas where donor skin is unavailable.

Sequential layered tangential excision of burned tissue is employed to reach viable tissue with visible punctate bleeding. While blood loss is greater with this method, cosmetic outcome is improved and the maximum amount of viable tissue is preserved. Excision to fascia is limited to large, full-thickness injuries, where the risks of blood loss and potential graft compromise from a suboptimal recipient bed may cause increased mortality.

Current research is directed at the development of dermal and epidermal substitutes. Cultured autografts may be grown from uninjured skin samples obtained after injury. This process takes several weeks and, to date, has produced grafts which are flawed by easy shear loss and relatively poor take. A collagen-based artificial dermis has been developed and marketed which may be used with ultrathin (3/1000 inch-thickness) skin grafts.

Burn Shock Resuscitation

Burn shock has both hypovolemic and cellular components. Mediator cascades and resuscitation strategies are based on fundamental observations of patients and animals following burn injury. The variety of resuscitation approaches available suggests the value of careful observation and adjustment of treatment based on patient clinical response (Table 5).

Increased capillary permeability is one of the key components of the burn shock response. In small burns, maximal edema is seen in as little as 8 to 12 hours after injury, while larger burns manifest edema in a period of 12 to 24 hours post-injury. The initial mediators seen after burn injury are histamine and bradykinin. Histamine release from mast cells in skin is seen early after injury but appears to be transient. The chief site of histamine action appears to be the venules. Blocker studies suggested that histamine explains only part of the early changes in burn wound permeability. Other mediators for vascular changes in burns include complement, prostaglandins, leukotrienes, stress hormones, and vasoactive amines.

- Prostaglandin (PG) E_2 and PGI_2 cause arterial dilation in burned tissue with increased blood and hydrostatic pressure favoring edema formation.
- Serotonin is released by platelet aggregation and serves to amplify the vasoconstrictive effect of norepinephrine and angiotensin II.
- Proteolytic cascades including coagulation, fibrinolysis, complement, and the kinin family have been found in activated states after burn injury.
- The end result of these changes is disruption of normal capillary barriers between interstitial and intravascular compartments with rapid equilibration between them.
- Plasma volume loss, manifested as hypovolemia, coincides with increased extracellular fluid.

Cellular Changes

Baxter (reviewed in references 14 and 15) described the cellular changes which provide the foundation of our present resuscitation strategies. He noted a decrease in cell membrane potential involving burned *and unburned* tissues.

This potential change is associated with increased intracellular sodium, probably due to a decrease in sodium ATP activity. Resuscitation only partly restores normal intracellular sodium and membrane potentials. Inadequate resuscitation leads to further decline in cell membrane potential and cell death. Later work on burn shock concluded that this phenomenon is due not only to intravascular hypovolemia but also extracellular sodium depletion.

Hemodynamic Response

Global hemodynamic changes include a decrease in extracellular fluid of as much as 30 to 50% in unresuscitated animal models by 18 hours after burn. In 1 study, cardiac output decreased to 25% of control at 4 hours after injury and increased to only 40% of control at 18 hours after a 30% TBSA injury. The principal site of volume loss was the functional extracellular intravascular fluid.

- Subsequent studies with salt solutions confirmed a variety of approaches to minimize extracellular fluid loss and maximize hemodynamic response in the first 24 hours after burn.
- During the first 24 hours, the work of Baxter showed that plasma volume changes were independent of the fluid type employed. Thus, colloids should not be used in the first 24 hours of burn resuscitation.
- After 24 hours, infused colloids can increase plasma volume by anticipated amounts as capillary integrity is restored.
- Peripheral vascular resistance was actually very high in the initial 24 hours after burn, but decreased as cardiac output improved to supranormal levels coincident with the end of plasma and blood volume losses.

Burn wound edema is caused by dilation of precapillary arterioles and increased extravascular osmotic activity due to various products of thermal injury. All elements in the vascular space, except red blood cells, can escape from this site during the initial period of increased permeability.

Burn Resuscitation Strategies

In burn injury, intracellular and interstitial volume increase at the expense of plasma and blood volume. Edema formation is affected by resuscitation fluid administration. Thus, 2 principles are agreed upon:

- Give the least amount of fluid necessary to maintain adequate organ perfusion (as determined by vital signs, urine output, or function studies).
- Replace extracellular salt lost into cells and burned tissue with crystalloids and lactated Ringer's solution.

Probably the most popular resuscitation approach utilizes a modified Parkland formula, giving 4 mL/kg/% TBSA burn of fluid (lactated Ringer's) with half of the 24-hour volume required given in the first 8 hours. A variety of other formulas have been described. All represent guidelines for the initiation of resuscitation. Continuation of this process requires perfusion as indicated by a urine output of 30 to 50 mL/hr in the adult. Hypoproteinemia and edema formation complicate the use of isotonic crystalloids for resuscitation. Hypertonic resuscitation solutions have the theoretical advantages of improved hemodynamic response and diminished overall fluid needs as intracellular water is shifted into the extracellular space by the hyperosmolar solution. A clear role for hypertonic resuscitation has not yet been defined. Some groups add colloid to resuscitation fluids as protein formulations or dextran after the first 8 hours when much of the capillary leak has subsided. Groups most likely to benefit from supplemental colloid are the elderly, those patients with large burns (> 50% TBSA), and/or patients who have inhalation injury. Inhalation injury increases the overall fluid requirement of the burned patient from volume and total salt requirement standpoints.

Overall, patients in good health with burns of < 40% TBSA can be resuscitated with crystalloids alone. Where coexistent injury, comorbid conditions, limited cardiac reserve, and inhalation injury complicate burn trauma, a combination of crystalloid and colloids may be optimally employed. The resuscitation target is generally 30 to 50 mL/hr of urine output with acceptable vital signs. In the patient with complicated trauma or thermal injury management, a pulmonary artery catheter may be needed.

Patients receiving crystalloid resuscitation will frequently require supplemental colloid during the second 24 hours after burn injury. Maintenance fluids must include allowance for evaporative losses. This fluid may come from intravenous repletion or enteral feeding. Evaporative losses = (25 + % TBSA burn) x BSA (in m^2) x 24 hours. Potassium, calcium, magnesium, and phosphorus losses should be monitored and aggressively replaced. After 24 to 48 hours, a urine output of 30 to 50 mL/hr is an inadequate guide to perfusion, due to relative osmotic diuresis with the metabolite loss of burns and deranged antidiuretic hormone metabolism. Adults require 1500 to 2000 mL/24 hours of urine output to excrete the osmolar products of large burns. Serum sodium concentration, weight change, intake and output records, and physical examination also guide ongoing fluid administration.

Inhalation Injury

Inhalation injury has emerged as a persisting cause of increased mortality in burn victims. Upper airway injury is frequently due to direct heat exposure, while laryngeal reflexes protect the lung from thermal injury in all cases except possibly high-pressure steam exposure. The upper airway is also an extremely efficient heat sink. Lower airway injury is predominantly due to chemical products of combustion carried to the lung on particles of soot (particle size 5 um).

Table 5. Resuscitation formulas

Formula	Calculation: First 24 Hours	Calculation: Thereafter
Parkland	4 L/kg/% TBSA burn lactated Ringer's solution Give 50% total volume during first 8 hours after burn and the remaining 50% over the subsequent 16 hours	% dextrose in water, K, plasma to maintain normal serum sodium and K levels and colloid oncotic pressure
Brooke	2 mL/kg/% TBSA burn lactated Ringer's solution Give 50% total volume during the first 8 hours after burn and the remaining 50% over the subsequent 16 hours	Maintain urine output 0.5 to 1.0 mL/kg/hr
Shrine	5000 mL/m^2 TBSA burn + 2000 mL/m^2 BSA lactated Ringer's solution Give 50% total volume during the first 8 hours after burn and the remaining 50% over the subsequent 16 hours	3750 mL/m^2 TBSA burn + 1500 mL/m^2 BSA. May replace intravenous fluid with enteral feedings if GI function is normal

TBSA, total body surface area; K, potassium; BSA, body surface area; GI, gastrointestinal.
Reproduced with permission from the Society of Critical Care Medicine.

To a degree that varies unpredictably among affected patients, inhalation injury causes several physiologic derangements, including:

- Loss of airway patency secondary to mucosal edema
- Bronchospasm secondary to inhaled irritants
- Intrapulmonary shunting from small airway occlusion caused by mucosal edema and sloughed endobronchial debris
- Diminished compliance secondary to alveolar flooding and collapse with mismatching of ventilation and perfusion
- Pneumonia and tracheobronchitis secondary to loss of ciliary clearance endotracheal bronchial epithelium
- Respiratory failure secondary to a combination of the above factors.

Injuries evolve over time and parenchymal lung dysfunction is often minimal for 24 to 72 hours.

- Aldehydes, oxides of sulfur and hydrochloric acid, combine with water in the lung to yield corrosive acids and oxygen radicals. Degradation of polyvinyl chloride, for example, yields up to 75 toxic compounds.
- Carbon monoxide exposure is also associated with inhalation injury but does *not* define this process as the true degree of exposure to carbon monoxide is frequently not detected. The half-life of carboxyhemoglobin in room air is 4 hours, 30 minutes at 100% oxygen. Therefore, increased carboxyhemoglobin levels are not often found.
- Diagnosis of inhalation injury is most commonly made with bronchoscopy,

which reveals airway edema, erythema, soot accumulation, and sometimes mucosal sloughing. This test picks up far more injuries than standard clinical criteria, including history of closed-space burn injury, facial burns *with* nasal hair singeing, wheezing, and soot in the sputum. Chest radiography is frequently normal on hospital admission, and hypoxia on blood gases is not frequently seen.

Chemical injury to the lung stimulates release of substances including histamine, serotonin, and kallikreins with recruitment of leukocytes to airways and lung parenchyma. Edema of airway mucosa and sloughing can combine with formation of plugs of fibrin and purulent material to create casts, which obstruct small airways. Neutrophils and other activated inflammatory cells also release oxygen radicals and lytic enzymes, which magnify tissue change. Pulmonary edema is also seen due to increased capillary permeability, which is magnified by cutaneous burns if present. Patients with cutaneous injury alone do not increase extravascular lung water.

Three stages of clinical inhalation injury have been identified. a) Acute hypoxia with asphyxia typically occurs at the fire scene, sometimes in association with high carbon monoxide exposure, and is followed by acute upper airway and pulmonary edema. b) Pulmonary edema with acute airway swelling usually resolves by the passage of the first several days after injury. c) Later complications are infections with the morbidity of pneumonia complicating that of inhalation exposure to heat and chemical irritants.

Optimal initial management of inhalation injury requires directed assessment and assurance of airway patency. Prophylactic intubation is not indicated for a diagnosis of inhalation injury alone. However, if there is concern over progressive edema, intubation should be strongly considered. Intubation is indicated if upper airway patency is threatened, gas exchange or compliance mandate mechanical ventilatory support, or mental status is inadequate for airway protection. Prophylactic use of steroids and antibiotics is not indicated in the initial management of inhalation injury. In patients requiring mechanical ventilatory support, transpulmonary inflating pressures over 40 cm H_2O should be avoided, except in exceptional circumstances (e.g., pH < 7.2 or PaO_2 < 60 torr), or if impaired chest wall compliance suggests that inflating pressures measured at the endotracheal tube did not reflect transpulmonary pressures. Any mode of mechanical ventilation consistent with these limits is appropriate. Survivors of inhalation injury may have permanent pulmonary dysfunction, late endobronchial bleeding from granulation tissue, and upper airway stenosis. While there is no specific therapy for inhalation injury, proper initial management can have a favorable influence on outcome. Management goals during the first 24 hours are to prevent suffocation by assuring airway patency, to assure adequate oxygenation and ventilation, to forego the use of agents that may complicate subsequent care, and to avoid ventilator-induced lung injury.

In any situation where carbon monoxide exposure is possible, 100% oxygen should be provided to eliminate carbon monoxide. Resuscitation fluid administration should not be delayed or withheld in inhalation injury patients. These individuals may, in fact, require additional fluid. Humidification of inhaled gases may help to reduce desiccation injury. The role of early hyperbaric oxygen is minimized in the burn care community but remains popular among pulmonologists; prospective randomized clinical data are not available. Heparin nebulization is now employed in some centers over the initial days after inhalation injury due to presumed mucolytic and anti-inflammatory effects. This process may stimulate expectoration of accumulated proteinaceous material.

Outcome

Currently, 2 papers have detailed the outcome for burn-injured patients. The first paper is from the American Burn Association Patient Registry, the largest and most well organized body of data on burn-injured patients. Between 1991 and 1993, > 6,000 patients were registered at 28 burn centers. The mean burn size was 14% of the TBSA. The overall survival rate was 95.9%. However, the mortality rate among patients with inhalation injury was 29.4%. In young adults, the size of burn that was felt to be lethal to 50% of these patients was 81% of TBSA. In the total population studied, mean length of hospital stay was 13.5 days.

A second review of > 1,600 patients admitted to Massachusetts General Hospital and the Schriners' Burn Institute in Boston was published in early 1998. Logistic progression analysis was employed to develop probability estimates for mortality based on a small set of well-defined variables. Mean burn size and survival were similar to the larger report above. The following 3 risk factors for death were identified:

- Age > 60 years
- TBSA burned, > 40%
- Inhalation injury

The mortality formula developed from these data predicts 0.3%, 3%, 33%, or 90% mortality depending on whether 0, 1, 2, or 3 risk factors are present.

SUGGESTED READINGS

General Trauma Management

1. Trunkey DD, Lewis FR (Eds): Current Therapy of Trauma. Fourth Edition. St Louis, MO, Mosby, 1999
2. Mattox KA, Feliciano DV, Moore EE (Eds): Trauma. Fourth Edition, New York, NY, McGraw-Hill, 2000

Head Injury

3. Letarte P: Brain and spinal cord injury. *In:* Multidisciplinary Critical Care Board Review Course. Roberts PR (Ed). Anaheim, CA, Society of Critical Care Medicine, 1998; pp 613–630
4. Bauer BL, Kuhn TJ (Eds): Severe Head Injuries: Pathology, Diagnosis and Treatment. Berlin, Springer-Verlag, 1993
5. Brain Trauma Foundation: Management and prognosis of severe traumatic brain injury. *J Neurotrauma* 2000; 17:449-627
6. Rosner MJ, Daughton S: Cerebral perfusion pressure in the management of head injury. *J Trauma* 1996; 30:933–941
7. Marion DW (Ed): Traumatic Brain Injury. New York, Thieme, 1999
8. Sarrafzadeh AS, Peltonen EE, Kaisers U, et al: Secondary insults in severe head injury-do multiply injured patients do worse? *Crit Care Med* 2001; 29:1116-1123

Management Guidelines for Common Problems in the Initial Care of Injury

9. Pasqulae M, Fabian TC, EAST *Ad Hoc* Committee on Practice Management Guideline Development: Practice management guidelines for trauma from Eastern Association for the Surgery of Trauma. *J Trauma* 1998; 44:941–957
10. Luchette FA, Borzotta AP, Croce MA, et al: Practice management guidelines for prophylactic antibiotic use in penetrating abdominal trauma: The EAST practice management guidelines workgroup. *J Trauma* 2000; 48:508-518

Chest Trauma

11. Miller PR, Croce MA, Bee TK, et al: ARDS after pulmonary contusion: accurate measurement of contusion volume identifies high risk patients. *J Trauma* 2001; 51:223-230
12. Malhotra AK, Fabian TC, Croce DS, et al: Minimal aortic injury: A lesion associated with advancing diagnostic techniques. *J Trauma* 2001; 51:1042-1048
13. Cohn SM: Pulmonary contusion: Review of the clinical entity. *J Trauma* 1997; 42:973-979

General Burn Management

14. Herndon DN (Ed): Total Burn Care, 2nd ed. London, WB Saunders, 2002
15. Monafo WW: Initial management of burns. *N Engl J Med* 1996; 335:1581–1586

Burn Outcome

16. Saffle JR, Davis B, Williams P: Recent outcomes in the treatment of burn injury in the United States: A report from the American Burn Association Patient Registry. *J Burn Care Rehabil* 1995; 16: 219–232
17. Ryan CM, Schoenfield DA, Thorpe WP, et al: Objective estimates of the probability of

death from burn injuries. *N Engl J Med* 1998; 338:362–366

Hyperbaric Oxygen

18. Tibbles PM, Edelsberg JS: Hyperbaric oxygen therapy. *N Engl J Med* 1996; 334:1642–1648

Abdominal Organ Injury

19. Bee TK, Croce MA, Miller PR, et al: Failures of splenic nonoperative management: is the glass half empty or half full? *J Trauma* 2001; 50:230-236
20. Peitzman AB, Heil B, Rivera L, et al: Blunt splenic injury in adults: Multi-institutional study. *J Trauma* 2000; 49:177-189
21. Richardson JD, Franklin GA, Lukan JK, et al: Evolution in the management of hepatic trauma: A 25-year perspective. *Ann Surg* 2000; 232:324-330
22. Malhotra AK, Fabian TC, Katsis SB, et al: Blunt bowel and mesenteric injuries: The role of screening computed tomography. *J Trauma* 2000; 49:991-1000
23. Killeen KL, Shanmuganathan K, Poletti PA, et al: Helical computed tomography of bowel and mesenteric injuries. *J Trauma* 2001; 51:26-36

Abdominal Compartment Syndrome

24. Schein M, Wittmann DH, Aprahamian C, Condon RE: The abdominal compartment syndrome: The physiological and clinical consequences of elevated intra-abdominal pressure. *J Am Coll Surg* 1995; 180:745-753
25. Chang MM, Miller PR, D'Agostino R Jr, Meredith JW: Effect of abdominal decompression on cardiopulmonary function and visceral perfusion in patients with intra-abdominal hypertension. *J Trauma* 1998; 44(3):440-445

PEDIATRIC SURGICAL CRITICAL CARE

Mary L. Brandt, MD

AIRWAY

Airway Anatomy

Nasopharynx. The nose is the site of over 33% of airway resistance at all ages. Although there is some controversy, infants are considered "obligate nasal breathers" [1]. The roof of the nasopharynx is flat, which accounts for the less resonant voice of childhood. This also means a smaller airway volume than seen in adults.

Oropharynx. In children, the mandible is smaller and the tongue is proportionally larger, with less forward displacement than in adults.

Larynx. The epiglottis in infants is elongated, omega-shaped (rather than rectangular), and more "floppy." The epiglottis is at the level of C1 at birth and overlaps the soft palate, effectively obstructing the oropharynx when in this position. It moves to the level of C3 by 6 months, and no longer overlaps the soft palate. In the adult, the epiglottis is located at C5-6.

Glottis. The glottis is funnel-shaped and angled posteriorly in the infant, compared with what is more of a straight column in the adult. **The cricoid is the narrowest part of the airway until age 8-10, then vocal cords are narrowest.**

Trachea. The trachea is one-third of adult diameter at birth. Since resistance can be estimated by the formula $R = 8l/r^4$, resistance is substantially higher in smaller airways. Clinically, this means that even small changes in radius (edema, secretions, foreign body) have much greater consequences in children than in adults.

Managing the Pediatric Airway [2]

As in adults, initial management of the airway consists in adequate positioning. In children, the "sniff position" is the most effective position to open the airway. Nasopharyngeal and oropharyngeal airways can also be used to aid in keeping the airway intact in a child who is otherwise able to support respirations.

Endotracheal intubation in children has 3 important physiologic effects. In infants who have a disproportionate parasympathetic tone, bradycardia is common. An anticholinergic agent, usually atropine, is given before intubation in all infants and small children for this reason. Endotracheal intubation also results in increased intracranial and intraocular pressures.

The technique of endotracheal intubation is different in children. The size of tube is most easily estimated by the size of the child's little finger. The mm of internal diameter can also be approximated by the formula mm I.D. = [age (yr)/4] + 4. Because the cricoid is the narrowest portion of the airway, an uncuffed tube is used until approximately age 6-8. Using the cricoid to create the snug fit allows the maximum diameter of tube to be used; adding a cuff decreases size you can use by 0.5, with a marked decrease of I.D. Because the epiglottis is omega-shaped and floppy, a straight blade (to actually lift the epiglottis up) is used on the laryngoscope. Nasotracheal intubations are rarely performed in children; because glottis is anterior and small, a blind nasotracheal intubation is next to impossible. Do not forget axial traction if cervical spine injury is suspected, even if initially radiographs are negative (Don't forget SCIWORA!) [3].

In children who cannot be intubated, a surgical airway is indicated. Although cricothyroidotomy is the most commonly used alternate airway in adults, this procedure is associated with an increased risk of injury in children who have a narrower airway. A needle cricothyroidotomy will allow oxygenation (but poor ventilation), and can be used for 30-45 minutes while preparation is made for a formal tracheostomy. Cricothyroidotomy should be avoided until after puberty, when at all possible. Tracheostomy in children is performed via a vertical tracheotomy (no flaps or cruciate incisions!). Postoperatively, displacement is much easier, and pneumothorax may occur more often than in adults. Stay sutures are essential, and most surgeons paralyze the children for 3 days while the site is healing [4].

Conditions Compromising the Airway

Pharynx. Choanal atresia is congenital obstruction of the posterior nares, with either a septum or bony structure. Macroglossia is most commonly associated with Beckwith-Wiedeman syndrome (large infant, macroglossia, umbilical anomalies [large hernia or omphalocele] pancreatic hyperplasia with postnatal hypoglycemia). If this constellation of findings are present, serum glucose should be checked to avoid developmental delay due to hypoglycemia. Children with Pierre-Robin syndrome have a recessed and hypoplastic mandible and glossoptosis (tongue falls back).

Larynx. Congenital or acquired obstructions of the larynx in children include subglottic stenosis and web formation. Epiglottitis, which was previously an important cause of airway obstruction in 2-6-year-old children is rare in the era of the *H. influenza* vaccine. This is caused by acute inflammation with swelling of the epiglottis and is nearly always caused by *H. influenza*. If this diagnosis is suspected, a lateral CXR/soft tissue neck film will usually demonstrate the swelling. The child should go STAT to the OR, with no largyngoscopy performed outside of the operating room. Laryngomalacia presents with inspiratory stridor in children 1-2 months of age. No treatment is required; as the airway increases in diameter, the symptoms disappear.

Trachea. Tracheoesophageal fistula with or without esophageal atresia (TEF) is discussed in the section on newborn surgical emergencies. Laryngotracheobronchitis (croup) is usually viral in origin, and is most commonly caused by parainfluenza A and B. This presents most commonly in children 3 months - 3 years of age. It is treated with humidified air/oxygen ("croup tent") and racemic epinephrine. Tracheomalacia is a congenital deficiency of supporting cartilage in the trachea. As with laryngomalacia, the majority of children outgrow the stridor as their airway increases in diameter. For those children with life-threatening airway compromise, an aortopexy (suspension of the anterior wall of the aorta to the posterior sternum) may be indicated. Extrinsic compression of the trachea can occur in childhood from an anomalous thyroid. thyroglossal duct cyst, cervical teratoma, cystic hygroma, or other more uncommon tumors.

BREATHING

Normal lung development. Lung development begins early; the bronchial tree is complete by the sixteenth week. Alveoli continue to develop up to 8 years of age. The lung is a solid organ initially, but begins to canalize around 20 weeks. The cellular development begins around 28 weeks. There are 2 important cells in the alveoli, which begin to develop during this period. Type 1 pneumocytes are flat cells with little cytoplasm, and are important in the regulation of gas diffusion. Type 2 pneumocytes have microvilli and inclusions and produce surfactant. Surfactant is composed of 85% phospholipid (phosphatidylcholine [70-80% of lipids] and phosphatidylglycerol [5-10% of lipids]), 5% neutral lipids, 5% carbohydrates, and 10% proteins. Between 28 and 32 weeks, there is rapid maturation and differentiation. This can be measured *in utero* by an L/S ratio. Lecithin increases with maturation and sphyingomyelin remains constant. An L/S ratio of 2:1 = relatively mature lung. This maturation can be accelerated by *in utero* steroids.

Neonatal respiratory physiology. The chest wall of infants is more compliant. The chest wall recoil is ZERO in mature infants. The intercostal muscles must be "set" to avoid movement of the chest wall with diaphragmatic excursion, i.e., fatigue will decompensate the whole system. The lungs, however, are less compliant. Infants have a low FRC. The passive FRC (inward force = outward force) gives a resting lung volume of 15% of lung volume (cf. 30% in an adult). Infants compensate for this by "inspiratory muscle braking" (i.e., starting inspiration before expiration is complete and by a high respiratory rate). The diaphragm in infants is different. There are more fast oxidative, fatigue-sensitive fibers (Type IIa) and fewer fatigue-resistant fibers (Type 1). The diaphragm is rounder and higher than adults, which gives a better length-tension ratio

(Laplace's law P=2T/r) and better contraction. This advantage, however, is negated with increased intrathoracic or intraabdominal pressure.

Airway resistance In adults, 50% of resistance is from the nose; in infants, this is only 33%. Obstruction of the nose can dramatically increase the work of breathing in infants (e.g., NG tubes, choanal atresia). The lower airways contribute more to resistance than in adults. Small airways contribute more to resistance in infants (50%) than adults. This infant pattern does not change until 5-6 years of age. Diseases affecting small airways (e.g., bronchiolitis) have a greater effect in children.

Diseases of the Respiratory System

Hyaline Membrane Disease (HMD) is a disorder of inadequate surfactant production, usually due to the immaturity of structural components of the airway. This leads to collapse of terminal respiratory units at end-expiration. Infants at risk include infants < 35 weeks gestation, or < 38 weeks gestation if mother is diabetic, and infants delivered by C section without prior labor. The treatment is artificial surfactant and ventilatory support. Complications of HMD include pneumothorax (30% of patients with HMD who require mechanical ventilation), pulmonary interstitial emphysema (P.I.E.), and bronchopulmonary dysplasia.

Apnea in newborns is usually idiopathic. Other causes of apnea include hypoxia, hypoglycemia, sepsis, meningitis, intraventricular hemorrhage, electrolyte imbalance, obstructive apnea, Pierre-Robin syndrome, and macroglossia. Monitoring is indicated in all newborns < 33-34 weeks gestation and all preterm (< 37 weeks gestation) infants after surgery (until 44-54 weeks postconceptional age). The treatment of apnea is tactile stimulation. If it is prolonged, empty stomach then bag with mask. These infants are given IV caffeine as well. In severe cases, intubation and mechanical ventilation may be necessary.

Transient tachypnea of the newborn is the most common lung disease of the newborn. It is due to inadequate removal of lung water from the interstitium during delivery and is more common after cesarean section. The gas exchange resolves after 24-48 hours and tachypnea in several days. The therapy is respiratory support only.

Meconium aspiration. Meconium is present in amniotic fluid in 10% of births. If there is fetal asphyxia prior to or near the time of delivery, the fetus develops "apnea," then "gasping" of amniotic fluid. After birth, there can be patchy bilateral airway obstruction (mechanical). There is a low correlation of x-ray findings with severity in the first 24 hours. Inflammation (especially to bile salts) increases during the second 24 hours and creates a VQ mismatch: > hypoxemia, > pulmonary hypertension, > R to L shunt (most important element of the pathophysiology). These infants probably have an underlying problem more significant than the mechanical aspiration of the meconium. This condition probably represents chronic hypoxia *in utero* as the muscular walls of the pulmonary arteries in these infants are hypertrophied (and therefore more sensitive to hypoxia). These infants are usually postmature (> 41 weeks) infants. The initial presentation may be mild and then deteriorate. The treatment is to: a) suction out meconium (this is probably not as important as once thought - the meconium is probably more a marker of chronic distress than the cause of acute distress); b) start mechanical ventilation. (PEEP [other than physiologic] is not of great benefit.) If the infant cannot be supported adequately with the ventilator, ECMO should be considered.

Congenital diaphragmatic hernia. The posterior (Bochdalek) is more common than anterior (Morgagni), and left is more common than right. The mortality is from pulmonary hypoplasia and PPHN, not the mechanical problem with the hernia. This is discussed in the section on newborn surgical emergencies.

Congenital lung malformations may create expanding air-filled lesions, which create the physiologic effect of a tension pneumothorax. These include congenital cysts of the lung, congenital adenomatoid malformation, and lobar empysema (most common in the LUL). All of these lesions may require emergent surgical resection if they become overexpanded. Pulmonary sequestrations consist of nonfunctioning lung tissue (does not communicate with tracheobronchial tree) and come in 2 varieties: intralobar versus extralobar. These lesions have a systemic blood supply, usually directly from the aorta.

Pediatric Ventilators

Physiology of Respiratory Support. The distribution of perfusion depends on gravity-dependent distribution of blood flow, lung volume, cardiac output, and the degree of alveolar hypoxia. The distribution of ventilation depends on compliance, resistance, time constants, the work of breathing, lung volumes, and airway closure and ventilation/perfusion matching. There are also developmental considerations: Respiratory rate is faster in infants and children, who also have a shorter inspiratory time. Tidal volume remains 6-8 ml/kg at all ages, although the absolute volume increases with age (18 ml/breath in newborn versus 500 ml/breath in adults) Inspiratory flow averages1.9 liters/min newborn (compared with 24 liters/min in the adult). Peak inspiratory flow is 20 liters/min in the newborn (300-600 liters/min adult). Respiratory compliance based on weight remains constant (0.06 ml/cm H_2O/ml lung volume), but the absolute value increases by 20 from newborn to adolescence.

Oxygen Therapy. Oxygen can be delivered by a variety of delivery systems: Venturi systems, simple face masks, nasal cannulae, reservoir systems, oxygen hoods, or oxygen tents. Oxygen toxicity is progressive, with early parenchymal changes, destruction of type I pneumocytes, decreased mucocilliary clearance, hyperplasia of type II pneumocytes, and fibrosis. In the premature infant, retinopathy of prematurity is added to this list.

Types of Mechanical Ventilation. Mechanical ventilation can be carried out by negative-pressure ventilation (still used in select cases) or, more commonly, positive-pressure ventilation. Ventilators can be classified by what initiates the breath (patient, ventilator, or combination), what terminates inspiration (time limited, pressure limited, volume limited, flow limited, or mixed), and what the pattern is of inspiratory flow (constant, sine wave, decelerating). The conventional modes of mechanical ventilation include control mode ventilation, assist-control mode ventilation, intermittent mandatory ventilation, pressure support ventilation, and mandatory minute ventilation. Unconventional modes of mechanical ventilation include inverse ratio ventilation and high-frequency ventilation.

Indications for Ventilation. Positive-pressure support is indicated when there is inadequate alveolar ventilation, failure of arterial oxygenation, to secure control of breathing, in patients with intracranial hypertension, when there is circulatory insufficiency, or to decrease the work of breathing.

Initiation of Mechanical Ventilation. To initiate ventilation for volume-controlled ventilation (used in older children), the rate should be set at the physiologic norm for age, the tidal volume at 12-15 ml/kg, the I/E ratio at usually 1:2, and PEEP as indicated. For the pressure-controlled ventilator (used in infants), **the rate again is set at the physiologic norm** for age. The PIP is increased to provide adequate ventilation, which can be judged by adequate chest excursion or tidal volume (usually 20-30 cm H_2O). Again, the I/E ratio is set at usually 1:2, and PEEP is adjusted as indicated [5].

Extubation. The criteria for extubation in children is a normal pCO_2, a crying vital capacity > 15 ml/kg, a maximum NIP > 45 cm H_2O, and adequate oxygenation[5].

Table 122-3   Normal Vital Signs in Children

Age	Heart Rate* (bpm)		Respiratory Rate (per min)
	Awake	Sleeping	
Infant	120-160	80-180	30-60
Toddler	90-140	70-120	24-40
Preschool age	80-110	60-90	22-34
School age	75-100	60-90	18-30
Adolescent	60-90	50-90	12-16

Age	Blood Pressure (mm Hg)†	
	Systolic	Diastolic
Neonate (1 mo)	85-100	51-65
Infant (6 mo)	87-105	53-66
Toddler (2 yr)	95-105	53-66
School age (7 yr)	97-112	57-71
Adolescent (15 yr)	112-128	66-80

Respiratory Monitoring

With increased morbidity from invasive monitoring, noninvasive monitoring takes on an even greater importance in infants and children [6].

Pulse Oximetry. Basic concept: reduced and oxygenated hemoglobin absorb light differently at specific wavelengths. The addition of plethysmography ensures that Hg is measured in a pulsatile flow. There are 2 light sources: red light and infrared light. It is important to know about the potential sources of error in ill children. There can be a difference in the calculated (pulse ox) versus measured (blood gas) paO2. The calculation of saturation by the pulse oximeter assumes normal, adult oxihemoglobin desaturation curve. A shift in the curve to the left will give falsely high values (e.g., deficiency of 2,3-DPG, transfusions, phosphate depletion due to malnutrition). A shift in the curve to the right will give falsely low values (e.g., increased 2,3-DPG from sickle cell anemia, chronic hypoxia, or high altitudes). Ambient light, particularly the infrared lights used in infant warmers, bilirubin lights, and fluorescent lights can cause errors in the readings. The 2 other important causes of error are venous pulsations (obstructed venous return, severe right heart failure, tricuspid regurgitation, measurement in a dependent area, wide swings of intrathoracic pressure) and motion artifact [7].

Abnormal Hemaglobins and the Effect on Pulse Oximetry. Fetal hemoglobin is the same as adult hemoglobin at the 2 wavelengths used in routine pulse oximeter [8]. There will be inaccurate measurements in the presence of HgF if 4 wavelength oximeter is used (wavelengths added for carboxyhemoglobin and methhemoglobin). Most clinically routine dyshemoglobins have similar wavelengths as HgA.

Capnography. If there is no VQ mismatch, $PaCO_2$ and the partial pressure of end-tidal CO_2 ($PetCO_2$) should be virtually equal. A normal capnogram is characaterized by zero baseline during early exhalation, a sharp upstroke during mid-exhalation, a relatively horizontal alveolar plateau, and a sharp downstroke and return to a zero baseline. There are 2 physiologic assumptions for capnography:

a) that ventilation and perfusion are matched, and b) that the lung units empty completely and will approximately equal time constants. An abnormal capnogram means 1 of 3 things: an anomaly in the patient's cardiopulmonary system, b) a malfunction in the airway, or c) a malfunction in the gas delivery system. A gradually decreasing end-tidal CO_2 may represent falling body temperature (decreased metabolism), a slowly decreasing pulmonary or systemic perfusion (mismatched V-Q), or hyperventilation (mismatched V-Q). A sustained low $etCO_2$ without good plateaus means that full exhalation is not occuring before the next breath (secretions in airway, bronchospasm, partial obstruction of ET tube or that the patient's TV is being diluted with fresh gas. In children with a small tidal volume, the sample collected may be so proportionally large that it is mixed with the incoming fresh gas. An exponential decrease in $etCO_2$ = BIG PROBLEM (sudden hypotension, circulatory arrest with continued ventilation, pulmonary embolism with thrombus or air).

Extracorporeal Membrane Oxygenation (ECMO)

There are 2 types of circuit for ECMO: venoarterial and venovenous. In venoarterial ECMO, the venous cannula is introduced via the internal jugular and positioned in the right atrium. Venous blood flows to the reservoir by gravity, so adequate venous volume must be maintained and other problems which limit right atrial filling (i.e., pneumothorax, pneumomediastinum) must be corrected. The blood flows to the membrane oxygenator and returns to the patient via a cannula in the carotid artery. Venovenous ECMO requires normal cardiac function. A double lumen venous catheter, placed in the internal jugular, is used in infants. The iliac vein and internal jugular are used (2 separate cannulae) in older children.

Oxygen exchange is carried out via 30% oxygen in membrane = 228 torr (at sea level). The PO2 of the blood is usually around 40 torr, but this varies with oxygen delivery and consumption. The driving pressure for gas exchange = 228 - 40, or 188 torr, which is adequate to saturate blood to 95% [9].

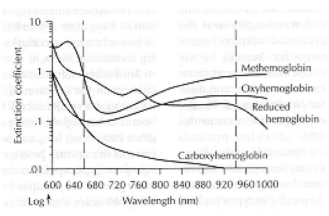

Carbon dioxide exchange is maintained by keeping the CO_2 in the membrane gas < 5%. The membrane coefficient for CO_2 is higher (x6) than oxygen; despite small differences in blood and membrane CO_2, there is easy diffusion [9].

The usual clinical problems which require ECMO include meconium aspiration syndrome, respiratory distress syndrome, sepsis, persistent pulmonary hypertension of the newborn, and congenital diaphragmatic hernia. The contraindications to ECMO are weight < 2000gm, intracranial hemorrhage > Grade I (confined to germinal matrix), and irreversible respiratory failure.

Selection criteria for infants is based on a predicted mortality rate > 80% [9]. These criteria are:

Alveolar-arterial oxygenation difference ($AaDO_2$) > 610 × 8 hours, or > 605 × 4 hours, if PIP >38 cm H_2O. ($AaDO_2$ = RAO_2 - RaO_2, PAO_2 = FIO_2 (760 - 47) - ($PaCO_2$/RQ), $AaDO_2$ = FIO_2 (760 -14) - ($PaCO_2$/RQ) - PaO_2)

Oxygenation index (OI) > 40. OI = (mean airway pressure × FIO_2 × 100)/postductal PaO_2

Acute deterioration with PaO_2 < 40 torr × 2 hours and/or pH < 7.15 × 2 hours

Unresponsiveness: PaO_2 < 55 torr and pH < 7.40 × 3 hours

Barotrauma (any 4 of 7 simultaneously): pneumothorax, pneumopericardium, pneumoperitoneum, pulmonary interstitial emphysema, persistent air leak > 24 hours, mean airway pressure > 15 cm H_2O, and subcutaneous emphysema.

To wean from ECMO, flow is decreased by 10 to 20 mL/min if PaO_2 > 60 torr and venous saturation > 65%. When ECMO flow reaches 60 to 70 mL/kg/min, the ventilator is increased to FIO_2 0.3 to 0.4 and IMV to 20 breath/min. If adequate PaO_2 and/or venous saturation is maintained, weaning is continued. A trial off pump is then attempted prior to removing the cannulae.

Complications of ECMO include bleeding (cannulation sites, chest tubes, etc., GI, pulmonary and intracranial bleeding, which occurs in 11% of patients and leads to death in 2%), infection, hypertension, and mechanical malfunction.

Outcome after ECMO. Overall, 83% of infants treated with ECMO survive. The average time on ECMO is 5 to 7 days. Sixty-six percent of infants are neurologically normal, 33% have damage (23% have sensorineural hearing loss, mild to severe deficits in motor or cognitive function). Although there is no immediate consequence of ligation of the carotid artery, there may be long-term effects that we do not know yet.

CIRCULATION

Hemodynamic Monitoring-Arterial Lines. Pediatric vessels react differently than adult vessels, which may affect monitoring of blood pressure. Impedance is the ratio of change in pressure to change in flow and is a function of resistance and reactance. Resistance is mostly affected by the length and caliber of the blood vessels and the viscosity of the blood. This may particularly play a role in newborn infants who have polycythemia. Reactance is a function of the complicance of the vessel and the inertia of the blood. Pediatric vessels are very elastic, therefore have higher reactance (and therefore higher impedance) than adult vessels. Arterial lines in children are most often placed in the radial artery. In newborn infants, the right radial is used if preductal blood sampling is indicated. Other sites for the placement of arterial lines includes the posterior tibial, dorsalis pedis, and axillary arteries. The femoral artery is avoided, if possible, due to risk of osteomyelitis (even single punctures!). Because of the risk of upper extremity ischemia, the brachial artery is essentially never used. The technique of placement is the same as adults but smaller; a 24-g catheter is used for newborns and a 22-g in children.

The complications of arterial lines in children include complications common to adults, such as infection and ischemia. Complications specific to the pediatric population include malfunction or overuse of the heparin flush with fluid overload or full heparinization . Arterial lines in children should never be flushed with a large, aggressive bolus. The monitor should be used when flushing the line to ensure that the pressure of the flush does not exceed the pulse pressure. An overly aggressive flush can lead to retrograde flow into the coronary or cerebral circulation. If this occurs, a small air bubble can be fatal or lead to coronary or cerebral infarct [10].

In newborn infants, during the first 7-10 days of life, the umbilical vessels can also be used for vascular access. There are usually 2 arteries and 1 vein. When introduced into the umbilical vessel, the arterial catheter will first pass caudally into the iliac vessels, then cranially into the aorta. The position of the tip of the catheter is very important; if not positioned properly, thrombotic complications can occur. There are 2 accepted positions: a) high (below ductus arteriosus but above celiac artery) and b) low (between IMA and aortic bifurcation). The fundamental concept is to avoid placing the tip near the SMA or renal arteries.

Hemodynamic Monitoring: Pulmonary Artery Catheters. With the exception of children with congenital heart disesase, underlying cardiac dysfunction is unusual in the pediatric population. Therefore, most pediatric patients do not benefit from the added information received from pulmonary artery catheters. For the rare patient that does need a PA catheter, there are smaller sizes available (5 Fr, 70 cm). In small children, these are usually placed via the femoral vein.

Venous Access in the Child. The smaller peripheral catheters which are necessary in children result in higher resistance and lower flows (Poiseuille-Hagen equation). $F = ([Pa - Pb] \times r^4 \times 3.14)/(8 \times n \times l)$ or $R = (8 \times n \times l)/(3.14 \times r^4)$ where F is flow rate, Pa - Pb is pressure gradient along the tube, r is tube radius, n is viscosity coefficient of the fluid, and R is resistance. In addition to peripheral IVs and cutdowns (typically the saphenous or basilica), vascular access can also be obtained via the interosseous route in children. The interosseous route allows rapid and nearly equivalent volume delivery. All resuscitation drugs can be given safely via this route. The only exception is Bretyllium; since it is fat soluble, it does not distribute into the systemic circulation. The only contraindications to using this technique are a known coagulopathy and the presence of a fracture in the bone being considered for infusion. The interosseous cannula, which is a bone marrow biopsy needle, is placed in the anterior tibia, 1 cm inferior and 1 cm medial to the tibial tubercle. Alternate sites include the midline of distal femur, 3 cm proximal to external condyles, the distal tibia just proximal to medial malleolus, and the anterior superior iliac spine. The technique is to insert the needle with the solid trocar in place, until a "give" is felt. A check is then made that the needle is lodged in the bone. The trocar is removed and the needle aspirated for return of marrow. It is then flushed with saline and the area inspected to assure that there is no soft tissue extravasation. This technique is absolutely effective in children less than 2, but may be possible (depending on bone density) in children up to age 6. Despite the fact that this is usually performed in a very ill child, in a stressful situation, It is very important that the technique be done deliberately and carefully, with a proper sterile field. The complications of this technique can mostly be prevented by careful attention to the preparation and insertion of the cannula. The complications include extravasation into subcutaneous tissue, extravasation into the muscular compartments with compartment syndrome, bone fracture, osteomyelitis. Although fat and bone marrow embolism was suggested as a potential complication, this has never been reported following use of an intraosseous cannula.

Endotracheal Access to the Circulation. In children, venous access is often the weakest link in the chain of resuscitation. In situations of extreme emergency, the "LEAN" drugs (Lidocaine, Epinephrine, Atropine, and Narcan) can be given via an endotracheal tube. The dose for these drugs is usually around 10 times the IV dose. The drugs should be delivered distally into the lung by passing small suction catheter to the tip of the ET tube, injecting, then bagging.

Central Venous Catheters. Central venous catheters are used routinely in children in the intensive care units. These are placed usually by the Seldinger technique or direct cut down. The tip is positioned in the SVC or proximal atrium, but not deep into the heart. Although rare, perforation of the heart has been reported following placement of central venous catheters [11]. Although traditionally these lines have been placed in the femoral vein or internal jugular vein, the subclavian can be used even in tiny infants if an appropriate size line is chosen.

Transition From Fetal to Postnatal Circulation. In utero, circulation is designed to bypass the lungs, and provide oxygenated blood from the placenta to the systemic circulation of the fetus. The right and left heart work as circuits in parallel, rather than circuits in series. Oxygenated blood from the placenta returns to the heart via the umbilical vein. Both the right and left ventricles pump blood into the descending thoracic aorta. Blood from the right ventricle enters the thoracic aorta via the patent ductus arteriosus. Only 7% of the cardiac output enters the pulmonary circulation. The single most important factor that keeps the blood from entering the pulmonary circulation is the elevated pulmonary resistance. At birth, the infant enters "transitional" circulation. **The first and critical event is a sudden fall in the pulmonary resistance as the baby takes his/her first breath.** Because of the initially high resistance, at birth, the flow in the PDA is right to left. As the pulmonary resistance falls, this shunt decreases. At the point when the pulmonary pressures fall below the systemic pressures, the shunt reverses and becomes left to right. The process of transition ultimately results in reversal of flow in the ductus arteriosus with subsequent closure, closure of ductus venosus, and closure of the foramen ovale. By the end of

24 hours, the ductus arteriosus functionally closes. However, the ductus arteriosus does not close completely until 10-14 days. **During this critical period, any stress which results in elevated pulmonary pressures can reopen the ductus arteriosus.** The pulmonary vasculature of infants has increased muscularity (i.e., is more sensitive to stimuli). This is clinically manifested by hypoxia, which is resistant to treatment and was previous called PFC (Persistent Fetal Circulation). Currently, this is refered to as PPHN (Persistent Pulmonary Hypertension of the Newborn).

Patent Ductus Arteriosus. The premature infant has a slightly different physiology; the pulmonary vasculature has less muscle in wall than the term infant, and is therefore less vasoreactive. Premature infants have lower pulmonary vascular pressure and more left-to-right shunting. The more premature the infant, the less likely the PDA will close. This results in a persistent left-to-right shunt with decreased peripheral perfusion (which can lead to renal and GI ischemia) and increased pulmonary congestion. The closure of the PDA becomes important to protect the marginal pulmonary function of these immature infants. **The treatment of infants with a PDA is fluid restriction (< 150ml/kg/day) and pharmacologic (indomethacin) or surgical closure of the ducuts. The contraindications to attempting closure with indomethicin include oliguria, thrombocytopenia, or an evolving hemorrhage.**

Oxygen delivery and consumption. Oxygen consumption in children, in general is higher than adults, primarily because of the metabolic demands of growth (175 ml/min/m^2 versus 100 ml/min/m^2). In young infants, 3-13% of O_2 consumption goes toward growth. In addition, temperature regulation and fever also places significant metabolic demands on children. Maintaining termperature is harder in children than adults, and a significant problem in infants, particularly premature infants. Fever, which is common and often high in children, increases oxygen consumption 10-13% for each degree C elevation. With increased oxygen consumption, the margin for supply-dependent oxygen consumption decreases ($VO_2 = Q$ x $[CaO_2 - CvO_2]$ x 0.01). At rest, in normal adults, the amount of oxygen delivered (DO_2) is greatly in excess of the oxygen consumed (VO_2). When oxygen delivery falls, a critical point is reached when oxygen delivery = oxygen consumption (critical SOT or Systemic Oxygen Transport). Any fall below this level leads to a fall in oxygen consumption - oxygen consumption then becomes a function not only of metabolic demands, but of oxygen delivery as well (i.e., "supply dependent oxygen consumption"). Because children have higher metabolic demands (i.e., higher oxygen consumption), they are more at risk of entering this portion of the curve with decreases in SOT. Oxygen delivery $\{(DO_2 = Q \times CaO_2 \times 0.01)$ with $(CaO_2 = (1.34 \times Hb \times SaO_2) + (PaO_2 \times 0.003)\}$ is affected by a decrease in O_2 saturation, a decrease in oxygen carrying capacity, and/or a decrease in cardiac output. One of the factors that affects oxygen carrying capacity is the amount and type of hemoglobin available. Because 80% of Hg is fetal at birth, newborn infants need a higher cardiac output to effectively deliver oxygen. This increased cardiac output persists for 4-6 weeks, until the levels of fetal hemoglobin decrease. Children not only have a physiologic anemia (nadir at 6 months with an increase to normal Hg levels by 12 months), but may have significant nutritional-based anemia as well. In addition, undiagnosed sickle cell anemia, thalessemia, or other hemoglobinemias may complicate oxygen delivery in children.

Cardiac output is a product of EDV (preload), ejection fraction, and heart rate. **Cardiac output is rate dependent in small children**. This is particularly true (and important) in newborns. The cutoff for rate dependency is around a size of 6 kg. Decreased cardiac output from decreased preload in children can be caused by hypovolemia, sepsis, severe pulmonary hypertension (with RV encroachment on LV filling), severe arrhythmias, or rapid pericardial effusion (septic pericarditis). Increased afterload may also affect cardiac output and can be the result of severe systemic hypertension, coarctation, or severe polycythemia. With the exception of congenital heart disease, children do not usually have any underlying cardiac disease which directly affects cardiac ontractility (ejection fraction). However, sepsis, acidosis, hypoglycemia, hypoxia, hyperkalemia,

hypocalcemia, cardiomyopathy, and myocarditis may result in decreased cardiac contractility.

Shock

The basic principles of treating shock are no different in children than adults. The fundamental goal is to increase oxygen delivery in order to assure that oxygen delivery is greater than oxygen consumption. Oxygen delivery is improved by maintaining arterial oxygen saturation, optimizing hemoglobin, and maintaining optimal cardiac output and systemic blood flow. This is usually accomplished by correcting acidosis (1-2 mEq NaBicarb/kg body weight for metabolic acidosis with pH < 7.2), and manipulating the components of cardiac output. Since the issue is oxygen delivery for a given level of oxygen consumption, it is also beneficial to decrease the amount of oxygen consumed by assisting ventilation, using muscle relaxants to paralyze the patient, controlling fever or hypothermia, and decreasing anxiety with appropriate drugs.

Hypovolemic Shock. As in adults, increasing loss of blood volume results in increasing levels of hypovolemic shock. The diagnosis of hypovolemic shock in children, however, may be more difficult because of the different physiology of children. Children can vasoconstrict much more effectively than adults, and therefore can maintain their blood pressure until very late. Hypotension is, for children, often a terminal event. Because pediatric heart rates are higher to begin with, and stress (e.g., pain, or being in the emergency room or ICU) can increase this even more, tachycardia may not be as reliable in children. Skin changes and mental status are the most reliable indicators of

SOT = Q x [(1.34 x Hb x O2 sat) + (.003 x PaO2)] x 0.01

A. HYPOXIC HYPOXIA

   DISTURBANCE: ↓ O2 sat, ↓ PaO2 → ↓ SOT

   ACUTE COMPENSATION: ↑ Q → ↑ SOT (NL)

   CHRONIC COMPENSATION: ↑ Hb → ↓ Q, ↔ SOT (NL)

B. ANEMIC HYPOXIA

   DISTURBANCE: ↓ Hb → ↓ SOT

   ACUTE AND CHRONIC COMPENSATION: ↑ Q, ↔ O2 sat → ↑ SOT (NL)

C. STAGNANT HYPOXIA

   DISTURBANCE: ↓ Q → ↓ SOT

   COMPENSATION: NONE (↔ Hb, ↔ O2 sat → ↓ SOT)

early shock. The initial response of the newborn to hypovolemia is tachycardia. But, as this response is quickly maximized, subsequent response is most often bradycardia and acidosis.

The blood volume in children, as in adults, is approximately 70-75 ml/kg. In term infants, blood volume is 80 ml/kg and in premature infants, 90-100 ml/kg. Therefore, in an average 10-kg toddler, the total blood volume will be around 700-750 ccs. A 10-15% blood volume loss (or 70-80 ccs in the average toddler) will result in mild to moderate tachycardia, and some cutaneous vasoconstriction. A 25% blood volume loss (or 175-187 ccs in the average toddler) will result in tachycardia, decreased pulse pressure, cutaneous vasoconstriction, +/- hypotension.

The etiology of hypovolemic shock in children is from whole blood loss, plasma loss, or fluid and electrolyte loss. Whole blood loss may occur from trauma or GI bleeding in children. Infants who have open fontanelles and cranial sutures that are not yet fixed can develop hypovolemic shock from intracranial bleeding. **This is the one exception to the surgical dictum that head trauma alone cannot cause hypotension.** Vasodilitation, which can occur in response to sepsis, spinal cord injury, sepsis, or anaphylaxis, may result in a relative loss of volume with resulting shock. Plasma loss can occur following burns, or in patients with capillary

leak syndrome from inflammation, sepsis, or anaphylaxis. Protein losing disease of childhood such as nephrotic syndrome or protein enteropathies can also result in significant plasma loss. Childhood viral illness, with vomiting and diarrhea, can result in significant fluid and electrolyte loss. Other less common causes of fluid and electrolyte loss include the use (or toxic ingestion) of diuretics, adrenal insufficiency, diabetes insipidus, and DKA. Adrenal insufficiency may occur from sudden withdrawal of glucosteroid therapy, destruction of adrenal tissue, autoimmune disease, meningococcus or other infection, or hemorrhage into the adrenal gland (particularly in infants). The classic findings which should suggest the diagnosis of acute adrenal insufficiency include hyponatremia, hyperkalemia, hypoglycemia, and evidence of hemoconcentration.

The treatment of hypovolemic shock in children is volume. The initial bolus should be an isotonic crystalloid bolus of 20ml/kg, which is repeated once. If there is inadequate response and patient has a low hemoglobin or has lost blood, 10-20 cc/kg of blood is given next. One of the hardest issues for surgeons who do not routinely treat children is estimating the weight of a child in shock. Although there is a formula for calculating the weight of children, in the shock room, it is probably more convenient to remember 3

Table 1. Basic Resuscitation Drugs in Children

Epinephrine	10 mcg/kg = 0.1ml/kg (1:10,000)	
atropine	0.02 mg/kg = .1 cc/kg	max 1 mg (child) max 2 mg (adolescent)
lidocaine	1mg/kg IV loading then 100 mg in 100 ml D5W	(wt in kg)ml/hr = 17 mcg/kg/min
Na bicarb	1 Meq/kg IV	
dopamine/dobutamine	60mg in 100 ml D5W	(wt in kg)ml/hr = 10mcg/kg/min
isoproterenol/epinephrine	1 mg in 100 ml D5W	(wt in kg) ml/hr = 0/167 mcg/kg/min
Defibrillation currents		
V fib.	start with 2 watt-sec/kg increase to 4 watt-sec/kg	
V. tach/ SVT	start with 1-2 watt-sec/kg	

numbers: A newborn weighs 3 kg, a 1-year-old child weighs 10 kg, and children reach 20 kg at about 5 years of age.

Cardiogenic Shock. Cardiogenic shock, particularly in infants may be difficult to diagnose. By history, these infants have some increase in respiratory effort, poor feeding and weight gain, and excessive sweating. The history of sweating during feedings should always lead to an evaluation of possible cardiac disease in an infant. On physical examination, the key finding, unlike adults, is hepatomegaly. In addition, arrhythmias (particularly tachycardia), a gallop, wheezing, or rales may be appreciated on physical examination. In older children, the history and physical exam is similar to adults. The etiology of cardiac insufficiency in childhood includes arrhythmias, cardiomyopathies, and congenital heart disease. The most common heart rate abnormalities are supraventricular tachycardia, ventricular dysrhythmias, and bradycardia. Cardiomyopathies can be hypoxic/ischemic in origin (such as following trauma or an arrest from other causes), metabolic (hypoglycemia, hypocalcemia, acidosis, thyroid disorders, hypothermia, glycogen storage disorders), infectious (generalized sepsis, myocarditis), vascular (Kawasaki's disease, polyarteritis nodosa, SLE, acute rheumatic fever), toxic (following accidental poisoning), or may be due to an underlying neuromuscular disease (muscular dystrophy). The treatment of cardiac insufficiency in childhood is tailored to the etiology. **However, because of the importance of rate in maintaining cardiac output, if you can only pick 1 cardiac drug in childhood - pick epinephrine {10 mcg/kg = 0.1ml/kg (1:10,000)}. The doses of other important resusciation drugs are given in Table 1.**

Obstructive Shock. Obstructive shock in children can be due to tension pneumothorax or dardiac tamponade. Infants with a coarctation or interrupted arch may present with obtructive shock. In these patients, prostaglandin E₁ is given to keep the PDA open prior to surgical correction of the aortic anomaly. Hypertensive emergencies in children, with subsequent shock, may be from a renal source, coarctation of the aorta, or excessive catecholamine production from a pheochromocytoma or neuroblastoma.

Septic shock. As in adults, most children with septic shock have a hyperdynamic initial state with fever and mental confusion being the predominant initial findings. Infants, who have a low cardiac reserve to start with, rarely, if ever, have this initial hyperdynamic stage. Hyperventilation, with hypocapnia and respiratory alkalosis may also be present and should always suggest sepsis as a source for shock when present. With progression, the patient may develop hemoynamic deterioration as the initially high cardiac output deteriorates. In addition, direct myocardial depression and a primary defect in tissue oxygen uptake may contribute to the overall deterioration of the patient.

Congenital Heart Disease

Congenital heart disease occurs commonly–about 1/140 births. It is often associated with other anomalies. In order of frequency, the anomalies seen in the newborn period include: PDA, transposition of the great vessels, VSD, complex heart disease, hypoplastic left heart syndrome, coarctation, and tetralogy of Fallot. In evaluating the newborn with suspected heart disease, it is easiest to first determine if they are cyanotic or not cyanotic.

Cyanotic Heart Disease. Important differential diagnosis is persistent pulmonary hypertension of the newborn. Otherwise, the defects which lead to cyantonic congenital heart disease can then further be divided on the basis of whether or not there is increased pulmonary vascularity on chest x-ray. The 3 cyanotic lesions associated with increased pulmonary vascularity on chest x-ray are transposition of the great vessel, truncus arteriosus, and total anomalous pulmonary venous return. The most common cyanotic lesion in this category is transposition of the great vessels. These are most commonly term babies, as this lesion is rare in premature infants. There is usually a systolic murmur. The immediate treatment is balloon atrial septostomy. Truncus arteriosus, in which the infant has a single ventricle or large VSD will also present as a cyanotic lesion with increased pulmonary vascularity. In infants with total anomalous pulmonary venous return, the pulmonary veins connect directly to the systemic

	CXR/exam	Murmur	Initial tx	Other info
		CYANOTIC LESIONS		
Transposition of the great vessels	Increased pulm vascularity, "egg-shaped heart with narrow base"	Systolic or none	Atrial septostomy and PGE1 initially, arterial switch in first 2 weeks of life	Most common cyanotic lesion
Truncus arteriosus	Increased pulm vascularity	Systolic upper stenum, diastolic rumble at apex	Treat failure (dig, diuretics), surgery before 3 months	Single vessel from heart
TAPVR	Increased pulm vascularity, hepatomegaly	Variable or absent	Surgical correction	Mimics RDS
Tetrology of Fallot	Decreased pulm vascularity	Loud systolic	Blalock-Taussig shunt, then correction 9-12 months	1. large, high VSD 2. pulm stenosis 3. overriding aorta "Tet spells"
Tricuspid atresia	Decreased pulm vascularity	Soft PDA murmur initially	PGE1, then pulm to systemic shunt. Fontan is definitive procedure-2 yearrs of age	
hypoplastic left heart syndrome	Nl pulm vascularity	Usually none	Defect incompatible with life for most. Norwood procedure for some	Acyanotic initially, become cyanotic in first days of life
Ebstein's anomaly	Decreased pulm vascular markings	Blowing systolic from tricuspid regurg	Medical support until improvement occurs	
		ACYANOTIC LESIONS		
VSD	Increased pulm vascularity	Holosystolic murmur	Small defects watched, large are closed	Ventricular L→R shunt
PDA	Increased pulm vascularity	Continuous or systolic "machinery" murmur	Indomethacin or surgical closure	Aortic L→R shunt, bounding peripheral pulses
AV canal	Increased pulm vascularity	Holosystolic murmur		Ventricular L→R shunt
partial anomalous venous return	Increased pulm vascularity	Short syst murmur in pulm window, wide S2		Atrial L→R shunt
ASD	Increased pulm vascularity	Short syst murmur in pulm window, wide S2		Atrial L→R shunt
Pulmonary stenosis	Decreased pulm vascularity , RH enlargement	Systolic ejection at LU sternum, radiates peripherally	PGE1 at birth if critical, balloon valvuloplasty	Often aysymptomatic until older
aortic stenosis	Nl pulm vascularity	May or may not have a murmur	PGE1 in infancy, balloon or surgical valvotomy	
aortic insufficiency	Nl pulm vascularity			
coarctation of the aorta	Nl pulm vascularity	May or may not have a murmure	PGE1 then surgery	One of most common causes of CHF in first week of life
congenital mitral stenosis	Nl pulm vascularity			

venous system via the right atrium, right SVC, or axygous veins. In this condition, a murmur may be variable or absent. Total anomalous pulmonary return is surgically corrected in infancy. The 3 cyanotic heart defects which have decreased pulmonary vascularity are Tetrology of Fallot, tricuspic atresia, and Ebstein's anomaly. The 4 components of the Tetrology of Fallot are a VSD, obstruction to RV outflow, overriding aorta, and RVH. A loud systolic murmur is usually present. In tricuspid atresia, a systolic murmur is usually present. This anomaly is treated with prostaglandin E_1. Ebstein's anomaly is a malformation of the tricuspid valve. There is severe regurgitation, and the right ventricle becomes "atrialized"

Acyanotic heart disease. As with cyanotic heart disease, these lesions can be further subdivided based on the state of the pulmonary vascularity seen on CXR (Table {Congenital heart disease}). The acyanotic lesions with increased pulmonary vascular markings are VSD, PDA, AV canal, partial anomalous venous return, and ASD. The only significant acyanotic lesion with decreased pulmonary markings is pulmonary stenosis. Acyanotic lesions which have normal appearing pulmonary vascular markings include: aortic stenosis, aortic insufficiency, coarctation of the aorta, hypoplastic left heart syndrome, and congenital mitral stenosis.

Temperature Regulation In Children [12]

Premature infants are particularly susceptible to heat loss because they have smaller subcutaneous fat stores, smaller mass-to-body surface ratio, a more open and exposed resting posture, and immature temperature regulating mechanism. Newborns do not shiver; temperature control is by "non-shivering thermogenesis." The control of hypothermia in infants is very important; calories used to maintain temperature are calories not used for growth. Severe hypothermia in infants can result in DIC. The goal in caring for infants is to create a Neutral Thermal Environment (NTE), which is defined as "the ambient temperature range in which an infant utilizes the fewest calories to maintain a normal and constant core temperature." NTE varies with size, postnatal and postconceptional age. Oxygen consumption increases above and below NTE.

There are 4 sources of heat loss in infants and children: a) Evaporation, which is caused by moisture on the skin of the child. This can be prevented by drying off any extraneous moisture, waterproof barriers under OR drapes, maintaining 50% relative humidity in incubators. b) Conduction, when the child is in direct contact with a cold surface. Warming blankets in the OR are an example of prevention. c) Convection, when air flows over the child. The incubators used for small infants, or directing heater or cooling ducts away from the child, are examples of prevention. d) Radiation, when the child radiates heat into cooler environment. This is probably the

single most important loss in infants. Controlling the temperature around the patient in the operating room, intensive care unit, or nursery is the most important control. Radiant loss can also be prevented by cotton batting around the extremities and plastic wrap around the head or body. The radiant warmers used in the neonatal intensive care unit also prevent radiant heat loss.

Fluid and Electrolytes: Pediatric Considerations

Anatomy of Body Fluid Compartments. Total body water, which averages 60% of weight for young men and 50% of weight for young women, is 75-80% of infants. Infants are born "fluid overloaded" and must undergo a physiologic diuresis in the first week of life. (Hence, maintenance fluids for a newborn are 70cc/kg/day and increase by 10cc/kg/day increments for each day of life until they are 100-120 cc/kg/day.) At 1 year of age, total body water is 65% of body weight. Intracellular fluid is roughly 30-40% of body weight and increases following birth as ECF increases. Extracellular fluid is roughly 20% of body weight (plasma = roughly 5% of body weight and interstitial fluid = roughly 15% of body weight). **The physiologic diuresis of the newborn comes from this compartment (ECF).**

Water Exchange. The adult normal daily intake of water is 2000 - 2500 mls/day. Adult daily loss includes 800 - 1500 mls in urine, 250 mls in stool, and 600 - 900 as insensible loss (75% from skin, which may increase as much as 250 ml for each degree of fever, and 25% from lungs.). An adult with an unhumidified tracheostomy can lose up to 1500 mls/day. Insensible losses in premature infants can reach extraordinary levels. Term infants lose 25% from lungs. Preemies lose proportionally less from the lungs because of high losses from the skin. The major determinants for the insensible loss from the skin are conceptional age and environmental (humidity, temperature). For infants < 30 weeks gestation, they will lose roughly 40 ml/kg/day at birth, 30 ml/kg/day at 1 week of age and 25 ml/kg/day at 1 month. For infants 30-36 weeks gestation, skin losses are 12 ml/kg/day at birth, 12 ml/kg/day at 1 week, and 7 ml/kg/day at 1 month. For infants > 36 weeks gestation, the loss is 7 ml/kg/day regardless of age. To these numbers, you should add 5 ml/kg/day if not mechanically ventilated. **Water loss increases by 50-140% under a radiant warmer and by 60% with phototherapy**. Water loss decreases by 50-70% if infant is covered with plastic.

Sodium Exchange. The normal daily intake of sodium in adults is 50 - 90 mEq (3-5 g). **In infants and small children, sodium requirements are 2-3 mEq/kg/24 hours**. Sodium is primarily lost through the kidneys, sweat, and GI losses. With reduced intake, the kidneys can retain sodium, excreting < 1 mEq/day. In salt-wasting diseases, losses may be > 100 mEq/liter of urine. Premature infants and critically ill infants (i.e., postop from major surgery) are "salt wasters" and need extra NaCl.

Volume changes. Volume deficit is the most common volume problem of surgical patients and is usually due to loss of GI fluids (e.g., vomiting, NG tube), and sequestration of fluids (peritonitis, burns). In children, this may be more difficult to diagnose: tachycardia in chilldren is less reliable, and hypotension occurs only very late. Children in the early stages of volume loss may manifest sleepiness, apathy, anorexia, a progressive decrease in food consumption, and decreased skin turgor. As the deficit becomes more severe, they will show nausea, vomiting, ileus, mottling, cold extremities, atonic muscles, sunken eyes, and marked hypothermia. Labratory values will usually show an elevated BUN, with minimal (or absent) increases in creatinine, and increased RBC, H/H, WBC, and platelets (concentrated). Sodium may be low, normal, or high. Oliguria may be one of the more reliable measures of volume status. **Oliguria is definded as < 2 ml/kg/hr urine output in newborns, < 1 ml/kg/hr in children, and < 0.5 ml/kg/hr in adults**. The kidney's response to volume loss can be seen in urine osmolality, NaCl (but remember infants are not able to concentrate their urine in response to hypovolemia). **The renal failure index and fractional excretion of filtered sodium are the most accurate tests in differentiating prerenal (hypovolemic) oliguria from renal failure - but these tests may not be accurate in infants.**

Concentration Changes. Because the osmolality is the same in all compartments, Na (the principle contributor to the osmolality of the extracellular compartment) is used to estimate osmolality of the body. Osmolality can be estimated by the formula $2(Na) + [Glucose/18] + [BUN/2.8]$. The physiology of the kidney is different in the newborn in order to permit the necessary postnatal diuresis. This postnatal shift in body fluids is mediated by water and sodium excretion in the kidney. **GFR is less in infants**. In adults, GFR is around 80-100 $ml/min/1.73m^2$. In the normal term infant, GFR is approximately 21 $ml/min/1.73^2$. In the premature infant, GFR is slightly less—around 16 $ml/min/1.73m^2$. Adult levels of GFR are reached around 18 months. **The key concept is that newborn kidneys have little ability to concentrate urine**. The maximum urine osmolality an adult can reach is approximately 1200 mOsm. The maximum urine osmolality for term infant is approximately 500-600 mOsm, Although normal levels of ADH are produced, the newborn tubules do not seem to respond. **Newborn kidneys are much more efficient at clearing free water than adults (i.e., can make very dilute urine)**. The lowest osmolality an adult can reach is approximately 70-100 mOsm, but an infant can achieve levels of 30-50 mOsm. **Newborns can retain sodium when in negative balance, but cannot excrete excessive sodium when in positive balance.**

TRAUMA

Closed Head Injury. The head is proportionally larger in small children, and closed head injuries are among the most common injuries seen after trauma. Children < 3 months have a more malleable skull (and therefore may have significant brain injury without external findings such as skull fractures), a quasi-gelatinous consistency of the brain, a larger subarachnoid space, and large basal cisterns. Skull fractures in children can be open versus closed, linear versus comminuted, depressed, or diastatic. Admission and observation are required is the fracture is: a) basilar, b) across dural venous sinus (especially transverse sinus and even if the CT is negative),

c) depressed, or d) associated with neurologic findings. Direct carotid injury is unusual but should be suspected in the presence of appropriate history (pencil-point injury, blunt trauma to the neck), symptoms out of proportion to CT findings, the finding of Horner's syndrome, or the presence of an orbital bruit. Younger children tend to experience more brain injury for a given force than older children or adults. Fifty percent of children with open fontanelles will suffer fracture from acceleration or deceleration injuries compared with 29% if fontanelles are closed. **There is a higher morbidity and mortality with CHI for patients < 1 to 2 years of age.** The higher metabolic rate of young children may lead to more swelling. Secondary brain injury can be caused by decreased cerebral perfusion pressure (hypotension or increased intracranial pressure), ischemia, hypoxia, hypercarbia, or hypothermia. The systemic responses to brain injury include initial hypertension with subsequent hypotension, neurogenic pulmonary edema, and DIC. DIC is probably due to release of brain stores of thromboplastin and is more frequent in children than adults. Seventy-five percent of children with CHI have some coagulopathy, and 32% have true DIC. Both diabetes insipidus and SIADH can occur after CHI.

Spinal cord injuries in children are a relatively rare injury, representing 0.65 to 9.5% of all spinal cord injuries. High cervical injuries more common in children (Atlanto-occipital fracture dislocation, odontoid fracture, C4 and above). **In addition, the unique anatomy of the pediatric spine predisposes children to SCIWORA, or spinal cord injury without radiologic abnormalities**. SCIWORA has a 15% to 20% incidence in adult spinal cord injuries, and a 36% to 67% incidence in children. This is due to the greater laxity of ligaments and immaturity of vasculature. In children, there is greater mobility of the vertebrae; the vertebral facets are shallowly angulated, and the vertebral bodies are wedge-shaped. There is a different fulcrum of neck motion (C2-3 in children versus C 5-6 in adults). Spinal shock, which occurs as sympathetic control is lost distal to injury and parasympathetic innervation dominates, is not as prominent in children, and, therefore, children

are much less likely than adults to need sympathomimetic agents. The diagnosis of spinal cord injury is more difficult in children than adults. As in adults, a C-spine series, with a good few of all 7 vertebrae is essential. However, these films are much harder to interpret in children. There may be a physiologic subluxation of C2 on C3 (normal until age 7), and growth centers may mimic fractures. An MRI may show the edema and/or hematoma even when plain films and CT are "normal," and should be considered in children with a mechanism of injury that places them at risk for spinal cord injury [13].

Thoracic injuries are uncommon in children and, when present, are indicative of major trauma with decreased prognosis. Anatomic and physiologic differences in children include increased compliance of the chest wall, increased mobility of the mediastinum, and greater elasticity of the great vessels. Rib fractures are much less common in children because of increased compliance of the thorax. For the same reason, rib fractures are a sign of more serious trauma in a child. Pulmonary contusion is more common in children than adults - again because of increased thoracic wall compliance.

Abdominal injuries. CT scan is the "golden standard" for diagnosis in children. DPLs are rarely performed in children, but may be indicated if perforation of a hollow viscus is the issue, if the child is being taken emergently to the OR for head injury, or to rule out the abdomen as the cause of hypotension in an unstable child with multiple sites for potential blood loss. If a DPL is performed, 10 mL/kg is infused. As in adults, ultrasound is now being used in children as a screening examination. The spleen is the most commonly injured abdominal organ in children. Nonoperative management is standard, as > 90% of children will stop bleeding from an injured spleen spontaneously. The indications for surgery include another reason for laparotomy, penetrating injury, instability after transfusion of 25% of blood volume, or total transfusions > 50% of blood volume (35-40ml/kg) [14]. If surgery is indicated, spleen-saving operations should be performed whenever possible. If splenectomy is performed, immunizations for pneumococcus,

Haemophilus influenzae B, and meningococcus should be given. In addition, the patient should be maintained on once-daily oral penicillin until age 7 to 12. Liver injuries, like the spleen, are often managed nonoperatively in children. Pancreatic injuries occur most classically after a fall onto the handlebars of a bicycle. However, any mechanism of injury which compresses the epigastrium into the spine (e.g., child abuse with a blow to the abdomen, MVA, fall onto an object from a height) can result in compression with injury to the pancreas and/or duodenum. Pancreatic injuries which result in pancreatic pseduocysts may still be managed nonopeatively. In children, pseudocysts drained percutaneously resolve in > 80% of cases.

Burns and Inhalational Injuries in Children [15]. Fluid resuscitation in children is more accurately calculated using body surface area (BSA). **The standard Parkland formula tends to overestimate fluid need in children.** In the first 24 hours - 2000ml/m^2 BSA + 5000 ml/m^2 BSA burned (give half in first 8 hours then give half in next 16 hours). Solutions which are recommended in children are: 950ml D$_5$LR + 50 ml 25% albumin (Na 132, Cl 109, K 3.8, glucose 47.5 g/L, albumin 12.5 g/L). **Because of the difference in renal physiology, it is important to decrease the sodium load for infants** (< 12 months): 930 ml D$_5$ 33%NaCl + 20 ml NaBicarb + 50 ml 25% albumin (Na 81, Cl 61, HCO3 20, glucose 46.5 g/L, albumin 12.5 g/L). The volume starting on day 2 of resuscitation should be 75% of the first 24 hours for subsequent days. In most children, the sodium should be decreased to the level of half normal saline (approx 75 mEq/L). Additional potassium may be needed during the diuretic phase (days 2-14). If the Parkland formula is used, it should be noted that the percentages are different in children— the head is proportionally more of the body surface area and the extremities proportionally less the younger the child. Nutritional support of these children is critical. Enteral feeding should be started at 24 hours if the patient is stable. **The calories needed/day can be calculated by 1800 kcal/m^2 + 2200 kcal/m^2 of burn.** Inhalation injury causes injury by heat damage, chemical damage (inhaled combustion products of plastics and rubber release strong alkali and acids when dissolved in the distal airways), and by production of carbon monoxide (which has 250 times the affinity of oxygen for hemoglobin).

NEWBORN SURGICAL EMERGENCIES

Upper airway obstruction. Masses at the base of the tongue can obstruct the airway. These include thyroglossal duct cyst and ectopic thyroid. In ectopic thyroid, this may be child's only thyroid tissue, i.e., aspirate before removal! You can temporize and control the airway with a suture through tongue to pull it forward. Lymphangioma (cystic hygroma) is a malformation of the lymphatics which presents as a mass, usually in the posterior cervical triangle, which has thin-walled cysts lined with flat endothelium. There are equivalent lesions in the chest (obstruction/malformation of thoracic duct) and abdomen (cisterna chylie), e.g., mesenteric cysts. Fifty percent of cystic hygromas are present at birth, and 90% are present before 2 years of age. Seventy-five percent are cervical, usually posterior triangle

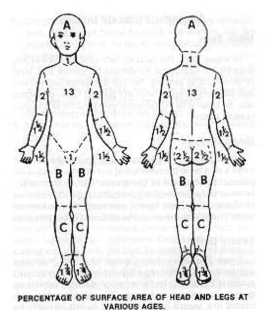

PERCENTAGE OF SURFACE AREA OF HEAD AND LEGS AT VARIOUS AGES.

AREA IN DIAGRAM	0	1	5	10	15
A = ½ of head	9½	8½	6½	5½	4½
B = ½ of one thigh	2¾	3¼	4	4¼	4½
C = ½ of one lower leg	2½	2½	2¾	3	3¼

(AGE IN YEARS)

FIGURE 44.3. This chart of body areas, together with the table showing the percentage of surface area of the head and legs at various ages, can be used to estimate the surface area burned in a child. (From Solomon JR. Pediatric burns. Crit Care Clin 1985;1:161.)

and may extend into mediastinum and axilla. These cervical lesions may also extend into tongue and larynx with respiratory compromise. The treatment is excision as soon as diagnosed, unless facial nerve is involved then wait 6 months. The goal is to operate before infection (30% become infected). Congenital lesions of the tongue may also cause airway obstruction. Hemangiomas of the tongue will regress with waiting, with involution starting by 2 to 3 years, and total disappearance by 5 or 6 years. Lymphangiomas of the tongue do not regress and are subject to multiple infections. These lesions may cause malformed teeth and mandible with growth of the child. Surgery may be necessary to reduce the size of the tongue (total resection always impossible). A ranula is a cyst of salivary glands which presents as a large, cystic lesion in the floor of the mouth. The treatment is marsupialization. Cervical teratomas are tumors which may cause respiratory compromise in the neonate. These lesions are usually associated with thyroid, and therefore, resection may result in injury to the recurrent laryngeal nerve(s). The chronic tracheal compression which these lesions cause predisposes the infant to tracheomalacia postop, i.e., need for long-term intubation.

Esophageal Atresia. Esophageal atresia can present with or without fistulae. The classification systems have become increasingly complex, and most pediatric surgeons now simply describe the anomaly. The most common (86%) anomaly is esophageal atresia with distal tracheoesophageal fistula. These infants have drooling at birth, and a KUB will show gas in the abdomen (from the distal fistula). The danger to these children is from aspiration of saliva from proximal pouch and aspiration of gastric contents from distal fistula. The preoperative treatment consists of aspirating the proximal pouch with Replogle tube, elevating the head of the bed, starting antibiotics (usually Amp and Gent to cover vaginal flora), and surgery when physiologically best. The fistula is usually 1 to 1.5 cm above carina. A second, proximal fistula is present in 7% of patients and is located in the neck. Atresia of esophagus without fistula is the next most common anomaly. The KUB will show no air in abdomen and the only risk of aspirating is from proximal

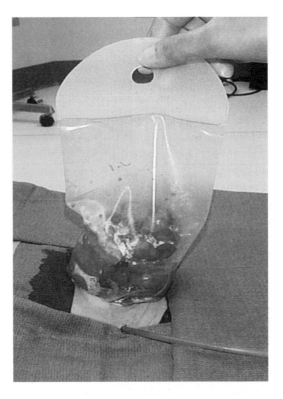

pouch (i.e., can avoid with proper nursing care). A feeding gastrostomy is placed as an initial procedure. Correction of the esophageal atresia is delayed for 2-3 months as the esophagus has a greater rate of growth than the infant (i.e., the 2 ends will become closer together). Tracheoesophageal fistula without atresia is the most difficult anomaly to diagnosis. This is misnamed "H fistula"—it is actually an "N" fistula, with fistula higher on trachea than esophagus. Because of this anatomy, aspiration occurs during reflux NOT swallowing. Fifty percent of children with TEF/EA have associated anomalies: 14% to 28% have cardiac anomalies (PDA, VSD, ASD, Right aortic arch).

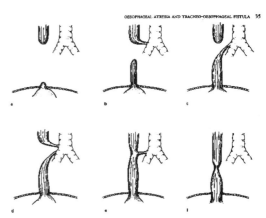

OESOPHAGEAL ATRESIA AND TRACHEO-OESOPHAGEAL FISTULA 35

TEF/EA is one of the components of the VACTERL complex: V=Vertebral anomalies (75% of infants, Hemivertebra, extra vertebrae), A=Imperforate Anus, C=Cardiac, TE=TE fistula, R=Renal, and L=Limb (usually radial anomalies).

Congenital Diaphragmatic Hernia. The most common is the Bochdalek hernia, which is a posterolateral defect in the diaphragm, representing a failure of closure of pleuroperitoneal canal. Eighty percent are on the left side. The Morgagni hernia is an anteromedial hernia, presents much later in life, and represents only 3% to 5% of all CDH. Associated defects are common. Pulmonary hypoplasia of some degree is almost universal. There is an arrest in bronchial branching with decreased bronchi, but an appropriate number of alveolae per bronchus. There is also thickening of the medium-sized bronchial arterioles. Other anomalies seen in association with CDH include pumonary sequestration, cardiac defects, and nonrotation. The preoperative management – and timing of surgery – is critical in the outcome for these infants. All infants are kept warm. All efforts to avoid distention of the GI tract are made with early intubation, placement of an NG tube, and no bagging. A right radial arterial line (preductal) is placed. These infants are at high risk for PPHN, so all efforts are made to avoid any sudden changes in hemodynamic or pulmonary status. Permissive hypercapnia is used to avoid excessive barotraumas or lung injury as long as accepatable oxygenation can be achieved. Extracorporeal Membrane Oxygenation (ECMO) is used prior to surgery if the patient has documented adequate lung mass (good initial gases) and then deteriorates.

Congenital Malformations of the Lungs. Congenital lung cysts are lined by ciliated pseudostratified columnar epithelium. The wall of the cyst contains smooth muscle, elastic tissue, and varying amounts of cartilage. The differential diagnosis includes postinfectious cysts, bronchogenic cyst (lung cyst in lung parenchyma, bronchogenic cyst is paratracheal or in the mediastinum), and CCAM. Congential cystic adenomatoid malformation (CCAM) differs from congenital lung cyst in that there is absence of bronchial cartilage, absence of bronchial tubular glands, presence of tall columnar, mucinous epithelium, and overproduction of terminal bronchiolar structures without alveolar differentiation. There can be massive enlargement of the affected lobe with displacement of other thoracic structures. This lesion is easy to confuse on CXR with diaphragmatic hernia — key is presence of stomach bubble beneath diaphragm. Congenital lobar emphysema is an important cause of respiratory distress in infancy. There is overinflation or severe distention of 1 lobe with compression of adjacent lobes and shift of the mediastinum. This is most commonly seen in the left upper lobe (47%), followed by the right middle (38%) and right upper lobe (20%). Only 5% occur in the lower lobes. The differential diagnosis includes CCAM, pulmonary overinflation from aberrant vessels, right lower lobe inflation in preemies who have required long term ventilatory support (bronchial obstruction secondary to repeated suctioning), and Swyer-James syndrome or unilateral hyperlucent lung syndrome secondary to decreased pulmonary flow. Cardiac defects are frequently associated with congential lobar emphysema (VSD, Coarctation, PDA). Bronchogenic cysts usually present with stridor and wheezing. These cysts are lined with respiratory epithelium and are usually located adjacent to the trachea or main stem bronchus. Pulmonary sequestrations are pulmonary tissue that has no connection with the bronchial vessels, i.e., receives its blood supply from systemic arteries. There are 2 types: a) extralobar (no connection to lung) and b) intralobar (within lung). Extralobar sequestrations occur most commonly in left costophrenic angle, with blood supply from thoracic or abdominal aorta. Intralobar sequestrations are most commonly found in the posterior basal segment of the lower lobe.

Abdominal Wall Defects. There are 2 kinds of congenital abdominal wall defects: omphalocele and gastroschisis. Omphaloceles have a defect at the base of umbilical cord. Associated anomalies are common (especially in giant omphaloceles), but intestinal anomalies are uncommon. Twenty percent of these children have cardiac defects, with Tetralogy of Fallot most common. Other associated anomalies include diaphragmatic hernia, meningocele, Trisomy syndromes, microcephaly, and Beckwith-Wideman syndrome (hypoglycemia, large tongue, umbilical anomaly). In gastroschisis, the defect is to the right of the umbilical cord. There is a 16% incidence of GI anomalies (usually atresia), but other associated anomalies are rare. Preoperatively, it is critical to avoid hypothermia from exposed intestine: the intestines are wrapped in Kerlex, moistened with warm saline, and covered with plastic. The infant is placed on his/her side, not back, in order to prevent any kink of the mesenteric vessels at the exit. The goal of surgical correction is to maximize space in the abdominal cavity to allow primary closure. A functioning NG tube is placed, and the surgeon does mechanical stretching of the abdominal wall. The factors which determine if primary closure is possible are the change in PIP, the hemodynamic response to tense abdomen, and the adequacy of intestinal perfusion. **If primary closure is not possible, a silo is placed and delayed closure undertaken 5-10 days later**. If an atresia is present, it is left alone and repaired during a subsequent procedure (usually 4 to 6 weeks later). Prolonged ileus is the norm, and a central line is placed for TPN.

Pyloric and Duodenal Obstruction. Pyloric atresia is very rare, but duodenal atresia is not. Duodenal atresia can vary from a web with a central open lumen to total disruption of the duodenum from the jejunum. Infants with duodenal obstruction will have a classic "double bubble" on radiograph. Fifty percent of patients with duodenal atresia have associated anomalies (Down's syndrome [40%], malrotation, congenital heart disease, TEF, renal anomalies, imperforate anus). Duodenal atresia is not a surgical emergency, but the difficulty is in distinguishing it from malrotation (which is an emergency). **Sixteen percent of duodenal atresias have an associated malrotation.** The surgical procedures are: Web, excision and duodenoplasty; Atresia, bypass with duodenoduodenostomy or duodenojejunostomy. Other causes of duodenal obstruction include annular pancreas, preduodenal portal vein, and malrotation. Annular pancreas is always associated with duodenal stenosis or atresia and has frequent associated anomalies (Down's syndrome, TEF, congenital heart disease).

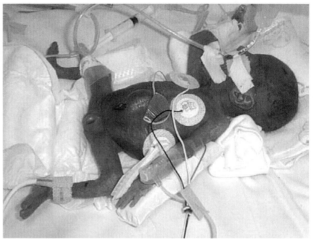

Malrotation. Malrotation can present in a variety of ways: Duodenal obstruction, volvulus, chronic pain, vomiting, and diarrhea. In the "classic" malrotation, the cecum is in the right upper quadrant, and there is abnormal fixation of cecum to RUQ abdominal wall = Ladd's bands (obstruct duodenum). **If volvulus is present the twist is in a clockwise direction (i.e., reduction is counterclockwise)**. The procedure to correct malrotation is a Ladd's procedure: Divide Ladd's bands, elongate the base of mesentery, put bowel in position of nonrotation (duodenum vertical down right abdomen, small bowel on right, colon on left, cecum ends up in left upper quadrant), appendectomy.

Jejunal and Ileal Atresia. There are 5 types of small bowel atresia: Type I: "web" — bowel and mesentery in continuity; Type II: bowel in continuity, mesenteric defect; Type III: defect in bowel and mesentery; Type IV: multiple atresias (string of sausages); Type V: "Christmas tree" or "apple peel" deformity — loss of entire mesentery of midgut = all distal bowel has single, ileocolic vessel as blood supply). Preoperatively, a contrast enema is indicated in order to eliminate Hirschsprung's, meconium ileus, small left colon syndrome, meconium plug, and to eliminate the rare associated colonic atresia. Associated anomalies are unusual. A localized volvulus with atresia is associated with CF.

Meconium Ileus, Meconium Plug and Meconium Peritonitis. Fifteen percent of children with CF have meconium ileus at birth. Meconium ileus has been reported in children without CF (rare). Obstruction is usually at the level of ileocecal valve. **On KUB there is a "soap bubble appearance" of proximal, dilated bowel (meconium mixed with air bubbles) and no air fluid levels.** Initial treatment is with water soluble contrast enema + Tween, which may loosen the meconium and resolve the obstruction. Surgery is reserved for enema failure. Complicated meconium ileus, i.e., perforation (prenatal perforation = meconium peritonitis), atresia requires surgery. Meconium plug syndrome has no relation to meconium ileus. It is caused by inspissated meconium in the colon and is associated with prematurity and maternal complications. These infants virtually never require surgery.

Hirschsprung's Disease is caused by a lack of ganglion cells in Meyerbach's and Meissner's plexuses of the colon. In the neonatal period, we now usually manage this condition without a colostomy (unless there has been significant enterocolitis), with the definitive pull-through performed in the newborn period. **Hirschsprung's enterocolitis can occur after the pull-through (even though there is no longer any obstruction).** They present with foul-smelling diarrhea, fever, and leukocytosis. Treatment is with antibiotics to cover bowel flora and frequent rectal irrigations.

Imperforate Anus. Imperforate anus in general is high in boys and low in girls. In high imperforate anus, there is usually a fistula to the GU tract. The morbidity from this lesion comes from this contamination of the GU system.

Necrotizing Enterocolitis (NEC). NEC is an acquired disease of newborns, particularly premature newborns. It is "caused" by a triad of variables: prematurity of the gut mucosal barrier; presence of substrate (i.e., feedings); presence of bacteria. Clinically, these infants develop feeding intolerance, apnea, and lethargy. This is followed by abdominal distention, blood in the stools, and temperature instability. Laboratory values may show leukocytosis, thrombocytopenia, and a metabolic acidosis. The diagnosis is made radiographically on plain films of the abdomen. **Radiographic signs of NEC include pneumatosis intestinalis and portal vein gas.** The treatment is initially nonoperative with OG suction (npo for 10 to 14 days), intravenous antibiotics, and TPN. Serial KUBs are used to follow the bowel gas pattern

and to help in determining the need for surgery. The only absolute indication for surgery is the presence of free air on the KUB. Other indications, all of which indicate irreversible damage to the bowel, include a persistent mass or distended loop, abdominal wall erythema, obstruction, or deteriorating clinical status.

CHILDHOOD POISONINGS [16]

Children put things in their mouths as part of exploring their world. Unfortunately, some fo these things are toxic. In a potential ingestion, a history should be taken as to possible agents and possible dose, and how long it has been since the exposure. Physical examination should look for decreased respiratory rate (narcotics, alcohol, barbiturates, sedatives) or increased repiratory rate (aspirin, ethylene glycol, methanol, cyanide). Bradycardia can be associated with ingestion of digitalis, cholinergics, clonidine, and beta blockers. SVT may suggest ingestion of aminophylline or PCP. PVCs and sinus tachycardia can be seen following ingestion of tricyclics or cocaine. The odor of the child's breath may provide a clue: bitter almonds = cyanide, garlic = arsenic, organophosphates. Other findings on physical examination that may suggest the toxic agent include a dry mouth (anticholinergics), excessive salivation (organophosphates, carbamate), cherry red skin (carbon monoxide), sweating (sympathomemetics, organophosphates), dry skin (anticholinergics), wheezing (organophosphates), and hyperperistaltic bowel sounds (cholinergics).

Organophosphate and Carbamate Poisoning. Insecticides come in 2 broad classes: a) organophostphate (e.g., Parathion, Malathion) and b) carbamate (e.g., Aldicarb, Carbaryl, Popoxur). This poising occurs because of binding to acetylcholinesterase receptors, which is irreversible for organophosphates and temporary for carbamates. This leads to accumulation of acetylcholine at receptors and increased neurotransmission. The clinical manifestations are respiratory initially (if the substance was inhaled), with bronchorrhea and wheezing. If the insecticide was absorbed through the skin, systemic signs will appear first with sweating and muscle fasiculations. If the substance was ingested, GI symptoms will be first: cramps, vomiting, diarrhea, and abdominal pain. The pneumonic "SLUDGE" can be used to remember the overall clinical picture: Salivation, Lacrimation, Urination, Defecation, Emesis. There may be an odor of garlic on the breath. The treatment is supportive care and immediate decontamination. Atropine, scopolamine, and glycopyrrolate can be given.

Tricyclic Antidepressant Poisoning. A dose of 10-20 mg/kg of tricyclid antidepressants will cause toxicity. There is a central and peripheral anticholinergic action with blockage of the amine pump, a decrease in reuptake of norepi, increased catecholamine action, and a "Quinidine-like" myocardial depression. Clinically, these patients have CNS disturbances with lethargy, coma, confusion, and agitation. There are peripheral anticholinergic effects with dry mucous membranes, flushed, warm, dry skin, and urinary retention. Cardiovascular disturbances may be the most clinically threatening with re-entry type arrythmias (e.g., PVCs, VT), ventricular fibrillation, and bradycardia. The treatment is supportive care, gastric lavage (the drugs are absorbed only in alkaline small bowel - delayed gastric emptying makes this worthwhile even 24 hours later), activated charcoal, cathartics, and antiarrhythmics.

Anticholinergic Poisoning. Examples of anticholinergics include antihistamines, anti-Parkinsonian drugs, GI and GU antispasmodics, and phenothiazines. These drugs block normal cholinergic nerve transmission. The clinical manifestations can be remembered by the phrase "Hot as a hare, blind as a bat, dry as a bone, red as a beet, mad as a hatter." Peripheral manifestations include tachycardia (earliest and most consistent), hypertension, dry mucous membranes, warm, red, dry skin, mydriasis, blurred vision, decreased bowel sounds, constipation, and urinary retention. Central manifestations include confusion, memory loss, hallucinations, agitation, coma, and convulsions. The treatment is physostigmine and supportive care.

Methanol Intoxication. Methanol is a frequent component of solvents and antifreeze. As little as 5 ml is toxic to a toddler. A dose of 1

mg/kg is lethal at all ages. It is metabolized to formaldehyde and causes an increased anion gap metabolic acidosis. Clinically, it initially affects the CNS with inebriation and drowsiness. Subsequently, patients manifest restlessness, headache, nausea, vomiting, abdominal pain, photophobia, and blurred vision. You may be able to smell formaldehyde on the breath and may note Kussmaul breathing. The permanent sequelae of this intoxication include blindness and a Parkinson-like syndrome. The treatment is supportive care, gastric lavage or emesis, charcoal (may not be effective), correction of metabolic acidosis with bicarb, dialysis to remove methanol and metabolites, and the administration of ethanol to block formation of metabolites.

Isopropyl Alcohol Intoxication. Isopropyl alcohol is less toxic than methanol, but more than ethanol. The toxic dose is 1 ml/kg of 70% alcohol. Clinical manifestations are similar to ethanol and the treatment is supportive care and gastric decontamination.

Ethylene Glycol Intoxication. Ethylene glycol is found in cosmetics and antifreeze. The T1/2 is normally 3 hours, but can be prolonged to 17 hours in the presence of ethanol. The metabolites of ethylene glycol include glycolaldehyde, glycolic acid, and glycoxylate. Initially, these patients appear drunk (30 minutes-12 hours after ingestion). They subsequently (12-18 hours) develop a metabolic acidosis, renal failure, and cardiorespiratory failure with pulmonary edema and cyanosis. Treatment is supportive care, gastric decontamination, sodium bicarb for acidosis, ethanol, and dialysis.

Opioid Intoxication. Narcotic toxicity is manifested by respiratory depression, miosis, impaired consciousness, and pulmonary edema. The treatment is airway control, gastric decontamination, and Narcan.

Cyanide Intoxication. Cyanide binds irreversibly with ferric iron of cytochrome oxidase and halts aerobic metabolism in the mitochondria. **Iatrogenic poisoning can occur with Nipride.** The clinical manifestations are nonspecific signs of cellular hypoxia: acute anxiety, dizziness, tachypnea, hypertension, palpitations, headache, and myocardial ischemia. There may be a bitter almond smell on breath, but the ability to smell this is genetically determined and present in only 20-40% of people. The treatment is supportive care, treat the acidosis, and attempt to produce methemoglobin, which has a high affinity for cyanide. Amyl nitrate can be inhaled while IV sodium nitrite is being prepared. **Methemoglobin toxicity is treated with methylene blue.**

Acetaminophen Intoxication. The toxic doses of acetaminophen are > 7.5 gms in adults and > 140 mg/kg in children. The toxic metabolites cause hepatocellular damage. In the first 12-24 hours, patients have nausea, anorexia, and vomiting. From 24-28 hours, these symptoms resolve and LFTs begin to rise. During day 3-4, the liver function abnormalities peak and the patient develops nausea and vomiting (symptoms of hepatitis). **Children are more resistant to liver failure than adults after ingestion of acetaminophen.** Treatment is emesis, catharsis, lavage, and **N-acetylcysteine.**

Salicylate Intoxication. Aspirin is a weak acid that is poorly absorbed in the stomach. It works by uncoupling oxidative phosphorylation. The clinical manifestations of a salicylate intoxication include, fever, tinnitus, tachycardia, hyperventilation, nausea, vomiting, lethargy, coma, and seizures. Aspirin has a profound affect on acid-base balance in the body. **Initially, there is direct stimulation of respiration, which leads to a respiratory alkalosis. As the drug affects oxidative phosphorylation, there is increased carbon dioxide with a resultant respiratory acidosis.** There is also a metabolic acidosis, but the age of the patient and the chronicity of intoxication determines the final acid-base pattern. **In infants and young children, metabolic acidosis predominates, while respiratory alkalosis is more common in older children and adults.** Other disturbances in metabolism are manfested by hyperglycemia, dehydration, hypernatremia, and hypokalemia. The treatment is ABCs, gastric decontamination, alkalinization and diuresis, and close monitoring of electrolytes and glucose.

Iron Intoxication. Iron intoxication can be mild (20-60 mg/kg elemental iron), moderate (> 60 mg/kg elemental iron), or lethal (200 mg/kg elemental iron). Clinically, these patients have gastointestinal (vomiting, diarrhea - often bloody, abdominal pain), cardiovascular (shock), coagulopathic (DIC, depressed production of hepatic factors), hepatic, and CNS manifestations. **These patients may present with perforation of the GI tract.** The treatment is gastric decontamination and chelation therapy with desferoxamine.

REFERENCES

1. Rodenstein, D, Perlmutter N, Stanescu D: Infants are not obligate nasal breathers. *An Rev Respir Dis*1985; 131:p 439
2. Thompson, A: Pediatric airway management in pediatric critical care. B Fuhrman and J Zimmerman (Eds). Mosby Year Book, St. Louis, 1992, p 111-128
3. Pang D, Wilberger J: Spinal cord injury without radiologic abnormalities in children. *J Neurosurg* 1982; 57: 114
4. Tepas JI, et al: Tracheostomy in neonates and small infants: Problems and pitfalls. *Surgery* 1981; 89: 635
5. Martin L, et al: Principles of respiratory support and mechanical ventilation. *In:* Textbook of Pediatric Intensive Care. M Rogers (Ed). Williams and Wilkins, Baltimore, 1992, p 134-203
6. Swedlow D: Noninvasive respiratory gas monitoring. *In:* Pediatric Critical Care. B Fuhrman, J Zimmerman (Eds). Mosby Year Book, St. Louis, 1992, p 99-110
7. Bowes W, Corke B, Hulka J: Pulse oximetry: A review of the theory, accuracy, and clinical applications. *Obstet Gynecol* 1989; 74: 541
8. Hay W, Brockway J, Eyzaguirre M: Neonatal pulse oximetry: Accuracy and reliability. *Pediatrics* 1989; 83: 717
9. Dalton H, Thompson A: Extracorporeal membrane oxygenation. *In: Pediatric Critical Care.* B Fuhrman, J Zimmerman (Eds). Mosby Year Book, St. Louis, 1992, p 545-558
10. Chang C, et al: Air embolism and the radial arterial line. *Crit Care Med* 1988; 16:141
11. Aldridge HJay A: Central venous catheters and heart perforation. *Can Med Assoc*1986; 135: 1082

12. Hodson WTruog W: Critical care of the newborn, Philadelphia, W.B. Saunders, 1989

13. Grabb P, Pang D: Magnetic resonance imaging in the evaluation of spinal cord injury without radiographic abnormality in children. *Neurosurgery* 1994; 35: 406

14. Schwartz M, Kangah R: Splenic injury in children after blunt trauma: Blood transfusion requirements and length of hospitalizaiton for laparotomy versus observation. *J Pediatr Surg* 1994; 29: 596

15. Carvajal H: Pediatric burns: Consideration in acute medical managment. *In:* Pediatric Critical Care Clinical Review Series: Part 3. Society of Critical Care Medicine, 1991

16. Berkowitz I, et al: Poisoning and the critically ill child. *In:* Textbook of Pediatric Intensive Care. R MC (Ed). Williams and Wilkins, Baltimore, 1992, p 1290-1356